Patient Safety in Developing Countries

Understanding the various aspects of patient safety education, practice, and research in developing countries is vital in preparing a plan to overcome the challenges of improving patient safety. This unique volume discusses patient safety in developing countries, and the achievements and challenges faced in those places when trying to improve patient safety education and practice. This book includes a compilation of over 100 case studies surrounding patient safety in all aspects of health care. Both real and simulated scenarios are provided to help medical students and professionals apply their knowledge to solve the cases and prepare for real practice.

Features

- Describes the achievements and challenges of patient safety in developing countries.

- Includes real and simulated case studies and key answers on patient safety issues.

- Prepares medical students and practitioners for real-life situations.

- Diverse audience including those in medication to safety testing, patient education, dispensing changes, and the design of health systems.

- Aids medical students and practitioners to improve their skills to solve cases.

Drugs and the Pharmaceutical Sciences

A Series of Textbooks and Monographs
Series Editor Anthony J. Hickey
RTI International, Research Triangle Park, USA

The Drugs and Pharmaceutical Sciences series is designed to enable the pharmaceutical scientist to stay abreast of the changing trends, advances and innovations associated with therapeutic drugs and that area of expertise and interest that has come to be known as the pharmaceutical sciences. The body of knowledge that those working in the pharmaceutical environment have to work with, and master, has been, and continues, to expand at a rapid pace as new scientific approaches, technologies, instrumentations, clinical advances, economic factors and social needs arise and influence the discovery, development, manufacture, commercialization and clinical use of new agents and devices.

Recent Titles in Series

Pharmaceutical Inhalation Aerosol Technology
Third Edition, Anthony J. Hickey and Sandro R. da Rocha

Good Manufacturing Practices for Pharmaceuticals
Seventh Edition, Graham P. Bunn

Pharmaceutical Extrusion Technology
Second Edition, Isaac Ghebre-Sellassie, Charles E. Martin, Feng Zhang, and James Dinunzio

Biosimilar Drug Product Development
Laszlo Endrenyi, Paul Declerck, and Shein-Chung Chow

High Throughput Screening in Drug Discovery
Amancio Carnero

Generic Drug Product Development: International Regulatory Requirements for Bioequivalence
Second Edition, Isadore Kanfer and Leon Shargel

Aqueous Polymeric Coatings for Pharmaceutical Dosage Forms
Fourth Edition, Linda A. Felton

Good Design Practices for GMP Pharmaceutical Facilities
Second Edition, Terry Jacobs and Andrew A. Signore

Handbook of Bioequivalence Testing
Second Edition, Sarfaraz K. Niazi

FDA Good Laboratory Practice Requirements
First Edition, Graham Bunn

Continuous Pharmaceutical Processing and Process Analytical Technology
Ajit Narang and Atul Dubey

Project Management for Drug Developers
Joseph P. Stalder

Emerging Drug Delivery and Biomedical Engineering Technologies: Transforming Therapy
Dimitrios Lamprou

RNA-seq in Drug Discovery and Development
Feng Cheng and Robert Morris

Patient Safety in Developing Countries: Education, Research, Case Studies
Yaser Al-Worafi

For more information about this series, please visit: www.routledge.com/Drugs-and-the-Pharmaceutical-Sciences/book-series/IHCDRUPHASCI

Patient Safety in Developing Countries
Education, Research, Case Studies

Yaser Al-Worafi

College of Pharmacy, University of Science and Technology of Fujairah,
Fujairah, UAE (also Azal University for Human Development,
Sana'a, Yemen)

CRC Press
Taylor & Francis Group
Boca Raton London New York

CRC Press is an imprint of the
Taylor & Francis Group, an **informa** business

Front cover image: Panchenko Vladimir/Shutterstock

First edition published 2024
by CRC Press
2385 NW Executive Center Drive, Suite 320, Boca Raton FL 33431

and by CRC Press
4 Park Square, Milton Park, Abingdon, Oxon, OX14 4RN

Library of Congress Cataloguing-in-Publication Data
Names: Al-Worafi, Yaser, author.
Title: Patient safety in developing countries : education, research, case studies / authored by Yaser Al-Worafi.
Other titles: Drugs and the pharmaceutical sciences.
Description: First edition. | Boca Raton : CRC Press, 2024. | Series: Drugs and the pharmaceutical sciences | Includes bibliographical references and index. |
Identifiers: LCCN 2023013801 (print) | LCCN 2023013802 (ebook) | ISBN 9781032136943 (hardback) | ISBN 9781032136974 (paperback) | ISBN 9781003230465 (ebook)
Subjects: MESH: Patient Safety | Medical Errors--prevention & control | Developing Countries
Classification: LCC R859.7.S43 (print) | LCC R859.7.S43 (ebook) | NLM WX 185 |
DDC 610.28/9--dc23/eng/20230706
LC record available at https://lccn.loc.gov/2023013801
LC ebook record available at https://lccn.loc.gov/2023013802

ISBN: 978-1-032-13694-3 (hbk)
ISBN: 978-1-032-13697-4 (pbk)
ISBN: 978-1-003-23046-5 (ebk)

DOI: 10.1201/9781003230465

Typeset in Palatino
by MPS Limited, Dehradun

To
My brothers:
Moammer Qahtan
Akram Qahtan
Ahmed Qahtan
Abdulrhman Alsaar
Mohammed Alkholany
Prof. Dr. Long Chiau Ming
Dr. Abdulkareem Al-Shami
Dr. Salman Al-Shami
Dr. Ammar Ali Jaber
Dr. Abdulsalam Abuelsamen
Dr. Belal Al-Najjar
Dr. Sami Alshakhshir
Dr. Ammar Al-Mortada
Adel Thalab
Dr. Mohammed Zeib
Dr. Saleh Al-Omary
Dr. Hamzah Al-Mowali
Dr. Adel Am-Moait (Late)

Table of Contents

Preface xi

Acknowledgment xiii

About the Author xv

Section 1: Patient Safety Education 1

  1. Patient Safety Education: History and Importance 2

  2. Patient Safety Education in Developing Countries 7

  3. Patient Safety Education: Competencies and Learning Outcomes 10

  4. Patient Safety Education: Teaching Strategies and Assessment Methods 14

Section 2: Patient Safety Practice 21

  5. Patient Safety-Related Issues: History and Importance 22

  6. Patient Safety-Related Issues: Patient Care Errors and Related Problems 24

  7. Patient Care Errors and Related Problems: Preventive Medicine Errors and Related Problems 34

  8. Patient Care Errors and Related Problems: Patient Assessment and Diagnostic Errors and Related Problems 42

  9. Patient Care Errors and Related Problems: Non-pharmacological Errors and Related Problems 52

  10. Patient Care Errors and Related Problems: Medical Errors and Related Problems 61

  11. Patient Care Errors and Related Problems: Surgical Errors and Related Problems 69

  12. Patient Care Errors and Related Problems: Complementary and Alternative Medicines (CAM) Errors and Related Problems 78

  13. Patient Care Errors and Related Problems: Nutrition Errors and Related Problems 92

  14. Patient Care Errors and Related Problems: Pharmacological Errors and Related Problems (Medication Errors and Related Problems) 101

  15. Patient Care Errors and Related Problems: Dispensing and Administration Errors and Related Problems 110

  16. Patient Care Errors and Related Problems: Monitoring Errors and Related Problems 119

  17. Patient Care Errors and Related Problems: Patient Education and Counseling Errors and Related Problems 129

  18. Patient Safety-Related Issues: Other Medication Safety Issues 138

  19. Patient Safety Culture 149

  20. Nosocomial Infections in Developing Countries 158

  21. Patient Safety in Laboratory Medicine 165

  22. Patient Safety in Radiology 174

23. Patient Safety in the Emergency Department (ED) 183

24. Patient Safety in Intensive Care Unit (ICU) 192

25. Patient Safety in Surgery 200

26. Patient Safety in Internal Medicine (IM) 208

27. Patient Safety in Oncology 216

28. Patient Safety in Pharmacies 225

29. Patient Safety for Special Populations: Geriatrics 235

30. Patient Safety for Special Populations: Pediatrics 243

31. Patient Safety for Special Populations: Pregnancy 252

32. Patient Safety for Special Populations: Lactation 261

33. Patient Safety for Special Populations: Adolescents 270

34. Patient Safety during Pandemics 278

35. Patient Safety Training 287

36. Patient Safety: Antimicrobial-Resistance and Interventions 298

37. Patient Safety: Dermatology, Beauty, and Cosmetic Medicine 308

38. Technology for Patient Safety 319

39. Evidence-Based Patient Safety 332

Section 3: Patient Safety Research 343

40. Patient Safety Research: History and Importance 344

41. Patient Safety Research: Literature Review 349

42. Patient Safety Research: Qualitative Methods 359

43. Patient Safety Research: Quantitative Methods 371

44. Patient Safety Research: Mixed Methods 384

45. Patient Safety Research: Clinical Trials 395

46. Patient Safety Research: Epidemiology and Pharmacoepidemiology 407

47. Patient Safety Research in Developing Countries: Achievements, Challenges, and
    Recommendations 417

Section 4: Patient Safety Case Studies 427

48. Patient Safety Case Studies: Patient Care Plan Errors and Related Problems (Part I) 428

49. Patient Safety Case Studies: Patient Care Plan Errors and Related Problems (Part II) 435

50. Patient Safety Case Studies: Nosocomial Infections Cases 442

51. Patient Safety Case Studies: Laboratory Medicine and Radiology 447

52. Patient Safety Case Studies: Emergency Department 452

53. Patient Safety Case Studies: Intensive Care Unit 456

54. Patient Safety Case Studies: Internal Medicine 461

55. Patient Safety Case Studies: Oncology 466

56. Patient Safety Case Studies: Antimicrobials 470

57. Patient Safety Case Studies: Special Population 474

58. Patient Safety Resources and Tools 479

Index 486

Preface

Patient safety education, practice, and research are very important for healthcare professionals, students, researchers, policymakers, patients, and the public. Preparing future healthcare professionals with the necessary competencies related to patient safety-related issues is the key to success in patient safety practice in the future. Improving the current healthcare professionals' patient safety competencies is very important in order to improve the patient's treatment outcomes in terms of efficacy and safety. Conducting research about the various patient safety issues are key to identifying the current practice, identifying the challenges and suggesting interventions to overcome the challenges and improve the practice, which leads to improving the patient's treatment clinical, economic, and humanistic outcomes. This book comprises four sections containing more than 50 chapters. The four sections are as follows: Section 1 will focus on Patient Safety Education-related issues; it includes four chapters describing how the history of patient safety education began in chapter 1. Moreover, chapters 2–4 describe the importance of patient safety education degrees, certificates, boards, curriculum-related issues, learning outcomes and competencies, and other education issues. Section 2 will focus on the patient safety practice-related issues. Further, it includes 19 chapters about the patient safety practice-related issues. It describes how the history of patient safety practice and other issues began, it covers the patient care errors and related problems new model, and patient safety practice issues through the chapters 5–38. Section 3 will focus on the patient safety research-related issues. Further, it includes eight chapters about the patient safety research-related issues. It describes how the history of patient safety research began in chapter 39, moreover, it describes the importance of patient safety research and other research-related issues in chapters 39–46 with a special focus on the situation in the developing countries. Section 4 will focus on the real and simulation cases about the patient care errors and related problems and other patient safety issues in chapters 47–56. I hope that this book can provide the pharmacy educators, students, partitioners, researchers, and other readers with the necessary information and practical guidelines about online pharmacy education, practice, research, teaching strategies, and assessment methods in pharmacy education.

Yaser Mohammed Al-Worafi
February 2023

Acknowledgment

It would have been difficult to write such a book without the help of:

My wife for providing me the time and support to work on the book and spend less time with the family.

Hilary LaFoe for her valuable guidance, advice, and help during the writing of this book.

Sukirti Singh and all the production team for their great efforts.

About the Author

Professor Yaser Mohammed Al-Worafi is a Professor of Clinical Pharmacy at the College of Pharmacy, University of Science and Technology of Fujairah, UAE (Previously known as Ajman University). He graduated with a bachelor's degree in Pharmacy (BPharm) from Sana'a University, Yemen, and obtained Master and PhD degree in Clinical Pharmacy from the Universiti Sains Malaysia (USM), Malaysia. Prof. Yaser has many postgraduate programs certificates including Training to Teach in Medicine 2023 from Harvard Medical School, Harvard University; Contemporary Approaches to University Teaching from The Council of Australasian University Leaders in Learning and Teaching (CAULLT). He has more than 20 years' experiences in education, practice, and research in Yemen, Saudi Arabia, United Arab Emirates, and Malaysia. He has held various academic and professional positions including Deputy Dean for Medical Sciences College; PharmD program director, Head of Clinical Pharmacy/Pharmacy Practice department; Head of Teaching & learning committee, Head of Training committee, head of curriculum committee and other committees. He has authored over 100 peer-reviewed papers in international journals, book chapters and editing more than 10 books by Springer, Elsevier, Taylors & Francis, USA. Prof. Yaser has supervised/co-supervised many PhD, Master, PharmD, and B-Pharm students. He is a reviewer for eight recognized international peer-reviewed journals. Prof. Yaser taught, prepared, designed, and wrote many pharmacy programs for many universities including Master of Clinical Pharmacy/Pharmacy Practice program; PharmD program and BPharm program; internship/clerkships for Master, PharmD, and BPharm programs; more than 30 courses related to Clinical Pharmacy, Pharmacy Practice, Social Pharmacy, and Patients care.

SECTION 1

PATIENT SAFETY EDUCATION

1 Patient Safety Education

History and Importance

1.1 BACKGROUND

The history of medical education goes back to ancient times, early medical traditions include those of Babylon, China, Egypt, India, Greeks, Persians, and Romans when official schools for training physicians were established in the early 16th Century. Medical education Between the 9th and 11th centuries flourish in the Muslim world at such centers as Baghdad, Cairo, and Córdoba. Throughout the Greek world, medical education was based more on experience than on book learning, practical training generally being acquired from a physician-father, or by an aspiring student apprenticing himself to a practitioner for a period of years. Books were used, but only as adjuncts, and they never replaced practical experience. The first school of medicine of medieval times came into existence, probably in the 9th century, on the shores of the Tyrrhenian Sea, in the town of Salerno. Tradition has it that the school was founded by representatives of the four cultural forces which had persisted through the Middle Ages—a Greek, a Latin, a Jew, and an Arab. Few traces now remain of this once a flourishing center of medical thought; however, its published texts, such as the Regimen of Health (Al-Worafi, 2022a,b; Fulton, 1953). World Health Organization described patient safety as "Patient Safety is a health care discipline that emerged with the evolving complexity in health care systems and the resulting rise of patient harm in health care facilities. It aims to prevent and reduce risks, errors, and harm that occur to patients during the provision of health care. A cornerstone of the discipline is a continuous improvement based on learning from errors and adverse events; Patient safety is fundamental to delivering quality essential health services" (WHO, 2019). Patient safety-related issues such as medications safety are a major concern in developing countries as well as developed countries; it is associated with treatment outcomes, increase morbidity and mortality, an increase in the cost of illness, an increase in the length of hospital stay, increase the admission to the emergency department as well as visiting the healthcare facilities; decrease the quality of life among patients and public, decrease the satisfaction toward the healthcare services and systems, increase the health expenditure (Al-Worafi, 2020a; WHO, 2019). Patient safety issues such as medical errors, medication errors, surgical errors, adverse drug reactions, and drug-related problems are affecting patients, patients' families, and the healthcare system, therefore, the collaboration between healthcare professionals, healthcare researchers, healthcare educators, healthcare colleges and centers and policymakers are very important and the key to success in improving the patient care, improving the patient safety practice and preventing harm due to patient safety issues such as medical errors, medication errors, and others (Al-Worafi, 2020a; WHO, 2019).

1.2 HISTORY OF PATIENT SAFETY EDUCATION

Drug safety education has been an important aspect of healthcare for centuries, with various approaches and strategies developed over time to ensure the safe and effective use of medications. In ancient times, healers relied on trial and error and traditional knowledge to develop remedies from plants and other natural sources. Over time, medical practitioners began to document their findings and develop more systematic approaches to drug use and safety. In the 19th century, advances in chemistry and pharmacology led to the development of synthetic drugs and more rigorous scientific methods for evaluating their safety and efficacy. In 1906, the United States passed the Pure Food and Drug Act, which established the FDA (Food and Drug Administration) and gave the government the power to regulate the safety and labeling of drugs and food products. During the mid-20th century, a number of major drug disasters highlighted the need for greater attention to drug safety. These included the thalidomide tragedy of the 1950s, in which a drug prescribed to pregnant women caused severe birth defects in thousands of babies; the DES (diethylstilbestrol) scandal of the 1960s and 1970s, in which a synthetic estrogen given to pregnant women was linked to cancer and other health problems in their offspring; and the Fen-Phen debacle of the 1990s, in which a weight-loss drug was linked to heart valve damage and other serious health problems. In response to these and other drug safety issues, governments and healthcare organizations around the world have developed a range of strategies and programs to promote safe and responsible drug use. These include regulations governing drug development, clinical trials, and labeling; patient education and advocacy programs; and initiatives to promote transparency and accountability in the pharmaceutical industry. It is reported that the term primum

DOI: 10.1201/9781003230465-2

non nocere (first, do no harm) is attributed by some historians to Galen and was introduced to American and British medical culture by Worthington Hooker in 1847 (Hooker, 1847; Ilan & Foweler, 2005). Dr Harvey Cushing, a pioneer in surgery and neurosurgery, published detailed descriptions of harm caused to his patients secondary to his own performance at the beginning of the 20th century (Ilan & Foweler, 2005; Pinkus, 2001). However, it is believed that Drug Related Problems had a very long history since ancient times (Al-Worafi, 2020b) and literature reported that during the Greek period "a court physician called Glaucos, who took care of a mad man named Hephaestus. According to Arries, Glaucos prescribed him a wrong medication, and Hephaestus died" (Siculus, 1933; Somville et al., 2010). Adverse drug reactions have been reported for more than 2,000 years (Al-Worafi, 2020c). The patient safety education history timeline can be summarized as follows (ISMP, 2020; Patient Safety History, 2023):

1850s
Florence Nightingale is the first to use charts and graphs to show the relationship between hygiene and patient outcomes during the Crimean War.

1900–1949
The American College of Surgeons (ACS) developed the first set of hospital standards, which was one page long, and began on-site inspections.

1950
The American College of Surgery and several other physician groups joined to become the Joint Commission for Accreditation of Hospitals (JCAH). The name changed later to JCAHO as the focus became on outpatient settings and is now known as TJC, or The Joint Commission.

1965–1966
The U.S. government institutes the Medicare program to insure those over 65 or with chronic conditions. Medicaid, a similar program run by states for low-income populations, begins a year later.

1970's
The Institute of Medicine (IoM) was founded under the National Academy of Sciences to address the concerns of medicine and healthcare. The IoM has now been renamed the National Academy of Medicine (NAM).

1975
ISMP's work officially begins with a continuing column on medication safety in *Hospital Pharmacy* (now published by Thomas Land Publishers).

1980's
The concept of Quality Improvement is more widely introduced in healthcare by Donabedian and others. Diagnostic-Related Groups (DRGs) are instituted in the United States, which reduces payment to hospitals from Medicare.

1981
First printing of *Medication Errors: Causes and Prevention*, a comprehensive book on the causes and prevention of drug mistakes, written by Michael Cohen and Neil Davis, ISMP cofounders.

1987
ISMP convenes national meeting that influences the United States Pharmacopeia (USP) and U.S. Food and Drug Administration (FDA) to require that potassium chloride concentrate for injection have black caps, closures, and warning statements to prevent mix-ups with other parenteral drugs.
First ISMP list of dangerous medical abbreviations published in Nursing '87 magazine.

1989
Walt Bogdanich in his Great White Lie book exposed many of the failings of our healthcare system that lead to preventable deaths, even care providers'.

1991
National, confidential, voluntary medication error reporting program (MERP) is created by ISMP in coordination with the United States Pharmacopeia (USP) to provide expert analysis of the system causes of medication errors.

1992
First scholarly publication in the medical literature about the dangers of free-flow infusion pumps appears with ISMP-authored article in Hospital Pharmacy.
November, 1999
Institute of Medicine releases report, To Err is Human: Building a Safer Health System, claims that as many as 98,000 people are dying in hospitals due to medical errors each year. Over the next decade, Founder Joe Kiani becomes passionate about how to significantly reduce this number.

2001
The World Health Organization (WHO) launches its World Alliance for Patient Safety, with the goal of improving patient safety worldwide.
Josie King passes away due to Sepsis at world-renowned The Johns Hopkins Hospital.
In response to Josie King's passing, John Hopkins intensive care specialist, Dr. Peter Pronovost, who cared for Josie King, developed a 5-item checklist to reduce central line infections and the infection rate within Johns Hopkins decreased from 11% to 0%.

2003
The U.S. government introduces "Core Measures" requirements for U.S. hospitals: the first publicly reported patient outcome data. The Joint Commission introduced the "National Patient Safety Goals" program which articulates steps for reducing medical error and is updated on an annual basis.

2005
The National Patient Safety Foundation (NPSF) launches Patient Safety Awareness Week, an annual campaign to raise awareness of patient safety issues.

2008
The World Alliance for Patient Safety launches the "Global Patient Safety Challenge," with the goal of reducing healthcare-associated infections worldwide.
The Association of American Medical Colleges (AAMC) created the Integrating Quality Initiative which focused on emphasizing patient safety in its medical schools and teaching hospitals' curriculum.

2010
The Affordable Care Act includes provisions to improve patient safety, such as requiring hospitals to report certain types of medical errors and infections.

2014
The WHO launches the third edition of its "Patient Safety Curriculum Guide" to promote patient safety education worldwide.

2016
The National Patient Safety Foundation merges with the Institute for Healthcare Improvement (IHI) to form the Institute for Healthcare Improvement/NPSF Patient Safety Awareness Week.

2019
The WHO launches the "Global Patient Safety Action Plan," a five-year initiative to improve patient safety worldwide.

1.3 IMPORTANCE OF PATIENT SAFETY EDUCATION

Patient safety education, practice, and research are very important for healthcare professionals, students, researchers, policymakers, patients, and the public. Preparing future healthcare professionals with the necessary competencies related to patient safety-related issues is the key to success in patient safety practice in the future. Improving the current healthcare professionals' patient safety competencies is very important in order to improve the patients' treatment outcomes in terms of efficacy and safety. Conducting research about the various patient safety issues is key to identifying the current practice, identifying the challenges and suggesting interventions to overcome the challenges and improve the practice, which leads to improving the patient's treatment clinical, economical, and humanistic outcomes.

Patient safety education is crucial for healthcare professionals and patients alike, as it plays a significant role in ensuring the delivery of safe and effective healthcare. The importance of patient safety education can be understood from the following perspectives:

1. Reducing Medical Errors: Patient safety education can help healthcare professionals to identify potential sources of error and equip them with skills to manage the risks associated with medical procedures. Educating healthcare professionals on patient safety can also help to reduce the frequency and severity of medical errors, which can cause harm to patients.

2. Improving Healthcare Outcomes: Patient safety education can improve healthcare outcomes by ensuring that healthcare professionals have the knowledge and skills necessary to provide high-quality care. It can also empower patients to take an active role in their own care, which can lead to better health outcomes.

3. Enhancing Patient Confidence: When patients are aware that healthcare professionals are trained in patient safety, they are more likely to have confidence in the healthcare system. This can lead to improved patient satisfaction and better healthcare experiences.

4. Promoting Professionalism: Patient safety education can help healthcare professionals to develop a sense of responsibility toward their patients, promoting professionalism and ethical behavior. Healthcare professionals who are trained in patient safety are more likely to prioritize patient well-being and to advocate for patient rights.

5. In conclusion, patient safety education is essential for ensuring that healthcare professionals are equipped with the knowledge and skills necessary to provide safe and effective care. It can also help patients to be more confident in the healthcare system, lead to better healthcare outcomes, and promote professionalism among healthcare professionals.

1.4 CONCLUSION

This chapter has discussed the history and importance of patient safety education. Collaboration between healthcare professionals, healthcare researchers, healthcare educators, healthcare colleges and centers, and policymakers is very important and the key to success in improving patient care, improving patient safety practice, and preventing harm due to patient safety issues such as medical errors, medication errors, and others. Preparing future healthcare professionals with the necessary competencies related to patient safety-related issues is the key to success in patient safety practice in the future. Improving the current healthcare professionals' patient safety competencies is very important in order to improve the patients' treatment outcomes in terms of efficacy and safety.

REFERENCES

Al-Worafi, Y.M. (Ed.). (2020a). Drug Safety in Developing Countries: Achievements and Challenges. Academic Press.

Al-Worafi, Y.M. (2020b). Drug-related problems. In Drug Safety in Developing Countries (pp. 105–117). Academic Press.

Al-Worafi, Y.M. (2020c). Adverse drug reactions. In Drug Safety in Developing Countries (pp. 39–57). Academic Press.

Al-Worafi, Y. (2022a). A Guide to Online Pharmacy Education: Teaching Strategies and Assessment Methods. CRC Press.

Al-Worafi, Y. (2022b). History and importance. In A Guide to Online Pharmacy Education: Teaching Strategies and Assessment Methods. CRC Press.

Fulton, J.F. (1953). History of medical education. British Medical Journal, 2(4834), 457.

Hooker W. (1847). Physician and patient. New York (NY)7 Baker and physician and patient. New York (NY): Baker and Scribner.

ISMP (2020). ISMP Historical Timeline. Available at: https://www.ismp.org/about/historical-timeline

Ilan, R., & Fowler, R. (2005). Brief history of patient safety culture and science. Journal of Critical Care, 20(1), 2–5.

Patient Safety History (2023). Available at: https://psmf.org/patient-safety/historical-timeline/

Pinkus, R.L.B. (2001). Mistakes as a social construct: An historical approach. Kennedy Institute of Ethics Journal, 11(2), 117–133.

Siculus, D. (1933). Diodorus Siculus. Life [edit], 7, p.2.

Somville, F.J.M.P., Broos, P.L.O., & Van Hee, R. (2010). Some notes on medical liability in ancient times. Acta Chirurgica Belgica, 110(3), 405–409.

World Health Organization (WHO). (2019). Available at: https://www.who.int/news-room/fact-sheets/detail/patient-safety

2 Patient Safety Education in Developing Countries

2.1 DEGREES AND PROGRAMS

2.1.1 Undergraduate Degrees and Programs

There is no specific patient safety degree at the level of undergraduate programs, however, the majority of undergraduate medical and health sciences programs (medicine, pharmacy, dentistry, nursing, public health, and others) contain many patients safety issues such as pharmacovigilance, adverse drug reactions, medication errors, drug-related problems, and other issues (Al-Worafi, 2020a-d). There is an opportunity to launch a bachelor's degree in patient safety in developing countries with a curriculum related to patient safety issues.

2.1.2 Postgraduate Degrees and Programs

There are many postgraduate programs related to patient safety in many developing countries, however, the majority of programs are by research and under the umbrella of other programs such as public health, clinical pharmacy, pharmacy practice, health care, and others (Al-Worafi, 2020a; Al-Worafi, 2022). There is an opportunity to launch many postgraduate programs as follows:

2.1.3 Postgraduate Diploma

To study for 1 to 2 years about patient safety issues. It can help students prepare for their master's studies.

2.1.4 At Master Level

To study about patient safety issues by course work or by research or mixed (courses and research).

2.1.5 At Doctorate/Ph.D. Level

To study about patient safety issues by research or mixed mode (courses and research).

2.1.6 Certificates

Healthcare professionals and students can obtain many certificates related to patient safety issues such as the Medication Safety Certificate, which is Organized by the American Society of Health-System Pharmacists (ASHP): 40 continuous education (CE) hours designed to enhance the skills and knowledge for pharmacy professionals, physicians, and nurses who lead medication safety improvements (ASHP, 2021). Moreover, there is an opportunity to launch many postgraduate certificate programs related to patient safety issues in developing countries.

2.2 ONLINE PATIENT SAFETY EDUCATION

There is little known about the availability of online patient safety programs by the medical and health schools in developing countries, however, as the nature of online education, there is an opportunity to launch many online programs related to patient safety issues in developing countries or attend the programs offered by the medical and health schools in the developed countries such as those offering in the United Kingdom (UK).

2.3 CURRICULUM

As mentioned above, there is an opportunity to launch many undergraduate and postgraduate programs related to patient safety issues in developing countries. The curriculum will be designed for specific programs based on many factors such as the name of the program as a patient safety program will include courses related to patient safety in general, while the pharmacovigilance will include courses related to the pharmacovigilance. Examples of courses, subjects, and topics related to patient safety are: pharmacovigilance; adverse drug reactions (ADRs); medication errors; medication abuse and misuse; drug-related problems (DRPs); counterfeit and substandard medications; counterfeit and substandard medical devices; counterfeit and substandard pharmaceutical products; medical errors; surgical errors; antimicrobial resistance and stewardship and others.

2.4 QUALITY AND ACCREDITATION

Quality of patient safety programs is very important to ensure that medical and health sciences schools are able to graduate students with the essential competencies to be able to provide effective patient care services with the best evidence-based patient safety practices. Accreditation systems, bodies, regulations, and standards could be different from one country to another and usually under the supervision of the Ministry of higher education.

2.5 CHALLENGES AND RECOMMENDATIONS

There are many challenges related to patient safety education in developing countries as follows:

2.5.1 Availability of Programs

The majority of developing countries' medical and health sciences schools don't have patient safety programs, therefore, launching patient safety programs is very important and highly recommended.

2.5.2 Patient Safety Topics

The majority of patient safety topics are not included in the majority of developing countries' medical and health sciences programs. Including patient safety topics in the medical and health sciences programs is very important and highly recommended.

2.5.3 Medical and Health Sciences Programs Curriculums

Update the pharmacy curriculum in medical and health sciences programs to meet the actual needs of patient care and patient safety evidence-based practice. Special attention should be given to the integration of patent safety topics into the program's curriculums. Integrating new teaching methods such as problem-based learning, team-based learning (TBL), case discussion (CD), and simulation-based education is very important and highly recommended. Collaboration with university teaching hospitals, government hospitals, private hospitals, community and hospital pharmacies, and other healthcare facilities is very important and highly recommended. and research.

2.5.4 Faculty Members

There is little known about the number of faculty members in developing countries' medical and health sciences schools with patient safety experience, therefore, hiring faculty members with experience in patient safety issues is very important and highly recommended.

2.5.5 Training

Training plays an important role in the preparation of medical and healthcare students about patient safety issues. Including training sessions as part of patient safety-related courses is very important and highly recommend, moreover, designing clerkships or at least part of clerkships about patient safety is very important and highly recommended.

2.5.6 Continuous Professional Development (CPD)

Launching Continuous Professional Development (CPD) about patient safety issues is very important to improve the knowledge and skills of current healthcare professionals about patient safety.

2.5.7 Online Education

Accreditation of online programs is very difficult in many developing countries, allowing students and healthcare professionals to pursue postgraduate degrees online from developed countries such as United Kingdom (UK); launching online programs in developing countries medical and health sciences schools are very important and highly recommended.

2.5.8 Research

There is little known about patient safety issues in the medical and health sciences schools due to a lack of research about it, conducting research about the various patient safety issues is key to identifying the current practice, identifying the challenges, and suggesting interventions to overcome the challenges and improve the practice, which lead to improving the education.

2.6 CONCLUSION

This chapter has discussed patient safety degrees, programs, and certificates. This chapter includes the different degrees offered by the medical and health sciences schools and also discusses the recommendations to launch new programs. This chapter described the challenges of patient safety education in developing countries and suggests recommendations to overcome them. Launching patient safety programs is very important and highly recommended.

REFERENCES

Al-Worafi, Y.M. (Ed.). (2020a). *Drug Safety in Developing Countries: Achievements and Challenges.*

Al-Worafi, Y.M. (2020b). Drug-related problems. In *Drug Safety in Developing Countries* (pp. 105–117). Academic Press.

Al-Worafi, Y.M. (2020c). Adverse drug reactions. In *Drug Safety in Developing Countries* (pp. 39–57). Academic Press.

Al-Worafi, Y.M. (2020d). *Medication errors. In Drug Safety in Developing Countries* (pp. 59–71). Academic Press.

Al-Worafi, Y. (2022). *A Guide to Online Pharmacy Education: Teaching Strategies and Assessment Methods.* CRC Press.

ASHP. (2021). Professional certificates. Available at; www.ashp.org/professional-development/professional-certificate-programs?loginreturnUrl=SSOCheckOnly

3 Patient Safety Education

Competencies and Learning Outcomes

3.1 BACKGROUND

Competencies (ability to do things well) are very important in medical education, all medical and health sciences education schools/departments (medicine, pharmacy, dentistry, nursing, public health, and others) designed the program's competencies based on the profession and community needs; moreover, update the competencies is very important and necessary every three to five years based on the development of the profession and patient care services. Frank et al., 2010 reported the following competencies-based education principles (Frank et al., 2010):

3.1.1 Focusing on Outcomes

To ensure that all graduates are competent in all essential domains. Prepare the graduates for efficient practice, and make them good professionals able to provide effective patient care services.

3.1.2 Emphasizing Abilities

Medical curricula must emphasize the abilities to be acquired. An emphasis on the abilities of learners should be derived from the needs of those served by graduates (i.e., societal needs).

3.1.3 De-emphasizing Time-Based Training

Medical education can shift from a focus on the time a learner spends on an educational unit to a focus on the learning attained. Greater emphasis should be placed on the developmental progression of abilities and on measures of performance.

3.1.4 Promoting Greater Learner-Centredness

Medical education can promote greater learner engagement in training. A curriculum of competencies provides clear goals for learners.

3.2 PATIENT SAFETY EDUCATION COMPETENCIES AND LEARNING OUTCOMES

Preparing future healthcare professionals with the necessary competencies related to the patient safety-related issues is the key to success in patient safety practice in the future. Improving the current healthcare professionals' patient safety competencies is very important in order to improve the patients' treatment outcomes in terms of efficacy and safety. Local and international accreditations agencies are responsible for the development, update, and approval of the competencies and learning outcomes for the medical and health sciences education programs (medicine, pharmacy, dentistry, nursing, public health, and others) to prepare future healthcare professionals to work locally and internationally, taking into consideration what the country needs as well as to be able to work outside the country. Nowadays, medical and health sciences education competencies and learning outcomes are well designed better than at any time in history. The following suggested patient safety competencies and learning outcomes are developed based on the literature, personal experience, and experts' opinion with three-round Delphi methods (ACPE, 2015; Al-Worafi, 2022; Al-Worafi, 2020; Levett-Jones et al., 2018; WHO, 2010):

The healthcare professionals and future healthcare professionals should be able to:

3.2.1 Knowledge (Learner, Educator and Health and Wellness Promoter, and Counselor)

- Describe the basics/principles/fundamentals of patient safety.
- Describe the patient safety issues to patients, the public, and healthcare professionals.
- Demonstrate ability to learn online when needed.

3.2.2 Cognitive (Thinker, Analyzer, Problem Solver, and Decision-maker)

- Apply patient safety knowledge in patient care services and activities.
- Apply critical thinking to identify and solve and minimize Drug Related Problems (DRPs) and other patient safety issues.

DOI: 10.1201/9781003230465-4

- Retrieve and evaluate drug information from pharmaceutical and biomedical science resources and reports for application in specific patient care situations to enhance clinical decision-making.

- Apply basic scientific pharmaceutical and clinical knowledge in calculations and solving clinical cases.

3.2.3 Communication, Education, and Collaboration (Communicator, Educator, and Collaborator)

- Demonstrate effective communication with patients, the public, healthcare professionals, students, organizations, and societies face-to-face or online if needed.

- Demonstrate ability to work effectively within teams (interprofessional and intraprofessional).

- Demonstrate ability to educate, and counsel patients, the public, healthcare professionals, and students about their diseases, conditions, medicines information, management plan, and other health-related issues face to face or online if needed.

3.2.4 Life-long Learning and Personal/Professional Development (Learner and Innovator)

- Demonstrate the ability to take responsibility for their learning.

- Demonstrate ability to engage in innovative activities by using creative thinking to envision better ways of accomplishing professional goals.

- Demonstrate ability to use online sources/resources for their learning.

3.2.5 Leadership and Management (Leader)

- Demonstrate ability to lead teams effectively (interprofessional and intraprofessional).

- Demonstrate leadership abilities in professional endeavors.

- Demonstrate effective leadership and management skills as part of the multi-disciplinary team

- Take appropriate actions to respond to complaints, incidents, or errors in a timely manner and to prevent them from happening again

- Demonstrate resilience and flexibility, and apply effective strategies to manage multiple priorities, uncertainty, complexity, and change

- Develop, lead, and apply effective strategies to improve the quality of care and safe use of medicines.

3.2.6 Patient Care (Care Provider and Innovator)

- Demonstrate ability to provide effective patient care services to patients, the public, students, and healthcare professionals face to face or online if needed.

- Apply evidence-based care to achieve and improve the clinical, economic, and humanistic outcomes for treating patients/public health diseases and conditions.

- Demonstrate the ability to recognize social determinants of health to diminish disparities and inequities in access to quality care.

- Demonstrate the ability to represent the patient's best interests.

- Demonstrate effective communication with patients, the public, and healthcare professionals during the pharmacist/patient care services.

- Demonstrate the ability to be creative and innovative toward patient care.

3.2.7 Medication Safety (Care Provider and Health Protector)

- Demonstrate ability to dispense medications, herbal medication, and other nutraceuticals appropriately, safely, and effectively to patients and the public.

- Demonstrate ability to perform pharmaceutical compounding and patient-specific calculations, including pharmacokinetic and other therapeutic calculations to individualize the dosage regimens for patients when needed.

- Demonstrate ability to identify the potential drug-related problems (DRPs) such as potential adverse drug reactions (ADRs), minimize them as well as the actual DRPs such as ADRs, and manage them.

- Demonstrate ability to work effectively with other healthcare professionals to minimize, prevent, and manage the actual medication errors, and prevent/minimize the potential medication errors.

- Demonstrate ability to improve knowledge and skills toward medication safety aspects

- Demonstrate ability to collaborate effectively in developing, implementing, and evaluating policies, procedures, and activities that promote quality and safety.

3.2.8 Patient Safety (Care Provider and Health Protector)

- Demonstrate ability to identify potential patient safety issues and risks, minimize them as well solve the actual problems and manage them.

- Demonstrate ability to work effectively with other healthcare professionals to minimize, prevent, and manage actual medical errors, and surgical errors and prevent/minimize potential errors.

- Demonstrate ability to improve knowledge and skills toward patient safety aspects

- Demonstrate ability to collaborate effectively in developing, implementing, and evaluating policies, procedures, and activities that promote quality and safety.

- Demonstrate ability to design and conduct patient safety research

3.2.9 Prescribing (Prescriber)

- Demonstrate ability to provide safe and effective prescribing based on evidence-based medicine.

- Demonstrate ability to develop a systematic, evidence-based, and reflective approach to prescribing practice.

- Demonstrate ability to provide safe and effective prescribing and consultations online.

3.2.10 Ethical, Legal, and Professional Responsibilities

- Demonstrate integrity, honesty, knowledge of ethical principles and the standards of professional conduct, and the ability to apply ethical principles in patient care, research, education, or community service.

- Demonstrate ability to work within country legal requirements

3.2.11 Health Promotion and Community Services (Health and Wellness Promoter and Counselor)

- Demonstrate ability to Engage in health promotion and community services activities face-to-face or online.

3.2.12 Research (Researcher)

- Demonstrate ability to design and conduct patient safety research

3.2.13 Technology (IT User)

- Demonstrate ability to use different software/programs, mobile applications, social media, online platforms, media technologies, and other technologies for the purpose of learning, research, and practice.

3.3 CONCLUSION

This chapter has discussed the development of patient safety competencies and learning outcomes based on the literature and experts' opinions. The developed competencies and learning outcomes are related to knowledge, cognition, communication, education and collaboration, life-long learning and personal/professional development, leadership and management, patient care, medication safety, patient safety, prescribing, ethical, legal, and professional responsibilities, health Promotion and community services, researcher and technology user. Preparing future healthcare professionals with the necessary competencies related to the patient safety issues is the key to success in patient safety practice.

REFERENCES

Accreditation Council for Pharmacy Education. (2015). Accreditation standards and key elements for the professional program in pharmacy leading to the doctor of pharmacy degree. *(Standards 2016)*. Available at: https://www.acpe-accredit.org/pdf/Standards2016FINAL.pdf

Al-Worafi, Y.M. (Ed.). (2020). Drug Safety in Developing Countries: Achievements and Challenges.

Al-Worafi, Y. (2022). *A Guide to Online Pharmacy Education: Teaching Strategies and Assessment Methods*. CRC Press.

Frank, J.R., Snell, L.S., Cate, O.T., Holmboe, E.S., Carraccio, C., Swing, S.R., Harris, P., Glasgow, N.J., Campbell, C., Dath, D., & Harden, R.M., 2010. Competency-based medical education: theory to practice. Medical teacher, 32(8), pp. 638–645.

Levett-Jones, T., Dwyer, T., Reid-Searl, K., Heaton, L., Flenady, T., Applegarth, J., & Andersen, P. (2018). The patient safety competency framework for nursing students.

World Health Organization. (2010). Development of the core competencies for Patient Safety Research. *Patient Safety Research Education and Training Working Group*. Geneva: WHO.

4 Patient Safety Education

Teaching Strategies and Assessment Methods

4.1 TEACHING STRATEGIES

There are many effective teaching strategies that can be used in patient safety education programs/ courses such as the following (Al-Worafi, 2022a-q; Al-Meman et al., 2014; McCoy et al., 2018; Stewart et al., 2011):

4.1.1 Interactive-Spaced Education

Use of repetition of content at spaced intervals combined with testing of that content; developed and used heavily within the context of medical education.

4.1.2 Interactive Web-Based Learning

Use of web-based modules to deliver content and assess student understanding in an interactive format.

4.1.3 Audience Response System/Clickers

Use of remote control devices by students to anonymously respond to multiple-choice questions posed by the instructor; can be integrated into traditional lectures, often termed "active lecture" Audience response: Individual students respond to the application of skill questions via an audience response system.

4.1.4 Discussion-Based Learning, Including Deliberative Discussion

The use of communication among learners (both synchronous and asynchronous) as a teaching modality; can be used with other strategies such as case studies.

4.1.5 Patient Simulation

Use of human patient simulators in a laboratory environment to teach providers to respond to a variety of physiological emergencies and situations.

4.1.6 Process-Oriented Guided Inquiry Learning (POGIL)/Discovery Learning

Use of exercises specifically designed to lead teams of students through the stages of exploring data, developing concepts based on that data, and applying the concepts.

4.1.7 Problem-Based Learning (PBL), Including Case-Based Learning

Use of cases or problem sets meant to be explored in self-managed teams of students (with a facilitator); PBL sessions precede any discussion of content by the instructor.

4.1.8 Team-Based Learning (TBL)

Use of small student groups to facilitate discussion, case study exploration, or other aspects of content; preparation required in advance and content integrated throughout the class by the facilitator (expert).

4.1.9 Traditional Laboratory Experiences

Use of traditional laboratory and benchtop experiences to provide hands-on learning experiences.

4.1.10 Vodcast + Pause Activities

A video podcast with pause activities, appended exercises, or practice questions.

4.1.11 Vodcast + Hyperlinks

A video podcast with no pause activities but includes hyperlinks to external or web media for enrichment.

4.1.12 Interactive Vodcast

A vodcast that requires students to physically click through questions or interactivities. (vodcasts using Flash).

DOI: 10.1201/9781003230465-5

4.1.13 Interactive Module

An electronic lesson, often audiovisual, that requires students to complete interactivities.

4.1.14 Case-Based Instruction

The use of patient cases to stimulate discussion, questioning, problem-solving, and reasoning on issues pertaining to the basic sciences and clinical disciplines.

4.1.15 Demonstration

A performance or explanation of a process, illustrated by examples, realia, observable action, specimens, etc.

4.1.16 Discussion or Debate

Instructors facilitate a structured or informal discussion or debate.

4.1.17 Game

An instructional method requiring the learner to participate in a competitive activity with Preset Rules.

4.1.18 Interview or Panel

Students interview standardized patients or experts to practice interviewing and history-taking skills.

4.1.19 Learning Station

Students rotate through learning stations, participating in performance exercises at each station.

4.1.20 Worksheet or Problem Set

Learners work in pairs or teams to solve problems or categorize information.

4.1.21 CP Scheme

An interactive exercise that encourages learners to make clinical decisions following a clinical presentation scheme (flowchart).

4.1.22 Simulation or Role Play

A method used to replace or amplify real patient encounters with scenarios designed to replicate real healthcare situations, using lifelike mannequins, physical models, or standardized patients.

4.1.23 Oral Presentation

Students present topics to their peers. Professors and peers evaluate the presentations using a specific rubric.

4.1.24 Team-Based Activity

A collaborative learning activity that fosters team discussion, thinking, or problem-solving.

4.1.25 Problem-Based Learning

Working in peer groups, students identify what they already know, what they need to know, and how and where to access new information that may lead to the resolution of the problem.

4.1.26 Lab or Studio

Students apply knowledge in the lab, by engaging in a hands-on or kinesthetic activity.

4.1.27 Formative Quizzes

The lesson includes a set of questions bundled together into a quiz, which allows learners to self-assess.

4.1.28 Technology-Enhanced Active Learning (TEAL)

An interactive lesson integrating educational technology, such as electronic games, mobile apps, virtual simulations, EHR, videoconferencing, web exercises, or bioinstruments38.

4.1.29 Flipped Classroom

The traditional lecture and homework elements of a course are reversed. Short video lectures or electronic handouts are viewed by students before class. In-class time is devoted to exercises, projects, or discussions. The flipped classroom (also called reverse, inverse, or backward classroom) is a pedagogical approach in which basic concepts are provided to students for pre-class learning so that class time can apply and build upon those basic concepts. The flipped classroom can be used to prepare the students to be lifelong learners and improve their self-reading skills. Furthermore, improve their basic and clinical knowledge and skills.

4.1.30 Interactive Lecture-Based Teaching Strategy

Pharmacy educators can make the lecture interactive in many ways such as asking students questions every five to ten minutes, presenting short videos/audios, rallies, and team share groups will make students attracted to the lectures. Link the theory part with life, share your practice experience with students with mini and long cases, and give students time to think about it, and solve it. Engage all students and remember that many students may be hesitant to participate, encourage all to participate. Remember as a pharmacy educator you are teaching the students, and assessing their needs, understanding can help also. Weekly and monthly feedback from students and colleagues can improve online teaching. Record the lectures and give them to students as well as to yourself, colleagues. Add many active teaching strategies to the lecture such as videos, cases, and others.

4.1.31 Blended Teaching Strategy

Traditionally, blended learning combines online educational materials and opportunities for interaction online with traditional place-based classroom methods.

4.1.32 Video-Based Learning

Short videos can be used as an effective teaching strategy for theory, practicals, and training.

4.1.33 Simulation

Role play and other simulation methods can be used with the help of new technologies as an effective online teaching strategy for theory.

4.1.34 Project-Based Learning

Project-Based Learning is a model that can be used to prepare students for real practice, Project-Based Education (PBL) gives students the opportunity to develop knowledge and skills through engaging projects set around challenges and problems they may face in the real world.

4.1.35 Journal Club

To critically evaluate recent articles in the academic literature.

4.1.36 Case Studies Discussion

It is a very important and effective teaching strategy, to encourage students to read the giving cases individually or as teams and solve it.

4.1.37 Self-directed Learning

This allows students, and improves their skills, toward self-learning.

4.1.38 Community Services-Based Learning

Many theory courses can be used this effective teaching strategy, which allows students to achieve the course learning outcomes while contributing to the patients, the public, and society.

4.1.39 Seminars

An effective strategy that can be used online to improve the students' presentation skills.

4.2 ASSESSMENT METHODS

There are many direct and indirect assessment methods that can be used in patient safety education programs/courses such as the following (Allen, 2004; Al-Worafi, 2022, r-v):

4.2.1 Direct Assessment Methods and Its Application

There are many direct assessment methods that can be used in patient safety education programs/courses such as the following:

4.2.1.1 Published/Standardized Tests

Published tests are published or standardized tests, that are instruments that have been commercially published by a test publisher. These instruments are administered and scored in a consistent, or "standard" manner. The validity and reliability of the instrument are two essential elements for defining the standard quality of the test. These tests are generally only available from the publisher and often come in the form of kits or multiple booklets. They can be very costly if purchased.

4.2.1.2 Locally Developed Tests

Faculty may decide to develop their own internal test that reflects the program's learning outcomes such as the Multiple Choices Questions (MCQs) and other questions developed by faculty in Pharmacotherapy modules.

4.2.1.3 Embedded Assignments and Course Activities

Embedded Assignments and Course Activities are assignments, activities, or exercises that are done as part of a class, but that are used to provide assessment data about a particular learning outcome.

4.2.1.4 Examples of Embedded Assignments and Course Activities in Pharmacy Education

- Community-service learning and other fieldwork activities such as awareness programs in the malls, among others.
- Culminating projects, such as papers in capstone courses
- Exams or parts of exams
- Group projects
- Homework assignments
- In-class presentations
- Student recitals and exhibitions
- Comprehensive exams, theses, dissertations, and defense interviews.

4.2.1.5 Portfolios

A portfolio can be generally defined as "a purposeful collection of student's work that exhibits the student's efforts, progress, and achievements in one or more areas. The collection must include student participation in selecting contents, the criteria for selection, the criteria for judging merit, and evidence of student self-reflection".

4.2.2 Indirect Assessment Methods and Its Application

There are many indirect assessment methods that can be used in patient safety education programs/courses such as the following:

4.2.2.1 Surveys

The survey is an examination of opinions, behavior, etc., made by asking people questions (Cambridge Dictionary).
  Point-of-contact surveys
  Online, e-mailed, registration, or grad check surveys
  Keep it simple!

4.2.2.2 Examples of Surveys

Surveys and Questionnaires to stakeholders to ask them about the graduates.
  Surveys & Questionnaires to (students, alumni, employers, public) about any issues.

4.2.2.3 *Interviews*

- Interviews can be conducted one-on-one, in small groups, or over the phone.

- Interviews can be structured (with specified questions) or unstructured (a more open process).

- Questions can be close-ended (e.g., multiple-choice style) or open-ended (respondents construct a response).

- Can target students, graduating seniors, alumni, employers, community members, faculty, etc.

- Can do exit interviews or pre-post interviews.

- Can focus on student experiences, concerns, or attitudes related to the program being assessed.

- Generally should be conducted by neutral parties to avoid bias and conflict of interest.

4.2.2.4 *Focus Groups*

- Traditional focus groups are free-flowing discussions among small, homogeneous groups (typically from 6 to 10 participants), guided by a skilled facilitator who subtly directs the discussion in accordance with pre-determined objectives. This process leads to in-depth responses to questions, generally with full participation from all group members. The facilitator departs from the script to follow promising leads that arise during the interaction.

- Structured group interviews are less interactive than traditional focus groups and can be facilitated by people with less training in group dynamics and traditional focus group methodology. The group interview is highly structured, and the report generally provides a few core findings, rather than an in-depth analysis.

4.3 OBJECTIVE STRUCTURED CLINICAL EXAMINATION (OSCE)

The objective structured clinical examination (OSCE) is a method of assessing a student's clinical competence which is objective rather than subjective, and in which the areas tested are carefully planned by the examiners. "Objective structured clinical examination (OSCE) is an approach to the assessment of clinical competence in which the components of competence are assessed in a planned or structured way with attention being paid to the objectivity of the examination." (Harden & Gleeson, 1979). The examination consists of multiple, standard stations at which students must complete 1 to 2 specific clinical tasks, often in an interactive environment involving patient actors such as standardized patients (Harden & Gleeson, 1979).

4.4 CONCLUSION

This chapter has discussed the effective teaching strategies and assessment methods that can be used in patient safety education programs/courses. This chapter covers team-based learning, problem-based learning, project-based learning, community service-based learning, and other active teaching strategies. It also includes the direct and indirect assessment methods and the OSCE.

REFERENCES

Al-Meman, A., Al-Worafi, Y.M., & Saeed, M.S., 2014. Team-based learning as a new learning strategy in pharmacy college, Saudi Arabia: Students' perceptions. *Universal Journal of Pharmacy*, 3(3), pp. 57–65.

Allen, M.J., 2004. Assessing academic programs in higher education. *Bolton, MA. Anker Publishing. Retrieved February*, 6, p. 2013.

Al-Worafi, Y. (2022a). *A Guide to Online Pharmacy Education: Teaching Strategies and Assessment Methods*. CRC Press.

Al-Worafi, Y. (2022b). Pharmacy Education: Learning Styles. In *A Guide to Online Pharmacy Education: Teaching Strategies and Assessment Methods*. CRC Press.

Al-Worafi, Y. (2022c). Competencies and Learning Outcomes. In *A Guide to Online Pharmacy Education: Teaching Strategies and Assessment Methods*. CRC Press.

Al-Worafi, Y. (2022d). Teaching the Theory. In *A Guide to Online Pharmacy Education: Teaching Strategies and Assessment Methods*. CRC Press.

Al-Worafi, Y. (2022e). Teaching the Practice and Tutorial. In *A Guide to Online Pharmacy Education: Teaching Strategies and Assessment Methods*. CRC Press.

Al-Worafi, Y. (2022f). Self-Learning and Self-Directed Learning. In *A Guide to Online Pharmacy Education: Teaching Strategies and Assessment Methods*. CRC Press.

Al-Worafi, Y. (2022g). Traditional and Active Strategies. In *A Guide to Online Pharmacy Education: Teaching Strategies and Assessment Methods*. CRC Press.

Al-Worafi, Y. (2022h). Team-Based Learning in Pharmacy Education. In *A Guide to Online Pharmacy Education: Teaching Strategies and Assessment Methods*. CRC Press.

Al-Worafi, Y. (2022i). Problem-Based Learning in Pharmacy Education. In *A Guide to Online Pharmacy Education: Teaching Strategies and Assessment Methods*. CRC Press.

Al-Worafi, Y. (2022j). Case-Based Learning in Pharmacy Education. In *A Guide to Online Pharmacy Education: Teaching Strategies and Assessment Methods*. CRC Press.

Al-Worafi, Y. (2022k). Simulation in Pharmacy Education. In *A Guide to Online Pharmacy Education: Teaching Strategies and Assessment Methods*. CRC Press.

Al-Worafi, Y. (2022l). Project-Based Learning in Pharmacy Education. In *A Guide to Online Pharmacy Education: Teaching Strategies and Assessment Methods*. CRC Press.

Al-Worafi, Y. (2022m). Flipped Classes in Pharmacy Education. In *A Guide to Online Pharmacy Education: Teaching Strategies and Assessment Methods*. CRC Press.

Al-Worafi, Y. (2022n). Educational Games in Pharmacy Education. In *A Guide to Online Pharmacy Education: Teaching Strategies and Assessment Methods*. CRC Press.

Al-Worafi, Y. (2022o). Web-Based Learning in Pharmacy Education. In *A Guide to Online Pharmacy Education: Teaching Strategies and Assessment Methods*. CRC Press.

Al-Worafi, Y. (2022p). Lecture-Based/Interactive Lecture-Based Learning in Pharmacy Education. In *A Guide to Online Pharmacy Education: Teaching Strategies and Assessment Methods*. CRC Press.

Al-Worafi, Y. (2022q). Blended Learning in Pharmacy Education. In *A Guide to Online Pharmacy Education: Teaching Strategies and Assessment Methods*. CRC Press.

Al-Worafi, Y. (2022r). Assessment Methods in Pharmacy Education: Strengths and Limitations. In *A Guide to Online Pharmacy Education: Teaching Strategies and Assessment Methods*. CRC Press.

Al-Worafi, Y. (2022s). Assessment Methods in Pharmacy Education: Direct Assessment. In *A Guide to Online Pharmacy Education: Teaching Strategies and Assessment Methods*. CRC Press.

Al-Worafi, Y. (2022t). Assessment Methods in Pharmacy Education: Indirect Assessment. In *A Guide to Online Pharmacy Education: Teaching Strategies and Assessment Methods*. CRC Press.

Al-Worafi, Y. (2022u). Assessment Methods in Pharmacy Education: Formative Assessment. In *A Guide to Online Pharmacy Education: Teaching Strategies and Assessment Methods*. CRC Press.

Al-Worafi, Y. (2022v). Objective Structured Clinical Examination (OSCE) in Pharmacy Education. In *A Guide to Online Pharmacy Education: Teaching Strategies and Assessment Methods*. CRC Press.

Harden, R.M., & Gleeson, F.A., 1979. Assessment of clinical competence using an objective structured clinical examination (OSCE). *Medical education*, 13(1), pp. 39–54.

McCoy, L., Pettit, R.K., Kellar, C., & Morgan, C., 2018. Tracking active learning in the medical school curriculum: A learning-centered approach. *Journal of Medical Education and Curricular Development*, 5, p. 2382120518765135.

Stewart, D.W., Brown, S.D., Clavier, C.W., & Wyatt, J. (2011). Active-learning processes used in US pharmacy education. *American Journal of Pharmaceutical Education*, 75(4).

SECTION 2
PATIENT SAFETY PRACTICE

5 Patient Safety-Related Issues

History and Importance

5.1 BACKGROUND

World Health Organization described "Patient Safety is a health care discipline that emerged with the evolving complexity in health care systems and the resulting rise of patient harm in health care facilities. It aims to prevent and reduce risks, errors, and harm that occur to patients during the provision of health care. A cornerstone of the discipline is a continuous improvement based on learning from errors and adverse events; Patient safety is fundamental to delivering quality essential health services" (WHO, 2019). Patient safety-related issues such as medications safety are a major concern in developing countries as well as developed countries; it is associated with treatment outcomes, an increase in morbidity and mortality, an increase in the cost of illness, an increase in the length of hospital stay, and an increase in the admission to the emergency department as well as visiting the healthcare facilities; decrease the quality of life among patients and public, decrease the satisfaction toward the healthcare services and systems, increase the health expenditure (Al-Worafi, 2020a; WHO, 2019). Patient safety issues such as medical errors, medication errors, surgical errors, adverse drug reactions, and drug-related problems are affecting patients, patients' families, and the healthcare system, therefore, the collaboration between healthcare professionals, healthcare researchers, healthcare educators, healthcare colleges and centers and policymakers are very important and the key to success in improving the patient care, improving the patient safety practice and prevent harm due to patient safety issues such as medical errors, medication errors, and others (Al-Worafi, 2020a; WHO, 2019).

5.2 HISTORY OF PATIENT SAFETY

It is reported that the term primum non nocere (first, do no harm) is attributed by some historians to Galen and was introduced to American and British medical culture by Worthington Hooker in 1847 (Hooker, 1847; Ilan & Foweler, 2005). Dr Harvey Cushing, a pioneer in surgery and neurosurgery, published detailed descriptions of harm caused to his patients secondary to his own performance at the beginning of the 20th century (Ilan & Foweler, 2005; Pinkus, 2001). However, it is believed that Drug Related Problems had a very long history since ancient times (Al-Worafi, 2020b) and literature reported that during the Greek period "a court physician called Glaucos, who took care of a mad man named Hephaestus. According to Arries, Glaucos prescribed him a wrong medication, and Hephaestus died" (Siculus, 1933; Somville et al., 2010). Adverse drug reactions have been reported for more than 2000 years (Al-Worafi, 2020c).

5.3 IMPORTANCE OF PATIENT SAFETY PRACTICE

Patient safety education, practice, and research are very important for healthcare professionals, students, researchers, policymakers, patients, and the public. Preparing future healthcare professionals with the necessary competencies related to patient safety-related issues is the key to success in patient safety practice in the future. Improving the current healthcare professionals' patient safety competencies is very important in order to improve the patients' treatment outcomes in terms of efficacy and safety. Conducting research about the various patient safety issues is key to identifying the current practice, identifying the challenges and suggesting interventions to overcome the challenges and improve the practice, which leads to improving the patient's treatment clinical, economical, and humanistic outcomes.

5.4 CONCLUSION

This chapter has discussed the history and importance of patient safety. Collaboration between healthcare professionals, healthcare researchers, healthcare educators, healthcare colleges and centers, and policymakers are very important and the key to success in improving patient care, improving patient safety practice, and preventing harm due to patient safety issues such as medical errors, medication errors, and others.

REFERENCES

Al-Worafi, Y.M. (Ed.). (2020a). Drug Safety in Developing Countries: Achievements and Challenges.

DOI: 10.1201/9781003230465-7

Al-Worafi, Y.M. (2020b). Drug-related problems. In *Drug Safety in Developing Countries* (pp. 105–117). Academic Press.

Al-Worafi, Y.M. (2020c). Adverse drug reactions. In *Drug Safety in Developing Countries* (pp. 39–57). Academic Press.

Hooker W. (1847). Physician and patient. New York (NY)7 Baker and physician and patient. New York (NY)7 Baker and Scribner.

Ilan, R., & Fowler, R. (2005). Brief history of patient safety culture and science. *Journal of critical care*, 20(1), 2–5.

Pinkus, R.L.B. (2001). Mistakes as a social construct: an historical approach. *Kennedy Institute of Ethics Journal*, 11(2), 117–133.

Siculus, D. (1933). Diodorus Siculus. *Life [edit]*, 7, p. 2.

Somville, F.J.M.P., Broos, P.L.O., & Van Hee, R. (2010). Some notes on medical liability in ancient times. *Acta Chirurgica Belgica*, 110(3), 405–409.

World Health Orgainization (WHO). (2019). Available at: https://www.who.int/news-room/fact-sheets/detail/patient-safety

6 Patient Safety-Related Issues

Patient Care Errors and Related Problems

6.1 BACKGROUND

Patient care is the optimal goal of all healthcare professionals. Physicians, pharmacists, dentists, nurses, and other healthcare professionals are providing great efforts to treat patients and improve their quality of life. Moreover, healthcare professionals play a very important role in diseases preventions. However, during the patient care process, unintentional errors and unexpected problems could occur due to many reasons; therefore, patient safety is very important in healthcare services and patient care. The history of patient care goes back to ancient times when people and therapists used herbs to treat and prevention of diseases and conditions in ancient's times, followed by complementary and alternative medicines (CAM) for centuries, and eventually by conventional medicine and complementary and alternative medicines (CAM) in modern history. The history of patient care errors and unexpected problems goes back to ancient times (Al-Worafi, 2020a-c); a patient died as a result of using the wrong medication, which was prescribed to him by a physician during the Greek period (Al-Worafi, 2020a-c; Siculus, 1933). It is reported that the term primum non nocere (first, do no harm) is attributed by some historians to Galen and was introduced to American and British medical culture by Worthington Hooker in 1847 (Hooker, 1847; Ilan & Foweler, 2005). Dr Harvey Cushing, a pioneer in surgery and neurosurgery, published detailed descriptions of harm caused to his patients secondary to his own performance at the beginning of the 20th century (Ilan & Foweler, 2005; Pinkus, 2001). However, it is believed that Drug Related Problems had a very long history since ancient times (Al-Worafi, 2020b) and literature reported that during the Greek period "a court physician called Glaucos, who took care of a mad man named Hephaestus. According to Arries, Glaucos prescribed him a wrong medication, and Hephaestus died" (Siculus, 1933; Somville et al, 2010). Adverse drug reactions have been reported for more than 2000 years (Al-Worafi, 2020c). It has been reported that chloroform-induced arrhythmia and death in England in 1848 (Al-Worafi, 2020a-c; Siculus, 1933). Literature reported that thalidomide-related congenital malformation in 1961 was the cornerstone and the basics for developing adverse drug reaction reporting systems (McBride, 1961; Routledge, 1998). Patient care errors and related problems are nowadays more than at any other time in history due to many reasons, such as the increase in the population worldwide, the increase in the prevalence of diseases, polypharmacy, self-care, and others (Al-Worafi, 2020a-c;). Patient care errors and problems are affecting patients, the public, healthcare professionals, healthcare systems, and the ministries of health worldwide; it could lead to failure in achieving the clinical, economic, and humanistic treatment desired outcomes (Al-Worafi, 2020a).

6.2 RATIONALITY OF THE PATIENT CARE ERRORS AND RELATED PROBLEMS MODEL

There is a gap between the literature and practice in terms of patient care errors and related problems; while a huge number of studies is about a few types of patient care errors and related problems, such as medication errors or prescribing errors, there is a dearth of the literature about the whole picture of patient care errors and related problems or at least all types of patient care errors and related problems. Many terminologies, definitions, and classifications related to patient care errors and related problems are confusing for healthcare professionals, students, and researchers; medication errors, prescribing errors, prescription writing errors, and drug-related problems are reported in the literature and used by researchers in many countries with almost same types of errors, therefore, what are the actual differences between the terminologies? There are many definitions for medication errors and adverse drug reactions. However, many definitions are not consistent with the practice and patient care. Achieving clinical, economic, and humanistic outcomes, including the safety of patients, are the key to the patient care process. Therefore, the development of patient care errors and related problems is very important to healthcare professionals, researchers, students, and policymakers.

6.3 DEVELOPMENT OF THE PATIENT CARE ERRORS AND RELATED PROBLEMS MODEL AND DEFINITIONS

A mixed-method study was conducted to develop and validate the patient care errors and related problems model and definitions, including an extensive literature review, experts' opinions, and the Delphi method.

DOI: 10.1201/9781003230465-8

6.3.1 Literature Review

An extensive literature review for more than two years (Alshahrani et al., 2019a,b; Al-Qahtani et al., 2015; Alshahrani et al., 2020a,b; Al-Worafi, 2014; Al-Worafi, 2015; Al-Worafi, 2016; Al-Worafi et al., 2017; Al-Worafi, 2018a-d; Al-Worafi et al., 2018a-b; Al-Worafi et al., 2019; Al-Worafi, 2020a-z; Al-Worafi et al., 2020a-b; Al-Worafi et al., 2021a,b; Al-Worafi, 2022a,b; Al-Worafi, 2023; Baig et al., 2020; Elkalmi et al., 2020; Elsayed & Al-Worafi, 2020; Hasan et al., 2019; Hassan et al., 2014; Izahar et al., 2017; Lee et al., 2017; Mahmoud et al., 2020; Manan et al., 2014; Manan et al., 2016; Ming et al., 2016; Ming et al., 2020; Othman et al., 2020; Saeed et al., 2014). The initial draft of the model and definitions waere developed in this step.

6.3.2 Experts Selection

Experts panel selection was based on their experience in patient care and patient safety field and experts were selected from different countries such as UK, USA, Canada, Europe, Asia, and the Middle East.

6.3.3 Qualitative Interview

Forty-three semi-structured online interviews were conducted for the face and content validation of the model and definitions. The expert panel consisted of 23 university professors with Ph.D. or PharmD degrees and 20 healthcare professionals The interview was conducted in English and Arabic languages with a period ranging from 20 minutes to 80 minutes from May 2021 to February 2022. The second draft of the model and four definitions were developed in this step.

6.3.4 Delphi Method

6.3.4.1 Sample Size

There is no standard size of the panel members. However, the literature recommended that the Delphi panels range between 10 and 1000 will be accepted (Akins et al., 2005). Therefore, a target of 100 experts was selected for this study.

6.3.4.2 Round 1

The invitation was sent to 130 experts from different developing and developed countries. However, only 60 university professors with Ph.D. or PharmD degrees and 30 healthcare professionals accepted the invitation to participate in this study. The experts were asked to respond to the appropriateness of model items and definitions by email, with (yes, no, I don't know or partially yes), and write suggestions about each item.

6.3.4.3 Round 2 and Round 3

The experts from Round 1 were invited to participate in this round. However, 10 experts did not respond to the invitation. The experts were asked to respond to the appropriateness of model items and definitions by email, with (coded 1 = Extremely Important, 2 = Very Important, 3 = Moderately Important, 4 = Neutral, 5 = Slightly Important, 6 = Not Very Important, 7 = Not At All Important) for the model items and indicate their extent of agreement with the proposed definition using a scale numbered from 1= strongly agree, 2 = agree, 3 = neither agree nor disagree, 4 = disagree, 5 = strongly disagree. The participants were also asked to write suggestions about each item and the proposed definitions. The survey was in English and conducted between April 2022 and October 2022.

6.3.4.4 Statistical Analysis

Data were entered and analyzed using SPSS version 21 (SPSS Statistics for Windows, version 21.0, IBM Corp., USA). Frequency and percentage were used for Round 1; items and definitions were included in the second round of the survey if 70% or more of the participants agreed about it. Likert questions were analyzed for the median, mode, and interquartile range (IQR). The consensus was considered achieved if the IQR was ≤1 and the median was ≤2 (Very Important) (Heiko, 2012) The qualitative part was manually analyzed, then summarized all transcripts.

6.4 PATIENT CARE ERRORS AND RELATED PROBLEMS MODEL

The patient care errors and related problems model are summarized in Fig. 6.1.

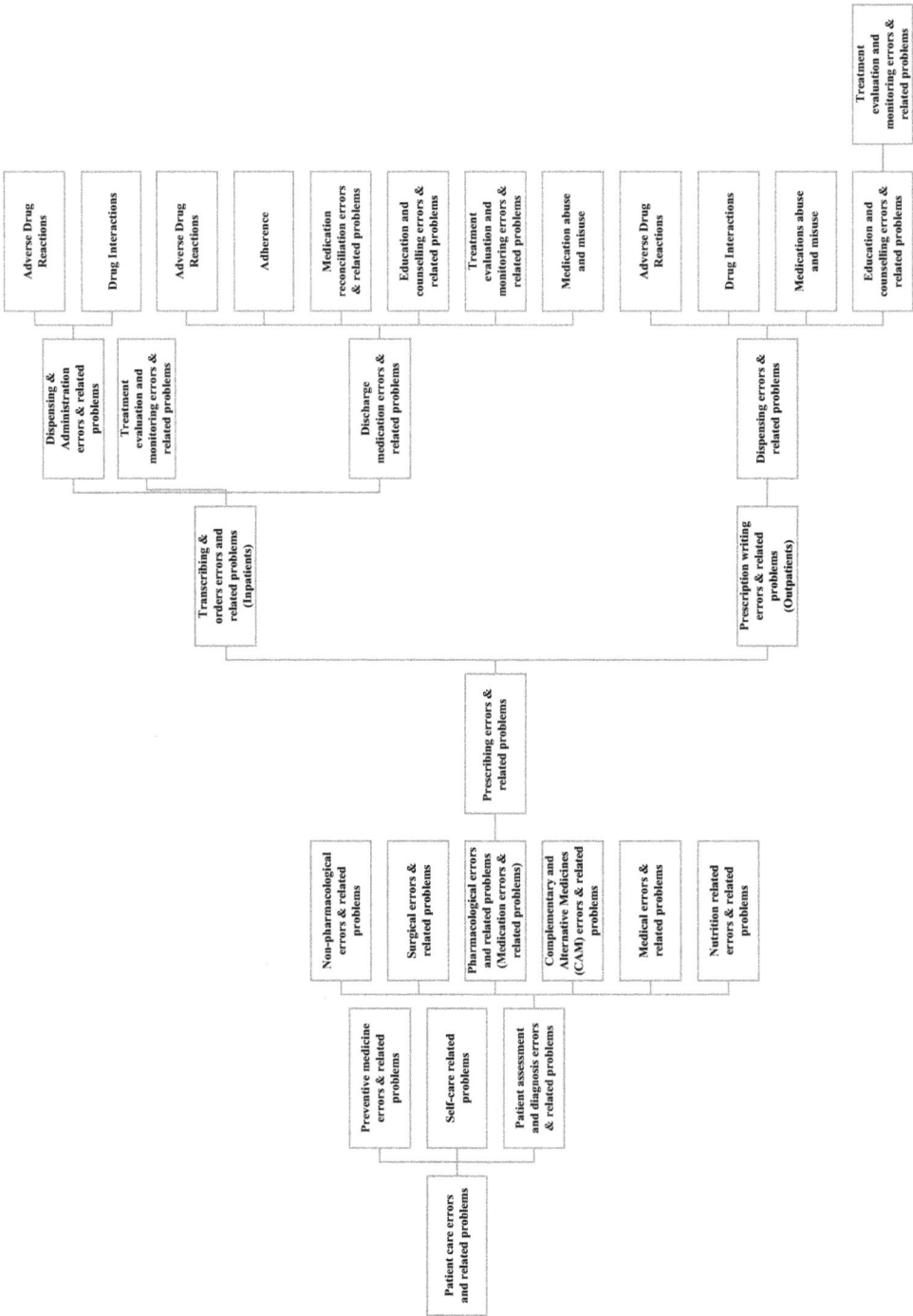

Figure 6.1 Patient care errors and related problems model.

6.5 PATIENT CARE ERRORS AND RELATED PROBLEMS RELATED DEFINITIONS

The patient care errors and related problems definitions are summarized as follows:

6.5.1 Patient Care Errors and Related Problems

It can be defined simply as any intentional or unintentional errors or problems occurring during the patient care process, such as health screening, patient assessment, diagnosis, management, etc.

6.5.2 Preventive Medicine Errors and Related Problems

Any intentional or unintentional errors or problems occurring during the preventive medicine practice, such as health screening or vaccination.

6.5.3 Self-care Related Problems

Any intentional or unintentional errors or problems occurring during the self-care practice, such as self-medications and self-diagnosis.

6.5.4 Patient Assessment and Diagnosis Errors and Related Problems

Any intentional or unintentional errors or problems occurring during the patient assessment and diagnosis.

6.5.5 Non-pharmacological Errors and Related Problems

Any intentional or unintentional errors or problems occurring during non-pharmacological therapy interventions such as diet, exercise, and lifestyle changes.

6.5.6 Surgical Errors and Related Problems

Any intentional or unintentional errors or problems occur during the surgical procedures.

6.5.7 Pharmacological Errors and Related Problems (Medication Errors and Related Problems)

Any intentional or unintentional errors or problems occur during the medication use cycle, such as prescribing, transcribing, dispensing, administration, etc.

6.5.8 Prescribing Errors and Related Problems

Any intentional or unintentional errors or problems occur during the prescribing process.

Any error related to the identification of patients relates problems; gathering patients related information; medical and medications histories; assessment; management plan which includes objective and desired outcomes, non-pharmacological recommendations such as weight control, appropriate and rational pharmacological recommendations with dose, dosage form route of administration, frequency, duration; time of taking medications and instructions; monitoring for the efficacy and safety as well as disease; patient education and counseling related to adherence toward the management plan, self-management, potential adverse drug effects and reactions, possible interactions, cautions and precautions, contraindications and warning, proper storage and disposal of medications.

6.5.9 Transcribing and Orders Errors and Related Problems (Inpatients)

Any intentional or unintentional errors or problems occur during the transcribing or orders.

6.5.10 Dispensing Errors and Related Problems

Any intentional or unintentional errors or problems occur during the dispensing process.

6.5.11 Administration Errors and Related Problems

Any intentional or unintentional errors or problems occur during the administration process.

6.5.12 Adverse Drug Reactions

Any reaction from using the medication could be reported before in the literature or a new reaction. This could occur for many reasons.

6.5.13 Drug Interactions

Any interaction between the medication and (medication, herbs, foods, disease, and others) could be pharmacokinetics or pharmacodynamic mechanism interactions. This could occur for many reasons.

6.5.14 Treatment Evaluation and Monitoring Errors and Related Problems

Any intentional or unintentional errors or problems occur during the evaluation of therapy outcomes and monitoring parameters.

6.5.15 Discharge Medication Errors and Related Problems

Any intentional or unintentional errors or problems occur during the discharge from the hospital or healthcare facilities.

6.5.16 Adherence

Not following the recommendations of the healthcare professionals regarding non-pharmacological or pharmacological interventions such as stopping taking medications, not taking medications as recommended, not doing exercises as recommended, etc.

6.5.17 Medication Reconciliation Errors and Related Problems

Any intentional or unintentional errors or problems occur during the medication reconciliation process, such as forgetting to update the list of medications, medication duplication, and others.

6.5.18 Education and Counseling Errors and Related Problems

Any intentional or unintentional errors or problems occur during the patient education and counseling process, such as not educating the patient about his/her disease, medications, and others.

6.5.19 Medication Abuse and Misuse

It can be defined simply as using medications wrongly for not what is prescribed, dispensed, and recommended by healthcare professionals or guidelines.

6.5.20 Prescription Writing Errors and Related Problems (Outpatients)

Any intentional or unintentional errors or problems occur during the prescription writing.

This type of error occurs when the prescription elements are either not written or written wrongly, which includes the following related errors: **1. errors related to a physician or authorized prescriber:** name, contact details, and signature. **2. errors related to patient information:** name, address, age, gender, and weight; **3. errors related to prescribed medications:** drug name, strength, dose units, dosage form, the number of medications, duration of therapy, route of administration, dose interval, instructions, drug abbreviation, unit abbreviation, and spelling. **4. errors related to prescription:** date of prescription, diagnosis, and clarity of prescription if the three pharmacists couldn't read the prescription.

6.5.21 Dispensing Errors and Related Problems

Any intentional or unintentional errors or problems occur during the medication dispensing process.

6.5.22 Dispensing Errors (For Dispensing Prescriptions and Orders)

Any error related to checking the appropriateness of the prescription for the prescribed medications such as dose, route of administration, frequency, duration, quantity, time of taking medications and instructions; monitoring for the efficacy and safety as well as disease; patient education and counseling related to adherence toward the management plan, self-management, potential adverse effects and reactions, possible interactions, cautions and precautions, contraindications and warning, proper storage and disposal of medications.

6.5.23 Dispensing Errors (For Patient's Self-medication, Prescribing and Dispensing Non-prescription Medications (OTC) Practice)

Any error related to gathering patients related information, medical and medications histories, allergies, chief complaints, history of present illness, assessment, management plan which includes objective and desired outcomes, non-pharmacological therapy and recommendations such as weight control, smoking cessation, appropriate and rational pharmacological therapy with dose, dosage form and route of administration, frequency, duration; time of taking medications and instructions; monitoring for the efficacy and safety as well as disease; patient education and counseling related to adherence toward the management plan, self-management, potential adverse effects and reactions, possible interactions, cautions and precautions, contraindications and warning, proper storage and disposal of medications; refer patients to physicians, clinics, hospitals.

6.5.24 Complementary and Alternative Medicines (CAM) Errors and Related Problems
Any intentional or unintentional errors or problems occur during the Complementary and Alternative Medicines (CAM) practice.

6.5.25 Medical Errors and Related Problems
Any intentional or unintentional errors or problems occur during the patient care process.

6.5.26 Nutrition-Related Errors and Related Problems
Any intentional or unintentional errors or problems occur during the nutrition care process, such as patient screening, patient assessment, nutrition care plan, etc.

6.6 CONCLUSION
This chapter has discussed patient care errors and related problem models and definitions which are very important to healthcare professionals, researchers, students, and policymakers.

REFERENCES

Akins, R.B., Tolson, H., & Cole, B.R. (2005). Stability of response characteristics of a Delphi panel: application of bootstrap data expansion. *BMC medical research methodology*, 5(1), 1–12.

Al-Qahtani, I., Almoteb, T.M., & Al-Warafi, Y. (2015). Competency of metered-dose inhaler use among Saudi community pharmacists: A Simulation method study. *RRJPPS*, 4(2), 37–31.

Alshahrani, S.M., Alakhali, K.M., & Al-Worafi, Y.M. (2019a). Medication errors in a health care facility in southern Saudi Arabia. *Tropical Journal of Pharmaceutical Research*, 18(5), pp. 1119–1122.

Alshahrani, S.M., Alavudeen, S.S., Alakhali, K.M., Al-Worafi, Y.M., Bahamdan, A.K., & Vigneshwaran, E., (2019b). Self-Medication Among King Khalid University Students. *Saudi Arabia. Risk Management and Healthcare Policy*, 12, pp. 243–249.

Alshahrani, S.M., Alakhali, K.M., Al-Worafi, Y.M., & Alshahrani, N.Z. (2020a). Awareness and use of over the counter analgesic medication: a survey in the Aseer region population, Saudi Arabia. *Int J Advan Appl Sci*, 7(3), 130–134.

Alshahrani, S.M., Alzahran, M., Alakhali, K., Vigneshwaran, E., Iqbal, M.J., Khan, N.A., … & Alavudeen, S.S. (2020b). Association Between Diabetes Consequences and Quality of Life Among Patients With Diabetes Mellitus in the Aseer Province of Saudi Arabia. *Open Access Macedonian Journal of Medical Sciences*, 8(E), 325–330.

Al-Worafi, Y.M. (2014). Prescription writing errors at a tertiary care hospital in Yemen: prevalence, types, causes and recommendations. *Am J Pharm Health Res*, 2, 134–140.

Al-Worafi, Y.M.A. (2015). Appropriateness of metered-dose inhaler use in the Yemeni community pharmacies. *Journal of Taibah University Medical Sciences*, 10(3), 353–358.

Al-Worafi, Y.M.A. (2016). Pharmacy practice in Yemen. In *Pharmacy Practice in Developing Countries* (pp. 267–287). Academic Press.

Al-Worafi, Y.M., Kassab, Y.W., Alseragi, W.M., Almutairi, M.S., Ahmed, A., Ming, L.C., Alkhoshaiban, A.S., & Hadi, M.A. (2017). Pharmacovigilance and adverse drg reaction reporting: a perspective of community pharmacists and pharmacy technicians in Sana'a, Yemen. *Therapeutics and clinical risk management*, 13, p. 1175.

Al-Worafi, Y.M. (2018a). Knowledge, Attitude and Practice of Yemeni Physicians Toward Pharmacovigilance: A Mixed Method Study. *International Journal of Pharmacy and Pharmaceutical Sciences*, 10 (10), 74–77.

Al-Worafi, Y. (2018b). Knowledge, attitude and practice of Yemeni physicians toward pharmacovigilance: A mixed method study. *Int. J. Pharm. Pharm. Sci*, 10, 74–77.

Al-Worafi, Y.M. (2018c). Dispensing errors observed by community pharmacy dispensers in IBB–YEMEN. *Asian J. Pharm. Clin. Res*, 11(11).

Al-Worafi, Y.M. (2018d). Evauation of inhaler technique among patients with asthma and COPD in Yemen. *Journal of Taibah University medical sciences*, 13(5), 488–490.

Al-Worafi, Y.M., Patel, R.P., Zaidi, S.T.R., Alseragi, W.M., Almutairi, M.S., Alkhoshaiban, A.S., & Ming, L.C. (2018a). Completeness and legibility of handwritten prescriptions in Sana'a, Yemen. *Medical Principles and Practice*, 27, 290–292.

Al-Worafi, Y.M., Alseragi, W.M., Seng, L.K., Kassab, Y.W., Yeoh, S.F., Chiau, L., ... & Husain, K. (2018b). Dispensing errors in community pharmacies: a prospective study in Sana'a, Yemen. *Arch Pharm Pract*, 9(4), 1–3.

Al-Worafi, Y.M., Alseragi, W.M., & Mahmoud, M.A. (2019). Competency of metered-dose inhaler use among community pharmacy dispensers in Ibb, Yemen: A simulation method study. *Latin American Journal of Pharmacy*, 38(3), 489–494.

Al-Worafi, Y.M. (Ed.). (2020a). Drug Safety in Developing Countries: Achievements and Challenges.

Al-Worafi, Y.M. (2020b). Drug-related problems. In *Drug Safety in Developing Countries* (pp. 105–117). Academic Press.

Al-Worafi, Y.M. (2020c). Adverse drug reactions. In *Drug Safety in Developing Countries* (pp. 39–57). Academic Press.

Al-Worafi, Y.M. (2020d). Medications registration and marketing: safety-related issues. In *Drug Safety in Developing Countries* (pp. 21–28). Academic Press.

Al-Worafi, Y.M. (2020e). Pharmacovigilance. In *Drug Safety in Developing Countries* (pp. 29–38). Academic Press.

Al-Worafi, Y.M. (2020f). Medication errors. In *Drug safety in developing countries* (pp. 59–71). Academic Press.

Al-Worafi, Y.M. (2020g). Medications safety-related terminology. In *Drug safety in developing countries* (pp. 7–19). Academic Press.

Al-Worafi, Y.M. (2020h). Self-medication. In *Drug Safety in Developing Countries* (pp. 73–86). Academic Press.

Al-Worafi, Y.M. (2020j). Antibiotics safety issues. In *Drug Safety in Developing Countries* (pp. 87–103). Academic Press.

Al-Worafi, Y.M. (2020k). Medications safety research issues. In *Drug Safety in Developing Countries* (pp. 213–227). Academic Press.

Al-Worafi, Y.M. (2020l). Counterfeit and substandard medications. In *Drug safety in developing countries* (pp. 119–126). Academic Press

Al-Worafi, Y.M. (2020m). Medication abuse and misuse. In *Drug safety in developing countries* (pp. 127–135). Academic Pres

Al-Worafi, Y.M. (2020n). Storage and disposal of medications. In *Drug Safety in Developing Countries* (pp. 137–142). Academic Press

Al-Worafi, Y.M. (2020o). Safety of medications in special population. In *Drug safety in developing countries* (pp. 143–162). Academic Press.

Al-Worafi, Y.M. (2020p). Herbal medicines safety issues. In *Drug Safety in developing countries* (pp. 163–178). Academic Press.

Al-Worafi, Y.M. (2020q). Medications safety pharmacoeconomics-related issues. In *Drug Safety in Developing Countries* (pp. 187–195). Academic Press.

Al-Worafi, Y.M. (2020r). Evidence-based medications safety practice. In *Drug Safety in Developing Countries* (pp. 197–201). Academic Press.

Al-Worafi, Y.M. (2020s). Quality indicators for medications safety. In *Drug safety in developing countries* (pp. 229–242). Academic Press.

Al-Worafi, Y.M. (2020t). Drug safety in Yemen. In *Drug Safety in Developing Countries* (pp. 391–405). Academic Press.

Al-Worafi, Y.M. (2020u). Drug safety in Saudi Arabia. In *Drug Safety in Developing Countries* (pp. 407–417). Academic Press.

Al-Worafi, Y.M. (2020v). Drug safety in United Arab Emirates. In *Drug Safety in Developing Countries* (pp. 419–428). Academic Press.

Al-Worafi, Y.M. (2020w). Drug safety in Indonesia. In *Drug Safety in Developing Countries* (pp. 279–285). Academic Press.

Al-Worafi, Y.M. (2020x). Drug safety in Palestine. In *Drug Safety in Developing Countries* (pp. 471–480). Academic Press.

Al-Worafi, Y.M. (2020y). Drug safety: comparison between developing countries. In *Drug Safety in Developing Countries* (pp. 603–611). Academic Press.

Al-Worafi, Y.M. (2020z). Drug safety in developing versus developed countries. In *Drug Safety in Developing Countries* (pp. 613–615). Academic Press.

Al-Worafi, Y.M., Alseragi, W.M., Ming, L.C., & Alakhali, K.M. (2020a). Drug safety in China. In *Drug Safety in Developing Countries* (pp. 381–388). Academic Press.

Al-Worafi, Y.M., Alseragi, W.M., Alakhali, K.M., Ming, L.C., Othman, G., Halboup, A.M., ... & Elkalmi, R.M. (2020b). Knowledge, beliefs and factors affecting the use of generic medicines among patients in Ibb, Yemen: a mixed-method study. *Journal of Pharmacy Practice and Community Medicine*, 6(4).

Al-Worafi, Y.M., Elkalmi, R.M., Ming, L.C., Othman, G., Halboup, A.M., Battah, M.M., ... & Mani, V. (2021a). Dispensing errors in hospital pharmacies: A prospective study in Yemen.

Al-Worafi, Y.M., Hasan, S., Hassan, N.M., & Gaili, A.A. (2021b). Knowledge, Attitude and Experience of Pharmacist in the UAE towards Pharmacovigilance. *Research Journal of Pharmacy and Technology*, 14(1), 265–269.

Al-Worafi, Y. (2022a). *A Guide to Online Pharmacy Education: Teaching Strategies and Assessment Methods*. CRC Press.

Al-Worafi, Y.M. (2022b). Patient care errors and related problems (part I): development and validation of the model.

Al-Worafi, Y.M. (Ed.). (2023). *Clinical Case Studies on medication Safety*. Academic Press.

Baig, M.R., Al-Worafi, Y.M., Alseragi, W.M., Ming, L.C., & Siddique, A. (2020). Drug safety in India. In *Drug Safety in Developing Countries* (pp. 327–334). Academic Press.

Elkalmi, R.M., Al-Worafi, Y.M., Alseragi, W.M., Ming, L.C., & Siddique, A. (2020). Drug safety in Malaysia. In *Drug Safety in Developing Countries* (pp. 245–253). Academic Press.

Elsayed, T., & Al-Worafi, Y.M. (2020). Drug safety in Egypt. In *Drug Safety in Developing Countries* (pp. 511–523). Academic Press.

Hasan, S., Al-Omar, M.J., AlZubaidy, H., & Al-Worafi, Y.M. (2019). Use of medications in Arab Countries. *Handbook of Healthcare in the Arab World*. Cham: Springer, 42.

Hassan, Y., Abd Aziz, N., Kassab, Y.W., Elgasim, I., Shaharuddin, S., Al-Worafi, Y.M.A., ... & Ming, L.C. (2014). How to help patients to control their blood pressure? Blood pressure control and its predictor. *Archives of Pharmacy Practice*, 5(4).

Heiko, A. V. D. G (2012). Consensus measurement in Delphi studies: review and implications for future quality assurance. *Technological forecasting and social change*, 79(8), 1525–1536.

Hooker W. (1847). Physician and patient. New York (NY)7 Baker and physician and patient. New York (NY)7 Baker and Scribner.

Ilan, R., & Fowler, R. (2005). Brief history of patient safety culture and science. *Journal of critical care*, 20(1), 2–5.

Izahar, S., Lean, Q.Y., Hameed, M.A., Murugiah, M.K., Patel, R.P., Al-Worafi, Y.M., ... & Ming, L.C. (2017). Content analysis of mobile health applications on diabetes mellitus. *Frontiers in Endocrinology*, 8, 318.

Lee, K.S., Yee, S.M., Zaidi, S.T.R., Patel, R.P., Yang, Q., Al-Worafi, Y.M. and Ming, L.C., 2017. Combating sale of counterfeit and falsified medicines online: a losing battle. *Frontiers in pharmacology*, 8, p. 268.

Mahmoud, M.A., Wajid, S., Naqvi, A.A., Samreen, S., Althagfan, S.S., & Al-Worafi, Y. (2020). Self-medication with antibiotics: A cross-sectional community-based study. *Latin American Journal Of Pharmacy*, 39(2), 348–353.

Manan, M.M., Rusli, R.A., Ang, W.C., Al-Worafi, Y.M., & Ming, L.C. (2014). Assessing the pharmaceutical care issues of antiepileptic drug therapy in hospitalised epileptic patients. *Journal of Pharmacy Practice and Research*, 44(3), 83–88.

Manan, M.M., Ibrahim, N.A., Aziz, N.A., Zulkifly, H.H., Al-Worafi, Y.M.A., & Long, C.M. (2016). Empirical use of antibiotic therapy in the prevention of early onset sepsis in neonates: a pilot study. *Archives of Medical Science*, 12(3), 603–613.

Ming, L.C., Hameed, M.A., Lee, D.D., Apidi, N.A., Lai, P.S.M., Hadi, M.A., Al-Worafi, Y.M.A., & Khan, T.M., (2016). Use of medical mobile applications among hospital pharmacists in Malaysia. *Therapeutic innovation & regulatory science*, 50(4), pp. 419–426.

Ming, L.C., Untong, N., Aliudin, N.A., Osili, N., Kifli, N., Tan, C.S. … & Goh, H.P. (2020). Mobile health apps on COVID-19 launched in the early days of the pandemic: content analysis and review. *JMIR mHealth and uHealth*, 8(9), e19796.

McBride, W.G., 1961. Thalidomide and congenital abnormalities. *Lancet*, 2(1358), pp. 90927–90928.

Othman, G., Ali, F., Ibrahim, M.I.M., Al-Worafi, Y.M., Ansari, M., & Halboup, A.M. (2020). Assessment of Anti-Diabetic Medications Adherence among Diabetic Patients in Sana'a City, Yemen: A Cross Sectional Study. *Journal of Pharmaceutical Research International*, 32(21), 114–122.

Pinkus, R.L.B. (2001). Mistakes as a social construct: an historical approach. *Kennedy Institute of Ethics Journal*, 11(2), 117–133.

Routledge, P., 1998. 150 years of pharmacovigilance. *Lancet (London, England)*, 351(9110), p. 1200.

Saeed, M.S., Alkhoshaiban, A.S., Al-Worafi, Y.M.A., & Long, C.M., (2014). Perception of self-medication among university students in Saudi Arabia. *Archives of Pharmacy Practice*, 5(4), p. 149.

Siculus, D., (1933). Diodorus Siculus. *Life [edit]*, 7, p. 2.

Somville, F.J.M.P., Broos, P.L.O., & Van Hee, R. (2010). Some notes on medical liability in ancient times. *Acta Chirurgica Belgica*, 110(3), 405–409.

7 Patient Care Errors and Related Problems

Preventive Medicine Errors and Related Problems

7.1 BACKGROUND

Preventive medicine is a branch of medicine that focuses on preventing diseases, injuries, and other health problems before they occur. This involves taking proactive measures to maintain and improve health, rather than simply treating illnesses and injuries after they have already developed. Preventive medicine encompasses a wide range of activities and strategies, including (Casens, 1992; Foege, 1994; Rakel & Minichiello, 2022):

1. Immunizations: Vaccinations are a key tool in preventing the spread of infectious diseases, such as influenza, measles, and polio.

2. Screening tests: Screening tests can help detect diseases in their early stages when they are most treatable. Examples include mammograms for breast cancer, colonoscopies for colon cancer, and blood tests for high cholesterol or diabetes.

3. Lifestyle modifications: Simple lifestyle changes, such as maintaining a healthy diet, exercising regularly, and not smoking, can have a big impact on preventing chronic diseases such as heart disease, diabetes, and certain cancers.

4. Environmental interventions: Preventive medicine also involves addressing environmental factors that contribute to poor health, such as pollution, unsafe drinking water, and hazardous working conditions.

5. Health education: Educating individuals and communities about healthy behaviors and disease prevention can also help reduce the incidence of illness and injury.

Overall, preventive medicine is an important aspect of healthcare that aims to promote health and prevent disease, ultimately improving the overall quality of life for individuals and communities.

7.2 IMMUNIZATION

Immunization, also known as vaccination, is the process of introducing a vaccine into the body to help the immune system develop protection against specific diseases. Vaccines are typically made from weakened or killed forms of the disease-causing microorganisms, or from fragments of the microorganisms. When the vaccine is administered, the immune system is stimulated to produce antibodies that can recognize and neutralize the microorganisms in case of exposure in the future. Immunization is a highly effective method of preventing infectious diseases and has been credited with the eradication of several diseases, including smallpox. In addition to preventing individual cases of the disease, immunization can also help protect entire populations from outbreaks of contagious diseases by creating herd immunity. Herd immunity occurs when a large portion of a population becomes immune to a disease, either through vaccination or natural infection, making it difficult for the disease to spread from person to person. This provides protection for those who are unable to be vaccinated, such as people with weakened immune systems, infants, and the elderly. Common vaccines include vaccines for measles, mumps, rubella, polio, influenza, and hepatitis. Immunization schedules may vary by country but generally involve a series of shots given during childhood, with additional booster shots recommended later in life.

7.3 HEALTH SCREENING

Health screening refers to the process of checking for a particular health condition or disease in an individual who may not be experiencing any symptoms. Health screening tests can help to identify potential health issues early on, which may allow for earlier intervention and better outcomes. Health screenings can include a range of tests and evaluations, such as blood tests, imaging studies, physical exams, and health questionnaires.

The specific health screening tests recommended will depend on factors such as age, sex, family history, and lifestyle factors such as smoking or alcohol use. Some examples of common health screening tests include:

1. Blood pressure measurement

2. Cholesterol testing

DOI: 10.1201/9781003230465-9

3. Blood glucose testing

4. Colon cancer screening

5. Breast cancer screening (mammography)

6. Prostate cancer screening

7. Skin cancer screening

8. Vision and hearing tests

It is important to note that not all screening tests are appropriate for all individuals, and the benefits and risks of specific tests should be discussed with a healthcare provider. Additionally, while screening tests can help identify potential health issues, they do not necessarily provide a definitive diagnosis and should be followed up with additional testing and evaluation as needed.

7.4 HEALTH EDUCATION

Health education is the process of educating individuals and communities about health-related topics with the goal of promoting healthy behaviors and preventing disease. Health education can take many forms, including classroom instruction, community outreach programs, and individual counseling. The ultimate goal of health education is to empower individuals with the knowledge, skills, and resources they need to make informed decisions about their health and well-being. Some examples of health education topics include:

1. Nutrition and healthy eating habits

2. Physical activity and exercise

3. Sexual health and contraception

4. Substance abuse prevention and treatment

5. Stress management and mental health

6. Chronic disease management

7. Environmental health and safety

8. First aid and emergency preparedness

Effective health education programs should be tailored to the specific needs and cultural context of the individuals and communities they serve. They should also be evidence-based, meaning that they are based on sound scientific research and have been shown to be effective in promoting healthy behaviors and preventing disease. Health education can be delivered in a variety of settings, including schools, healthcare facilities, community centers, and online platforms.

7.5 PREVENTIVE MEDICINES ERRORS AND RELATED PROBLEMS

Patient care errors and related problems can be defined simply as any intentional or unintentional errors or problems occurring during the patient care process, such as health screening, patient assessment, diagnosis, management, etc. While, preventive medicine errors and related problems can be defined as any intentional or unintentional errors or problems occurring during the preventive medicine practice, such as health screening or vaccination. Vaccines safety are very important to ensure that the public will be safe after receiving vaccination for the prevention of diseases, therefore, vaccine pharmacovigilance is very important to ensure the safety of vaccines and minimize negative effects on the health of individuals and lessen the potential negative impact on immunization of population (CIOMS, 2012). The most common safety issues reported in the literature and pharmacovigilance centers worldwide are vaccine adverse reactions. Patient care is the optimal goal of all healthcare professionals. Physicians, pharmacists, dentists, nurses, and other healthcare professionals are providing great efforts to treat patients and improve their quality of life. Moreover, healthcare professionals play a very important role in diseases preventions. However, during the patient care process, unintentional errors and unexpected problems could occur due to many reasons; therefore, patient safety is very important in healthcare services and patient care.

7.6 PREVENTIVE MEDICINES ERRORS AND RELATED PROBLEMS IN DEVELOPING COUNTRIES

Preventive medicine errors and related problems are a major concern in developing countries. These errors can lead to serious health problems, disability, and even death. Some of the common issues related to preventive medicine errors in developing countries are:

1. Lack of proper healthcare infrastructure: Developing countries often lack proper healthcare infrastructure, including hospitals, clinics, and diagnostic facilities. This can result in errors due to inadequate monitoring and limited access to medical resources.

2. Limited access to medicines: Access to medicines is often limited in developing countries due to factors such as affordability, availability, and distribution. This can lead to errors related to incorrect dosages, administration, and substitutions.

3. Poor training and education: Healthcare workers in developing countries may have limited access to training and education programs, resulting in errors related to inadequate knowledge and skills.

4. Inadequate regulatory framework: Many developing countries have inadequate regulatory frameworks for ensuring the safety and efficacy of medicines. This can result in errors related to the use of substandard or counterfeit medicines.

5. Cultural and language barriers: Cultural and language barriers can also contribute to preventive medicine errors in developing countries. These barriers can lead to misunderstandings and miscommunication between healthcare providers and patients, resulting in errors related to medication use.

6. Lack of patient education: Patients in developing countries may have limited knowledge about their health conditions and the medications they are taking. This can result in errors related to non-adherence to treatment regimens, incorrect self-medication, and medication interactions.

To address these issues, it is important to implement comprehensive strategies that include improving healthcare infrastructure, providing adequate training and education to healthcare workers, strengthening regulatory frameworks, promoting patient education, and addressing cultural and language barriers (Alshahrani et al., 2019a,b; Al-Qahtani et al., 2015; Alshahrani et al., 2020a,b; Al-Worafi, 2014; Al-Worafi, 2015; Al-Worafi, 2016; Al-Worafi et al., 2017; Al-Worafi, 2018a-d; Al-Worafi et al., 2018a-b; Al-Worafi et al., 2019; Al-Worafi, 2020a-z; Al-Worafi et al., 2020a-b; Al-Worafi et al., 2021a,b; Al-Worafi, 2022a-b; Al-Worafi, 2023; Baig et al., 2020; Elkalmi et al., 2020; Elsayed & Al-Worafi, 2020; Hasan et al., 2019; Hassan et al., 2014; Izhar et al., 2017; Lee et al., 2017; Mahmoud et al., 2020; Manan et al., 2014; Manan et al., 2016; Ming et al., 2016; Ming et al., 2020; Othman et al., 2020; Saeed et al., 2014).

Preventive medicine in developing countries faces many challenges, including limited resources, inadequate infrastructure, and high disease burden. However, there are several facilitators and recommendations that can help to improve preventive medicine in these settings:
Facilitators:

1. Public Health Infrastructure: The establishment of public health infrastructure, including healthcare facilities, laboratories, and surveillance systems, can help to identify and respond to disease outbreaks and other public health threats.

2. Education and Awareness: Education and awareness campaigns can help to promote healthy behaviors and practices, such as vaccination, hand hygiene, and safe food and water practices.

3. International Partnerships: International partnerships and collaborations can help to build capacity and provide resources and expertise to support preventive medicine efforts in developing countries.

4. Political Commitment: Political commitment and investment in public health programs can help to improve access to preventive services and reduce the burden of disease.

Recommendations:
Preventive medicine is an essential component of public health in developing countries. Here are some recommendations for preventive medicine in developing countries:

1. Immunization: Immunization is one of the most cost-effective ways to prevent diseases in developing countries. Governments should provide access to free or low-cost vaccines to children and adults, as well as educate the public about the importance of vaccination.

2. Vector Control: Developing countries should prioritize efforts to control vector-borne diseases, such as malaria, dengue fever, and Zika virus, through mosquito control measures and other interventions.

3. Access to clean water and sanitation: Access to clean water and sanitation is critical for preventing waterborne diseases such as cholera, typhoid, and diarrhea. Governments should invest in infrastructure to improve access to clean water and sanitation facilities, as well as educate the public on proper hygiene practices.

4. Health education: Health education is crucial in preventing diseases and promoting healthy lifestyles. Governments should invest in health education programs to educate the public on topics such as nutrition, hygiene, and sexual health.

5. Chronic Disease Prevention: Developing countries should prioritize efforts to prevent and manage chronic diseases, such as diabetes and hypertension, through lifestyle interventions, early detection, and appropriate treatment.

6. Disease surveillance and control: Developing countries should establish disease surveillance and control programs to monitor and prevent the spread of communicable diseases. This includes investing in public health infrastructure, such as laboratories, and developing systems to track and respond to disease outbreaks.

7. Primary healthcare: Primary healthcare services should be accessible and affordable to all. Governments should invest in primary healthcare infrastructure, such as clinics and community health workers, to provide basic health services to the population.

8. Community Engagement: Community engagement is essential for successful preventive medicine efforts. Developing countries should involve local communities in the planning, implementation, and evaluation of public health programs to ensure that they are culturally appropriate and effective.

9. Capacity Building: Developing countries should prioritize efforts to build the capacity of their healthcare workforce, including training in disease surveillance, diagnosis, and management,

10. Environmental health: Environmental factors such as air pollution, climate change, and exposure to toxic substances can have significant impacts on public health. Governments should invest in environmental health programs to address these issues and protect public health.

11. Addressing social determinants of health: Social determinants of health, such as poverty, education, and employment, can significantly impact public health. Governments should work to address these issues through policies and programs that improve access to education, job opportunities, and social safety nets.

In summary, preventive medicine in developing countries should focus on immunization, access to clean water and sanitation, health education, disease surveillance and control, primary healthcare, environmental health, and addressing social determinants of health.

7.7 CONCLUSION

This chapter has discussed preventive medicine errors and related problems, the facilitators, barriers, and recommendations for best practices in developing countries. Preventive medicine is a branch of medicine that focuses on preventing diseases, injuries, and other health problems before they occur. This involves taking proactive measures to maintain and improve health, rather than simply treating illnesses and injuries after they have already developed. Preventive medicine encompasses a wide range of activities and strategies, including immunization, health screening, and health education.

REFERENCES

Al-Qahtani, I., Almoteb, T.M., & Al-Warafi, Y. (2015). Competency of metered-dose inhaler use among Saudi community pharmacists: A Simulation method study. *RRJPPS*, 4(2), 37–31.

Alshahrani, S.M., Alakhali, K.M., & Al-Worafi, Y.M. (2019a). Medication errors in a health care facility in southern Saudi Arabia. *Tropical Journal of Pharmaceutical Research*, 18(5), pp. 1119–1122.

Alshahrani, S.M., Alavudeen, S.S., Alakhali, K.M., Al-Worafi, Y.M., Bahamdan, A.K., & Vigneshwaran, E. (2019b). Self-Medication Among King Khalid University Students, Saudi Arabia. *Risk Management and Healthcare Policy*, 12, pp. 243–249.

Alshahrani, S.M., Alakhali, K.M., Al-Worafi, Y.M., & Alshahrani, N.Z. (2020a). Awareness and use of over the counter analgesic medication: a survey in the Aseer region population, Saudi Arabia. *Int J Advan Appl Sci*, 7(3), 130–134.

Alshahrani, S.M., Alzahran, M., Alakhali, K., Vigneshwaran, E., Iqbal, M.J., Khan, N.A., ... & Alavudeen, S.S. (2020b). Association Between Diabetes Consequences and Quality of Life Among Patients With Diabetes Mellitus in the Aseer Province of Saudi Arabia. *Open Access Macedonian Journal of Medical Sciences*, 8(E), 325–330.

Al-Worafi, Y.M. (2014). Prescription writing errors at a tertiary care hospital in Yemen: prevalence, types, causes and recommendations. *Am J Pharm Health Res*, 2, 134–140.

Al-Worafi, Y.M.A. (2015). Appropriateness of metered-dose inhaler use in the Yemeni community pharmacies. *Journal of Taibah University Medical Sciences*, 10(3), 353–358.

Al-Worafi, Y.M.A. (2016). Pharmacy practice in Yemen. In *Pharmacy Practice in Developing Countries* (pp. 267–287). Academic Press.

Al-Worafi, Y.M., Kassab, Y.W., Alseragi, W.M., Almutairi, M.S., Ahmed, A., Ming, L.C., Alkhoshaiban, A.S., & Hadi, M.A. (2017). Pharmacovigilance and adverse drg reaction reporting: a perspective of community pharmacists and pharmacy technicians in Sana'a, Yemen. *Therapeutics and clinical risk management*, 13, p. 1175.

Al-Worafi, Y.M. (2018a). Knowledge, Attitude and Practice of Yemeni Physicians Toward Pharmacovigilance: A Mixed Method Study. *International Journal of Pharmacy and Pharmaceutical Sciences*, 10 (10), 74–77.

Al-Worafi, Y. (2018b). Knowledge, attitude and practice of Yemeni physicians toward pharmacovigilance: A mixed method study. *Int. J. Pharm. Pharm. Sci*, 10, 74–77.

Al-Worafi, Y.M. (2018c). Dispensing errors observed by community pharmacy dispensers in IBB–YEMEN. *Asian J. Pharm. Clin. Res*, 11(11).

Al-Worafi, Y.M. (2018d). Evauation of inhaler technique among patients with asthma and COPD in Yemen. *Journal of Taibah University medical sciences*, 13(5), 488–490.

Al-Worafi, Y.M., Patel, R.P., Zaidi, S.T.R., Alseragi, W.M., Almutairi, M.S., Alkhoshaiban, A.S., & Ming, L.C. (2018a). Completeness and legibility of handwritten prescriptions in Sana'a, Yemen. *Medical Principles and Practice*, 27, 290–292.

Al-Worafi, Y.M., Alseragi, W.M., Seng, L.K., Kassab, Y.W., Yeoh, S.F., Chiau, L., ... & Husain, K. (2018b). Dispensing errors in community pharmacies: a prospective study in Sana'a, Yemen. *Arch Pharm Pract*, 9(4), 1–3.

Al-Worafi, Y.M., Alseragi, W.M., & Mahmoud, M.A. (2019). Competency of metered-dose inhaler use among community pharmacy dispensers in Ibb, Yemen: A simulation method study. *Latin American Journal of Pharmacy*, 38(3), 489–494.

Al-Worafi, Y.M. (Ed.). (2020a). *Drug Safety in Developing Countries: Achievements and Challenges*.

Al-Worafi, Y.M. (2020b). Drug-related problems. In *Drug Safety in Developing Countries* (pp. 105–117). Academic Press.

Al-Worafi, Y.M. (2020c). Adverse drug reactions. In *Drug Safety in Developing Countries* (pp. 39–57). Academic Press.

Al-Worafi, Y.M. (2020d). Medications registation and marketing: safety-related issues. In *Drug Safety in Developing Countries* (pp. 21–28). Academic Press.

Al-Worafi, Y.M. (2020e). Pharmacovigilance. In *Drug Safety in Developing Countries* (pp. 29–38). Academic Press.

Al-Worafi, Y.M. (2020f). Medication errors. In *Drug safety in developing countries* (pp. 59–71). Academic Press.

Al-Worafi, Y.M. (2020g). Medications safety-related terminology. In *Drug safety in developing countries* (pp. 7–19). Academic Press.

Al-Worafi, Y.M. (2020h). Self-medication. In *Drug Safety in Developing Countries* (pp. 73–86). Academic Press.

Al-Worafi, Y.M. (2020j). Antibiotics safety issues. In *Drug Safety in Developing Countries* (pp. 87–103). Academic Press.

Al-Worafi, Y.M. (2020k). Medications safety research issues. In *Drug Safety in Developing Countries* (pp. 213–227). Academic Press.

Al-Worafi, Y.M. (2020l). Counterfeit and substandard medications. In *Drug safety in developing countries* (pp. 119–126). Academic Press.

Al-Worafi, Y.M. (2020m). Medication abuse and misuse. In *Drug safety in developing countries* (pp. 127–135). Academic Press

Al-Worafi, Y.M. (2020n). Storage and disposal of medications. In *Drug Safety in Developing Countries* (pp. 137–142). Academic Press.

Al-Worafi, Y.M. (2020o). Safety of medications in special population. In *Drug safety in developing countries* (pp. 143–162). Academic Press.

Al-Worafi, Y.M. (2020p). Herbal medicines safety issues. In *Drug Safety in developing countries* (pp. 163–178). Academic Press.

Al-Worafi, Y.M. (2020q). Medications safety pharmacoeconomics-related issues. In *Drug Safety in Developing Countries* (pp. 187–195). Academic Press.

Al-Worafi, Y.M. (2020r). Evidence-based medications safety practice. In *Drug Safety in Developing Countries* (pp. 197–201). Academic Press.

Al-Worafi, Y.M. (2020s). Quality indicators for medications safety. In *Drug safety in developing countries* (pp. 229–242). Academic Press.

Al-Worafi, Y.M. (2020t). Drug safety in Yemen. In *Drug Safety in Developing Countries* (pp. 391–405). Academic Press.

Al-Worafi, Y.M. (2020u). Drug safety in Saudi Arabia. In *Drug Safety in Developing Countries* (pp. 407–417). Academic Press.

Al-Worafi, Y.M. (2020v). Drug safety in United Arab Emirates. In *Drug Safety in Developing Countries* (pp. 419–428). Academic Press.

Al-Worafi, Y.M. (2020w). Drug safety in Indonesia. In *Drug Safety in Developing Countries* (pp. 279–285). Academic Press.

Al-Worafi, Y.M. (2020x). Drug safety in Palestine. In *Drug Safety in Developing Countries* (pp. 471–480). Academic Press.

Al-Worafi, Y.M. (2020y). Drug safety: comparison between developing countries. In *Drug Safety in Developing Countries* (pp. 603–611). Academic Press.

Al-Worafi, Y.M. (2020z). Drug safety in developing versus developed countries. In *Drug Safety in Developing Countries* (pp. 613–615). Academic Press.

Al-Worafi, Y.M., Alseragi, W.M., Ming, L.C., & Alakhali, K.M. (2020a). Drug safety in China. In *Drug Safety in Developing Countries* (pp. 381–388). Academic Press.

Al-Worafi, Y.M., Alseragi, W.M., Alakhali, K.M., Ming, L.C., Othman, G., Halboup, A.M., … & Elkalmi, R.M. (2020b). Knowledge, beliefs and factors affecting the use of generic medicines among patients in Ibb, Yemen: a mixed-method study. *Journal of Pharmacy Practice and Community Medicine*, 6(4).

Al-Worafi, Y.M., Elkalmi, R.M., Ming, L.C., Othman, G., Halboup, A.M., Battah, M.M., … & Mani, V. (2021a). Dispensing errors in hospital pharmacies: A prospective study in Yemen.

Al-Worafi, Y.M., Hasan, S., Hassan, N.M., & Gaili, A.A. (2021b). Knowledge, Attitude and Experience of Pharmacist in the UAE towards Pharmacovigilance. *Research Journal of Pharmacy and Technology*, 14(1), 265–269.

Al-Worafi, Y. (2022a). *A Guide to Online Pharmacy Education: Teaching Strategies and Assessment Methods*. CRC Press.

Al-Worafi, Y.M. (2022). Patient care errors and related problems (part I): development and validation of the model. https://orcid.org/0000-0002-5752-2913

Al-Worafi, Y.M. (Ed.). (2023). *Clinical Case Studies on medication Safety*. Academic Press.

Baig, M.R., Al-Worafi, Y.M., Alseragi, W.M., Ming, L.C., & Siddique, A. (2020). Drug safety in India. In *Drug Safety in Developing Countries* (pp. 327–334). Academic Press.

Cassens, B.J. (Ed.). (1992). *Preventive medicine and public health*. Lippincott Williams & Wilkins.

Council for International Organizations of Medical Sciences (CIOMS) (2012). Definition and application of terms for vaccine pharmacovigilance. Report of CIOMS/WHO Working Group on Vaccine Pharmacovigilance. *Geneva: Council for International Organizations of Medical Sciences*.

Elkalmi, R.M., Al-Worafi, Y.M., Alseragi, W.M., Ming, L.C., & Siddique, A. (2020). Drug safety in Malaysia. In *Drug Safety in Developing Countries* (pp. 245–253). Academic Press.

Elsayed, T., & Al-Worafi, Y.M. (2020). Drug safety in Egypt. In *Drug Safety in Developing Countries* (pp. 511–523). Academic Press.

Foege, W. (1994). Preventive medicine and public health. *JAMA*, 271(21), 1704–1705.

Hasan, S., Al-Omar, M.J., AlZubaidy, H., & Al-Worafi, Y.M. (2019). Use of medications in Arab Countries. *Handbook of Healthcare in the Arab World*. Cham: Springer, 42.

Hassan, Y., Abd Aziz, N., Kassab, Y.W., Elgasim, I., Shaharuddin, S., Al-Worafi, Y.M.A., … & Ming, L.C. (2014). How to help patients to control their blood pressure? Blood pressure control and its predictor. *Archives of Pharmacy Practice*, 5(4).

Izahar, S., Lean, Q.Y., Hameed, M.A., Murugiah, M.K., Patel, R.P., Al-Worafi, Y.M., … & Ming, L.C. (2017). Content analysis of mobile health applications on diabetes mellitus. *Frontiers in Endocrinology*, 8, 318.

Lee, K.S., Yee, S.M., Zaidi, S.T.R., Patel, R.P., Yang, Q., Al-Worafi, Y.M., & Ming, L.C., 2017. Combating sale of counterfeit and falsified medicines online: a losing battle. *Frontiers in pharmacology*, 8, p. 268.

Mahmoud, M.A., Wajid, S., Naqvi, A.A., Samreen, S., Althagfan, S.S., & Al-Worafi, Y. (2020). Self-medication with antibiotics: A cross-sectional community-based study. *Latin American Journal of Pharmacy*, 39(2), 348–353.

Manan, M.M., Rusli, R.A., Ang, W.C., Al-Worafi, Y.M., & Ming, L.C. (2014). Assessing the pharmaceutical care issues of antiepileptic drug therapy in hospitalised epileptic patients. *Journal of Pharmacy Practice and Research*, 44(3), 83–88.

Manan, M.M., Ibrahim, N.A., Aziz, N.A., Zulkifly, H.H., Al-Worafi, Y.M.A., & Long, C.M. (2016). Empirical use of antibiotic therapy in the prevention of early onset sepsis in neonates: a pilot study. *Archives of Medical Science*, 12(3), 603–613.

Ming, L.C., Hameed, M.A., Lee, D.D., Apidi, N.A., Lai, P.S.M., Hadi, M.A., Al-Worafi, Y.M.A., & Khan, T.M., (2016). Use of medical mobile applications among hospital pharmacists in Malaysia. *Therapeutic innovation & regulatory science*, 50(4), pp. 419–426.

Ming, L.C., Untong, N., Aliudin, N.A., Osili, N., Kifli, N., Tan, C.S., … & Goh, H.P. (2020). Mobile health apps on COVID-19 launched in the early days of the pandemic: content analysis and review. *JMIR mHealth and uHealth*, 8(9), e19796.

Othman, G., Ali, F., Ibrahim, M.I.M., Al-Worafi, Y.M., Ansari, M., & Halboup, A.M. (2020). Assessment of Anti-Diabetic Medications Adherence among Diabetic Patients in Sana'a City, Yemen: A Cross Sectional Study. *Journal of Pharmaceutical Research International*, 32(21), 114–122.

Rakel, D., & Minichiello, V. (Eds.). (2022). *Integrative Medicine, E-Book*. Elsevier health sciences.

Saeed, M.S., Alkhoshaiban, A.S., Al-Worafi, Y.M.A., & Long, C.M., (2014). Perception of self-medication among university students in Saudi Arabia. *Archives of Pharmacy Practice*, 5(4), p. 149.

8 Patient Care Errors and Related Problems

Patient Assessment and Diagnostic Errors and Related Problems

8.1 BACKGROUND

Patient assessment is critical in the patient care process; it is the first and most crucial to identify the patient's needs, identify their health problems to confirm the diagnosis, and design the appropriate management plan (Al-Worafi, 2020a). Patient assessment and diagnostic errors refer to mistakes made in the process of evaluating a patient's condition and reaching a diagnosis. These errors can occur at any stage of the process, from the initial patient interview and physical examination to the interpretation of test results and formulation of a treatment plan. There are several factors that can contribute to patient assessment and diagnostic errors, including:

1. Miscommunication: Miscommunication between healthcare providers, patients, and their families can lead to errors in patient assessment and diagnosis. This can occur when important information is not accurately conveyed or when assumptions are made based on incomplete or incorrect information.

2. Bias and stereotyping: Healthcare providers may unconsciously hold biases and stereotypes that influence their assessment and diagnosis of patients. This can lead to incorrect assumptions about a patient's condition or the interpretation of test results.

3. Inadequate training: Inadequate training or lack of experience can lead to errors in patient assessment and diagnosis. Healthcare providers may not be familiar with all of the signs and symptoms of a particular condition, or they may not be familiar with the latest diagnostic tools and techniques.

4. Time constraints: Healthcare providers often work under time constraints and may not have enough time to conduct a thorough assessment or review all of the available information before making a diagnosis. This can lead to errors in judgment and misdiagnosis.

5. Limited access to information: Healthcare providers may not have access to all of the information needed to make an accurate diagnosis. This can occur when patients are unable to provide a complete medical history or when test results are delayed or incomplete.

To reduce patient assessment and diagnostic errors, healthcare providers can take several steps, including:

1. Improving communication: Healthcare providers can work to improve communication with patients and their families, as well as between healthcare providers. This can include using plain language, asking open-ended questions, and listening actively.

2. Addressing biases and stereotypes: Healthcare providers can work to become more aware of their own biases and stereotypes and take steps to address them. This can include seeking out diversity training and actively seeking out patient perspectives.

3. Increasing training and experience: Healthcare providers can seek out additional training and experience to improve their knowledge and skills. This can include attending conferences and workshops, seeking out mentorship and collaboration opportunities, and pursuing advanced degrees or certifications.

4. Managing time constraints: Healthcare providers can work to manage their time more effectively, prioritizing patient care and ensuring that they have enough time to conduct a thorough assessment and review all of the available information.

5. Improving access to information: Healthcare providers can work to improve access to information, such as by using electronic health records and sharing information between healthcare providers. This can help ensure that all relevant information is available when making a diagnosis.

8.2 TERMINOLOGIES

There are many important terminologies related to patient assessment that could help healthcare professionals which are as follows.

DOI: 10.1201/9781003230465-10

8.2.1 Initial Assessment

The process used to identify and treat life-threatening problems concentrates on the Level of Consciousness, Cervical Spinal Stabilization, Airway, Breathing, and Circulation. You will also be forming a General Impression of the patient to determine the priority of care based on your immediate assessment and determining if the patient is a medical or trauma patient. The components of the initial assessment may be altered based on the patient's presentation (NYH, 2022).

8.2.2 Focused History and Physical Exam

In this step, you will reconsider the mechanism of injury, determine if a Rapid Trauma Assessment or a Focused Assessment is needed assess the patient's chief complaint, assess medical patients complaints and signs and symptoms using OPQRST, obtain a baseline set of vital signs, and perform a SAMPLE history. The components of this step may be altered based on the patient's presentation (NYH, 2022).

OPQRST: A mnemonic used to evaluate a patient's chief complaint and signs and symptoms: O = onset, P = provocation, Q = quality, R = radiation, S = severity, T = time.

SAMPLE A mnemonic for the history of a patient's condition to determine: · Signs & Symptoms, Allergies, Medications, Pertinent past history, Last oral intake, Events leading up to the illness/injury

8.2.3 Rapid Trauma Assessment

This is performed on patients with significant mechanisms of injury to determine potential life-threatening injuries. In the conscious patient, symptoms should be sought before and during the Rapid Trauma assessment. You will estimate the severity of the injuries, re-consider your transport decision, reconsider Advanced Life Support, consider the platinum 10 minutes and the Golden Hour, rapidly assess the patient from head to toe using DCAP-BTLS, obtain a baseline set of vital signs, and perform a SAMPLE history (NYH, 2022).

DCAP-BTLS: A mnemonic for EMT assessment in which each area of the body is evaluated for: Deformities, Contusions, Abrasions, Punctures/Penetrations, Burns, Tenderness, Lacerations, Swelling

SAMPLE A mnemonic for the history of a patient's condition to determine: Signs and Symptoms, Allergies, Medications, Pertinent past history, Last oral intake, Events leading up to the illness/injury

8.2.4 Rapid Medical Assessment

This is performed on medical patients who are unconscious, confused, or unable to adequately relate their chief complaint. This assessment is used to quickly identify existing or potentially life-threatening conditions. You will perform a head-to-toe rapid assessment using DACP-BTLS, obtain a baseline set of vital signs, and perform a SAMPLE history (NYH, 2022).

8.2.5 Detailed Physical Exam

This is a more in-depth assessment that builds on the Focused Physical Exam. Many of your patients may not require a Detailed Physical Exam because it is either irrelevant or there is not enough time to complete it. This assessment will only be performed while en route to the hospital or if there is time on-scene while waiting for an ambulance to arrive. Patients who will have this assessment completed are patients with significant mechanism of injury, unconscious, confused, or unable to adequately relate their chief complaint. In the Detailed Physical Exam, you will perform a head-to-toe assessment using DCAP-BTLS to find isolated and non-life-threatening problems that were not found in the Rapid Assessment and also to further explore what you learned during the Rapid Assessment (NYH, 2022).

8.2.6 Chief Complaint (CC)

The chief complaint is a brief statement of the reason why the patient consulted the physician, stated in the patient's own words (Schwinghammer & Koehler, 2009).

8.2.7 History of Present Illness (HPI)

The history of the present illness is a more complete description of the patient's symptom(s) (Schwinghammer & Koehler, 2009).

8.2.8 Past Medical History

The past medical history includes serious illnesses, surgical procedures, and injuries the patient has experienced previously (Schwinghammer & Koehler, 2009).

8.2.9 Past Medications History

The medication history should include an accurate record of the patient's current use of prescription medications, nonprescription products, and dietary supplements (Schwinghammer & Koehler, 2009).

8.2.10 Family History

The family history includes the age and health of parents, siblings, and children. For deceased relatives, the age and cause of death are recorded. In particular, heritable diseases and those with a hereditary tendency are noted (e.g., diabetes mellitus, cardiovascular disease, malignancy, rheumatoid arthritis, obesity) (Schwinghammer & Koehler, 2009).

8.2.11 Social History

The social history includes the social characteristics of the patient as well as the environmental factors and behaviors that may contribute to the development of the disease. Items that may be listed are the patient's marital status; number of children; educational background; occupation; physical activity; hobbies; dietary habits; and use of tobacco, alcohol, or other drugs. (Schwinghammer & Koehler, 2009).

8.2.12 Allergies

Allergies to drugs, food, pets, and environmental factors (e.g., grass, dust, pollen) are recorded. An accurate description of the reaction that occurred should also be included. Care should be taken to distinguish adverse drug effects ("upset stomach") from true allergies ("hives") (Schwinghammer & Koehler, 2009).

8.2.13 Physical Examination

The exact procedures performed during the physical examination vary depending on the chief complaint and the patient's medical history. In some practice settings, only a limited and focused physical examination is performed. In psychiatric practice, greater emphasis is usually placed on the type and severity of the patient's symptoms than on physical findings (Schwinghammer & Koehler, 2009).

8.2.14 Patient Assessment Errors

Patient assessment errors can be defined as any error that occurs during the patient assessment process, such as during the identification of patients related problems, gathering patient-related information, medical and medications histories, and body system assessment/head-to-toe assessment (Al-Worafi, 2020a). Patient assessment is a very important step in the patient care process; without this step, the management plan will not be appropriate, and the treating outcomes will not be achieved. Good prescribing requires good assessment, which has a good impact on the patient's health as well as the healthcare system. A good assessment will help in achieving the treating outcomes; decrease the admission rate to hospitals; decrease morbidity and mortality; decrease the cost of therapy, improve the quality of life, and improve patient satisfaction toward health care (Al-Worafi, 2020b-f).

8.2.15 Diagnosis Errors

A diagnostic error can be defined as a diagnosis that is missed, wrong, or delayed, as detected by some subsequent definitive test or finding (John Hopkins, 2013).

Diagnosis errors can be defined as any errors occurred during the diagnosis.

8.3 PATIENT ASSESSMENT TOOLS

There are many tools used during patient assessment in different healthcare settings and situations such as:

The AG assessment tool (Airway, Breathing, Circulation, Disability, Exposure, Further information and Goals) (Benson, 2017).

The Airway, Breathing, Circulation, Disability, Exposure (ABCDE) approach (Jevon, 2010).

8.3.1 Head to Toe Assessment

Gen (general appearance)

VS (vital signs)—blood pressure, pulse, respiratory rate, and temperature.

In hospital settings, the presence and severity of pain are included as "the fifth vital sign." For ease of use and consistency in this casebook, weight and height are included in the vital signs section, but they are not technically considered to be vital signs.

Skin (integumentary)

HEENT (head, eyes, ears, nose, and throat)

Lungs/Thorax (pulmonary)

Cor or CV (cardiovascular)

Abd (abdomen)

Genit/Rect (genitalia/rectal)

MS/Ext (musculoskeletal and extremities)

Neuro (neurologic) (Schwinghammer & Koehler, 2009).

8.3.2 Body System Approach

- **General presentation of symptoms:** Fever, chills, malaise, pain, sleep patterns, fatigability

- **Diet:** Appetite, likes and dislikes, restrictions, written dairy of food intake

- **Skin, hair, and nails:** rash or eruption, itching, color or texture change, excessive sweating, abnormal nail or hair growth

- **Musculoskeletal:** Joint stiffness, pain, restricted motion, swelling, redness, heat, deformity

- **Head and neck:**

Eyes: visual acuity, blurring, diplopia, photophobia, pain, the recent change in vision
Ears: Hearing loss, pain, discharge, tinnitus, vertigo
Nose: Sense of smell, frequency of colds, obstruction, epistaxis, sinus pain, or postnasal discharge
Throat and mouth: Hoarseness or change in voice, frequent sore throat, bleeding o swelling, of gums, recent tooth abscesses or extractions, soreness of tongue or mucosa.

- **Endocrine and genital reproductive:** Thyroid enlargement or tenderness, heat or cold intolerance, unexplained weight change, polyuria, polydipsia, changes in the distribution of facial hair; *Males:* Puberty onset, difficulty with erections, testicular pain, libido, infertility; *Females:* Menses (onset, regularity, duration and amount), Dysmenorrhea, last menstrual period, frequency of intercourse, age at menopause, pregnancies (number, miscarriage, abortions) type of delivery, complications, use of contraceptives; breasts (pain, tenderness, discharge, lumps)

- **Chest and lungs:** Pain related to respiration, dyspnea, cyanosis, wheezing, cough, sputum (character, and quantity), exposure to tuberculosis (TB), last chest X-ray

- **Heart and blood vessels:** Chest pain or distress, precipitating causes, timing and duration, relieving factors, dyspnea, orthopnea, edema, hypertension, exercise tolerance

- **Gastrointestinal:** Appetite, digestion, food intolerance, dysphagia, heartburn, nausea or vomiting, bowel regularity, change in stool color, or contents, constipation or diarrhea, flatulence or hemorrhoids

- **Genitourinary:** Dysuria, flank or suprapubic pain, urgency, frequency, nocturia, hematuria, polyuria, hesitancy, loss in force of stream, edema, sexually transmitted disease

- **Neurological:** Syncope, seizures, weakness or paralysis, abnormalities of sensation or coordination, tremors, loss of memory

- **Psychiatric:** Depression, mood changes, difficulty concentrating, nervousness, tension, suicidal thoughts, irritability.

- **Pediatrics:** Along with the systemic approach in the case of pediatrics, measure anthropometric measurement and neuromuscular assessment.

8.4 ASSESSMENT TECHNIQUES

The assessment techniques are (Seidel et al., 2010):

Inspection-observing, listening or smelling to gather data

Palpation assessment that uses the sense of touch
Percussion-act of striking one object against another to produce a sound
Auscultation-act of listening with a stethoscope to sounds produced within the body.

8.5 DIAGNOSIS

Appropriate diagnosis is based on the appropriate patient assessment and laboratory tests in addition to other diagnosis criteria, which are different from one disease to another (DiPiro et al., 2017).

8.6 EVIDENCE-BASED PATIENT ASSESSMENT AND DIAGNOSIS ERRORS PREVENTION

The best practices for preventing assessment and diagnosis errors are: have national medication errors (which include patient assessment and diagnosis errors) reporting system supervising all the medication errors systems or programs in the country; the existence of medication errors reporting system in hospitals; engage healthcare professionals to adhere to the good prescribing and practice and this is can be done by training; engage healthcare centers to report the suspected medication errors to the national medication errors reporting system which can be done through training, workshops, and other educational interventions; engage healthcare professionals to report the suspected medication errors to the national medication errors reporting system which can be done through training, workshops, and other educational interventions; communication and collaboration between the healthcare professionals and patients is the key of success in this practice (Al-Worafi, 2020a-z).

8.7 PATIENT ASSESSMENT AND DIAGNOSTIC ERRORS IN DEVELOPING COUNTRIES: Challenges and Recommendations

Despite there are many studies about medication errors in developing countries, there are few studies about patient assessment and diagnosis in developing countries; however, there are many challenges facing patient assessment and diagnosis in developing countries and they are as (Alshahrani et al., 2019a,b; Al-Qahtani et al., 2015; Alshahrani et al., 2020a,b; Al-Worafi, 2014; Al-Worafi, 2015; Al-Worafi, 2016; Al-Worafi et al., 2017; Al-Worafi, 2018a-d; Al-Worafi et al., 2018a-b; Al-Worafi et al., 2019; Al-Worafi, 2020a-z; Al-Worafi et al., 2020a-b; Al-Worafi et al., 2021a,b; Al-Worafi, 2022; Al-Worafi, 2023; Baig et al., 2020; Elkalmi et al., 2020; Elsayed & Al-Worafi, 2020; Hasan et al., 2019; Hassan et al., 2014; Izhar et al., 2017; Lee et al., 2017; Mahmoud et al., 2020; Manan et al., 2014; Manan et al., 2016; Ming et al., 2016; Ming et al., 2020; Othman et al., 2020; Saeed et al., 2014) follows.

8.7.1 Healthcare Systems

The quality of healthcare systems and healthcare services are the cornerstone in providing the most effective and safe patient care services; healthcare systems in many developing countries, especially low-income countries, are weak, with inadequate budgets and infrastructures, which affect patient safety in many ways. Therefore, strengthening the healthcare systems in developing countries is very important and highly recommended to improve patient safety practice, including patient assessment and diagnosis practice.

8.7.2 Financial Challenges

Patient assessment and diagnosis need financial support in the public healthcare sectors as well as private healthcare sectors, which is missing in many developing countries, especially low-income countries. Without support from the ministries of health or having good health insurance to be able to pay for the appropriate patient assessment and diagnosis, many healthcare professionals were/ are estimating the diagnosis from the symptoms only without the necessary laboratory tests and other assessment and diagnosis investigations. Therefore, increasing the health expenditure and the public healthcare budget is very important and highly recommended. Increasing the contribution from the private and charity sectors is very important and highly recommended.

8.7.3 Workforce Challenges

The inadequate number of healthcare professionals throughout the public as well as private healthcare facilities is a major barrier affecting the quality of healthcare services throughout developing countries, especially low-income countries; therefore, hiring more healthcare professionals is very important and highly recommended.

8.7.4 Migration of Healthcare Professionals

Migration of healthcare professionals has increased during the last two decades from many developing countries, especially low and middle-income countries, due to many reasons, such as the lack of jobs in healthcare facilities, low salaries, the attraction of jobs overseas, political and war issues, and others. Designing long-term plans and short-term plans to overcome this challenge is very important and highly recommended.

8.7.5 Reporting Challenges

Reporting patient assessment errors and diagnosis errors is very important to know the reasons and design the necessary interventions to overcome this challenge.

8.7.6 Research

There is little known about patient assessment errors and diagnosis errors in developing countries due to many reasons. Support from the Health Ministries, universities, pharmaceutical companies, organizations, and policymakers can overcome this challenge.

8.7.7 Technology Challenges

New technologies, applications, and social media can play an important role in patient care and safety, including patient assessment and diagnosis.

8.8 CONCLUSION

This chapter discusses the patient assessment and diagnosis practice based on evidence-based practice, patient assessment errors, and patient diagnosis errors. This chapter summarized the challenges of patient assessment and diagnosis in developing countries and suggested recommendations to overcome them. Patient assessment and diagnosis errors lead to an increase in admission rates to hospitals and healthcare facilities; an increase in morbidity and mortality; an increase in the cost of therapy, and a decrease in the quality of life and satisfaction with healthcare services.

REFERENCES

Al-Qahtani, I., Almoteb, T.M., & Al-Warafi, Y. (2015). Competency of metered-dose inhaler use among Saudi community pharmacists: A Simulation method study. *RRJPPS*, 4(2), 37–31.

Al-Worafi, Y. (2018b). Knowledge, attitude and practice of Yemeni physicians toward pharmacovigilance: A mixed method study. *Int. J. Pharm. Pharm. Sci*, 10, 74–77.

Al-Worafi, Y. (2022). *A Guide to Online Pharmacy Education: Teaching Strategies and Assessment Methods*. CRC Press.

Al-Worafi, Y.M. (2014). Prescription writing errors at a tertiary care hospital in Yemen: prevalence, types, causes and recommendations. *Am J Pharm Health Res*, 2, 134–140.

Al-Worafi, Y.M. (2018a). Knowledge, Attitude and Practice of Yemeni Physicians Toward Pharmacovigilance: A Mixed Method Study. *International Journal of Pharmacy and Pharmaceutical Sciences*, 10 (10), 74–77.

Al-Worafi, Y.M. (2018d). Evauation of inhaler technique among patients with asthma and COPD in Yemen. *Journal of Taibah University medical sciences*, 13(5), 488–490.

Al-Worafi, Y.M. (Ed.). (2020a). Drug Safety in Developing Countries: Achievements and Challenges.

Al-Worafi, Y.M. (2020b). Drug-related problems. In *Drug Safety in Developing Countries* (pp. 105–117). Academic Press.

Al-Worafi, Y.M. (2020c). Adverse drug reactions. In *Drug Safety in Developing Countries* (pp. 39–57). Academic Press.

Al-Worafi, Y.M. (2020d). Medications registation and marketing: safety-related issues. In *Drug Safety in Developing Countries* (pp. 21–28). Academic Press.

Al-Worafi, Y.M. (2020e). Pharmacovigilance. In *Drug Safety in Developing Countries* (pp. 29–38). Academic Press.

Al-Worafi, Y.M. (2020f). Medication errors. In *Drug safety in developing countries* (pp. 59–71). Academic Press.

Al-Worafi, Y.M. (2020g). Medications safety-related terminology. In *Drug safety in developing countries* (pp. 7–19). Academic Press.

Al-Worafi, Y.M. (2020h). Self-medication. In *Drug Safety in Developing Countries* (pp. 73–86). Academic Press.

Al-Worafi, Y.M. (2020j). Antibiotics safety issues. In *Drug Safety in Developing Countries* (pp. 87–103). Academic Press.

Al-Worafi, Y.M. (2020k). Medications safety research issues. In *Drug Safety in Developing Countries* (pp. 213–227). Academic Press.

Al-Worafi, Y.M. (2020l). Counterfeit and substandard medications. In *Drug safety in developing countries* (pp. 119–126). Academic Press.

Al-Worafi, Y.M. (2020m). Medication abuse and misuse. In *Drug safety in developing countries* (pp. 127–135). Academic Press.

Al-Worafi, Y.M. (2020n). Storage and disposal of medications. In *Drug Safety in Developing Countries* (pp. 137–142). Academic Press.

Al-Worafi, Y.M. (2020o). Safety of medications in special population. In *Drug safety in developing countries* (pp. 143–162). Academic Press.

Al-Worafi, Y.M. (2020p). Herbal medicines safety issues. In *Drug Safety in developing countries* (pp. 163–178). Academic Press.

Al-Worafi, Y.M. (2020q). Medications safety pharmacoeconomics-related issues. In *Drug Safety in Developing Countries* (pp. 187–195). Academic Press.

Al-Worafi, Y.M. (2020r). Evidence-based medications safety practice. In *Drug Safety in Developing Countries* (pp. 197–201). Academic Press.

Al-Worafi, Y.M. (2020s). Quality indicators for medications safety. In *Drug safety in developing countries* (pp. 229–242). Academic Press.

Al-Worafi, Y.M. (2020t). Drug safety in Yemen. In *Drug Safety in Developing Countries* (pp. 391–405). Academic Press.

Al-Worafi, Y.M. (2020u). Drug safety in Saudi Arabia. In *Drug Safety in Developing Countries* (pp. 407–417). Academic Press.

Al-Worafi, Y.M. (2020v). Drug safety in United Arab Emirates. In *Drug Safety in Developing Countries* (pp. 419–428). Academic Press.

Al-Worafi, Y.M. (2020w). Drug safety in Indonesia. In *Drug Safety in Developing Countries* (pp. 279–285). Academic Press.

Al-Worafi, Y.M. (2020x). Drug safety in Palestine. In *Drug Safety in Developing Countries* (pp. 471–480). Academic Press.

Al-Worafi, Y.M. (2020y). Drug safety: comparison between developing countries. In *Drug Safety in Developing Countries* (pp. 603–611). Academic Press.

Al-Worafi, Y.M. (2020z). Drug safety in developing versus developed countries. In *Drug Safety in Developing Countries* (pp. 613–615). Academic Press.

Al-Worafi, Y.M. (2022). Patient care errors and related problems (part I): development and validation of the model. https://orcid.org/0000-0002-5752-2913

Al-Worafi, Y.M. (Ed.). (2023). *Clinical Case Studies on medication Safety*. Academic Press.

Al-Worafi, Y.M., Kassab, Y.W., Alseragi, W.M., Almutairi, M.S., Ahmed, A., Ming, L.C., Alkhoshaiban, A.S., & Hadi, M.A. (2017). Pharmacovigilance and adverse drg reaction reporting: a perspective of community pharmacists and pharmacy technicians in Sana'a, Yemen. *Therapeutics and clinical risk management*, 13, 1175.

Al-Worafi, Y.M., Patel, R.P., Zaidi, S.T.R., Alseragi, W.M., Almutairi, M.S., Alkhoshaiban, A.S., & Ming, L.C. (2018a). Completeness and legibility of handwritten prescriptions in Sana'a, Yemen. *Medical Principles and Practice*, 27, 290–292.

Al-Worafi, Y.M., Alseragi, W.M., Seng, L.K., Kassab, Y.W., Yeoh, S.F., Chiau, L., … & Husain, K. (2018b). Dispensing errors in community pharmacies: a prospective study in Sana'a, Yemen. *Arch Pharm Pract*, 9(4), 1–3.

Al-Worafi, Y.M., Alseragi, W.M., & Mahmoud, M.A. (2019). Competency of metered-dose inhaler use among community pharmacy dispensers in Ibb, Yemen: A simulation method study. *Latin American Journal of Pharmacy*, 38(3), 489–494.

Al-Worafi, Y.M., Alseragi, W.M., Ming, L.C., & Alakhali, K.M. (2020a). Drug safety in China. In *Drug Safety in Developing Countries* (pp. 381–388). Academic Press.

Al-Worafi, Y.M., Alseragi, W.M., Alakhali, K.M., Ming, L.C., Othman, G., Halboup, A.M., … & Elkalmi, R.M. (2020b). Knowledge, beliefs and factors affecting the use of generic medicines among patients in Ibb, Yemen: a mixed-method study. *Journal of Pharmacy Practice and Community Medicine*, 6(4).

Al-Worafi, Y.M., Elkalmi, R.M., Ming, L.C., Othman, G., Halboup, A.M., Battah, M.M., … & Mani, V. (2021a). Dispensing errors in hospital pharmacies: A prospective study in Yemen.

Al-Worafi, Y.M.A. (2015). Appropriateness of metered-dose inhaler use in the Yemeni community pharmacies. *Journal of Taibah University Medical Sciences*, 10(3), 353–358.

Al-Worafi, Y.M.A. (2016). Pharmacy practice in Yemen. In *Pharmacy Practice in Developing Countries* (pp. 267–287). Academic Press.

Al-Worafi, Y.M. (2018c). Dispensing errors observed by community pharmacy dispensers in IBB–YEMEN. *Asian J. Pharm. Clin. Res*, 11(11).

Al-Worafi, Y.M., Hasan, S., Hassan, N.M., & Gaili, A.A. (2021b). Knowledge, Attitude and Experience of Pharmacist in the UAE towards Pharmacovigilance. *Research Journal of Pharmacy and Technology*, 14(1), 265–269.

Alshahrani, S.M., Alakhali, K.M., & Al-Worafi, Y.M. (2019a). Medication errors in a health care facility in southern Saudi Arabia. *Tropical Journal of Pharmaceutical Research*, 18(5), 1119–1122.

Alshahrani, S.M., Alavudeen, S.S., Alakhali, K.M., Al-Worafi, Y.M., Bahamdan, A.K., & Vigneshwaran, E. (2019b). Self-Medication Among King Khalid University Students. *Saudi Arabia. Risk Management and Healthcare Policy*, 12, 243–249.

Alshahrani, S.M., Alzahran, M., Alakhali, K., Vigneshwaran, E., Iqbal, M.J., Khan, N.A., ... & Alavudeen, S.S. (2020a). Association Between Diabetes Consequences and Quality of Life Among Patients With Diabetes Mellitus in the Aseer Province of Saudi Arabia. *Open Access Macedonian Journal of Medical Sciences*, 8(E), 325–330.

Alshahrani, S.M., Alakhali, K.M., Al-Worafi, Y.M., & Alshahrani, N.Z. (2020b). Awareness and use of over the counter analgesic medication: a survey in the Aseer region population. *Saudi Arabia. Int J Advan Appl Sci*, 7(3), 130–134.

Baig, M.R., Al-Worafi, Y.M., Alseragi, W.M., Ming, L.C., & Siddique, A. (2020). Drug safety in India. In *Drug Safety in Developing Countries* (pp. 327–334). Academic Press.

Benson, A. (2017). *The AG assessment tool (Airway, Breathing, Circulation, Disability, Exposure, Further information and Goals)*. Clinical Skills. Net Clinical Skills Limited.

DiPiro, J.T., Talbert, R.L., Yee, G.C., Matzke, G.R., Wells, B.G., & Posey, L. (2017). *Pharmacotherapy A Pathophysiologic Approach, 10e. Pharmacotherapy: A Pathophysiologic Approach. 10e.* New York: McGraw-Hill Education, 255–258.

Elkalmi, R.M., Al-Worafi, Y.M., Alseragi, W.M., Ming, L.C., & Siddique, A. (2020). Drug safety in Malaysia. In *Drug Safety in Developing Countries* (pp. 245–253). Academic Press.

Elsayed, T., & Al-Worafi, Y.M. (2020). Drug safety in Egypt. In *Drug Safety in Developing Countries* (pp. 511–523). Academic Press.

Hasan, S., Al-Omar, M.J., AlZubaidy, H., & Al-Worafi, Y.M. (2019). Use of medications in Arab Countries. *Handbook of Healthcare in the Arab World*. Cham: Springer, 42.

Hassan, Y., Abd Aziz, N., Kassab, Y.W., Elgasim, I., Shaharuddin, S., Al-Worafi, Y.M.A., ... & Ming, L.C. (2014). How to help patients to control their blood pressure? Blood pressure control and its predictor. *Archives of Pharmacy Practice*, 5(4).

Izahar, S., Lean, Q.Y., Hameed, M.A., Murugiah, M.K., Patel, R.P., Al-Worafi, Y.M., ... & Ming, L.C. (2017). Content analysis of mobile health applications on diabetes mellitus. *Frontiers in Endocrinology*, 8, 318.

Jevon, P. (2010). Assessment of critically ill patients: the ABCDE approach. *British Journal of Healthcare Assistants*, 4(8), 404–407.

John Hopkins (2013). Diagnostic Errors More Common, Costly And Harmful Than Treatment Mistakes. Available at: https://www.hopkinsmedicine.org/news/media/releases/diagnostic_errors_more_common_costly_and_harmful_than_treatment_mistakes#:~:text=Diagnostic%20error%20can%20be%20defined,subsequent%20definitive%20test%20or%20finding.

Lee, K.S., Yee, S.M., Zaidi, S.T.R., Patel, R.P., Yang, Q., Al-Worafi, Y.M., & Ming, L.C., 2017.

Combating sale of counterfeit and falsified medicines online: a losing battle. *Frontiers in pharmacology*, 8, p. 268.

Mahmoud, M.A., Wajid, S., Naqvi, A.A., Samreen, S., Althagfan, S.S., & Al-Worafi, Y. (2020). Self-medication with antibiotics: A cross-sectional community-based study. *Latin American Journal of Pharmacy*, 39(2), 348–353.

Manan, M.M., Rusli, R.A., Ang, W.C., Al-Worafi, Y.M., & Ming, L.C. (2014). Assessing the pharmaceutical care issues of antiepileptic drug therapy in hospitalised epileptic patients. *Journal of Pharmacy Practice and Research*, 44(3), 83–88.

Manan, M.M., Ibrahim, N.A., Aziz, N.A., Zulkifly, H.H., Al-Worafi, Y.M.A., & Long, C.M. (2016). Empirical use of antibiotic therapy in the prevention of early onset sepsis in neonates: a pilot study. *Archives of Medical Science*, 12(3), 603–613.

Ming, L.C., Hameed, M.A., Lee, D.D., Apidi, N.A., Lai, P.S.M., Hadi, M.A., Al-Worafi, Y.M.A., & Khan, T.M. (2016). Use of medical mobile applications among hospital pharmacists in Malaysia. *Therapeutic innovation & regulatory science*, 50(4), 419–426.

Ming, L.C., Untong, N., Aliudin, N.A., Osili, N., Kifli, N., Tan, C.S., … & Goh, H.P. (2020). Mobile health apps on COVID-19 launched in the early days of the pandemic: content analysis and review. *JMIR mHealth and uHealth*, 8(9), e19796.

New York Health Department (NYH), (2022). Available at: https://www.health.ny.gov/professionals/ems/pdf/srgpadefinitions.pdf

Othman, G., Ali, F., Ibrahim, M.I.M., Al-Worafi, Y.M., Ansari, M., & Halboup, A.M. (2020). Assessment of Anti-Diabetic Medications Adherence among Diabetic Patients in Sana'a City, Yemen: A Cross Sectional Study. *Journal of Pharmaceutical Research International*, 32(21), 114–122.

Saeed, M.S., Alkhoshaiban, A.S., Al-Worafi, Y.M.A., & Long, C.M. (2014). Perception of self-medication among university students in Saudi Arabia. *Archives of Pharmacy Practice*, 5(4), 149.

Schwinghammer, T.L., & Koehler, J. (2009). *Pharmacotherapy casebook: A Patient-Focused Approach*, 7e McGraw-Hill Professional Publishing.

Seidel, H.M., Stewart, R.W., Ball, J.W., Dains, J.E., Flynn, J.A., & Solomon, B.S. (2010). *Mosby's Guide to Physical Examination-E-Book*. Elsevier Health Sciences.

9 Patient Care Errors and Related Problems

Non-pharmacological Errors and Related Problems

9.1 BACKGROUND

Non-pharmacological interventions refer to any therapy, treatment, or approach that does not involve the use of medication or drugs. These interventions are often used in the treatment of a variety of conditions and can be highly effective in improving symptoms and overall quality of life. Here are some examples of non-pharmacological interventions (Ninot, 2021): Lifestyle changes refer to modifications that individuals make to their daily habits and routines in order to improve their overall health and well-being. Some common lifestyle changes include:

1. Healthy eating: Eating a balanced diet that includes plenty of fruits and vegetables, whole grains, lean protein, and healthy fats can help reduce the risk of chronic diseases and improve overall health.

2. Regular exercise: Engaging in regular physical activity, such as brisk walking, jogging, cycling, or strength training, can help improve cardiovascular health, increase muscle strength and endurance, and reduce the risk of chronic diseases.

3. Adequate sleep: Getting enough sleep is essential for physical and mental health. Adults should aim for 7–9 hours of sleep per night, while children and teenagers need more.

4. Stress management: Chronic stress can have negative effects on physical and mental health. Engaging in stress-reducing activities such as yoga, meditation, deep breathing, or spending time in nature can help reduce stress levels.

5. Smoking cessation: Quitting smoking is one of the most important lifestyle changes a person can make to improve their health. Smoking increases the risk of cancer, heart disease, stroke, and other chronic conditions.

6. Limiting alcohol consumption: Drinking alcohol in moderation, or not at all, can help reduce the risk of liver disease, certain cancers, and other health problems.

7. Maintaining a healthy weight: Being overweight or obese can increase the risk of a variety of health conditions, including diabetes, heart disease, and certain cancers. Maintaining a healthy weight through healthy eating and regular exercise can help reduce the risk of these conditions.

8. Cognitive Behavioral Therapy (CBT): CBT is a form of psychotherapy that aims to change negative thought patterns and behaviors. It has been shown to be effective in the treatment of anxiety disorders, depression, and other mental health conditions.

9. Mindfulness-based interventions: These interventions involve various mindfulness practices, such as meditation, breathing exercises, and yoga, which can be helpful in reducing stress, anxiety, and depression.

10. Exercise: Regular physical activity has been shown to improve mood, reduce stress, and improve overall health. Exercise can include any physical activity that gets the heart rate up, such as walking, running, or strength training.

11. Dietary changes: Changes in diet, such as increasing intake of fruits and vegetables and reducing processed foods, can have a positive impact on overall health and well-being.

12. Sleep hygiene: Establishing healthy sleep habits, such as maintaining a regular sleep schedule, avoiding caffeine and alcohol before bedtime, and creating a comfortable sleep environment, can improve sleep quality and reduce insomnia.

13. Occupational therapy: Occupational therapy focuses on helping individuals to perform daily activities and tasks, such as self-care, work, and leisure activities, more easily and effectively. It can be helpful for individuals with physical or cognitive impairments, as well as those with mental health conditions.

14. Social support: Social support from family, friends, and community can be an important factor in mental and physical health. Building and maintaining strong social connections can help reduce stress, promote healthy behaviors, and improve overall well-being.

DOI: 10.1201/9781003230465-11

9.2 NON-PHARMACOLOGICAL ERRORS AND RELATED PROBLEMS

Patient care errors and related problems can be defined simply as any intentional or unintentional errors or problems occurring during the patient care process, such as health screening, patient assessment, diagnosis, management, etc. While non-pharmacological errors and related problems can be defined as any intentional or unintentional errors or problems occurring during non-pharmacological therapy interventions such as diet, exercise, and lifestyle changes. and are as follows.

1. Diet errors and problems: One common problem with diets is that people may choose restrictive or fad diets that eliminate certain food groups or severely limit calorie intake. These types of diets can be difficult to maintain over time and may lead to nutrient deficiencies or unhealthy weight loss. Another issue is that some people may not consume enough fiber, which can lead to constipation and other digestive problems.

2. Exercise errors and problems: One common error with exercise is doing too much too soon. This can lead to injuries such as strains, sprains, and fractures. Another problem is not getting enough rest and recovery time between workouts, which can also increase the risk of injury. Additionally, some people may not exercise at a high enough intensity to achieve health benefits, while others may push themselves too hard and experience burnout or exhaustion.

3. Weight management errors and problems: One common problem with weight management is that people may focus too much on the number on the scale and not enough on overall health. This can lead to unhealthy weight loss practices such as crash diets or excessive exercise. Additionally, some people may struggle with weight gain or obesity due to genetic factors or other underlying health conditions, which can make it more difficult to achieve and maintain a healthy weight.

4. Smoking cessation errors and problems: One common problem with smoking cessation is that some people may not be fully committed to quitting. This can lead to relapses and a continued dependence on nicotine. Additionally, some people may not seek out appropriate resources or support to help them quit, which can make the process more difficult. Finally, some people may experience withdrawal symptoms such as anxiety or depression, which can make it difficult to stay motivated to quit.

9.3 FACILITATORS AND BARRIERS FOR NON-PHARMACOLOGICAL THERAPIES AND INTERVENTIONS

Facilitators and barriers to non-pharmacological therapies and interventions can be influenced by various factors. Here are some common facilitators and barriers to non-pharmacological therapies and interventions:

9.3.1 Facilitators

1. Evidence-based research: Evidence-based research and scientific studies that support the effectiveness of non-pharmacological therapies and interventions can be a facilitator for their adoption and integration into clinical practice.

2. Patient preference: When patients prefer non-pharmacological therapies and interventions over pharmacological ones, it can be a facilitator for their adoption and integration into clinical practice.

3. Provider training and education: Adequate training and education of healthcare providers can be a facilitator for the use of non-pharmacological therapies and interventions. When healthcare providers have the necessary knowledge and skills, they are more likely to offer these therapies and interventions to their patients.

4. Availability of resources: Availability of resources, such as equipment and trained personnel, can be a facilitator for the use of non-pharmacological therapies and interventions.

5. Collaborative care: Collaborative care among healthcare providers, such as coordination between physical therapists, occupational therapists, and physicians, can be a facilitator for the use of non-pharmacological therapies and interventions.

9.3.2 Barriers

1. Lack of knowledge and training: Healthcare providers may not have the necessary knowledge and training to provide non-pharmacological therapies and interventions, which can be a barrier to their adoption and integration into clinical practice.

2. Insurance coverage: Limited insurance coverage for non-pharmacological therapies and interventions can be a barrier to their adoption and integration into clinical practice, as patients may not be able to afford these therapies and interventions.

3. Patient access: Lack of patient access to non-pharmacological therapies and interventions, such as limited availability or long wait times, can be a barrier to their adoption and integration into clinical practice.

4. Skepticism and resistance: Skepticism and resistance from healthcare providers and patients can be a barrier to the adoption and integration of non-pharmacological therapies and interventions.

5. Limited research: Limited evidence-based research and scientific studies that support the effectiveness of non-pharmacological therapies and interventions can be a barrier to their adoption and integration into clinical practice.

9.4 FACILITATORS AND BARRIERS FOR NON-PHARMACOLOGICAL THERAPIES AND INTERVENTIONS IN DEVELOPING COUNTRIES

Facilitators and barriers to non-pharmacological therapies and interventions in developing countries can be influenced by various factors. Here are some common facilitators and barriers for non-pharmacological therapies and interventions in developing countries:

9.4.1 Facilitators

1. Traditional healing practices: In many developing countries, traditional healing practices are common and may include non-pharmacological therapies and interventions, such as acupuncture, herbal medicine, and massage. These practices may be more readily accepted and integrated into clinical practice.

2. Community health workers: Community health workers can play an important role in the delivery of non-pharmacological therapies and interventions in developing countries, particularly in remote and rural areas where access to healthcare may be limited.

3. Culturally appropriate interventions: Non-pharmacological therapies and interventions that are culturally appropriate and relevant to local customs and beliefs may be more readily accepted and integrated into clinical practice.

4. Low cost: Non-pharmacological therapies and interventions that are low cost and require minimal resources can be more easily implemented in resource-limited settings.

5. Holistic approach: Non-pharmacological therapies and interventions that take a holistic approach to health and wellbeing, addressing physical, emotional, and spiritual aspects of health, maybe more acceptable and integrated into clinical practice in developing countries.

9.4.2 Barriers

1. Limited resources: Limited resources, such as equipment, trained personnel, and funding, can be a significant barrier to the adoption and integration of non-pharmacological therapies and interventions in developing countries.

2. Lack of training and education: Healthcare providers may lack the necessary training and education to provide non-pharmacological therapies and interventions, which can be a significant barrier to their adoption and integration into clinical practice.

3. Limited research: Limited evidence-based research and scientific studies that support the effectiveness of non-pharmacological therapies and interventions may be a barrier to their adoption and integration into clinical practice in developing countries.

4. Cultural beliefs and practices: Cultural beliefs and practices may be a barrier to the adoption and integration of non-pharmacological therapies and interventions in developing countries, particularly if they conflict with traditional healing practices or beliefs.

5. Limited access: Limited access to non-pharmacological therapies and interventions, such as limited availability or long wait times, maybe a barrier to their adoption and integration into clinical practice in developing countries, particularly in remote and rural areas.

9.5 CHALLENGES OF NON-PHARMACOLOGICAL THERAPIES AND INTERVENTIONS IN DEVELOPING COUNTRIES

There are many challenges to patient care in general as well as non-pharmacological therapies and interventions as follows (Alshahrani et al., 2019a,b; Al-Qahtani et al., 2015; Alshahrani et al., 2020a,b; Al-Worafi, 2014; Al-Worafi, 2015; Al-Worafi, 2016; Al-Worafi et al., 2017; Al-Worafi, 2018a-d; Al-Worafi et al., 2018a-b; Al-Worafi et al., 2019; Al-Worafi, 2020a-z; Al-Worafi et al., 2020a-b; Al-Worafi et al., 2021a,b; Al-Worafi, 2022a,b; Al-Worafi, 2023; Baig et al., 2020; Elkalmi et al., 2020; Elsayed & Al-Worafi, 2020; Hasan et al., 2019; Hassan et al., 2014; Izhar et al., 2017; Lee et al., 2017; Mahmoud et al., 2020; Manan et al., 2014; Manan et al., 2016; Ming et al., 2016; Ming et al., 2020; Othman et al., 2020; Saeed et al., 2014).

9.5.1 Diet Challenges

In many developing countries, access to nutritious food can be limited. Some regions may have a high prevalence of food insecurity, which can lead to malnutrition and stunted growth. Additionally, traditional diets in some areas may be high in salt, sugar, and fat, which can contribute to the development of chronic diseases such as diabetes and heart disease.

Exercise challenges: In many developing countries, access to safe and affordable exercise facilities can be limited. This can make it difficult for people to engage in regular physical activity. Additionally, cultural norms may discourage women from participating in exercise, which can further limit opportunities for physical activity.

9.5.2 Weight Management Challenges

In many developing countries, the prevalence of obesity is increasing. This may be due in part to changes in lifestyle and diet as well as a lack of access to health education and resources. Additionally, weight management programs and resources may not be widely available or affordable, which can make it difficult for people to receive the support they need.

9.5.3 Smoking Cessation Challenges

Tobacco use is a major public health issue in many developing countries, and smoking cessation can be particularly challenging in these areas. This may be due in part to limited access to cessation resources such as nicotine replacement therapy and counseling. Additionally, social norms around smoking may make it difficult for people to quit, and tobacco companies may target developing countries with aggressive marketing campaigns.

9.5.4 Healthcare Systems

The quality of healthcare systems and healthcare services are the cornerstone in providing the most effective and safe patient care services; healthcare systems in many developing countries, especially low-income countries, are weak, with inadequate budgets and infrastructures, which affect patient safety in many ways. Therefore, strengthening the healthcare systems in developing countries is very important and highly recommended to improve patient care practice.

9.5.5 Financial Challenges

Patient care needs financial support in the public healthcare sectors as well as private healthcare sectors, which is missing in many developing countries, especially low-income countries. Therefore, increasing the health expenditure and the public healthcare budget is very important and highly recommended. Increasing the contribution from the private and charity sectors is very important and highly recommended.

9.5.6 Workforce Challenges

The inadequate number of healthcare professionals throughout the public as well as private healthcare facilities is a major barrier affecting the quality of healthcare services throughout developing countries, especially low-income countries; therefore, hiring more healthcare professionals is very important and highly recommended.

9.5.7 Migration of Healthcare Professionals

Migration of healthcare professionals has increased during the last two decades from many developing countries, especially low and middle-income countries, due to many reasons, such as the lack of jobs in healthcare facilities, low salaries, the attraction of jobs overseas, political and war issues, and others. Designing long-term plans and short-term plans to overcome this challenge is very important and highly recommended.

9.5.8 Reporting Challenges

Reporting patient care errors and related problems is very important to know the reasons and design the necessary interventions to overcome this challenge.

9.5.9 Research

There is little known about patient care errors and related problems in developing countries due to many reasons. Support from the Health Ministries, universities, pharmaceutical companies, organizations, and policymakers can overcome this challenge.

9.5.10 Technology Challenges

New technologies, applications, and social media can play an important role in the patient process.

9.5.11 Diet Recommendations

- Promote and support the development of local agriculture and food systems to increase access to fresh and nutritious food.

- Provide education and resources to help individuals make informed choices about their diets, including the benefits of a balanced and varied diet.

- Encourage policies that promote food safety and reduce the availability of unhealthy foods.

9.5.12 Exercise Recommendations

- Promote and support the development of safe and accessible exercise facilities, such as parks and community centers.

- Encourage physical education in schools and the promotion of physical activity in the workplace.

- Raise awareness of the benefits of regular physical activity through community events and campaigns.

9.5.13 Weight Management Recommendations

- Increase access to weight management programs and resources, such as counseling, support groups, and weight loss medications.

- Promote healthy lifestyle behaviors, such as regular physical activity and a balanced diet.

- Advocate for policies that support healthy food environments, such as food labeling and regulation of food marketing.

9.5.14 Smoking Cessation Recommendations

- Increase access to smoking cessation resources such as nicotine replacement therapy and counseling.

- Implement policies such as smoke-free environments and tobacco taxation to reduce tobacco use.

- Raise awareness of the dangers of tobacco use and the benefits of quitting through education and public health campaigns.

9.6 CONCLUSION

This chapter has discussed the non-pharmacological errors and related problems, the facilitators, barriers, and recommendations for best practices in developing countries. Non-pharmacological interventions refer to any therapy, treatment, or approach that does not involve the use of medication or drugs. These interventions are often used in the treatment of a variety of conditions and can be highly effective in improving symptoms and overall quality of life. Non-pharmacological errors and related problems can be defined as any intentional or unintentional errors or problems occurring during non-pharmacological therapy interventions such as diet, exercise, and lifestyle changes.

REFERENCES

Al-Qahtani, I., Almoteb, T.M., & Al-Warafi, Y. (2015). Competency of metered-dose inhaler use among Saudi community pharmacists: A Simulation method study. *RRJPPS*, 4(2), 37–31.

Alshahrani, S.M., Alakhali, K.M., & Al-Worafi, Y.M. (2019a). Medication errors in a health care facility in southern Saudi Arabia. *Tropical Journal of Pharmaceutical Research*, 18(5), 1119–1122.

Alshahrani, S.M., Alavudeen, S.S., Alakhali, K.M., Al-Worafi, Y.M., Bahamdan, A.K., & Vigneshwaran, E. (2019b). Self-Medication Among King Khalid University Students. *Saudi Arabia. Risk Management and Healthcare Policy*, 12, 243–249.

Alshahrani, S.M., Alakhali, K.M., Al-Worafi, Y.M., & Alshahrani, N.Z. (2020a). Awareness and use of over the counter analgesic medication: a survey in the Aseer region population. *Saudi Arabia. Int J Advan Appl Sci*, 7(3), 130–134.

Alshahrani, S.M., Alzahran, M., Alakhali, K., Vigneshwaran, E., Iqbal, M.J., Khan, N.A., … & Alavudeen, S.S. (2020b). Association Between Diabetes Consequences and Quality of Life Among Patients With Diabetes Mellitus in the Aseer Province of Saudi Arabia. *Open Access Macedonian Journal of Medical Sciences*, 8(E), 325–330.

Al-Worafi, Y.M. (2014). Prescription writing errors at a tertiary care hospital in Yemen: prevalence, types, causes and recommendations. *Am J Pharm Health Res*, 2, 134–140.

Al-Worafi, Y.M.A. (2015). Appropriateness of metered-dose inhaler use in the Yemeni community pharmacies. *Journal of Taibah University Medical Sciences*, 10(3), 353–358.

Al-Worafi, Y.M.A. (2016). Pharmacy practice in Yemen. In *Pharmacy Practice in Developing Countries* (pp. 267–287). Academic Press.

Al-Worafi, Y.M., Kassab, Y.W., Alseragi, W.M., Almutairi, M.S., Ahmed, A., Ming, L.C., Alkhoshaiban, A.S., & Hadi, M.A. (2017). Pharmacovigilance and adverse drg reaction reporting: a perspective of community pharmacists and pharmacy technicians in Sana'a, Yemen. *Therapeutics and clinical risk management*, 13, 1175.

Al-Worafi, Y.M. (2018a). Knowledge, Attitude and Practice of Yemeni Physicians Toward Pharmacovigilance: A Mixed Method Study. *International Journal of Pharmacy and Pharmaceutical Sciences*, 10 (10), 74–77.

Al-Worafi, Y. (2018b). Knowledge, attitude and practice of Yemeni physicians toward pharmacovigilance: A mixed method study. *Int. J. Pharm. Pharm. Sci*, 10, 74–77.

Al-Worafi, Y.M. (2018c). Dispensing errors observed by community pharmacy dispensers in IBB–YEMEN. *Asian J. Pharm. Clin. Res*, 11(11).

Al-Worafi, Y.M. (2018d). Evauation of inhaler technique among patients with asthma and COPD in Yemen. *Journal of Taibah University medical sciences*, 13(5), 488–490.

Al-Worafi, Y.M., Patel, R.P., Zaidi, S.T.R., Alseragi, W.M., Almutairi, M.S., Alkhoshaiban, A.S., & Ming, L.C. (2018a). Completeness and legibility of handwritten prescriptions in Sana'a, Yemen. *Medical Principles and Practice*, 27, 290–292.

Al-Worafi, Y.M., Alseragi, W.M., Seng, L.K., Kassab, Y.W., Yeoh, S.F., Chiau, L., ... & Husain, K. (2018b). Dispensing errors in community pharmacies: a prospective study in Sana'a, Yemen. *Arch Pharm Pract*, 9(4), 1–3.

Al-Worafi, Y.M., Alseragi, W.M., & Mahmoud, M.A. (2019). Competency of metered-dose inhaler use among community pharmacy dispensers in Ibb, Yemen: A simulation method study. *Latin American Journal of Pharmacy*, 38(3), 489–494.

Al-Worafi, Y.M. (Ed.). (2020a). Drug Safety in Developing Countries: Achievements and Challenges.

Al-Worafi, Y.M. (2020b). Drug-related problems. In *Drug Safety in Developing Countries* (pp. 105–117). Academic Press.

Al-Worafi, Y.M. (2020c). Adverse drug reactions. In *Drug Safety in Developing Countries* (pp. 39–57). Academic Press.

Al-Worafi, Y.M. (2020d). Medications registation and marketing: safety-related issues. In *Drug Safety in Developing Countries* (pp. 21–28). Academic Press.

Al-Worafi, Y.M. (2020e). Pharmacovigilance. In *Drug Safety in Developing Countries* (pp. 29–38). Academic Press.

Al-Worafi, Y.M. (2020f). Medication errors. In *Drug safety in developing countries* (pp. 59–71). Academic Press.

Al-Worafi, Y.M. (2020g). Medications safety-related terminology. In *Drug safety in developing countries* (pp. 7–19). Academic Press.

Al-Worafi, Y.M. (2020h). Self-medication. In *Drug Safety in Developing Countries* (pp. 73–86). Academic Press.

Al-Worafi, Y.M. (2020j). Antibiotics safety issues. In *Drug Safety in Developing Countries* (pp. 87–103). Academic Press.

Al-Worafi, Y.M. (2020k). Medications safety research issues. In *Drug Safety in Developing Countries* (pp. 213–227). Academic Press.

Al-Worafi, Y.M. (2020l). Counterfeit and substandard medications. In *Drug safety in developing countries* (pp. 119–126). Academic Press.

Al-Worafi, Y.M. (2020m). Medication abuse and misuse. In *Drug safety in developing countries* (pp. 127–135). Academic Press.

Al-Worafi, Y.M. (2020n). Storage and disposal of medications. In *Drug Safety in Developing Countries* (pp. 137–142). Academic Press.

Al-Worafi, Y.M. (2020o). Safety of medications in special population. In *Drug safety in developing countries* (pp. 143–162). Academic Press.

Al-Worafi, Y.M. (2020p). Herbal medicines safety issues. In *Drug Safety in developing countries* (pp. 163–178). Academic Press.

Al-Worafi, Y.M. (2020q). Medications safety pharmacoeconomics-related issues. In *Drug Safety in Developing Countries* (pp. 187–195). Academic Press.

Al-Worafi, Y.M. (2020r). Evidence-based medications safety practice. In *Drug Safety in Developing Countries* (pp. 197–201). Academic Press.

Al-Worafi, Y.M. (2020s). Quality indicators for medications safety. In *Drug safety in developing countries* (pp. 229–242). Academic Press.

Al-Worafi, Y.M. (2020t). Drug safety in Yemen. In *Drug Safety in Developing Countries* (pp. 391–405). Academic Press.

Al-Worafi, Y.M. (2020u). Drug safety in Saudi Arabia. In *Drug Safety in Developing Countries* (pp. 407–417). Academic Press.

Al-Worafi, Y.M. (2020v). Drug safety in United Arab Emirates. In *Drug Safety in Developing Countries* (pp. 419–428). Academic Press.

Al-Worafi, Y.M. (2020w). Drug safety in Indonesia. In *Drug Safety in Developing Countries* (pp. 279–285). Academic Press.

Al-Worafi, Y.M. (2020x). Drug safety in Palestine. In *Drug Safety in Developing Countries* (pp. 471–480). Academic Press.

Al-Worafi, Y.M. (2020y). Drug safety: comparison between developing countries. In *Drug Safety in Developing Countries* (pp. 603–611). Academic Press.

Al-Worafi, Y.M. (2020z). Drug safety in developing versus developed countries. In *Drug Safety in Developing Countries* (pp. 613–615). Academic Press.

Al-Worafi, Y.M., Alseragi, W.M., Ming, L.C., & Alakhali, K.M. (2020a). Drug safety in China. In *Drug Safety in Developing Countries* (pp. 381–388). Academic Press.

Al-Worafi, Y.M., Alseragi, W.M., Alakhali, K.M., Ming, L.C., Othman, G., Halboup, A.M., … & Elkalmi, R.M. (2020b). Knowledge, beliefs and factors affecting the use of generic medicines among patients in Ibb, Yemen: a mixed-method study. *Journal of Pharmacy Practice and Community Medicine*, 6(4).

Al-Worafi, Y.M., Elkalmi, R.M., Ming, L.C., Othman, G., Halboup, A.M., Battah, M.M., … & Mani, V. (2021a). Dispensing errors in hospital pharmacies: A prospective study in Yemen.

Al-Worafi, Y.M., Hasan, S., Hassan, N.M., & Gaili, A.A. (2021b). Knowledge, Attitude and Experience of Pharmacist in the UAE towards Pharmacovigilance. *Research Journal of Pharmacy and Technology*, 14(1), 265–269.

Al-Worafi, Y. (2022a). *A Guide to Online Pharmacy Education: Teaching Strategies and Assessment Methods*. CRC Press.

Al-Worafi, Y.M. (2022b). Patient care errors and related problems (part I): development and validation of the model. https://orcid.org/0000-0002-5752-2913

Al-Worafi, Y.M. (Ed.). (2023). *Clinical Case Studies on medication Safety*. Academic Press.

Baig, M.R., Al-Worafi, Y.M., Alseragi, W.M., Ming, L.C., & Siddique, A. (2020). Drug safety in India. In *Drug Safety in Developing Countries* (pp. 327–334). Academic Press.

Elkalmi, R.M., Al-Worafi, Y.M., Alseragi, W.M., Ming, L.C., & Siddique, A. (2020). Drug safety in Malaysia. In *Drug Safety in Developing Countries* (pp. 245–253). Academic Press.

Elsayed, T., & Al-Worafi, Y.M. (2020). Drug safety in Egypt. In *Drug Safety in Developing Countries* (pp. 511–523). Academic Press.

Hasan, S., Al-Omar, M.J., AlZubaidy, H., & Al-Worafi, Y.M. (2019). Use of medications in Arab Countries. *Handbook of Healthcare in the Arab World*. Cham: Springer, 42.

Hassan, Y., Abd Aziz, N., Kassab, Y.W., Elgasim, I., Shaharuddin, S., Al-Worafi, Y.M.A., ... & Ming, L.C. (2014). How to help patients to control their blood pressure? Blood pressure control and its predictor. *Archives of Pharmacy Practice*, 5(4).

Izahar, S., Lean, Q.Y., Hameed, M.A., Murugiah, M.K., Patel, R.P., Al-Worafi, Y.M., ... & Ming, L.C. (2017). Content analysis of mobile health applications on diabetes mellitus. *Frontiers in Endocrinology*, 8, 318.

Lee, K.S., Yee, S.M., Zaidi, S.T.R., Patel, R.P., Yang, Q., Al-Worafi, Y.M., & Ming, L.C., 2017. Combating sale of counterfeit and falsified medicines online: a losing battle. *Frontiers in pharmacology*, 8, p. 268.

Mahmoud, M.A., Wajid, S., Naqvi, A.A., Samreen, S., Althagfan, S.S., & Al-Worafi, Y. (2020). Self-medication with antibiotics: A cross-sectional community-based study. *Latin American Journal of Pharmacy*, 39(2), 348–353.

Manan, M.M., Rusli, R.A., Ang, W.C., Al-Worafi, Y.M., & Ming, L.C. (2014). Assessing the pharmaceutical care issues of antiepileptic drug therapy in hospitalised epileptic patients. *Journal of Pharmacy Practice and Research*, 44(3), 83–88.

Manan, M.M., Ibrahim, N.A., Aziz, N.A., Zulkifly, H.H., Al-Worafi, Y.M.A., & Long, C.M. (2016). Empirical use of antibiotic therapy in the prevention of early onset sepsis in neonates: a pilot study. *Archives of Medical Science*, 12(3), 603–613.

Ming, L.C., Hameed, M.A., Lee, D.D., Apidi, N.A., Lai, P.S.M., Hadi, M.A., Al-Worafi, Y.M.A., & Khan, T.M. (2016). Use of medical mobile applications among hospital pharmacists in Malaysia. *Therapeutic innovation & regulatory science*, 50(4), 419–426.

Ming, L.C., Untong, N., Aliudin, N.A., Osili, N., Kifli, N., Tan, C.S., ... & Goh, H.P. (2020). Mobile health apps on COVID-19 launched in the early days of the pandemic: content analysis and review. *JMIR mHealth and uHealth*, 8(9), e19796.

Ninot, G. (2021). *Defining Non-pharmacological Interventions (NPIs)* (pp. 1–46). Springer International Publishing.

Othman, G., Ali, F., Ibrahim, M.I.M., Al-Worafi, Y.M., Ansari, M., & Halboup, A.M. (2020). Assessment of Anti-Diabetic Medications Adherence among Diabetic Patients in Sana'a City, Yemen: A Cross Sectional Study. *Journal of Pharmaceutical Research International*, 32(21), 114–122.

Saeed, M.S., Alkhoshaiban, A.S., Al-Worafi, Y.M.A., & Long, C.M. (2014). Perception of self-medication among university students in Saudi Arabia. *Archives of Pharmacy Practice*, 5(4), 149.

10 Patient Care Errors and Related Problems

Medical Errors and Related Problems

10.1 BACKGROUND

Medical errors can be defined as any intentional or unintentional errors or problems that occur during the patient care process. Medical errors can occur in any healthcare setting, including hospitals, clinics, pharmacies, and nursing homes, among others. Medical errors can lead to serious consequences, such as prolonged hospitalization, disability, or even death. Medical errors are a significant public health concern, and they can result from a variety of factors, including miscommunication among healthcare providers, inadequate training or supervision, lack of access to patient information, and system-level issues such as poorly designed medical equipment or insufficient staffing. To prevent medical errors, healthcare organizations must implement strategies that promote patient safety, such as improving communication among healthcare providers, enhancing the accuracy and accessibility of patient information, and implementing robust quality improvement programs. Patients can also play a role in preventing medical errors by advocating for their own healthcare, asking questions, and ensuring that they understand their diagnosis and treatment plan. There are several types of clinical errors, including (Al-Worafi, 2020a-z; Lachman et al., 2022):

1. Diagnostic errors: These occur when a healthcare professional makes an incorrect diagnosis or fails to make a diagnosis in a timely manner.

2. Medication errors: These occur when a healthcare professional prescribes the wrong medication or the wrong dose, or administers the medication incorrectly.

3. Surgical errors: These occur during surgical procedures, such as performing the wrong procedure, operating on the wrong body part, or leaving surgical instruments inside the patient.

4. Communication errors: These occur when there is a breakdown in communication between healthcare professionals, patients, and their families, which can lead to misunderstandings and mistakes.

5. Systemic errors: These occur due to problems within the healthcare system, such as inadequate staffing, lack of resources, or faulty equipment.

6. Documentation errors: These occur when healthcare professionals fail to document important information, which can lead to confusion, errors in treatment, and legal issues.

7. Procedural errors: These occur when healthcare professionals fail to follow established procedures, such as infection control procedures, which can lead to patient harm.

10.2 MEDICAL ERRORS PREVENTION

Medical errors are a significant issue in the healthcare industry, and they can have serious consequences for patients. There are several strategies that can be implemented to help prevent medical errors (Al-Worafi, 2020a; Lachman et al., 2022), and are as follows.

1. Improved communication: Effective communication is crucial in healthcare, particularly between healthcare providers and patients. Clear and concise communication can help prevent errors related to miscommunication, such as incorrect medication dosages.

2. Proper training and education: Healthcare providers should receive regular training and education to stay up-to-date on the latest medical practices and procedures. This can help prevent errors related to outdated or incorrect information.

3. Standardized procedures: Standardized procedures can help reduce the likelihood of errors by ensuring that all healthcare providers follow the same protocols.

4. Use of technology: Technology can help prevent errors by providing accurate and up-to-date information on patients and their medical histories. Electronic health records (EHRs), for example, can help ensure that healthcare providers have access to all necessary information and can track medication orders and dosages.

DOI: 10.1201/9781003230465-12

5. Medication safety: Medication errors are a common cause of medical errors. Measures such as double-checking medication orders, using barcoding systems, and implementing medication reconciliation processes can help reduce the risk of medication errors.

6. Patient involvement: Patients can play an important role in preventing medical errors by communicating clearly with their healthcare providers and being active participants in their own care. Patients should be encouraged to ask questions and speak up if they have concerns.

Overall, preventing medical errors requires a multi-faceted approach that involves healthcare providers, patients, and technology. By implementing these strategies, healthcare organizations can help ensure that patients receive safe and effective care.

10.3 FACILITATORS AND BARRIERS FOR MEDICAL ERRORS PREVENTION
Facilitators and barriers to medical error prevention can be diverse and complex, depending on the context and circumstances of the healthcare system. Here are some examples of facilitators and barriers:
Facilitators:

1. Leadership commitment: Strong leadership and commitment to patient safety and quality improvement can facilitate the implementation of medical error prevention strategies.

2. Teamwork and collaboration: Collaboration among healthcare providers, patients, and families can facilitate effective communication and teamwork, which are essential for preventing medical errors.

3. Staff training and education: Providing regular training and education to healthcare staff can facilitate the adoption of best practices and new technologies for medical error prevention.

4. Patient involvement: Engaging patients in their care can facilitate the detection and reporting of medical errors, as well as the identification of areas for improvement.

5. Information technology: The use of information technology, such as electronic health records and decision support systems, can facilitate the timely and accurate exchange of patient information and decision-making.

Barriers:

1. Limited resources: Limited resources, including funding, equipment, and personnel, can create barriers to the implementation of medical error prevention strategies.

2. Resistance to change: Resistance to change, including new technologies or practices, can be a significant barrier to preventing medical errors.

3. Cultural and language barriers: Cultural and language barriers between healthcare providers and patients can create communication challenges and contribute to medical errors.

4. Lack of accountability: A lack of accountability and consequences for medical errors can create a culture of blame, fear, and secrecy, which can hinder reporting and learning from mistakes.

5. Regulatory barriers: Regulatory barriers, such as inadequate laws and regulations, can create obstacles to implementing medical error prevention strategies.

Overall, addressing these facilitators and barriers will require a multifaceted approach that involves a range of stakeholders, including healthcare providers, patients, families, policymakers, and regulatory bodies. It will also require ongoing commitment, collaboration, and investment in patient safety and quality improvement.

10.4 CHALLENGES OF MEDICAL ERRORS PREVENTION IN DEVELOPING COUNTRIES
There are many challenges to patient care in general as well as medical errors preventions as follows (Alshahrani et al., 2019a,b; Al-Qahtani et al., 2015; Alshahrani et al., 2020a,b; Al-Worafi, 2014; Al-Worafi, 2015; Al-Worafi, 2016; Al-Worafi et al., 2017; Al-Worafi, 2018a-d; Al-Worafi et al., 2018a-b; Al-Worafi et al., 2019; Al-Worafi, 2020a-z; Al-Worafi et al., 2020a-b; Al-Worafi et al., 2021a,b; Al-Worafi, 2022a,b; Al-Worafi, 2023; Baig et al., 2020; Elkalmi et al., 2020; Elsayed & Al-Worafi, 2020; Hasan et al., 2019; Hassan et al., 2014; Izhar et al., 2017; Lee et al., 2017; Mahmoud

et al., 2020; Manan et al., 2014; Manan et al., 2016; Ming et al., 2016; Ming et al., 2020; Othman et al., 2020; Saeed et al., 2014).

10.5 HEALTHCARE SYSTEMS

The quality of healthcare systems and healthcare services are the cornerstone in providing the most effective and safe patient care services; healthcare systems in many developing countries, especially low-income countries, are weak, with inadequate budgets and infrastructures, which affect patient safety in many ways. Therefore, strengthening the healthcare systems in developing countries is very important and highly recommended to improve patient care practice.

10.6 FINANCIAL CHALLENGES

Patient care needs financial support in the public healthcare sectors as well as private healthcare sectors, which is missing in many developing countries, especially low-income countries. Therefore, increasing the health expenditure and the public healthcare budget is very important and highly recommended. Increasing the contribution from the private and charity sectors is very important and highly recommended.

10.7 WORKFORCE CHALLENGES

The inadequate number of healthcare professionals throughout the public as well as private healthcare facilities is a major barrier affecting the quality of healthcare services throughout developing countries, especially low-income countries; therefore, hiring more healthcare professionals is very important and highly recommended.

10.8 MIGRATION OF HEALTHCARE PROFESSIONALS

Migration of healthcare professionals has increased during the last two decades from many developing countries, especially low and middle-income countries, due to many reasons, such as the lack of jobs in healthcare facilities, low salaries, the attraction of jobs overseas, political and war issues, and others. Designing long-term plans and short-term plans to overcome this challenge is very important and highly recommended.

10.9 REPORTING CHALLENGES

Reporting patient care errors and related problems is very important to know the reasons and design the necessary interventions to overcome this challenge.

10.10 RESEARCH

There is little known about patient care errors and related problems in developing countries due to many reasons. Support from the Health Ministries, universities, pharmaceutical companies, organizations, and policymakers can overcome this challenge.

10.11 TECHNOLOGY CHALLENGES

New technologies, applications, and social media can play an important role in the patient process. Medical errors prevention can be summarized as:

1. Improving Communication: Improving communication between healthcare professionals and patients can help prevent medical errors. This includes taking the time to explain medical procedures, providing clear instructions for medication use, and ensuring that patients have a way to ask questions and get clarification.

2. Electronic Medical Records: Electronic medical records can help prevent medical errors by ensuring that all healthcare professionals involved in a patient's care have access to the same information.

3. Medication Safety: Medication errors are a common cause of medical errors. To prevent medication errors, healthcare professionals should check and double-check medication orders, verify the patient's identity, and ensure that the medication is appropriate for the patient's condition and other medications they are taking.

4. Training and Education: Healthcare professionals should receive ongoing training and education to stay up-to-date on the latest medical procedures and technologies. This can help prevent errors caused by outdated or incorrect information.

5. Standardization: Standardizing processes and procedures can help prevent errors caused by inconsistencies or miscommunications between healthcare professionals. This can include standardizing medication administration processes, surgical procedures, and patient handoffs.

6. Quality Improvement Programs: Quality improvement programs can help healthcare organizations identify areas for improvement and implement changes to prevent medical errors.

7. Reporting and Learning: Encouraging healthcare professionals to report errors and near-misses can help organizations learn from mistakes and make changes to prevent future errors.

8. Patient Involvement: Patients should be encouraged to be active participants in their own care. This includes asking questions, providing information about their medical history and current medications, and reporting any concerns or changes in their condition to healthcare professionals.

10.12 CONCLUSION

This chapter has discussed medical errors and related problems, the facilitators, barriers, prevention, and recommendations for best practices in developing countries. Medical errors can be defined as any intentional or unintentional errors or problems that occur during the patient care process. Medical errors can occur in any healthcare setting, including hospitals, clinics, pharmacies, and nursing homes, among others. Medical errors can lead to serious consequences, such as prolonged hospitalization, disability, or even death. Medical errors are a significant public health concern, and they can result from a variety of factors, including mis-communication among healthcare providers, inadequate training or supervision, lack of access to patient information, and system-level issues such as poorly designed medical equipment or insufficient staffing.

REFERENCES

Al-Qahtani, I., Almoteb, T.M., & Al-Warafi, Y. (2015). Competency of metered-dose inhaler use among Saudi community pharmacists: A Simulation method study. *RRJPPS*, 4(2), 37–31.

Alshahrani, S.M., Alakhali, K.M., & Al-Worafi, Y.M. (2019a). Medication errors in a health care facility in southern Saudi Arabia. *Tropical Journal of Pharmaceutical Research*, 18(5), 1119–1122.

Alshahrani, S.M., Alavudeen, S.S., Alakhali, K.M., Al-Worafi, Y.M., Bahamdan, A.K., & Vigneshwaran, E. (2019b). Self-Medication Among King Khalid University Students, Saudi Arabia. *Risk Management and Healthcare Policy*, 12, 243–249.

Alshahrani, S.M., Alakhali, K.M., Al-Worafi, Y.M., & Alshahrani, N.Z. (2020a). Awareness and use of over the counter analgesic medication: a survey in the Aseer region population, Saudi Arabia. *Int J Advan Appl Sci*, 7(3), 130–134.

Alshahrani, S.M., Alzahran, M., Alakhali, K., Vigneshwaran, E., Iqbal, M.J., Khan, N.A., ... & Alavudeen, S.S. (2020b). Association Between Diabetes Consequences and Quality of Life Among Patients With Diabetes Mellitus in the Aseer Province of Saudi Arabia. *Open Access Macedonian Journal of Medical Sciences*, 8(E), 325–330.

Al-Worafi, Y.M. (2014). Prescription writing errors at a tertiary care hospital in Yemen: prevalence, types, causes and recommendations. *Am J Pharm Health Res*, 2, 134–140.

Al-Worafi, Y.M.A. (2015). Appropriateness of metered-dose inhaler use in the Yemeni community pharmacies. *Journal of Taibah University Medical Sciences*, 10(3), 353–358.

Al-Worafi, Y.M.A. (2016). Pharmacy practice in Yemen. In *Pharmacy Practice in Developing Countries* (pp. 267–287). Academic Press.

Al-Worafi, Y.M., Kassab, Y.W., Alseragi, W.M., Almutairi, M.S., Ahmed, A., Ming, L.C., Alkhoshaiban, A.S., & Hadi, M.A. (2017). Pharmacovigilance and adverse drg reaction reporting: a perspective of community pharmacists and pharmacy technicians in Sana'a, Yemen. *Therapeutics and clinical risk management*, 13, 1175.

Al-Worafi, Y.M. (2018a). Knowledge, Attitude and Practice of Yemeni Physicians Toward Pharmacovigilance: A Mixed Method Study. *International Journal of Pharmacy and Pharmaceutical Sciences*, 10 (10), 74–77.

Al-Worafi, Y. (2018b). Knowledge, attitude and practice of Yemeni physicians toward pharmacovigilance: A mixed method study. *Int. J. Pharm. Pharm. Sci*, 10, 74–77.

Al-Worafi, Y.M. (2018c). Dispensing errors observed by community pharmacy dispensers in IBB–YEMEN. *Asian J. Pharm. Clin. Res*, 11(11).

Al-Worafi, Y.M. (2018d). Evauation of inhaler technique among patients with asthma and COPD in Yemen. *Journal of Taibah University medical sciences*, 13(5), 488–490.

Al-Worafi, Y.M., Patel, R.P., Zaidi, S.T.R., Alseragi, W.M., Almutairi, M.S., Alkhoshaiban, A.S., & Ming, L.C. (2018a). Completeness and legibility of handwritten prescriptions in Sana'a, Yemen. *Medical Principles and Practice*, 27, 290–292.

Al-Worafi, Y.M., Alseragi, W.M., Seng, L.K., Kassab, Y.W., Yeoh, S.F., Chiau, L., … & Husain, K. (2018b). Dispensing errors in community pharmacies: a prospective study in Sana'a, Yemen. *Arch Pharm Pract*, 9(4), 1–3.

Al-Worafi, Y.M., Alseragi, W.M., & Mahmoud, M.A. (2019). Competency of metered-dose inhaler use among community pharmacy dispensers in Ibb, Yemen: A simulation method study. *Latin American Journal of Pharmacy*, 38(3), 489–494.

Al-Worafi, Y.M. (Ed.). (2020a). *Drug Safety in Developing Countries: Achievements and Challenges*.

Al-Worafi, Y.M. (2020b). Drug-related problems. In *Drug Safety in Developing Countries* (pp. 105–117). Academic Press.

Al-Worafi, Y.M. (2020c). Adverse drug reactions. In *Drug Safety in Developing Countries* (pp. 39–57). Academic Press.

Al-Worafi, Y.M. (2020d). Medications registation and marketing: safety-related issues. In *Drug Safety in Developing Countries* (pp. 21–28). Academic Press.

Al-Worafi, Y.M. (2020e). Pharmacovigilance. In *Drug Safety in Developing Countries* (pp. 29–38). Academic Press.

Al-Worafi, Y.M. (2020f). Medication errors. In *Drug safety in developing countries* (pp. 59–71). Academic Press.

Al-Worafi, Y.M. (2020g). Medications safety-related terminology. In *Drug safety in developing countries* (pp. 7–19). Academic Press.

Al-Worafi, Y.M. (2020h). Self-medication. In *Drug Safety in Developing Countries* (pp. 73–86). Academic Press.

Al-Worafi, Y.M. (2020j). Antibiotics safety issues. In *Drug Safety in Developing Countries* (pp. 87–103). Academic Press.

Al-Worafi, Y.M. (2020k). Medications safety research issues. In *Drug Safety in Developing Countries* (pp. 213–227). Academic Press.

Al-Worafi, Y.M. (2020l). Counterfeit and substandard medications. In *Drug safety in developing countries* (pp. 119–126). Academic Press.

Al-Worafi, Y.M. (2020m). Medication abuse and misuse. In *Drug safety in developing countries* (pp. 127–135). Academic Press.

Al-Worafi, Y.M. (2020n). Storage and disposal of medications. In *Drug Safety in Developing Countries* (pp. 137–142). Academic Press.

Al-Worafi, Y.M. (2020o). Safety of medications in special population. In *Drug safety in developing countries* (pp. 143–162). Academic Press.

Al-Worafi, Y.M. (2020p). Herbal medicines safety issues. In *Drug Safety in developing countries* (pp. 163–178). Academic Press.

Al-Worafi, Y.M. (2020q). Medications safety pharmacoeconomics-related issues. In *Drug Safety in Developing Countries* (pp. 187–195). Academic Press.

Al-Worafi, Y.M. (2020r). Evidence-based medications safety practice. In *Drug Safety in Developing Countries* (pp. 197–201). Academic Press.

Al-Worafi, Y.M. (2020s). Quality indicators for medications safety. In *Drug safety in developing countries* (pp. 229–242). Academic Press.

Al-Worafi, Y.M. (2020t). Drug safety in Yemen. In *Drug Safety in Developing Countries* (pp. 391–405). Academic Press.

Al-Worafi, Y.M. (2020u). Drug safety in Saudi Arabia. In *Drug Safety in Developing Countries* (pp. 407–417). Academic Press.

Al-Worafi, Y.M. (2020v). Drug safety in United Arab Emirates. In *Drug Safety in Developing Countries* (pp. 419–428). Academic Press.

Al-Worafi, Y.M. (2020w). Drug safety in Indonesia. In *Drug Safety in Developing Countries* (pp. 279–285). Academic Press.

Al-Worafi, Y.M. (2020x). Drug safety in Palestine. In *Drug Safety in Developing Countries* (pp. 471–480). Academic Press.

Al-Worafi, Y.M. (2020y). Drug safety: comparison between developing countries. In *Drug Safety in Developing Countries* (pp. 603–611). Academic Press.

Al-Worafi, Y.M. (2020z). Drug safety in developing versus developed countries. In *Drug Safety in Developing Countries* (pp. 613–615). Academic Press.

Al-Worafi, Y.M., Alseragi, W.M., Ming, L.C., & Alakhali, K.M. (2020a). Drug safety in China. In *Drug Safety in Developing Countries* (pp. 381–388). Academic Press.

Al-Worafi, Y.M., Alseragi, W.M., Alakhali, K.M., Ming, L.C., Othman, G., Halboup, A.M., ... & Elkalmi, R.M. (2020b). Knowledge, beliefs and factors affecting the use of generic medicines among patients in Ibb, Yemen: a mixed-method study. *Journal of Pharmacy Practice and Community Medicine*, 6(4).

Al-Worafi, Y.M., Elkalmi, R.M., Ming, L.C., Othman, G., Halboup, A.M., Battah, M.M., ... & Mani, V. (2021a). *Dispensing errors in hospital pharmacies: A prospective study in Yemen*.

Al-Worafi, Y.M., Hasan, S., Hassan, N.M., & Gaili, A.A. (2021b). Knowledge, Attitude and Experience of Pharmacist in the UAE towards Pharmacovigilance. *Research Journal of Pharmacy and Technology*, 14(1), 265–269.

Al-Worafi, Y. (2022a). *A Guide to Online Pharmacy Education: Teaching Strategies and Assessment Methods*. CRC Press.

Al-Worafi, Y.M. (2022b). Patient care errors and related problems (part I): development and validation of the model. https://orcid.org/0000-0002-5752-2913

Al-Worafi, Y.M. (Ed.). (2023). *Clinical Case Studies on medication Safety*. Academic Press.

Baig, M.R., Al-Worafi, Y.M., Alseragi, W.M., Ming, L.C., & Siddique, A. (2020). Drug safety in India. In *Drug Safety in Developing Countries* (pp. 327–334). Academic Press.

Elkalmi, R.M., Al-Worafi, Y.M., Alseragi, W.M., Ming, L.C., & Siddique, A. (2020). Drug safety in Malaysia. In *Drug Safety in Developing Countries* (pp. 245–253). Academic Press.

Elsayed, T., & Al-Worafi, Y.M. (2020). Drug safety in Egypt. In *Drug Safety in Developing Countries* (pp. 511–523). Academic Press.

Hasan, S., Al-Omar, M.J., AlZubaidy, H., & Al-Worafi, Y.M. (2019). Use of medications in Arab Countries. *Handbook of Healthcare in the Arab World*. Cham: Springer, 42.

Hassan, Y., Abd Aziz, N., Kassab, Y.W., Elgasim, I., Shaharuddin, S., Al-Worafi, Y.M.A., ... & Ming, L.C. (2014). How to help patients to control their blood pressure? Blood pressure control and its predictor. *Archives of Pharmacy Practice*, 5(4).

Izahar, S., Lean, Q.Y., Hameed, M.A., Murugiah, M.K., Patel, R.P., Al-Worafi, Y.M., ... & Ming, L.C. (2017). Content analysis of mobile health applications on diabetes mellitus. *Frontiers in Endocrinology*, 8, 318.

Lachman, P., Runnacles, J., Jayadev, A., Jayadev, C.R.P.A., Brennan, J., & Fitzsimons, J. (Eds.). (2022). *Oxford Professional Practice: Handbook of Patient Safety*. Oxford University Press.

Lee, K.S., Yee, S.M., Zaidi, S.T.R., Patel, R.P., Yang, Q., Al-Worafi, Y.M. and Ming, L.C., 2017. Combating sale of counterfeit and falsified medicines online: a losing battle. *Frontiers in pharmacology*, 8, p. 268.

Mahmoud, M.A., Wajid, S., Naqvi, A.A., Samreen, S., Althagfan, S.S., & Al-Worafi, Y. (2020). Self-medication with antibiotics: A cross-sectional community-based study. *LATIN American Journal of Pharmacy*, 39(2), 348–353.

Manan, M.M., Rusli, R.A., Ang, W.C., Al-Worafi, Y.M., & Ming, L.C. (2014). Assessing the pharmaceutical care issues of antiepileptic drug therapy in hospitalised epileptic patients. *Journal of Pharmacy Practice and Research*, 44(3), 83–88.

Manan, M.M., Ibrahim, N.A., Aziz, N.A., Zulkifly, H.H., Al-Worafi, Y.M.A., & Long, C.M. (2016). Empirical use of antibiotic therapy in the prevention of early onset sepsis in neonates: a pilot study. *Archives of Medical Science*, 12(3), 603–613.

Ming, L.C., Hameed, M.A., Lee, D.D., Apidi, N.A., Lai, P.S.M., Hadi, M.A., Al-Worafi, Y.M.A., & Khan, T.M. (2016). Use of medical mobile applications among hospital pharmacists in Malaysia. *Therapeutic innovation & regulatory science*, 50(4), 419–426.

Ming, L.C., Untong, N., Aliudin, N.A., Osili, N., Kifli, N., Tan, C.S., ... & Goh, H.P. (2020). Mobile health apps on COVID-19 launched in the early days of the pandemic: content analysis and review. *JMIR mHealth and uHealth*, 8(9), e19796.

Othman, G., Ali, F., Ibrahim, M.I.M., Al-Worafi, Y.M., Ansari, M., & Halboup, A.M. (2020). Assessment of Anti-Diabetic Medications Adherence among Diabetic Patients in Sana'a City, Yemen: A Cross Sectional Study. *Journal of Pharmaceutical Research International*, 32(21), 114–122.

Saeed, M.S., Alkhoshaiban, A.S., Al-Worafi, Y.M.A., & Long, C.M. (2014). Perception of self-medication among university students in Saudi Arabia. *Archives of Pharmacy Practice*, 5(4), 149.

11 Patient Care Errors and Related Problems

Surgical Errors and Related Problems

11.1 BACKGROUND

Surgery is a complex and highly technical medical procedure that carries risks of complications and errors. Here are some common surgical problems that can occur:

- Surgical site infections: Surgical site infections (SSIs) can occur when bacteria enter the surgical site during or after the operation. SSIs can cause pain, prolonged hospital stays, and in severe cases, can lead to sepsis or even death.

- Anesthesia complications: Anesthesia is a critical component of surgery, but it can also cause complications such as allergic reactions, breathing difficulties, and nerve damage.

- Bleeding: Surgery can cause bleeding, which can be a significant problem if it is not adequately controlled. Uncontrolled bleeding can lead to shock, organ damage, and death.

- Blood clots: Surgery can increase the risk of blood clots forming in the veins, which can be life-threatening if they break loose and travel to the lungs.

- Organ damage: Surgery can sometimes result in inadvertent damage to organs, such as the bladder, bowel, or blood vessels.

- Wrong-site surgery: Wrong-site surgery occurs when the surgery is performed on the wrong body part or even the wrong patient. This type of error is preventable with proper preoperative verification and communication.

- Equipment failure: Surgical equipment, such as surgical instruments or devices, can malfunction, causing harm to the patient.

- Poor communication: Communication breakdowns among healthcare providers, patients, and families can lead to surgical errors, such as incorrect procedures, missed steps, or medication errors.

Preventing surgical problems requires a comprehensive approach that includes careful preoperative planning, effective communication among healthcare providers, rigorous infection control measures, and continuous quality improvement programs. Additionally, patients should be informed about the risks and benefits of surgery and participate in decision-making regarding their care. Surgical errors can be defined as any intentional or unintentional errors or problems that occur during surgical procedures. Surgical errors refer to mistakes made during a surgical procedure that can cause harm to the patient. These errors can occur for a variety of reasons, including human error, equipment failure, miscommunication among medical staff, and other factors. Some examples of surgical errors include performing surgery on the wrong body part, leaving surgical instruments inside the patient, causing damage to surrounding tissues or organs during surgery, administering the wrong type or dosage of anesthesia, and other mistakes that can result in harm to the patient. To prevent surgical errors, medical professionals and hospitals follow strict protocols and procedures to ensure that surgeries are performed safely and efficiently. These protocols include double-checking the patient's medical history and surgical plan, verifying the patient's identity and the surgical site, and using the proper equipment and techniques to minimize the risk of complications. If a surgical error does occur, it is important for medical professionals to take immediate action to correct the mistake and minimize harm to the patient. Patients who have suffered harm due to a surgical error may be entitled to compensation for their injuries and other damages (Lachman et al., 2022; Maerz, 2006).

11.2 SURGICAL ERRORS POTENTIAL CAUSES AND FACTORS

Surgical errors can be caused by a variety of factors, including:

1. Human error: Mistakes made by surgeons, nurses, anesthesiologists, or other members of the surgical team, such as misreading charts, administering the wrong medication or dosage, or failing to follow proper surgical procedures.

2. Communication breakdowns: Miscommunication between team members, including failure to pass along important information or misunderstandings about the surgical plan.

DOI: 10.1201/9781003230465-13

3. Equipment failure: Malfunctioning surgical equipment, such as faulty surgical tools, anesthesia equipment, or monitoring devices.

4. Inadequate preoperative planning: Poorly designed surgical plans, incomplete or inaccurate patient information, or inadequate training or supervision of surgical staff.

5. Fatigue or stress: Surgical teams working long hours or under high-stress conditions may experience fatigue or stress, which can increase the risk of errors.

6. Poor surgical technique: Inexperienced surgeons, or those who lack the necessary skills or training, may make mistakes during surgery.

7. Patient-related factors: The patient's health condition or anatomy may make surgery more difficult, increasing the risk of errors.

8. Infection control: Poor adherence to infection control procedures, such as inadequate sterilization of surgical equipment or failure to follow proper hand hygiene protocols, can lead to surgical errors.

There are several risk factors that can increase the likelihood of surgical errors. Some of the most common factors include:

1. Inadequate preoperative planning and preparation: Failure to properly plan and prepare for surgery can increase the likelihood of errors during the procedure. This may include inadequate preoperative evaluation, incomplete or inaccurate medical records, and insufficient communication among medical staff.

2. Surgeon fatigue or stress: Surgeons who are overworked, fatigued, or experiencing high levels of stress may be more prone to making errors during surgery.

3. Lack of experience or training: Surgeons who lack experience or training in a particular procedure may be more likely to make errors during the surgery.

4. Equipment malfunctions: Malfunctioning equipment, such as surgical instruments, can increase the risk of errors during surgery.

5. Communication breakdowns: Miscommunication among medical staff, such as misunderstandings about the surgical plan or failure to relay critical information, can increase the risk of errors during surgery.

6. Patient factors: Patients who are elderly, have multiple medical conditions, or are undergoing complex surgeries may be at a higher risk of surgical errors.

It is important for medical professionals and hospitals to take steps to minimize these risk factors and ensure that surgeries are performed safely and efficiently. This may include implementing strict protocols and procedures, providing ongoing training and education for medical staff, and using advanced technology and equipment to minimize the risk of errors.

11.3 SURGICAL ERRORS PREVENTION

Preventing surgical errors requires a comprehensive approach that involves careful planning, communication, and adherence to established protocols and procedures. Some strategies that can help prevent surgical errors include:

There are several strategies that can be employed to help prevent surgical errors:

1. Proper communication: Effective communication between members of the surgical team can help ensure that everyone is on the same page and has a clear understanding of the surgical plan. This includes preoperative planning, team huddles, and postoperative debriefings.

2. Standardized procedures: Developing and implementing standardized procedures can help ensure that surgical protocols are followed consistently, minimizing the risk of errors.

3. Checklists: The use of checklists can help ensure that all necessary steps are taken before, during, and after surgery, reducing the risk of errors.

4. Preoperative planning: Adequate preoperative planning, including thorough patient assessments and medical history reviews, can help identify and address potential complications before surgery.

5. Proper training and education: Ensuring that surgical staff members have the necessary training and education can help prevent errors due to a lack of knowledge or skills.

6. Adequate staffing: Ensuring that there are enough staff members to handle the workload can help reduce the risk of errors due to fatigue or stress.

7. Use of technology: The use of technology, such as electronic health records and surgical imaging systems, can help improve accuracy and reduce the risk of errors.

8. Continuous quality improvement: Regular monitoring and evaluation of surgical processes can help identify areas for improvement and prevent future errors.

By implementing these strategies, surgical teams can help reduce the risk of errors and improve patient outcomes.

11.4 FACILITATORS AND BARRIERS TO SURGICAL ERRORS PREVENTION

Facililtators for Surgical Errors Prevention:

1. Communication and Teamwork: Effective communication between team members can help prevent errors, reduce complications, and improve outcomes. Team members should work together and share information to ensure everyone is on the same page.

2. Standard Operating Procedures: Standard Operating Procedures (SOPs) can help reduce errors by providing clear instructions for surgical procedures, protocols, and steps to follow. SOPs can also help improve the consistency of surgical procedures, which can lead to better outcomes.

3. Continuous Education and Training: Ongoing education and training can help healthcare professionals keep up to date with the latest surgical techniques, equipment, and procedures. Continuous education can also help improve communication and teamwork, and foster a culture of safety.

4. Checklists: Checklists are useful tools to prevent errors during surgery. They can help ensure that all necessary steps are taken and that the correct equipment and supplies are available.

5. Quality Improvement Programs: Quality improvement programs can help identify areas where errors are more likely to occur and develop strategies to prevent them. These programs can also provide feedback on surgical outcomes, allowing healthcare professionals to make adjustments and improve patient safety.

Barriers to Surgical Errors Prevention:

1. Time Pressure: Time pressure can be a major barrier to preventing surgical errors. Healthcare professionals may feel rushed to complete procedures quickly, which can increase the risk of mistakes.

2. Lack of Resources: Lack of resources, such as adequate staffing, equipment, and supplies, can make it difficult to provide safe and effective surgical care.

3. Communication Problems: Communication problems, such as language barriers or ineffective communication between team members, can lead to misunderstandings and errors.

4. Resistance to Change: Resistance to change can be a significant barrier to preventing surgical errors. Healthcare professionals may be resistant to new protocols or procedures, even if they have been shown to improve patient safety.

5. Human Error: Despite efforts to prevent errors, human error is still a significant risk factor for surgical errors. Mistakes can occur due to fatigue, distraction, or other factors, and even the most experienced healthcare professionals can make errors.

11.5 CHALLENGES OF SURGICAL ERRORS PREVENTION IN DEVELOPING COUNTRIES

There are many challenges to patient care in general as well as surgical errors prevention which are as follows (Alshahrani et al., 2019a,b; Al-Qahtani et al., 2015; Alshahrani et al., 2020a,b; Al-Worafi, 2014; Al-Worafi, 2015; Al-Worafi, 2016; Al-Worafi et al., 2017; Al-Worafi, 2018a-d; Al-Worafi et al., 2018a-b; Al-Worafi et al., 2019; Al-Worafi, 2020a-z; Al-Worafi et al., 2020a-b; Al-Worafi et al., 2021a,b; Al-Worafi, 2022a,b; Al-Worafi, 2023; Baig et al., 2020; Elkalmi et al., 2020; Elsayed & Al-Worafi, 2020; Hasan et al., 2019; Hassan et al., 2014; Izhar et al., 2017; Lee et al., 2017; Mahmoud et al., 2020; Manan et al., 2014; Manan et al., 2016; Ming et al., 2016; Ming et al., 2020; Othman et al., 2020; Saeed et al., 2014):

11.5.1 Healthcare Systems

The quality of healthcare systems and healthcare services are the cornerstone in providing the most effective and safe patient care services; healthcare systems in many developing countries, especially low-income countries, are weak, with inadequate budgets and infrastructures, which affect patient safety in many ways. Therefore, strengthening the healthcare systems in developing countries is very important and highly recommended to improve patient care practice.

11.5.2 Financial Challenges

Patient care needs financial support in the public healthcare sectors as well as private healthcare sectors, which is missing in many developing countries, especially in low-income countries. Therefore, increasing health expenditure and the public healthcare budget is very important and highly recommended. Increasing the contribution from the private and charity sectors is very important and highly recommended.

11.5.3 Workforce Challenges

The inadequate number of healthcare professionals throughout the public as well as private healthcare facilities is a major barrier affecting the quality of healthcare services throughout developing countries, especially low-income countries; therefore, hiring more healthcare professionals is very important and highly recommended.

11.5.4 Migration of Healthcare Professionals

Migration of healthcare professionals has increased during the last two decades from many developing countries, especially low and middle-income countries, due to many reasons, such as the lack of jobs in healthcare facilities, low salaries, the attraction of jobs overseas, political and war issues, and others. Designing long-term plans and short-term plans to overcome this challenge is very important and highly recommended.

11.5.5 Reporting Challenges

Reporting patient care errors and related problems is very important to know the reasons and design the necessary interventions to overcome this challenge.

11.5.6 Research

There is little known about patient care errors and related problems in developing countries due to many reasons. Support from the Health Ministries, universities, pharmaceutical companies, organizations, and policymakers can overcome this challenge.

11.5.7 Technology Challenges

New technologies, applications, and social media can play an important role in the patient process. Surgical errors prevention challenges can be summarized as:

1. Technical difficulties: Surgeries are complex procedures that require specialized skills, knowledge, and equipment. Technical difficulties such as equipment failure, poor visibility, or anatomical variations can lead to surgical errors.

2. Human error: Healthcare professionals are susceptible to making errors due to fatigue, stress, or distraction. Surgical errors can occur when healthcare professionals fail to follow proper protocols, misinterpret data, or make incorrect decisions.

3. Communication breakdown: Communication is critical in any healthcare setting. When there is a breakdown in communication between healthcare professionals, patients can suffer from surgical errors or complications. Examples of communication breakdowns include misunderstandings, language barriers, or incomplete transfer of patient information.

4. Systemic factors: Healthcare organizations and systems can play a role in surgical errors and problems. For example, a lack of resources, inadequate staffing, or high patient volume can increase the likelihood of surgical errors.

5. Patient factors: Patient characteristics, such as age, medical history, or obesity, can also impact surgical outcomes. Some patients may be at higher risk of complications due to their health status, which can increase the likelihood of surgical errors.

Overall, preventing surgical errors and problems requires a multifaceted approach that addresses the complex factors that contribute to these issues. This can involve improving communication and collaboration between healthcare professionals, investing in training and education programs, implementing technology and safety measures, and enhancing patient engagement and involvement in their care which are as follows:

1. Promote a Culture of Safety: Healthcare organizations should prioritize patient safety by promoting a culture of safety that encourages reporting of errors, near misses, and hazards. This can help identify areas for improvement and prevent future errors.

2. Standardize Processes: Standardizing processes, such as surgical procedures, equipment and supplies, and medication administration, can help reduce errors and improve outcomes. Organizations should develop and implement standardized procedures and protocols that are evidence-based and reviewed regularly.

3. Enhance Communication and Collaboration: Healthcare professionals should communicate effectively and work collaboratively as a team to prevent errors. This includes sharing information, clarifying roles and responsibilities, and using effective communication strategies such as closed-loop communication and readbacks.

4. Implement Quality Improvement Programs: Quality improvement programs can help identify areas for improvement, monitor outcomes, and implement changes to prevent errors. Organizations should develop and implement quality improvement programs that focus on patient safety and reducing surgical errors.

5. Provide Ongoing Education and Training: Healthcare professionals should receive ongoing education and training on new surgical techniques, equipment, and procedures, as well as communication and teamwork skills. This can help ensure that healthcare professionals are up-to-date and skilled in providing safe and effective care.

6. Enhance Patient and Family Engagement: Patients and their families should be engaged in their care and encouraged to participate in decision-making. This can help improve communication, enhance patient safety, and reduce the risk of errors.

7. Address Systemic Barriers: Healthcare organizations should address systemic barriers to preventing surgical errors, such as inadequate staffing, lack of resources, and poor infrastructure. This requires a commitment to investing in healthcare systems and improving the overall quality of care.

11.6 CONCLUSION

This chapter has discussed surgical errors and related problems, the facilitators, barriers, prevention, and recommendations for best practices in developing countries. Preventing surgical errors and related problems requires a comprehensive approach that includes careful preoperative planning, effective communication among healthcare providers, rigorous infection control measures, and continuous quality improvement programs. Additionally, patients should be informed about the risks and benefits of surgery and participate in decision-making regarding their care. Surgical errors can be defined as any intentional or unintentional errors or problems that occur during surgical procedures.

REFERENCES

Al-Qahtani, I., Almoteb, T.M., & Al-Warafi, Y. (2015). Competency of metered-dose inhaler use among Saudi community pharmacists: A Simulation method study. *RRJPPS*, 4(2), 37–31.

Alshahrani, S.M., Alakhali, K.M., & Al-Worafi, Y.M. (2019a). Medication errors in a health care facility in southern Saudi Arabia. *Tropical Journal of Pharmaceutical Research*, 18(5), 1119–1122.

Alshahrani, S.M., Alavudeen, S.S., Alakhali, K.M., Al-Worafi, Y.M., Bahamdan, A.K., & Vigneshwaran, E. (2019b). Self-medication among King Khalid University Students, Saudi Arabia. *Risk Management and Healthcare Policy*, 12, 243–249.

Alshahrani, S.M., Alakhali, K.M., Al-Worafi, Y.M., & Alshahrani, N.Z. (2020a). Awareness and use of over the counter analgesic medication: a survey in the Aseer region population, Saudi Arabia. *International Journal of Advances in Applied Sciences*, 7(3), 130–134.

Alshahrani, S.M., Alzahran, M., Alakhali, K., Vigneshwaran, E., Iqbal, M.J., Khan, N.A., … & Alavudeen, S.S. (2020b). Association Between Diabetes Consequences and Quality of Life Among Patients With Diabetes Mellitus in the Aseer Province of Saudi Arabia. *Open Access Macedonian Journal of Medical Sciences*, 8(E), 325–330.

Al-Worafi, Y.M. (2014). Prescription writing errors at a tertiary care hospital in Yemen: prevalence, types, causes and recommendations. *American Journal of Pharmacy and Health Research*, 2, 134–140.

Al-Worafi, Y.M.A. (2015). Appropriateness of metered-dose inhaler use in the Yemeni community pharmacies. *Journal of Taibah University Medical Sciences*, 10(3), 353–358.

Al-Worafi, Y.M.A. (2016). Pharmacy practice in Yemen. In *Pharmacy Practice in Developing Countries* (pp. 267–287). Academic Press.

Al-Worafi, Y.M., Kassab, Y.W., Alseragi, W.M., Almutairi, M.S., Ahmed, A., Ming, L.C., Alkhoshaiban, A.S., & Hadi, M.A. (2017). Pharmacovigilance and adverse drg reaction reporting: a perspective of community pharmacists and pharmacy technicians in Sana'a, Yemen. *Therapeutics and clinical risk management*, 13, 1175.

Al-Worafi, Y.M. (2018a). Knowledge, Attitude and Practice of Yemeni Physicians Toward Pharmacovigilance: A Mixed Method Study. *International Journal of Pharmacy and Pharmaceutical Sciences*, 10 (10), 74–77.

Al-Worafi, Y. (2018b). Knowledge, attitude and practice of Yemeni physicians toward pharmacovigilance: A mixed method study. *International Journal of Pharmacy and Pharmaceutical Sciences*, 10, 74–77.

Al-Worafi, Y.M. (2018c). Dispensing errors observed by community pharmacy dispensers in IBB–YEMEN. *Asian Journal of Pharmaceutical and Clinical Research*, 11(11).

Al-Worafi, Y.M. (2018d). Evauation of inhaler technique among patients with asthma and COPD in Yemen. *Journal of Taibah University medical sciences*, 13(5), 488–490.

Al-Worafi, Y.M., Patel, R.P., Zaidi, S.T.R., Alseragi, W.M., Almutairi, M.S., Alkhoshaiban, A.S., & Ming, L.C. (2018a). Completeness and legibility of handwritten prescriptions in Sana'a, Yemen. *Medical Principles and Practice*, 27, 290–292.

Al-Worafi, Y.M., Alseragi, W.M., Seng, L.K., Kassab, Y.W., Yeoh, S.F., Chiau, L., … & Husain, K. (2018b). Dispensing errors in community pharmacies: a prospective study in Sana'a, Yemen. *Archives of Pharmacy Practice*, 9(4), 1–3.

Al-Worafi, Y.M., Alseragi, W.M., & Mahmoud, M.A. (2019). Competency of metered-dose inhaler use among community pharmacy dispensers in Ibb, Yemen: A simulation method study. *Latin American Journal of Pharmacy*, 38(3), 489–494.

Al-Worafi, Y.M. (Ed.). (2020a). *Drug Safety in Developing Countries: Achievements and Challenges.*

Al-Worafi, Y.M. (2020b). Drug-related problems. In *Drug Safety in Developing Countries* (pp. 105–117). Academic Press.

Al-Worafi, Y.M. (2020c). Adverse drug reactions. In *Drug Safety in Developing Countries* (pp. 39–57). Academic Press.

Al-Worafi, Y.M. (2020d). Medications registation and marketing: safety-related issues. In *Drug Safety in Developing Countries* (pp. 21–28). Academic Press.

Al-Worafi, Y.M. (2020e). Pharmacovigilance. In *Drug Safety in Developing Countries* (pp. 29–38). Academic Press.

Al-Worafi, Y.M. (2020f). Medication errors. In *Drug safety in developing countries* (pp. 59–71). Academic Press.

Al-Worafi, Y.M. (2020g). Medications safety-related terminology. In *Drug safety in developing countries* (pp. 7–19). Academic Press.

Al-Worafi, Y.M. (2020h). Self-medication. In *Drug Safety in Developing Countries* (pp. 73–86). Academic Press.

Al-Worafi, Y.M. (2020j). Antibiotics safety issues. In *Drug Safety in Developing Countries* (pp. 87–103). Academic Press.

Al-Worafi, Y.M. (2020k). Medications safety research issues. In *Drug Safety in Developing Countries* (pp. 213–227). Academic Press.

Al-Worafi, Y.M. (2020l). Counterfeit and substandard medications. In *Drug safety in developing countries* (pp. 119–126). Academic Press.

Al-Worafi, Y.M. (2020m). Medication abuse and misuse. In *Drug safety in developing countries* (pp. 127–135). Academic Press.

Al-Worafi, Y.M. (2020n). Storage and disposal of medications. In *Drug Safety in Developing Countries* (pp. 137–142). Academic Press.

Al-Worafi, Y.M. (2020o). Safety of medications in special population. In *Drug safety in developing countries* (pp. 143–162). Academic Press.

Al-Worafi, Y.M. (2020p). Herbal medicines safety issues. In *Drug Safety in developing countries* (pp. 163–178). Academic Press.

Al-Worafi, Y.M. (2020q). Medications safety pharmacoeconomics-related issues. In *Drug Safety in Developing Countries* (pp. 187–195). Academic Press.

Al-Worafi, Y.M. (2020r). Evidence-based medications safety practice. In *Drug Safety in Developing Countries* (pp. 197–201). Academic Press.

Al-Worafi, Y.M. (2020s). Quality indicators for medications safety. In *Drug safety in developing countries* (pp. 229–242). Academic Press.

Al-Worafi, Y.M. (2020t). Drug safety in Yemen. In *Drug Safety in Developing Countries* (pp. 391–405). Academic Press.

Al-Worafi, Y.M. (2020u). Drug safety in Saudi Arabia. In *Drug Safety in Developing Countries* (pp. 407–417). Academic Press.

Al-Worafi, Y.M. (2020v). Drug safety in United Arab Emirates. In *Drug Safety in Developing Countries* (pp. 419–428). Academic Press.

Al-Worafi, Y.M. (2020w). Drug safety in Indonesia. In *Drug Safety in Developing Countries* (pp. 279–285). Academic Press.

Al-Worafi, Y.M. (2020x). Drug safety in Palestine. In *Drug Safety in Developing Countries* (pp. 471–480). Academic Press.

Al-Worafi, Y.M. (2020y). Drug safety: comparison between developing countries. In *Drug Safety in Developing Countries* (pp. 603–611). Academic Press.

Al-Worafi, Y.M. (2020z). Drug safety in developing versus developed countries. In *Drug Safety in Developing Countries* (pp. 613–615). Academic Press.

Al-Worafi, Y.M., Alseragi, W.M., Ming, L.C., & Alakhali, K.M. (2020a). Drug safety in China. In *Drug Safety in Developing Countries* (pp. 381–388). Academic Press.

Al-Worafi, Y.M., Alseragi, W.M., Alakhali, K.M., Ming, L.C., Othman, G., Halboup, A.M., … & Elkalmi, R.M. (2020b). Knowledge, beliefs and factors affecting the use of generic medicines among patients in Ibb, Yemen: a mixed-method study. *Journal of Pharmacy Practice and Community Medicine*, 6(4), 53–56.

Al-Worafi, Y.M., Elkalmi, R.M., Ming, L.C., Othman, G., Halboup, A.M., Battah, M.M., … & Mani, V. (2021a). Dispensing errors in hospital pharmacies: A prospective study in Yemen. AlQalam Journal of Medical and Applied Sciences, 4(2), 13–17.

Al-Worafi, Y.M., Hasan, S., Hassan, N.M., & Gaili, A.A. (2021b). Knowledge, attitude and experience of pharmacist in the UAE towards Pharmacovigilance. *Research Journal of Pharmacy and Technology*, 14(1), 265–269.

Al-Worafi, Y. (2022a). *A Guide to Online Pharmacy Education: Teaching Strategies and Assessment Methods*. CRC Press.

Al-Worafi, Y.M. (2022b). Patient care errors and related problems (part I): development and validation of the model. https://orcid.org/0000-0002-5752-2913

Al-Worafi, Y.M. (Ed.). (2023). *Clinical Case Studies on medication Safety*. Academic Press.

Baig, M.R., Al-Worafi, Y.M., Alseragi, W.M., Ming, L.C., & Siddique, A. (2020). Drug safety in India. In *Drug Safety in Developing Countries* (pp. 327–334). Academic Press.

Elkalmi, R.M., Al-Worafi, Y.M., Alseragi, W.M., Ming, L.C., & Siddique, A. (2020). Drug safety in Malaysia. In *Drug Safety in Developing Countries* (pp. 245–253). Academic Press.

Elsayed, T., & Al-Worafi, Y.M. (2020). Drug safety in Egypt. In *Drug Safety in Developing Countries* (pp. 511–523). Academic Press.

Hasan, S., Al-Omar, M.J., AlZubaidy, H., & Al-Worafi, Y.M. (2019). Use of medications in Arab Countries. *Handbook of Healthcare in the Arab World*. Cham: Springer, 42.

Hassan, Y., Abd Aziz, N., Kassab, Y.W., Elgasim, I., Shaharuddin, S., Al-Worafi, Y.M.A., … & Ming, L.C. (2014). How to help patients to control their blood pressure? Blood pressure control and its predictor. *Archives of Pharmacy Practice*, 5(4), 153–161.

Izahar, S., Lean, Q.Y., Hameed, M.A., Murugiah, M.K., Patel, R.P., Al-Worafi, Y.M., … & Ming, L.C. (2017). Content analysis of mobile health applications on diabetes mellitus. *Frontiers in Endocrinology*, 8, 318.

Lachman, P., Runnacles, J., Jayadev, A., Jayadev, C.R.P.A., Brennan, J., & Fitzsimons, J. (Eds.). (2022). Oxford Professional Practice: Handbook of Patient Safety. Oxford University Press.

Lee, K.S., Yee, S.M., Zaidi, S.T.R., Patel, R.P., Yang, Q., Al-Worafi, Y.M., & Ming, L.C., 2017. Combating sale of counterfeit and falsified medicines online: a losing battle. *Frontiers in pharmacology*, 8, 268.

Mahmoud, M.A., Wajid, S., Naqvi, A.A., Samreen, S., Althagfan, S.S., & Al-Worafi, Y. (2020). Self-medication with antibiotics: A cross-sectional community-based study. *Latin American Journal of Pharmacy*, 39(2), 348–353.

Maerz, L.L. (2006). Avoiding common surgical errors. *Annals of Surgery*, 244(5), 837.

Manan, M.M., Rusli, R.A., Ang, W.C., Al-Worafi, Y.M., & Ming, L.C. (2014). Assessing the pharmaceutical care issues of antiepileptic drug therapy in hospitalised epileptic patients. *Journal of Pharmacy Practice and Research*, 44(3), 83–88.

Manan, M.M., Ibrahim, N.A., Aziz, N.A., Zulkifly, H.H., Al-Worafi, Y.M.A., & Long, C.M. (2016). Empirical use of antibiotic therapy in the prevention of early onset sepsis in neonates: a pilot study. *Archives of Medical Science*, 12(3), 603–613.

Ming, L.C., Hameed, M.A., Lee, D.D., Apidi, N.A., Lai, P.S.M., Hadi, M.A., Al-Worafi, Y.M.A., & Khan, T.M. (2016). Use of medical mobile applications among hospital pharmacists in Malaysia. *Therapeutic Innovation & Regulatory Science*, 50(4), 419–426.

Ming, L.C., Untong, N., Aliudin, N.A., Osili, N., Kifli, N., Tan, C.S., … & Goh, H.P. (2020). Mobile health apps on COVID-19 launched in the early days of the pandemic: content analysis and review. *JMIR mHealth and uHealth*, 8(9), e19796.

Othman, G., Ali, F., Ibrahim, M.I.M., Al-Worafi, Y.M., Ansari, M., & Halboup, A.M. (2020). Assessment of Anti-Diabetic Medications Adherence among Diabetic Patients in Sana'a City, Yemen: A Cross Sectional Study. *Journal of Pharmaceutical Research International*, 32(21), 114–122.

Saeed, M.S., Alkhoshaiban, A.S., Al-Worafi, Y.M.A., & Long, C.M. (2014). Perception of self-medication among university students in Saudi Arabia. *Archives of Pharmacy Practice*, 5(4), 149.

12 Patient Care Errors and Related Problems

Complementary and Alternative Medicines (CAM) Errors and Related Problems

12.1 BACKGROUND

Complementary and Alternative Medicine (CAM) refers to a diverse range of medical and healthcare practices, products, and systems that are not considered part of conventional Western medicine. These practices are used in conjunction with or in place of conventional medical treatments. CAM includes a wide range of modalities, such as herbal medicine, acupuncture, massage therapy, chiropractic, homeopathy, energy therapies, and mind-body practices. Many CAM therapies have been used for centuries in traditional healing systems around the world.

While some CAM therapies have been rigorously studied and shown to be effective, many have not been subjected to the same scientific scrutiny as conventional medical treatments. As a result, the safety and effectiveness of CAM therapies can be uncertain (MSD Manual, 2022).

Five categories of complementary or alternative medicine are generally recognized:

12.1.1 Whole Medical Systems

Whole medical systems are complete systems with a defined philosophy and explanation of disease, diagnosis, and therapy. They include the following:

Ayurveda
Homeopathy
Naturopathy
Traditional Chinese medicine

12.1.2 Mind-Body Medicine

Mind-body medicine is based on the theory that mental and emotional factors regulate physical health through a system of interdependent neuronal, hormonal, and immunologic connections throughout the body. Behavioral, psychological, social, and spiritual techniques are used to enhance the mind's capacity to affect the body and thus to preserve health and to prevent or cure disease.

Because scientific evidence supporting the benefits of mind-body medicine is abundant, many of these approaches are now considered mainstream. For example, the following techniques are used in the treatment of chronic pain, coronary artery disease, headaches, insomnia, and menopausal symptoms, and as aids during childbirth:

Biofeedback
Guided imagery
Hypnotherapy
Meditation including mindfulness
Relaxation

These techniques are also used to help patients cope with disease-related and treatment-related symptoms of cancer and to prepare patients for surgery.

12.1.3 Biologically-Based Practices

Biologically-based practices use naturally occurring substances to affect health. These practices include the following:

Botanical medicine and natural products
Chelation therapy
Diet therapies

12.1.4 Manipulative and Body-Based Practices

Manipulative and body-based practices focus primarily on the body's structures and systems (e.g., bones, joints, soft tissues). These practices are based on the belief that the body can regulate and heal itself and that its parts are interdependent. They include

DOI: 10.1201/9781003230465-14

Chiropractic
Massage
Reflexology
Cupping
Gua sha (e.g., scraping, coining, spooning)
Moxibustion
Acupuncture—sometimes considered a manipulative therapy.

Some of these therapies (cupping, scraping, and moxibustion) result in lesions that may be mistaken for signs of trauma or abuse. These therapies are thought to stimulate the body's energy and enable toxins to leave the body. However, only studies of mixed quality have assessed their efficacy, and more research is needed.

12.1.5 Energy Medicine

Energy medicine intends to manipulate subtle energy fields (also called biofields) thought to exist in and around the body and thus affect health. All energy therapies are based on the belief that a universal life force (qi) or subtle energy resides in and around the body. Historically, a vital force was posited to explain biological processes that were not yet understood. As biological science progressed, this force was dismissed. Some investigators continue to explore the existence of the biofield and subtle energies.

Energy medicine is a component of several therapies, including the following:

Acupuncture
Magnets
Therapeutic touch
Reiki

Qi gong and Tai chi—components of traditional Chinese medicine using gentle postures, mindful movement, and breath to bring the patient's energy into better balance.

12.1.6 Terminologies

Complementary, alternative, and integrative medicine are terms often used interchangeably, but their meanings are different.

12.1.7 Complementary Medicine

Refers to non-mainstream practices used together with conventional medicine.

12.1.8 Alternative Medicine

Refers to non-mainstream practices used instead of conventional medicine.

12.1.9 Integrative Medicine

Integrative medicine is health care that uses all appropriate therapeutic approaches—conventional and non-mainstream—within a framework that focuses on health, the therapeutic relationship, and the whole person.

12.2 PATIENT CARE ERRORS AND RELATED PROBLEMS

It can be defined simply as any intentional or unintentional errors or problems occurring during the patient care process, such as health screening, patient assessment, diagnosis, management, etc.

12.3 COMPLEMENTARY AND ALTERNATIVE MEDICINES (CAM) ERRORS AND RELATED PROBLEMS

CAM refer to a wide range of healthcare practices that are not considered part of conventional medicine. CAM errors and related problems can be defined as any intentional or unintentional errors or problems that occur during the CAM practice. While some CAM practices can be effective, there are also potential errors and problems associated with their use. Some of these include:

1. Lack of scientific evidence: Many CAM practices lack scientific evidence to support their effectiveness, and in some cases, they may even be harmful. Patients who rely solely on 1CAM therapies may be putting themselves at risk by not seeking conventional medical treatment.

2. Interactions with conventional medicines: Some CAM therapies can interact with conventional medicines, leading to potentially dangerous side effects. Patients who are taking prescription medications should consult with their doctor before starting any CAM therapies.

3. Misdiagnosis: Patients who rely solely on CAM therapies may not receive a proper diagnosis for their condition. This can lead to delays in treatment and potentially worsen the condition.

4. Unregulated practices: Many CAM practices are not regulated by government agencies, which means that there are no standards for safety, efficacy, or quality control. This can put patients at risk of receiving ineffective or even harmful treatments.

5. False claims: Some CAM practitioners make false claims about their treatments, which can mislead patients into thinking that they are receiving effective treatment when they are not.

6. Financial burden: CAM therapies are often not covered by insurance, which means that patients may have to pay out-of-pocket for these treatments. This can be a financial burden, especially for patients with chronic or serious medical conditions.

It is important for patients to be informed about the potential risks and benefits of CAM therapies and to work with their healthcare provider to develop a comprehensive treatment plan that includes both conventional and complementary therapies.

12.3.1 Whole Medical Systems Errors and Related Problems

Whole medical systems are alternative healthcare practices that are based on a complete system of theory and practice, such as traditional Chinese medicine or Ayurveda. While some of these practices can be effective, there are potential errors and problems associated with their use. Some of these include:

1. Lack of scientific evidence: Many whole medical systems lack scientific evidence to support their effectiveness, and in some cases, they may even be harmful. Patients who rely solely on whole medical systems may be putting themselves at risk by not seeking conventional medical treatment.

2. Misdiagnosis: Practitioners of whole medical systems may not have the same level of training and knowledge as medical doctors, which can lead to misdiagnosis of medical conditions.

3. Ineffective treatments: Some whole medical systems may not be effective for certain medical conditions. Patients who rely solely on these treatments may be putting themselves at risk by not seeking conventional medical treatment.

4. False claims: Some practitioners of whole medical systems make false claims about the effectiveness of their treatments, which can mislead patients into thinking that they are receiving effective treatment when they are not.

5. Lack of regulation: Some whole medical systems are not regulated by government agencies, which means that there are no standards for safety, efficacy, or quality control. This can put patients at risk of receiving ineffective or even harmful treatments.

6. Delayed treatment: Patients who rely solely on whole medical systems may delay seeking conventional medical treatment for serious medical conditions, which can worsen the condition and make it more difficult to treat.

7. Financial burden: Whole medical systems may not be covered by insurance, which means that patients may have to pay out-of-pocket for these treatments. This can be a financial burden, especially for patients with chronic or serious medical conditions.

It is important for patients to be informed about the potential risks and benefits of whole medical systems and to work with their healthcare provider to develop a comprehensive treatment plan that includes both conventional and complementary therapies. Patients should also ensure that their practitioner is properly trained and licensed.

Ayurveda:

- Lack of standardization: Ayurveda has a wide variety of treatments and practices, which makes it difficult to standardize the treatments across practitioners. There is also a lack of regulation in the industry, which can lead to the use of low-quality herbs and treatments.

- Misuse of toxic substances: Some Ayurvedic remedies use toxic substances, such as heavy metals, which can be harmful if not used correctly.

- Lack of scientific evidence: While Ayurveda has been used for thousands of years, there is a lack of scientific evidence to support its effectiveness in treating certain conditions.

Homeopathy:

- Lack of scientific evidence: Homeopathy is based on the principle of "like cures like" and uses highly diluted substances. However, there is a lack of scientific evidence to support its effectiveness in treating illnesses.

- Potential for harmful interactions: Homeopathic remedies can interact with other medications and cause adverse reactions.

- Misuse of remedies: Some homeopathic remedies may contain ingredients that are not listed on the label, and some may not be prepared according to proper guidelines.

Naturopathy:

- Lack of regulation: Naturopathy is not regulated in all countries, which can lead to unqualified practitioners and unsafe treatments.

- Lack of scientific evidence: While some naturopathic treatments have been shown to be effective in certain conditions, many others have not been scientifically proven.

- Overreliance on supplements: Some naturopaths may prescribe excessive amounts of supplements, which can lead to harmful interactions with other medications and health issues.

Traditional Chinese Medicine:

- Quality control issues: Traditional Chinese Medicine uses a wide variety of herbs and substances, some of which may be contaminated or of poor quality.

- Misuse of remedies: Some Traditional Chinese Medicine remedies may contain toxic substances or contaminants, which can be harmful if not used correctly.

- Lack of scientific evidence: While Traditional Chinese Medicine has been used for thousands of years, there is a lack of scientific evidence to support its effectiveness in treating certain conditions.

12.3.2 Mind Body System Errors and Related Problems

The mind-body system is a complex network that involves the interactions between the brain, nervous system, immune system, endocrine system, and psychological and social factors. There are several errors and problems that can arise within this system, including:

- Chronic stress: Chronic stress can disrupt the balance between the nervous system and the immune system, leading to increased inflammation and a weakened immune response.

- Psychological factors: Negative emotions such as anxiety, depression, and stress can have a negative impact on physical health and lead to conditions such as hypertension, cardiovascular disease, and chronic pain.

- Placebo effect: The placebo effect occurs when a patient experiences a positive response to a treatment that has no active ingredients. While the placebo effect can be beneficial, it can also lead to the overuse of ineffective treatments.

- Mind-body interventions: While mind-body interventions such as meditation, yoga, and tai chi can be effective in improving mental and physical health, there is a lack of standardization and regulation in the industry.

- Psychosomatic disorders: Psychosomatic disorders occur when psychological factors such as stress, anxiety, or depression cause physical symptoms such as pain, fatigue, or digestive issues.

- Limited understanding: Despite significant progress in our understanding of the mind-body system, there is still much we do not know, and research in this area is ongoing.

Biofeedback:

- Lack of standardization: There is a lack of standardization in the biofeedback industry, which can lead to inconsistencies in treatment across practitioners.

- Limited effectiveness for certain conditions: While biofeedback has been shown to be effective for certain conditions, such as migraines and urinary incontinence, there is limited evidence to support its use for other conditions.

- Cost: Biofeedback can be expensive, and insurance may not cover the cost of treatment.

Guided imagery:

- Limited scientific evidence: While guided imagery has been shown to be effective in reducing anxiety and pain, there is limited scientific evidence to support its use for other conditions.

- Difficulty in accessing the technique: Guided imagery requires a trained practitioner, and it may not be available in all locations or covered by insurance.

- Lack of standardization: There is a lack of standardization in guided imagery techniques, which can lead to inconsistencies in treatment across practitioners.

Hypnotherapy:

- Lack of regulation: Hypnotherapy is not regulated in all countries, which can lead to unqualified practitioners and unsafe treatments.

- Limited scientific evidence: While hypnotherapy has been shown to be effective in treating certain conditions such as anxiety and irritable bowel syndrome, there is limited scientific evidence to support its use for other conditions.

- Potential for false memories: Hypnotherapy can potentially create false memories or suggestibility in some patients, leading to ethical concerns.

Meditation, including mindfulness:

- Lack of standardization: There is a lack of standardization in meditation techniques, which can lead to inconsistencies in treatment across practitioners.

- Limited effectiveness for certain conditions: While meditation has been shown to be effective in reducing stress, anxiety, and depression, there is limited evidence to support its use for other conditions.

- Difficulty in accessing the technique: Meditation requires time and practice, and it may not be accessible or suitable for all individuals.

Relaxation:

- Limited effectiveness for certain conditions: While relaxation techniques such as deep breathing and progressive muscle relaxation can be effective in reducing stress and anxiety, there is limited evidence to support their use for other conditions.

- Difficulty in accessing the technique: Relaxation techniques require time and practice, and they may not be accessible or suitable for all individuals.

- Lack of standardization: There is a lack of standardization in relaxation techniques, which can lead to inconsistencies in treatment across practitioners.

12.3.3 Biologically-Based Practices Errors and Related Problems

Biologically-based practices are alternative healthcare practices that involve the use of natural substances such as herbs, vitamins, and dietary supplements. While some of these practices can be effective, there are potential errors and problems associated with their use. Some of these include:

1. Lack of scientific evidence: Many biologically-based practices lack scientific evidence to support their effectiveness, and in some cases, they may even be harmful. Patients who rely solely on biologically-based therapies may be putting themselves at risk by not seeking conventional medical treatment.

2. Interactions with conventional medicines: Some biologically-based therapies can interact with conventional medicines, leading to potentially dangerous side effects. Patients who are taking prescription medications should consult with their doctor before starting any biologically-based therapies.

3. Mislabeling: Some biologically-based products may be mislabeled, which can lead to incorrect dosing or exposure to harmful substances.

4. Contamination: Some biologically-based products may be contaminated with harmful substances such as heavy metals, pesticides, or bacteria. Patients who use these products may be putting themselves at risk of serious health problems.

5. False claims: Some manufacturers of biologically-based products make false claims about their products, which can mislead patients into thinking that they are receiving effective treatment when they are not.

6. Lack of regulation: Biologically-based products are not regulated by government agencies in the same way that prescription drugs are regulated, which means that there are no standards for safety, efficacy, or quality control. This can put patients at risk of receiving ineffective or even harmful treatments.

It is important for patients to be informed about the potential risks and benefits of biologically-based practices and to work with their healthcare provider to develop a comprehensive treatment plan that includes both conventional and complementary therapies. Patients should also ensure that the products they are using are properly labeled and have been tested for safety and efficacy.

Botanical medicine and natural products:

■ Lack of regulation: Botanical medicine and natural products are not regulated in all countries, which can lead to inconsistent quality and potential for contamination.

■ Limited scientific evidence: While some natural products have been shown to be effective in treating certain conditions, there is limited scientific evidence to support their use for other conditions.

■ Potential for adverse effects: Natural products can cause adverse effects, especially if taken inappropriately or in combination with other medications.

Chelation therapy:

■ Lack of regulation: Chelation therapy is not regulated in all countries, which can lead to inconsistent quality and potential for contamination.

■ Limited scientific evidence: While chelation therapy has been shown to be effective in treating heavy metal poisoning, there is limited scientific evidence to support its use for other conditions.

■ Potential for adverse effects: Chelation therapy can cause adverse effects, especially if performed by an inexperienced practitioner or inappropriately applied.

Diet therapies:

■ Lack of standardization: There is a lack of standardization in diet therapies, which can lead to inconsistencies in treatment across practitioners.

■ Limited scientific evidence: While some diet therapies have been shown to be effective in treating certain conditions, there is limited scientific evidence to support their use for other conditions.

■ Potential for adverse effects: Diet therapies can cause adverse effects, especially if followed inappropriately or without proper guidance.

■ Difficulty in adherence: Diet therapies can be difficult to adhere to, especially if they require significant changes in eating habits or restrict certain foods.

12.3.4 Manipulative and Body-Based Practices Errors and Related Problems

Manipulative and body-based practices are alternative healthcare practices that involve the manipulation or movement of the body. While some of these practices can be effective, there are potential errors and problems associated with their use. Some of these include:

1. Misdiagnosis: Practitioners of manipulative and body-based practices may not have the same level of training and knowledge as medical doctors, which can lead to misdiagnosis of medical conditions.

2. Ineffective treatments: Some manipulative and body-based practices may not be effective for certain medical conditions. Patients who rely solely on these treatments may be putting themselves at risk by not seeking conventional medical treatment.

3. Injury: Some manipulative and body-based practices involve the manipulation of the spine, which can lead to injury if not performed properly. Patients who undergo these treatments should be aware of the potential risks.

4. False claims: Some practitioners of manipulative and body-based practices make false claims about the effectiveness of their treatments, which can mislead patients into thinking that they are receiving effective treatment when they are not.

5. Lack of regulation: Some manipulative and body-based practices are not regulated by government agencies, which means that there are no standards for safety, efficacy, or quality control. This can put patients at risk of receiving ineffective or even harmful treatments.

6. Financial burden: Some manipulative and body-based practices may not be covered by insurance, which means that patients may have to pay out-of-pocket for these treatments. This can be a financial burden, especially for patients with chronic or serious medical conditions.

It is important for patients to be informed about the potential risks and benefits of manipulative and body-based practices and to work with their healthcare provider to develop a comprehensive treatment plan that includes both conventional and complementary therapies. Patients should also ensure that their practitioner is properly trained and licensed.

Chiropractic:

- Risk of injury: Chiropractic adjustments can lead to injury, especially if performed by an inexperienced practitioner or inappropriately applied.

- Limited scientific evidence: While chiropractic care has been shown to be effective in treating certain conditions such as back pain, there is limited scientific evidence to support its use for other conditions.

- Potential for over-treatment: Some chiropractors may recommend frequent and ongoing treatment, which can be costly and potentially unnecessary.

Massage:

- Lack of standardization: There is a lack of standardization in massage techniques, which can lead to inconsistencies in treatment across practitioners.

- Risk of injury: Deep tissue massage can cause bruising and soreness, and inappropriate massage techniques can cause injury.

- Limited effectiveness for certain conditions: While massage therapy has been shown to be effective in reducing stress and anxiety and improving circulation, there is limited evidence to support its use for other conditions.

Reflexology:

- Limited scientific evidence: While reflexology has been shown to be effective in reducing stress and anxiety, there is limited scientific evidence to support its use for other conditions.

- Potential for harm: Reflexology can potentially cause harm, especially if pressure is applied too firmly or inappropriately.

- Lack of standardization: There is a lack of standardization in reflexology techniques, which can lead to inconsistencies in treatment across practitioners.

Cupping:

- Risk of injury: Cupping can cause bruising and soreness, and inappropriate cupping techniques can cause injury.

- Limited scientific evidence: While cupping has been shown to be effective in reducing pain, there is limited scientific evidence to support its use for other conditions.

- Potential for over-treatment: Some practitioners may recommend frequent and ongoing cupping treatment, which can be costly and potentially unnecessary.

Gua sha:

- Risk of injury: Gua sha can cause bruising and soreness, and inappropriate techniques can cause injury.

- Limited scientific evidence: While gua sha has been shown to be effective in reducing pain, there is limited scientific evidence to support its use for other conditions.

- Potential for over-treatment: Some practitioners may recommend frequent and ongoing gua sha treatment, which can be costly and potentially unnecessary.

Moxibustion:

- Risk of injury: Moxibustion can cause burns and inappropriate techniques can cause injury.

- Limited scientific evidence: While moxibustion has been shown to be effective in reducing pain and improving digestive function, there is limited scientific evidence to support its use for other conditions.

- Potential for over-treatment: Some practitioners may recommend frequent and ongoing moxibustion treatment, which can be costly and potentially unnecessary.

12.3.5 Energy Medicine Errors and Related Problems

Energy medicine is an alternative healthcare practice that involves the use of energy fields to promote health and healing. While some of these practices can be effective, there are potential errors and problems associated with their use. Some of these include:

1. Lack of scientific evidence: Many energy medicine practices lack scientific evidence to support their effectiveness, and in some cases, they may even be harmful. Patients who rely solely on energy medicine practices may be putting themselves at risk by not seeking conventional medical treatment.

2. Misdiagnosis: Practitioners of energy medicine may not have the same level of training and knowledge as medical doctors, which can lead to misdiagnosis of medical conditions.

3. False claims: Some practitioners of energy medicine make false claims about the effectiveness of their treatments, which can mislead patients into thinking that they are receiving effective treatment when they are not.

4. Lack of regulation: Some energy medicine practices are not regulated by government agencies, which means that there are no standards for safety, efficacy, or quality control. This can put patients at risk of receiving ineffective or even harmful treatments.

5. Delayed treatment: Patients who rely solely on energy medicine practices may delay seeking conventional medical treatment for serious medical conditions, which can worsen the condition and make it more difficult to treat.

6. Financial burden: Energy medicine practices may not be covered by insurance, which means that patients may have to pay out-of-pocket for these treatments. This can be a financial burden, especially for patients with chronic or serious medical conditions.

It is important for patients to be informed about the potential risks and benefits of energy medicine practices and to work with their healthcare provider to develop a comprehensive treatment plan that includes both conventional and complementary therapies. Patients should also ensure that their practitioner is properly trained and licensed

Acupuncture:

- Risk of injury: Acupuncture can lead to injury, especially if performed by an inexperienced practitioner or inappropriately applied.

- Limited scientific evidence: While acupuncture has been shown to be effective in treating certain conditions such as pain and nausea, there is limited scientific evidence to support its use for other conditions.

- Potential for over-treatment: Some acupuncturists may recommend frequent and ongoing treatment, which can be costly and potentially unnecessary.

Magnets:

- Limited scientific evidence: While magnets have been shown to be effective in reducing pain and inflammation in some cases, there is limited scientific evidence to support their use for other conditions.

- Potential for over-treatment: Some practitioners may recommend frequent and ongoing use of magnets, which can be costly and potentially unnecessary.

Therapeutic touch:

- Limited scientific evidence: While therapeutic touch has been shown to be effective in reducing anxiety and promoting relaxation, there is limited scientific evidence to support its use for other conditions.

- Potential for harm: Therapeutic touch can potentially cause harm, especially if practiced by an inexperienced practitioner or inappropriately applied.

Reiki:

- Limited scientific evidence: While Reiki has been shown to be effective in reducing anxiety and promoting relaxation, there is limited scientific evidence to support its use for other conditions.

- Potential for harm: Reiki can potentially cause harm, especially if practiced by an inexperienced practitioner or inappropriately applied.

Qi gong and Tai chi:

- Limited scientific evidence: While Qi gong and Tai chi have been shown to be effective in reducing stress and promoting relaxation, there is limited scientific evidence to support their use for other conditions.

- Potential for over-treatment: Some practitioners may recommend the frequent and ongoing practice of Qi gong and Tai chi, which can be costly and potentially unnecessary.

12.4 CHALLENGES OF COMPLEMENTARY AND ALTERNATIVE MEDICINES ERRORS PREVENTION IN DEVELOPING COUNTRIES

There are many challenges to patient care in general as well as surgical errors prevention which are as follows (Alshahrani et al., 2019a,b; Al-Qahtani et al., 2015; Alshahrani et al., 2020a,b; Al-Worafi, 2014; Al-Worafi, 2015; Al-Worafi, 2016; Al-Worafi et al., 2017; Al-Worafi, 2018a-d; Al-Worafi et al., 2018a-b; Al-Worafi et al., 2019; Al-Worafi, 2020a-z; Al-Worafi et al., 2020a-b; Al-Worafi et al., 2021a,b; Al-Worafi, 2022a,b; Al-Worafi, 2023; Baig et al., 2020; Elkalmi et al., 2020; Elsayed & Al-Worafi, 2020; Hasan et al., 2019; Hassan et al., 2014; Izhar et al., 2017; Lee et al., 2017; Mahmoud et al., 2020; Manan et al., 2014; Manan et al., 2016; Ming et al., 2016; Ming et al., 2020; Othman et al., 2020; Saeed et al., 2014).

12.4.1 Healthcare Systems

The quality of healthcare systems and healthcare services are the cornerstone in providing the most effective and safe patient care services; healthcare systems in many developing countries, especially low-income countries, are weak, with inadequate budgets and infrastructures, which affect patient safety in many ways. Therefore, strengthening the healthcare systems in developing countries is very important and highly recommended to improve patient care practice.

12.4.2 Financial Challenges

Patient care needs financial support in the public healthcare sectors as well as private healthcare sectors, which is missing in many developing countries, especially low-income countries. Therefore, increasing the health expenditure and the public healthcare budget is very important and highly recommended. Increasing the contribution from the private and charity sectors is very important and highly recommended.

12.4.3 Workforce Challenges

The inadequate number of healthcare professionals throughout the public as well as private healthcare facilities is a major barrier affecting the quality of healthcare services throughout developing countries, especially low-income countries; therefore, hiring more healthcare professionals is very important and highly recommended.

12.4.4 Migration of Healthcare Professionals

Migration of healthcare professionals has increased during the last two decades from many developing countries, especially low and middle-income countries, due to many reasons, such as the lack of jobs in healthcare facilities, low salaries, the attraction of jobs overseas, political and war issues, and others. Designing long-term plans and short-term plans to overcome this challenge is very important and highly recommended.

12.4.5 Reporting Challenges

Reporting patient care errors and related problems is very important to know the reasons and design the necessary interventions to overcome this challenge.

12.4.6 Research

There is little known about patient care errors and related problems in developing countries due to many reasons. Support from the Health Ministries, universities, pharmaceutical companies, organizations, and policymakers can overcome this challenge.

12.4.7 Technology Challenges

New technologies, applications, and social media can play an important role in patient process.

CAM are widely used in developing countries, and their popularity continues to grow. While CAM can offer many benefits, there are also risks associated with its use, particularly in developing countries where regulations and quality control measures may be lacking. Here are some ways to prevent errors and promote the safe use of CAM in developing countries:

1. Education and awareness: Increase public and healthcare provider education and awareness about CAM and its potential risks and benefits. This can be done through training programs, public education campaigns, and outreach to healthcare professionals.

2. Regulation: Develop and enforce regulations that ensure quality control and safety standards for CAM products. This includes requirements for labeling, manufacturing, and distribution.

3. Monitoring and reporting: Establish a system for monitoring adverse reactions and reactions to CAM products and reporting these incidents to regulatory authorities. This can help identify potential problems and prevent future harm.

4. Integration with conventional medicine: Encourage the integration of CAM with conventional medicine, where appropriate. This can improve patient outcomes and reduce the potential for harmful interactions between CAM and conventional treatments.

5. Research: Support research on the safety and efficacy of CAM products, particularly in developing countries. This can help identify effective treatments and prevent the use of harmful products.

6. Collaboration: Foster collaboration between healthcare providers, regulators, and CAM practitioners to develop safe and effective CAM practices that meet the needs of patients in developing countries.

Overall, preventing errors and promoting the safe use of CAM in developing countries requires a multi-faceted approach that involves education, regulation, monitoring, research, and collaboration. By working together, stakeholders can ensure that CAM products are safe and effective and that patients have access to the care they need.

12.5 CONCLUSION

This chapter has discussed CAM errors and related problems, prevention, and recommendations for best practices in developing countries. CAM refer to a wide range of healthcare practices that are not considered part of conventional medicine. CAM errors and related problems can be defined as any intentional or unintentional errors or problems that occur during the CAM practice. While some CAM practices can be effective, there are also potential errors and problems associated with their use.

REFERENCES

Al-Qahtani, I., Almoteb, T.M., & Al-Warafi, Y. (2015). Competency of metered-dose inhaler use among Saudi community pharmacists: A Simulation method study. *RRJPPS*, 4(2), 37–31.

Alshahrani, S.M., Alakhali, K.M., & Al-Worafi, Y.M. (2019a). Medication errors in a health care facility in southern Saudi Arabia. *Tropical Journal of Pharmaceutical Research*, 18(5), 1119–1122.

Alshahrani, S.M., Alavudeen, S.S., Alakhali, K.M., Al-Worafi, Y.M., Bahamdan, A.K., & Vigneshwaran, E. (2019b). Self-Medication Among King Khalid University Students, Saudi Arabia. *Risk Management and Healthcare Policy*, 12, 243–249.

Alshahrani, S.M., Alakhali, K.M., Al-Worafi, Y.M., & Alshahrani, N.Z. (2020a). Awareness and use of over the counter analgesic medication: a survey in the Aseer region population, Saudi Arabia. *Int J Advan Appl Sci*, 7(3), 130–134.

Alshahrani, S.M., Alzahran, M., Alakhali, K., Vigneshwaran, E., Iqbal, M.J., Khan, N.A., … & Alavudeen, S.S. (2020b). Association Between Diabetes Consequences and Quality of Life Among Patients With Diabetes Mellitus in the Aseer Province of Saudi Arabia. *Open Access Macedonian Journal of Medical Sciences*, 8(E), 325–330.

Al-Worafi, Y.M. (2014). Prescription writing errors at a tertiary care hospital in Yemen: prevalence, types, causes and recommendations. *Am J Pharm Health Res*, 2, 134–140.

Al-Worafi, Y.M.A. (2015). Appropriateness of metered-dose inhaler use in the Yemeni community pharmacies. *Journal of Taibah University Medical Sciences*, 10(3), 353–358.

Al-Worafi, Y.M.A. (2016). Pharmacy practice in Yemen. In *Pharmacy Practice in Developing Countries* (pp. 267–287). Academic Press.

Al-Worafi, Y.M., Kassab, Y.W., Alseragi, W.M., Almutairi, M.S., Ahmed, A., Ming, L.C., Alkhoshaiban, A.S., & Hadi, M.A. (2017). Pharmacovigilance and adverse drg reaction reporting: a perspective of community pharmacists and pharmacy technicians in Sana'a, Yemen. *Therapeutics and clinical risk management*, 13, 1175.

Al-Worafi, Y.M. (2018a). Knowledge, Attitude and Practice of Yemeni Physicians Toward Pharmacovigilance: A Mixed Method Study. *International Journal of Pharmacy and Pharmaceutical Sciences*. 10 (10), 74–77

Al-Worafi, Y. (2018b). Knowledge, attitude and practice of Yemeni physicians toward pharmacovigilance: A mixed method study. *Int. J. Pharm. Pharm. Sci*, 10, 74–77.

Al-Worafi, Y.M. (2018c). Dispensing errors observed by community pharmacy dispensers in IBB–YEMEN. *Asian J. Pharm. Clin. Res*, 11(11).

Al-Worafi, Y.M. (2018d). Evauation of inhaler technique among patients with asthma and COPD in Yemen. *Journal of Taibah University medical sciences*, 13(5), 488–490.

Al-Worafi, Y.M., Patel, R.P., Zaidi, S.T.R., Alseragi, W.M., Almutairi, M.S., Alkhoshaiban, A.S., & Ming, L.C. (2018a). Completeness and legibility of handwritten prescriptions in Sana'a, Yemen. *Medical Principles and Practice*, 27, 290–292.

Al-Worafi, Y.M., Alseragi, W.M., Seng, L.K., Kassab, Y.W., Yeoh, S.F., Chiau, L., … & Husain, K. (2018b). Dispensing errors in community pharmacies: a prospective study in Sana'a, Yemen. *Arch Pharm Pract*, 9(4), 1–3.

Al-Worafi, Y.M., Alseragi, W.M., & Mahmoud, M.A. (2019). Competency of metered-dose inhaler use among community pharmacy dispensers in Ibb, Yemen: A simulation method study. *Latin American Journal of Pharmacy*, 38(3), 489–494.

Al-Worafi, Y.M. (Ed.). (2020a). *Drug Safety in Developing Countries: Achievements and Challenges*.

Al-Worafi, Y.M. (2020b). Drug-related problems. In *Drug Safety in Developing Countries* (pp. 105–117). Academic Press.

Al-Worafi, Y.M. (2020c). Adverse drug reactions. In *Drug Safety in Developing Countries* (pp. 39–57). Academic Press.

Al-Worafi, Y.M. (2020d). Medications registation and marketing: safety-related issues. In *Drug Safety in Developing Countries* (pp. 21–28). Academic Press.

Al-Worafi, Y.M. (2020e). Pharmacovigilance. In *Drug Safety in Developing Countries* (pp. 29–38). Academic Press.

Al-Worafi, Y.M. (2020f). Medication errors. In *Drug safety in developing countries* (pp. 59–71). Academic Press.

Al-Worafi, Y.M. (2020g). Medications safety-related terminology. In *Drug safety in developing countries* (pp. 7–19). Academic Press.

Al-Worafi, Y.M. (2020h). Self-medication. In *Drug Safety in Developing Countries* (pp. 73–86). Academic Press.

Al-Worafi, Y.M. (2020j). Antibiotics safety issues. In *Drug Safety in Developing Countries* (pp. 87–103). Academic Press.

Al-Worafi, Y.M. (2020k). Medications safety research issues. In *Drug Safety in Developing Countries* (pp. 213–227). Academic Press.

Al-Worafi, Y.M. (2020l). Counterfeit and substandard medications. In *Drug safety in developing countries* (pp. 119–126). Academic Press.

Al-Worafi, Y.M. (2020m). Medication abuse and misuse. In *Drug safety in developing countries* (pp. 127–135). Academic Press.

Al-Worafi, Y.M. (2020n). Storage and disposal of medications. In *Drug Safety in Developing Countries* (pp. 137–142). Academic Press.

Al-Worafi, Y.M. (2020o). Safety of medications in special population. In *Drug safety in developing countries* (pp. 143–162). Academic Press.

Al-Worafi, Y.M. (2020p). Herbal medicines safety issues. In *Drug Safety in developing countries* (pp. 163–178). Academic Press.

Al-Worafi, Y.M. (2020q). Medications safety pharmacoeconomics-related issues. In *Drug Safety in Developing Countries* (pp. 187–195). Academic Press.

Al-Worafi, Y.M. (2020r). Evidence-based medications safety practice. In *Drug Safety in Developing Countries* (pp. 197–201). Academic Press.

Al-Worafi, Y.M. (2020s). Quality indicators for medications safety. In *Drug safety in developing countries* (pp. 229–242). Academic Press.

Al-Worafi, Y.M. (2020t). Drug safety in Yemen. In *Drug Safety in Developing Countries* (pp. 391–405). Academic Press.

Al-Worafi, Y.M. (2020u). Drug safety in Saudi Arabia. In *Drug Safety in Developing Countries* (pp. 407–417). Academic Press.

Al-Worafi, Y.M. (2020v). Drug safety in United Arab Emirates. In *Drug Safety in Developing Countries* (pp. 419–428). Academic Press.

Al-Worafi, Y.M. (2020w). Drug safety in Indonesia. In *Drug Safety in Developing Countries* (pp. 279–285). Academic Press.

Al-Worafi, Y.M. (2020x). Drug safety in Palestine. In *Drug Safety in Developing Countries* (pp. 471–480). Academic Press.

Al-Worafi, Y.M. (2020y). Drug safety: comparison between developing countries. In *Drug Safety in Developing Countries* (pp. 603–611). Academic Press.

Al-Worafi, Y.M. (2020z). Drug safety in developing versus developed countries. In *Drug Safety in Developing Countries* (pp. 613–615). Academic Press.

Al-Worafi, Y.M., Alseragi, W.M., Ming, L.C., & Alakhali, K.M. (2020a). Drug safety in China. In *Drug Safety in Developing Countries* (pp. 381–388). Academic Press.

Al-Worafi, Y.M., Alseragi, W.M., Alakhali, K.M., Ming, L.C., Othman, G., Halboup, A.M., … & Elkalmi, R.M. (2020b). Knowledge, beliefs and factors affecting the use of generic medicines among patients in Ibb, Yemen: a mixed-method study. *Journal of Pharmacy Practice and Community Medicine*, 6(4).

Al-Worafi, Y.M., Elkalmi, R.M., Ming, L.C., Othman, G., Halboup, A.M., Battah, M.M., … & Mani, V. (2021a). Dispensing errors in hospital pharmacies: A prospective study in Yemen.

Al-Worafi, Y.M., Hasan, S., Hassan, N.M., & Gaili, A.A. (2021b). Knowledge, Attitude and Experience of Pharmacist in the UAE towards Pharmacovigilance. *Research Journal of Pharmacy and Technology*, 14(1), 265–269.

Al-Worafi, Y. (2022a). *A Guide to Online Pharmacy Education: Teaching Strategies and Assessment Methods*. CRC Press.

Al-Worafi, Y.M. (2022b). Patient care errors and related problems (part I): development and validation of the model. https://orcid.org/0000-0002-5752-2913

Al-Worafi, Y.M. (Ed.). (2023). *Clinical Case Studies on medication Safety*. Academic Press.

Baig, M.R., Al-Worafi, Y.M., Alseragi, W.M., Ming, L.C., & Siddique, A. (2020). Drug safety in India. In *Drug Safety in Developing Countries* (pp. 327–334). Academic Press.

Elkalmi, R.M., Al-Worafi, Y.M., Alseragi, W.M., Ming, L.C., & Siddique, A. (2020). Drug safety in Malaysia. In *Drug Safety in Developing Countries* (pp. 245–253). Academic Press.

Elsayed, T., & Al-Worafi, Y.M. (2020). Drug safety in Egypt. In *Drug Safety in Developing Countries* (pp. 511–523). Academic Press.

Hasan, S., Al-Omar, M.J., AlZubaidy, H., & Al-Worafi, Y.M. (2019). Use of medications in Arab Countries. *Handbook of Healthcare in the Arab World*. Cham: Springer, 42.

Hassan, Y., Abd Aziz, N., Kassab, Y.W., Elgasim, I., Shaharuddin, S., Al-Worafi, Y.M.A., ... & Ming, L.C. (2014). How to help patients to control their blood pressure? Blood pressure control and its predictor. *Archives of Pharmacy Practice*, 5(4).

Izahar, S., Lean, Q.Y., Hameed, M.A., Murugiah, M.K., Patel, R.P., Al-Worafi, Y.M., ... & Ming, L.C. (2017). Content analysis of mobile health applications on diabetes mellitus. *Frontiers in Endocrinology*, 8, 318.

Lee, K.S., Yee, S.M., Zaidi, S.T.R., Patel, R.P., Yang, Q., Al-Worafi, Y.M., & Ming, L.C., 2017. Combating sale of counterfeit and falsified medicines online: a losing battle. *Frontiers in pharmacology*, 8, p. 268.

Mahmoud, M.A., Wajid, S., Naqvi, A.A., Samreen, S., Althagfan, S.S., & Al-Worafi, Y. (2020). Self-medication with antibiotics: A cross-sectional community-based study. *Latin American Journal of Pharmacy*, 39(2), 348-35.

Manan, M.M., Rusli, R.A., Ang, W.C., Al-Worafi, Y.M., & Ming, L.C. (2014). Assessing the pharmaceutical care issues of antiepileptic drug therapy in hospitalised epileptic patients. *Journal of Pharmacy Practice and Research*, 44(3), 83–88.

Manan, M.M., Ibrahim, N.A., Aziz, N.A., Zulkifly, H.H., Al-Worafi, Y.M.A., & Long, C.M. (2016). Empirical use of antibiotic therapy in the prevention of early onset sepsis in neonates: a pilot study. *Archives of Medical Science*, 12(3), 603–613.

Ming, L.C., Hameed, M.A., Lee, D.D., Apidi, N.A., Lai, P.S.M., Hadi, M.A., Al-Worafi, Y.M.A. and Khan, T.M., (2016). Use of medical mobile applications among hospital pharmacists in Malaysia. *Therapeutic innovation & regulatory science*, 50(4), pp. 419–426.

Ming, L.C., Untong, N., Aliudin, N.A., Osili, N., Kifli, N., Tan, C.S., ... & Goh, H.P. (2020). Mobile health apps on COVID-19 launched in the early days of the pandemic: content analysis and review. *JMIR mHealth and uHealth*, 8(9), e19796.

MSD Manual (2022). Complementary and Alternative Medicine (CAM). Available at: https://www.msdmanuals.com/

Othman, G., Ali, F., Ibrahim, M.I.M., Al-Worafi, Y.M., Ansari, M., & Halboup, A.M. (2020). Assessment of Anti-Diabetic Medications Adherence among Diabetic Patients in Sana'a City, Yemen: A Cross Sectional Study. *Journal of Pharmaceutical Research International*, 32(21), 114–122.

Saeed, M.S., Alkhoshaiban, A.S., Al-Worafi, Y.M.A., & Long, C.M. (2014). Perception of self-medication among university students in Saudi Arabia. *Archives of Pharmacy Practice*, 5(4), 149.

13 Patient Care Errors and Related Problems

Nutrition Errors and Related Problems

13.1 BACKGROUND

Nutrition is the study of how food affects the body and its functions. It encompasses all aspects of food, including its composition, preparation, consumption, and digestion, as well as the nutrients and other substances that it provides. Good nutrition is essential for maintaining good health, and a balanced diet can help prevent many chronic diseases, such as heart disease, diabetes, and cancer. There are six main classes of nutrients that are essential for human health: carbohydrates, proteins, fats, vitamins, minerals, and water (Krause & Mahan, 2021). Each of these nutrients plays a unique role in the body, and a healthy diet should include appropriate amounts of each. Carbohydrates are the body's primary source of energy, and they come in two forms: simple and complex. Simple carbohydrates, such as sugar, are easily digested and provide a quick source of energy, while complex carbohydrates, such as whole grains, provide sustained energy and are rich in fiber. Proteins are the building blocks of the body, and they are essential for the growth, repair, and maintenance of tissues. They are made up of amino acids, which are used by the body to create new proteins and other essential molecules. Fats are also an important source of energy and are necessary for many body functions, such as insulation, cell structure, and hormone production. However, it is important to consume the right types of fats, such as unsaturated fats found in nuts, seeds, and fish, while limiting saturated and trans fats found in processed foods. Vitamins and minerals are micronutrients that are necessary for many body processes, such as bone health, immune function, and energy metabolism. They are found in many foods, but some people may need to supplement their diet with vitamins and minerals to meet their daily requirements. Water is essential for many body functions, such as regulating body temperature, transporting nutrients, and eliminating waste. It is important to drink enough water to stay hydrated, especially during physical activity or in hot weather. Overall, a balanced diet that includes a variety of nutrient-rich foods is essential for good health and well-being (Krause & Mahan, 2021).

13.2 NUTRITION SUPPORT

Nutrition support is the provision of nutrients to individuals who are unable to meet their nutritional needs through oral intake or who have a clinical condition that requires additional nutritional support. Nutrition support can be provided through various methods, including enteral nutrition (feeding through a tube that goes into the stomach or small intestine) and parenteral nutrition (feeding through a vein). The goal of nutrition support is to prevent malnutrition, promote healing, and improve clinical outcomes. It is commonly used in individuals with chronic illnesses, such as cancer or gastrointestinal disorders, or in those who have undergone surgery or have been hospitalized for an extended period. Nutrition support may involve the use of specialized formulas that provide specific nutrients, such as high protein or low carbohydrate formulas. It may also involve the use of supplements, such as vitamins and minerals, to help meet an individual's nutritional needs. Nutrition support is typically managed by a registered dietitian or a healthcare provider with expertise in nutrition. The management of nutrition support requires ongoing monitoring of an individual's clinical status, as well as their nutritional needs and response to therapy.

13.3 ROUTES OF NUTRITION

Nutrition can be obtained through various routes. Here are the common routes of nutrition:

1. Oral Route: This is the most common route of nutrition intake, where food is taken through the mouth and broken down by enzymes in the digestive system. The nutrients are then absorbed into the bloodstream and transported to the cells of the body.

2. Intravenous Route: This route involves injecting nutrients directly into a vein. This is often used when a person is unable to consume food orally or absorb nutrients through their digestive system.

3. Topical Route: This route involves applying nutrients directly to the skin, where they are absorbed into the body. This is commonly used for topical medications and supplements.

DOI: 10.1201/9781003230465-15

4. Inhalation Route: This route involves inhaling nutrients, such as oxygen and other gases, into the lungs. This is commonly used for medical treatments that require oxygen therapy.

5. Transdermal Route: This route involves applying nutrients directly to the skin through a patch, where they are absorbed into the bloodstream. This method is commonly used for delivering medications and supplements.

6. Subcutaneous Route: This route involves injecting nutrients into the fatty tissue under the skin, where they are slowly absorbed into the bloodstream. This method is commonly used for insulin injections and other medications.

7. Enteral nutrition is a method of feeding that involves delivering nutrients directly into the digestive system through a feeding tube. This can include tube feeding through a nasogastric, nasojejunal, gastrostomy, or jejunostomy tube. Enteral nutrition is typically used for patients who are unable to eat or swallow, or who have a medical condition that affects their ability to digest food properly.

8. Parenteral nutrition, on the other hand, involves delivering nutrients directly into the bloodstream through an IV (intravenous) line. This method is used for patients who are unable to tolerate or absorb enteral nutrition, or who have a medical condition that prevents them from eating or digesting food properly. Parenteral nutrition is typically used for patients who require a more specialized and customized nutrition plan, such as those with severe malnutrition, gastrointestinal disorders, or certain types of cancer. Both enteral and parenteral nutrition can provide patients with the necessary nutrients to maintain their health and support their recovery from illness or injury. However, each method has its own benefits and risks, and the choice of which method to use depends on the patient's individual needs and medical condition.

13.4 NUTRITION CARE PROCESS

The Nutrition Care Process (NCP) is a systematic approach to providing high-quality nutrition care. It is a four-step model that includes assessment, diagnosis, intervention, and monitoring/evaluation. The NCP is widely used by registered dietitian nutritionists (RDNs) and other healthcare professionals to provide evidence-based nutrition care to patients and clients.

Here are the four steps of the Nutrition Care Process:

1. Assessment: This involves gathering and analyzing information about a patient's or client's nutrition status, medical history, lifestyle, and food habits. This information is used to identify nutrition-related problems, determine the patient's or client's nutrition needs, and develop an individualized nutrition plan.

2. Diagnosis: Based on the information gathered during the assessment, the RDN will identify and label the patient's or client's nutrition-related problems. These labels are standardized and categorized according to the International Classification of Diseases, Tenth Revision, Clinical Modification (ICD-10-CM).

3. Intervention: Once the diagnosis has been made, the RDN will develop an intervention plan that addresses the patient's or client's nutrition-related problems. The intervention plan will include specific goals, actions, and outcomes that are designed to improve the patient's or client's nutrition status.

4. Monitoring/Evaluation: The RDN will continuously monitor and evaluate the patient's or client's progress toward achieving the intervention goals. The RDN will make adjustments to the intervention plan as needed, based on the patient's or client's progress.

Overall, the NCP is a systematic and evidence-based approach to providing high-quality nutrition care. It ensures that the RDN and other healthcare professionals are providing individualized nutrition care that is tailored to the patient's or client's specific needs and goals.

13.5 NUTRITION CARE PLAN

A nutrition care plan is a document developed by a registered dietitian nutritionist (RDN) that outlines specific dietary recommendations and interventions to meet the individualized nutrition needs of a patient or client. The nutrition care plan is developed based on the information gathered during the NCP, which includes assessment, diagnosis, intervention, and monitoring/evaluation.

Here are some key elements that are typically included in a nutrition care plan:

1. Goals: The nutrition care plan will outline specific goals that the patient or client should strive to achieve. These goals may include weight loss, improved blood sugar control, increased nutrient intake, or improved digestion.

2. Dietary recommendations: The RDN will provide specific recommendations for the patient or client's diet, based on their individualized nutrition needs. This may include recommendations for specific foods, meal plans, or dietary supplements.

3. Lifestyle modifications: The nutrition care plan may also include recommendations for lifestyle modifications, such as increasing physical activity, reducing stress, or getting more sleep.

4. Follow-up and monitoring: The nutrition care plan will outline a schedule for follow-up and monitoring to assess the patient's or client's progress toward achieving their goals. The RDN may make adjustments to the plan as needed based on the patient's or client's progress.

5. Education: The nutrition care plan may also include education on nutrition and lifestyle modifications to empower the patient or client to take an active role in their own care.

Overall, a nutrition care plan is a critical component of providing high-quality, individualized nutrition care. It ensures that the patient or client receives the specific dietary recommendations and interventions they need to improve their health and well-being.

13.6 NUTRITION ERRORS AND RELATED PROBLEMS

Nutrition errors and related problems can have significant negative impacts on a patient's health and well-being. Here are some examples of common nutrition errors and related problems:

1. Malnutrition: Malnutrition occurs when the body does not receive adequate amounts of essential nutrients. This can be caused by a variety of factors, such as inadequate dietary intake, gastrointestinal disorders, chronic diseases, or medication interactions.

2. Overnutrition: Overnutrition occurs when the body receives an excessive amount of nutrients, typically due to excessive calorie intake or overconsumption of specific nutrients, such as fat or sugar. Overnutrition can lead to obesity, diabetes, and other chronic health conditions.

3. Drug-nutrient interactions: Certain medications can interfere with the body's ability to absorb, metabolize, or utilize nutrients, leading to nutrient deficiencies or toxicity. For example, some medications used to treat acid reflux can interfere with the absorption of vitamin B12.

4. Food allergies and intolerances: Food allergies and intolerances can cause a variety of symptoms, such as nausea, vomiting, diarrhea, abdominal pain, or skin rashes. These conditions can make it difficult to consume a balanced and varied diet.

5. Inadequate hydration: Inadequate hydration can lead to dehydration, which can cause symptoms such as fatigue, dizziness, confusion, and low blood pressure. Chronic dehydration can also contribute to the development of kidney stones and other urinary tract problems.

6. Foodborne illnesses: Foodborne illnesses are caused by consuming contaminated food or beverages. These can range from mild symptoms such as nausea and vomiting to severe and life-threatening conditions such as botulism or *E. coli* infection.

13.7 ENTERAL AND PARENTERAL NUTRITION-RELATED PROBLEMS

Enteral and parenteral nutrition are two different methods of providing nutrition to patients who cannot meet their nutritional needs through regular oral intake. Enteral nutrition involves providing nutrition directly into the gastrointestinal tract, while parenteral nutrition involves providing nutrition directly into the bloodstream.

Here are some common problems associated with enteral and parenteral nutrition:

1. **Enteral nutrition-related problems:**

    a. Tube-related complications such as tube dislodgement, blockage, infection, or skin irritation around the tube insertion site.

b. Gastrointestinal complications such as diarrhea, constipation, abdominal distention, and vomiting.

c. Aspiration pneumonia, a condition in which food or liquid enters the lungs, leading to infection.

d. Malabsorption of nutrients due to underlying gastrointestinal issues such as inflammatory bowel disease or radiation enteritis.

2. **Parenteral nutrition-related problems:**

a. Catheter-related bloodstream infections, which occur when bacteria enter the bloodstream through the catheter site.

b. Electrolyte imbalances such as hyperglycemia, hypokalemia, or hypernatremia.

c. Hepatobiliary complications such as liver dysfunction or gallstones due to excessive lipid administration.

d. Metabolic complications such as hyperglycemia, hypoglycemia, or hypertriglyceridemia.

It is important for healthcare providers to closely monitor patients receiving enteral or parenteral nutrition to prevent and manage these potential complications

13.8 CHALLENGES OF NUTRITION ERRORS PREVENTION IN DEVELOPING COUNTRIES

Preventing nutrition errors and problems in developing countries is a complex challenge that requires a multi-faceted approach. Here are some challenges and recommendations for addressing this issue: There are many challenges to patient care in general as well as nutrition errors prevention as follows (Alshahrani et al., 2019a,b; Al-Qahtani et al., 2015; Alshahrani et al., 2020a,b; Al-Worafi, 2014; Al-Worafi, 2015; Al-Worafi, 2016; Al-Worafi et al., 2017; Al-Worafi, 2018a-d; Al-Worafi et al., 2018a-b; Al-Worafi et al., 2019; Al-Worafi, 2020a-z; Al-Worafi et al., 2020a-b; Al-Worafi et al., 2021a,b; Al-Worafi, 2022a,b; Al-Worafi, 2023; Baig et al., 2020; Elkalmi et al., 2020; Elsayed & Al-Worafi, 2020; Hasan et al., 2019; Hassan et al., 2014; Izhar et al., 2017; Lee et al., 2017; Mahmoud et al., 2020; Manan et al., 2014; Manan et al., 2016; Ming et al., 2016; Ming et al., 2020; Othman et al., 2020; Saeed et al., 2014).

13.8.1 Healthcare Systems

The quality of healthcare systems and healthcare services are the cornerstone in providing the most effective and safe patient care services; healthcare systems in many developing countries, especially low-income countries, are weak, with inadequate budgets and infrastructures, which affect patient safety in many ways. Therefore, strengthening the healthcare systems in developing countries is very important and highly recommended to improve patient care practice.

13.8.2 Financial Challenges

Patient care needs financial support in the public healthcare sectors as well as private healthcare sectors, which is missing in many developing countries, especially low-income countries. Therefore, increasing health expenditures and the public healthcare budget is very important and highly recommended. Increasing the contribution from the private and charity sectors is very important and highly recommended.

13.8.3 Workforce Challenges

The inadequate number of healthcare professionals throughout the public as well as private healthcare facilities is a major barrier affecting the quality of healthcare services throughout developing countries, especially low-income countries; therefore, hiring more healthcare professionals is very important and highly recommended.

13.8.4 Migration of Healthcare Professionals

Migration of healthcare professionals has increased during the last two decades from many developing countries, especially low and middle-income countries, due to many reasons, such as the lack of jobs in healthcare facilities, low salaries, the attraction of jobs overseas, political and war issues, and others. Designing long-term plans and short-term plans to overcome this challenge is very important and highly recommended.

13.8.5 Reporting Challenges

Reporting patient care errors and related problems is very important to know the reasons and design the necessary interventions to overcome this challenge.

13.8.6 Research

There is little known about patient care errors and related problems in developing countries due to many reasons. Support from the Health Ministries, universities, pharmaceutical companies, organizations, and policymakers can overcome this challenge.

13.8.7 Technology Challenges

New technologies, applications, and social media can play an important role in the patient process.

13.8.8 Limited Access to Nutritious Food

In many developing countries, access to nutritious food is limited due to factors such as poverty, **Lack of infrastructure, and environmental issues.**

13.8.9 Lack of Awareness about Proper Nutrition

Many people in developing countries may not be aware of the importance of proper nutrition and the consequences of malnutrition.

13.8.10 Poor Sanitation and Hygiene

Poor sanitation and hygiene can increase the risk of malnutrition due to waterborne diseases.

13.8.11 Limited Resources

Developing countries often have limited resources to address nutrition problems and may prioritize other pressing issues.

Recommendations:

1. Increase awareness: Education campaigns can be implemented to raise awareness about the importance of proper nutrition and the consequences of malnutrition. This can include community-based interventions, media campaigns, and school-based programs.

2. Improve access to nutritious food: Policies can be put in place to increase access to fresh fruits, vegetables, and other nutrient-rich foods. This can include initiatives such as food subsidies, community gardens, and public markets.

3. Fortify food: Fortifying staple foods with essential nutrients like vitamins and minerals can help address deficiencies and prevent malnutrition. This can be done through public-private partnerships and government-led initiatives.

4. Improve sanitation and hygiene: Efforts to improve access to clean water and sanitation facilities can help prevent waterborne diseases that can cause malnutrition. This can include initiatives such as providing access to clean water sources, improving waste management systems, and promoting good hygiene practices.

5. Address poverty and inequality: Policies that address poverty and inequality can help reduce malnutrition in developing countries. This can include initiatives such as income support programs, job creation programs, and social protection programs.

6. Strengthen health systems: Strong health systems can help prevent and address malnutrition. This can include initiatives such as training health workers, improving access to health services, and investing in health infrastructure.

7. Foster partnerships: Partnerships between governments and the private sector can help address nutrition challenges in developing countries. This can include initiatives such as public-private partnerships, collaborations, and partnerships with local communities.

13.9 CONCLUSION

This chapter has discussed nutrition errors and related problems, prevention, and recommendations for best practices in developing countries. Nutrition support is the provision of nutrients to individuals who are unable to meet their nutritional needs through oral intake or who have a clinical condition that requires additional nutritional support. Nutrition support can be provided through various methods, including enteral nutrition (feeding through a tube that goes into the stomach or small intestine) and parenteral nutrition (feeding through a vein). The goal of nutrition support is to prevent malnutrition, promote healing, and improve clinical outcomes. Nutrition errors and related problems can have significant negative impacts on a patient's health and well-being.

REFERENCES

Al-Qahtani, I., Almoteb, T.M., & Al-Warafi, Y. (2015). Competency of metered-dose inhaler use among Saudi community pharmacists: A Simulation method study. *RRJPPS*, 4(2), 37–31.

Alshahrani, S.M., Alakhali, K.M., & Al-Worafi, Y.M. (2019a). Medication errors in a health care facility in southern Saudi Arabia. *Tropical Journal of Pharmaceutical Research*, 18(5), 1119–1122.

Alshahrani, S.M., Alavudeen, S.S., Alakhali, K.M., Al-Worafi, Y.M., Bahamdan, A.K., & Vigneshwaran, E. (2019b). Self-Medication Among King Khalid University Students, Saudi Arabia. *Risk Management and Healthcare Policy*, 12, 243–249.

Alshahrani, S.M., Alakhali, K.M., Al-Worafi, Y.M., & Alshahrani, N.Z. (2020a). Awareness and use of over the counter analgesic medication: a survey in the Aseer region population, Saudi Arabia. *Int J Advan Appl Sci*, 7(3), 130–134.

Alshahrani, S.M., Alzahran, M., Alakhali, K., Vigneshwaran, E., Iqbal, M.J., Khan, N.A., ... & Alavudeen, S.S. (2020b). Association Between Diabetes Consequences and Quality of Life Among Patients With Diabetes Mellitus in the Aseer Province of Saudi Arabia. *Open Access Macedonian Journal of Medical Sciences*, 8(E), 325–330.

Al-Worafi, Y.M. (2014). Prescription writing errors at a tertiary care hospital in Yemen: prevalence, types, causes and recommendations. *Am J Pharm Health Res*, 2, 134–140.

Al-Worafi, Y.M.A. (2015). Appropriateness of metered-dose inhaler use in the Yemeni community pharmacies. *Journal of Taibah University Medical Sciences*, 10(3), 353–358.

Al-Worafi, Y.M.A. (2016). Pharmacy practice in Yemen. In *Pharmacy Practice in Developing Countries* (pp. 267–287). Academic Press.

Al-Worafi, Y.M., Kassab, Y.W., Alseragi, W.M., Almutairi, M.S., Ahmed, A., Ming, L.C., Alkhoshaiban, A.S., & Hadi, M.A. (2017). Pharmacovigilance and adverse drg reaction reporting: a perspective of community pharmacists and pharmacy technicians in Sana'a, Yemen. *Therapeutics and clinical risk management*, 13, 1175.

Al-Worafi, Y.M. (2018a). Knowledge, Attitude and Practice of Yemeni Physicians Toward Pharmacovigilance: A Mixed Method Study. *International Journal of Pharmacy and Pharmaceutical Sciences*, 10 (10), 74–77

Al-Worafi, Y. (2018b). Knowledge, attitude and practice of Yemeni physicians toward pharmacovigilance: A mixed method study. *Int. J. Pharm. Pharm. Sci*, 10, 74–77.

Al-Worafi, Y.M. (2018c). Dispensing errors observed by community pharmacy dispensers in IBB–YEMEN. *Asian J. Pharm. Clin. Res*, 11(11).

Al-Worafi, Y.M. (2018d). Evauation of inhaler technique among patients with asthma and COPD in Yemen. *Journal of Taibah University medical sciences*, 13(5), 488–490.

Al-Worafi, Y.M., Patel, R.P., Zaidi, S.T.R., Alseragi, W.M., Almutairi, M.S., Alkhoshaiban, A.S., & Ming, L.C. (2018a). Completeness and legibility of handwritten prescriptions in Sana'a, Yemen. *Medical Principles and Practice*, 27, 290–292.

Al-Worafi, Y.M., Alseragi, W.M., Seng, L.K., Kassab, Y.W., Yeoh, S.F., Chiau, L., … & Husain, K. (2018b). Dispensing errors in community pharmacies: a prospective study in Sana'a, Yemen. *Arch Pharm Pract*, 9(4), 1–3.

Al-Worafi, Y.M., Alseragi, W.M., & Mahmoud, M.A. (2019). Competency of metered-dose inhaler use among community pharmacy dispensers in Ibb, Yemen: A simulation method study. *Latin American Journal of Pharmacy*, 38(3), 489–494.

Al-Worafi, Y.M. (Ed.). (2020a). *Drug Safety in Developing Countries: Achievements and Challenges*.

Al-Worafi, Y.M. (2020b). Drug-related problems. In *Drug Safety in Developing Countries* (pp. 105–117). Academic Press.

Al-Worafi, Y.M. (2020c). Adverse drug reactions. In *Drug Safety in Developing Countries* (pp. 39–57). Academic Press.

Al-Worafi, Y.M. (2020d). Medications registation and marketing: safety-related issues. In *Drug Safety in Developing Countries* (pp. 21–28). Academic Press.

Al-Worafi, Y.M. (2020e). Pharmacovigilance. In *Drug Safety in Developing Countries* (pp. 29–38). Academic Press.

Al-Worafi, Y.M. (2020f). Medication errors. In *Drug safety in developing countries* (pp. 59–71). Academic Press.

Al-Worafi, Y.M. (2020g). Medications safety-related terminology. In *Drug safety in developing countries* (pp. 7–19). Academic Press.

Al-Worafi, Y.M. (2020h). Self-medication. In *Drug Safety in Developing Countries* (pp. 73–86). Academic Press.

Al-Worafi, Y.M. (2020j). Antibiotics safety issues. In *Drug Safety in Developing Countries* (pp. 87–103). Academic Press.

Al-Worafi, Y.M. (2020k). Medications safety research issues. In *Drug Safety in Developing Countries* (pp. 213–227). Academic Press.

Al-Worafi, Y.M. (2020l). Counterfeit and substandard medications. In *Drug safety in developing countries* (pp. 119–126). Academic Press.

Al-Worafi, Y.M. (2020m). Medication abuse and misuse. In *Drug safety in developing countries* (pp. 127–135). Academic Press.

Al-Worafi, Y.M. (2020n). Storage and disposal of medications. In *Drug Safety in Developing Countries* (pp. 137–142). Academic Press.

Al-Worafi, Y.M. (2020o). Safety of medications in special population. In *Drug safety in developing countries* (pp. 143–162). Academic Press.

Al-Worafi, Y.M. (2020p). Herbal medicines safety issues. In *Drug Safety in developing countries* (pp. 163–178). Academic Press.

Al-Worafi, Y.M. (2020q). Medications safety pharmacoeconomics-related issues. In *Drug Safety in Developing Countries* (pp. 187–195). Academic Press.

Al-Worafi, Y.M. (2020r). Evidence-based medications safety practice. In *Drug Safety in Developing Countries* (pp. 197–201). Academic Press.

Al-Worafi, Y.M. (2020s). Quality indicators for medications safety. In *Drug safety in developing countries* (pp. 229–242). Academic Press.

Al-Worafi, Y.M. (2020t). Drug safety in Yemen. In *Drug Safety in Developing Countries* (pp. 391–405). Academic Press.

Al-Worafi, Y.M. (2020u). Drug safety in Saudi Arabia. In *Drug Safety in Developing Countries* (pp. 407–417). Academic Press.

Al-Worafi, Y.M. (2020v). Drug safety in United Arab Emirates. In *Drug Safety in Developing Countries* (pp. 419–428). Academic Press.

Al-Worafi, Y.M. (2020w). Drug safety in Indonesia. In *Drug Safety in Developing Countries* (pp. 279–285). Academic Press.

Al-Worafi, Y.M. (2020x). Drug safety in Palestine. In *Drug Safety in Developing Countries* (pp. 471–480). Academic Press.

Al-Worafi, Y.M. (2020y). Drug safety: comparison between developing countries. In *Drug Safety in Developing Countries* (pp. 603–611). Academic Press.

Al-Worafi, Y.M. (2020z). Drug safety in developing versus developed countries. In *Drug Safety in Developing Countries* (pp. 613–615). Academic Press.

Al-Worafi, Y.M., Alseragi, W.M., Ming, L.C., & Alakhali, K.M. (2020a). Drug safety in China. In *Drug Safety in Developing Countries* (pp. 381–388). Academic Press.

Al-Worafi, Y.M., Alseragi, W.M., Alakhali, K.M., Ming, L.C., Othman, G., Halboup, A.M., ... & Elkalmi, R.M. (2020b). Knowledge, beliefs and factors affecting the use of generic medicines among patients in Ibb, Yemen: a mixed-method study. *Journal of Pharmacy Practice and Community Medicine*, 6(4).

Al-Worafi, Y.M., Elkalmi, R.M., Ming, L.C., Othman, G., Halboup, A.M., Battah, M.M., ... & Mani, V. (2021a). *Dispensing errors in hospital pharmacies: A prospective study in Yemen*.

Al-Worafi, Y.M., Hasan, S., Hassan, N.M., & Gaili, A.A. (2021b). Knowledge, Attitude and Experience of Pharmacist in the UAE towards Pharmacovigilance. *Research Journal of Pharmacy and Technology*, 14(1), 265–269.

Al-Worafi, Y. (2022a). *A Guide to Online Pharmacy Education: Teaching Strategies and Assessment Methods*. CRC Press.

Al-Worafi, Y.M. (2022b). Patient care errors and related problems (part I): development and validation of the model. https://orcid.org/0000-0002-5752-2913

Al-Worafi, Y.M. (Ed.). (2023). *Clinical Case Studies on medication Safety*. Academic Press.

Baig, M.R., Al-Worafi, Y.M., Alseragi, W.M., Ming, L.C., & Siddique, A. (2020). Drug safety in India. In *Drug Safety in Developing Countries* (pp. 327–334). Academic Press.

Elkalmi, R.M., Al-Worafi, Y.M., Alseragi, W.M., Ming, L.C., & Siddique, A. (2020). Drug safety in Malaysia. In *Drug Safety in Developing Countries* (pp. 245–253). Academic Press.

Elsayed, T., & Al-Worafi, Y.M. (2020). Drug safety in Egypt. In *Drug Safety in Developing Countries* (pp. 511–523). Academic Press.

Hasan, S., Al-Omar, M.J., AlZubaidy, H., & Al-Worafi, Y.M. (2019). Use of medications in Arab Countries. *Handbook of Healthcare in the Arab World*. Cham: Springer, 42.

Hassan, Y., Abd Aziz, N., Kassab, Y.W., Elgasim, I., Shaharuddin, S., Al-Worafi, Y.M.A., ... & Ming, L.C. (2014). How to help patients to control their blood pressure? Blood pressure control and its predictor. *Archives of Pharmacy Practice*, 5(4).

Izahar, S., Lean, Q.Y., Hameed, M.A., Murugiah, M.K., Patel, R.P., Al-Worafi, Y.M., ... & Ming, L.C. (2017). Content analysis of mobile health applications on diabetes mellitus. *Frontiers in Endocrinology*, 8, 318.

Krause, M.V., & Mahan, L.K. (2021). *Krause and Mahan's Food & the Nutrition Care Process*. Elsevier.

Lee, K.S., Yee, S.M., Zaidi, S.T.R., Patel, R.P., Yang, Q., Al-Worafi, Y.M., & Ming, L.C., 2017. Combating sale of counterfeit and falsified medicines online: a losing battle. *Frontiers in pharmacology*, 8, p. 268.

Mahmoud, M.A., Wajid, S., Naqvi, A.A., Samreen, S., Althagfan, S.S., & Al-Worafi, Y. (2020). Self-medication with antibiotics: A cross-sectional community-based study. *Latin American Journal of Pharmacy*, 39(2), 348–353.

Manan, M.M., Rusli, R.A., Ang, W.C., Al-Worafi, Y.M., & Ming, L.C. (2014). Assessing the pharmaceutical care issues of antiepileptic drug therapy in hospitalised epileptic patients. *Journal of Pharmacy Practice and Research*, 44(3), 83–88.

Manan, M.M., Ibrahim, N.A., Aziz, N.A., Zulkifly, H.H., Al-Worafi, Y.M.A., & Long, C.M. (2016). Empirical use of antibiotic therapy in the prevention of early onset sepsis in neonates: a pilot study. *Archives of Medical Science*, 12(3), 603–613.

Ming, L.C., Hameed, M.A., Lee, D.D., Apidi, N.A., Lai, P.S.M., Hadi, M.A., Al-Worafi, Y.M.A., & Khan, T.M. (2016). Use of medical mobile applications among hospital pharmacists in Malaysia. *Therapeutic innovation & regulatory science*, 50(4), 419–426.

Ming, L.C., Untong, N., Aliudin, N.A., Osili, N., Kifli, N., Tan, C.S., ... & Goh, H.P. (2020). Mobile health apps on COVID-19 launched in the early days of the pandemic: content analysis and review. *JMIR mHealth and uHealth*, 8(9), e19796.

Othman, G., Ali, F., Ibrahim, M.I.M., Al-Worafi, Y.M., Ansari, M., & Halboup, A.M. (2020). Assessment of Anti-Diabetic Medications Adherence among Diabetic Patients in Sana'a City, Yemen: A Cross Sectional Study. *Journal of Pharmaceutical Research International*, 32(21), 114–122.

Saeed, M.S., Alkhoshaiban, A.S., Al-Worafi, Y.M.A., & Long, C.M. (2014). Perception of self-medication among university students in Saudi Arabia. *Archives of Pharmacy Practice*, 5(4), 149.

14 Patient Care Errors and Related Problems

Pharmacological Errors and Related Problems (Medication Errors and Related Problems)

14.1 BACKGROUND

Pharmacological errors or medication errors are mistakes that occur in the prescribing, dispensing, administering, or monitoring of medication. These errors can happen at any point in the medication use process and can lead to harmful outcomes for patients. There are many different types of medication errors, including:

1. Prescribing errors—These occur when the wrong medication or dose is prescribed, or when the prescription is written illegibly or incorrectly.

2. Dispensing errors—These occur when the wrong medication or dose is dispensed by a pharmacist.

3. Administration errors—These occur when the wrong medication or dose is given to a patient, or when it is given through the wrong route or at the wrong time.

4. Monitoring errors—These occur when a patient's medication therapy is not monitored properly, leading to adverse reactions or other negative outcomes.

Medication errors can have serious consequences for patients, including adverse drug reactions, hospitalization, and even death. To prevent medication errors, healthcare providers should follow established protocols for medication use, double-check prescriptions and doses, and communicate clearly with patients about their medications. Patients should also be aware of their medications and their potential side effects and should communicate any concerns or questions to their healthcare providers (ASHP, 1993; Al-Worafi, 2020a,b; Billstei-Leber et al., 2018).

14.2 PHARMACOLOGICAL ERRORS POTENTIAL CAUSES AND FACTORS

The top 10 causes of medication errors identified by the United States Pharmacopoeia (USP) (Al-Worafi, 2020a,b; Cowley et al, 2001) are:

1. Performance deficit

2. Procedure or protocol not followed

3. Miscommunication

4. Inaccurate or omitted transcription

5. Improper documentation

6. Drug distribution system error

7. Knowledge deficit,

8. Calculation error

9. Computer entry errors and

10. Lack of system safeguards.

The Institute of Safe Medicine Practices (ISMP) identifies the following areas as potential causes of medication error (Reason, 1990):

- Failed communication

- Handwriting and oral communication

- Drugs with similar names

- Missing or misplaced zero and decimal points,

- Use of non-standard abbreviations,

- Poor drug distribution practices,

- Complex or poorly designed technology,

- Access to drugs by no pharmacy personnel,

- Workplace environmental problem that leads to increased job stress

- Dose miscalculations

- Lack of patient information

- Lack of patient understanding of their therapy.

14.3 PHARMACOLOGICAL ERRORS PREVENTION

Literature reported (ASHP, 1993; Al-Worafi, 2020a,b; Billstein-Leber et al., 2018) many recommendations in order to prevent medication errors as following:

- Drug manufacturers and the Food and Drug Administration are urged to involve pharmacists, nurses, and physicians in decisions about drug names, labeling, and packaging.

- Look-alike or sound-alike trademarked names and generic names should be avoided.

- Organizational policies and procedures should be established to prevent medication errors. Development of the policies and procedures should involve multiple departments, including pharmacy, medicine, nursing, risk management, legal counsel, and organizational administration. The system should ensure adequate written and oral communications among personnel involved in the medication use process to optimize therapeutic appropriateness and to enable medications to be prescribed, dispensed, and administered in a timely fashion.

- To determine appropriate drug therapy, prescribers should stay abreast of the current state of knowledge through literature review, consultation with pharmacists, consultation with other physicians, participation in continuing professional education programs, and other means.

- Written drug or prescription orders (including signatures) should be legible. Prescribers with poor handwriting should print or type medication or prescription orders if direct order entry capabilities for computerized systems are unavailable. A handwritten order should be completely readable.

- Pharmacists should participate in drug therapy monitoring (including the following when indicated: the assessment of therapeutic appropriateness, medication administration appropriateness, and possible duplicate therapies; review for possible interactions; and evaluation of pertinent clinical and laboratory data) and Drug Use Evaluation (DUE) activities to help achieve a safe, effective, and rational use of drugs.

- To recommend and recognize appropriate drug therapy, pharmacists should stay abreast of the current state of knowledge through familiarity with literature, consultation with colleagues and other healthcare providers, participation in continuing professional education programs, and other means.

- Pharmacists should make themselves available to prescribers and nurses to offer information and advice about therapeutic drug regimens and the correct use of medications.

- Pharmacists should be familiar with the medication ordering system and drug distribution policies.

- Before dispensing medication in nonemergency situations, the pharmacist should review an original copy of the written medication order.

- When dispensing medications to patients, pharmacists should counsel patients or caregivers and verify that they understand why a medication was prescribed and dispensed, its intended use, any special precautions that might be observed, and other needed information. For inpatients, pharmacists should make their services available to counsel patients, families, or other caregivers when appropriate.

- Nurses should review patients' medications with respect to desired patient outcomes, therapeutic duplications, and possible drug interactions. Adequate drug information (including information on medication administration and product compatibilities) should be obtained from pharmacists, nurses, other healthcare providers, the literature, and other means when there are questions. There should be appropriate follow-up communication with the prescriber when this is indicated.

■ All drug orders should be verified before medication administration. Nurses should carefully review original medication orders before administration of the first dose and compare them with medications dispensed.

■ Patient identity should be verified before the administration of each prescribed dose. When appropriate, the patient should be observed after administration of the drug product to ensure that the doses were administered as prescribed and have the intended effect.

■ All doses should be administered at scheduled times unless there are questions or problems to be resolved.

■ Patients should inform appropriate direct healthcare providers (e.g., physicians, nurses, and pharmacists) about all known symptoms, allergies, sensitivities, and current medication use. Patients should communicate their actual self-medication practices, even if they differ from the prescribed directions.

■ Patients should be educated and counseled about their medications.

14.4 CHALLENGES OF PHARMACOLOGICAL ERRORS PREVENTION IN DEVELOPING COUNTRIES

Pharmacological errors are common in developing countries, however, there are many challenges which are as follows (Alshahrani et al., 2019a,b; Al-Qahtani et al., 2015; Alshahrani et al., 2020a,b; Al-Worafi, 2014; Al-Worafi, 2015; Al-Worafi, 2016; Al-Worafi et al., 2017; Al-Worafi, 2018a-d; Al-Worafi et al., 2018a-b; Al-Worafi et al., 2019; Al-Worafi, 2020a-z; Al-Worafi et al., 2020a-b; Al-Worafi et al., 2021a,b; Al-Worafi, 2022a,b; Al-Worafi, 2023; Baig et al., 2020; Elkalmi et al., 2020; Elsayed & Al-Worafi, 2020; Hasan et al., 2019; Hassan et al., 2014; Izhar et al., 2017; Lee et al., 2017; Mahmoud et al., 2020; Manan et al., 2014; Manan et al., 2016; Ming et al., 2016; Ming et al., 2020; Othman et al., 2020; Saeed et al., 2014).

14.4.1 Healthcare Systems

The quality of healthcare systems and healthcare services are the cornerstone in providing the most effective and safe patient care services; healthcare systems in many developing countries, especially low-income countries, are weak, with inadequate budgets and infrastructures, which affect patient safety in many ways. Therefore, strengthening the healthcare systems in developing countries is very important and highly recommended to improve patient care practice.

14.4.2 Financial Challenges

Patient care needs financial support in the public healthcare sectors as well as private healthcare sectors, which is missing in many developing countries, especially low-income countries. Therefore, increasing the health expenditure and the public healthcare budget is very important and highly recommended. Increasing the contribution from the private and charity sectors is very important and highly recommended. Lack of financial support is the main challenge for medication error reporting systems in developing countries. In order to run a comprehensive, effective, and high-quality system, and infrastructures, hiring highly qualified and trained healthcare professionals and staff is required, therefore, support from the policymakers, pharmaceutical industries and companies, and international organizations is highly recommended.

14.4.3 Workforce Challenges

The inadequate number of healthcare professionals throughout the public as well as private healthcare facilities is a major barrier affecting the quality of healthcare services throughout developing countries, especially low-income countries; therefore, hiring more healthcare professionals is very important and highly recommended. The lack of human resources and experts is a major challenge for medication error reporting systems in developing countries. In order to run a comprehensive, effective, and high-quality system, hiring highly qualified and trained healthcare professionals and staff are required, therefore, support from the policymakers, pharmaceutical industries and companies, and international organizations is highly recommended.

14.4.4 Migration of Healthcare Professionals

Migration of healthcare professionals has increased during the last two decades from many developing countries, especially low- and middle-income countries, due to many reasons, such as the lack of jobs in healthcare facilities, low salaries, the attraction of jobs overseas, political and war issues, and others. Designing long-term plans and short-term plans to overcome this challenge is very important and highly recommended.

14.4.5 Reporting Challenges

Reporting patient care errors and related problems is very important to know the reasons and design the necessary interventions to overcome this challenge.

14.4.6 Research

There is little known about patient care errors and related problems in developing countries due to many reasons. Support from the Health Ministries, universities, pharmaceutical companies, organizations, and policymakers can overcome this challenge.

14.4.7 System Challenges

- Despite the efforts from the drug authorities in many developing countries toward the safety of medications by establishing pharmacovigilance systems in many developing countries but in general they are focusing on Adverse Drug reactions (ADRs) and ignoring medication errors, medication error reporting systems are either not available or very weak and centralized, all healthcare centers in general or a majority of them don't have medication errors reporting programs in developing countries. Therefore, establishing medication errors reporting systems in all developing countries is highly recommended, and launching medication errors reporting programs in all developing countries is highly recommended.

14.4.8 Education and Training

Introducing the pharmacovigilance issues such as medication errors and its reporting to all medical and health sciences curriculums is highly recommended. Training the current healthcare professionals about pharmacovigilance issues is highly recommended. Launching postgraduate programs is also recommended.

14.4.9 Knowledge and Attitude

Improving the knowledge and attitude of healthcare professionals and patients and the public regarding medication errors and their reporting is highly recommended and can be done through media, workshops, general lectures, brochures, and distribution of educational material which is needed to increase the awareness of healthcare professionals.

14.4.10 Reporting Challenges

Reporting medication errors, the absence of medication errors reporting is the major challenge in developing countries, and difficulties in reporting procedures are also another challenge. Therefore, designing the necessary interventions to overcome the barriers is very important and highly recommended. Mandatory reporting could help overcome this barrier.

14.4.11 Research

Lack of research about different issues of medication errors in the majority of developing countries due to lack of funds and other reasons. Support from the Health Ministries, universities, pharmaceutical companies, organizations, and policymakers can overcome this challenge. Collaborative research with researchers from developed countries could overcome this barrier.

14.4.12 International Collaboration

Collaborating with international organizations is highly recommended in order to share experiences, training, and research about medication errors and their reporting and various medication safety issues.

14.4.13 Quality and Accreditations of Pharmacovigilance Systems and Programs

This important concept should be implemented to measure the quality of the system in developing countries as well as in all healthcare settings in developing countries. Take the necessary actions towards it in order to improve the medication safety practice in all healthcare settings. Establishing a medication safety accreditation in developing countries and perhaps in the world is highly recommended in order to measure the safety of medication safety practice systems in the countries as well as in the healthcare settings, this could motivate the countries to improve their medication safety practice.

14.4.14 Technology Challenges

New technologies, applications, and social media could play an important role in the success of reporting, adapting such technologies could improve the pharmacovigilance practice.

14.4.15 Regulations and Guidelines Challenges

Developing and adapting regulations and guidelines related to medication safety issues such as mandatory reporting of medication errors is highly recommended in developing countries.

14.4.16 Documentation Challenges

Documenting the reporting and other activities is very important for the policymakers, healthcare professionals, researchers, and medical and health sciences students in order to develop the necessary interventions and improve the practice.

14.5 CONCLUSION

This chapter has discussed the pharmacological errors, causes, prevention, and recommendations for the best practice in developing countries. Pharmacological errors or medication errors are mistakes that occur in the prescribing, dispensing, administering, or monitoring of medication. These errors can happen at any point in the medication use process and can lead to harmful outcomes for patients. There are many different types of medication errors such as prescribing and dispensing errors. Medication errors can have serious consequences for patients.

REFERENCES

Al-Qahtani, I., Almoteb, T.M., & Al-Warafi, Y. (2015). Competency of metered-dose inhaler use among Saudi community pharmacists: A Simulation method study. *RRJPPS*, 4(2), 37–31.

Alshahrani, S.M., Alakhali, K.M., & Al-Worafi, Y.M. (2019a). Medication errors in a health care facility in southern Saudi Arabia. *Tropical Journal of Pharmaceutical Research*, 18(5), 1119–1122.

Alshahrani, S.M., Alavudeen, S.S., Alakhali, K.M., Al-Worafi, Y.M., Bahamdan, A.K., & Vigneshwaran, E. (2019b). Self-Medication Among King Khalid University Students, Saudi Arabia. *Risk Management and Healthcare Policy*, 12, 243–249.

Alshahrani, S.M., Alakhali, K.M., Al-Worafi, Y.M., & Alshahrani, N.Z. (2020a). Awareness and use of over the counter analgesic medication: a survey in the Aseer region population, Saudi Arabia. *Int J Advan Appl Sci*, 7(3), 130–134.

Alshahrani, S.M., Alzahran, M., Alakhali, K., Vigneshwaran, E., Iqbal, M.J., Khan, N.A., … & Alavudeen, S.S. (2020b). Association Between Diabetes Consequences and Quality of Life Among Patients With Diabetes Mellitus in the Aseer Province of Saudi Arabia. *Open Access Macedonian Journal of Medical Sciences*, 8(E), 325–330.

Al-Worafi, Y.M. (2014). Prescription writing errors at a tertiary care hospital in Yemen: prevalence, types, causes and recommendations. *Am J Pharm Health Res*, 2, 134–140.

Al-Worafi, Y.M.A. (2015). Appropriateness of metered-dose inhaler use in the Yemeni community pharmacies. *Journal of Taibah University Medical Sciences*, 10(3), 353–358.

Al-Worafi, Y.M.A. (2016). Pharmacy practice in Yemen. In *Pharmacy Practice in Developing Countries* (pp. 267–287). Academic Press.

Al-Worafi, Y.M., Kassab, Y.W., Alseragi, W.M., Almutairi, M.S., Ahmed, A., Ming, L.C., Alkhoshaiban, A.S., & Hadi, M.A. (2017). Pharmacovigilance and adverse drg reaction reporting: a perspective of community pharmacists and pharmacy technicians in Sana'a, Yemen. *Therapeutics and clinical risk management*, 13, 1175.

Al-Worafi, Y.M. (2018a). Knowledge, Attitude and Practice of Yemeni Physicians Toward Pharmacovigilance: A Mixed Method Study. *International Journal of Pharmacy and Pharmaceutical Sciences*, 10 (10), 74–77

Al-Worafi, Y. (2018b). Knowledge, attitude and practice of Yemeni physicians toward pharmacovigilance: A mixed method study. *Int. J. Pharm. Pharm. Sci*, 10, 74–77.

Al-Worafi, Y.M. (2018c). Dispensing errors observed by community pharmacy dispensers in IBB–YEMEN. *Asian J. Pharm. Clin. Res*, 11(11).

Al-Worafi, Y.M. (2018d). Evauation of inhaler technique among patients with asthma and COPD in Yemen. *Journal of Taibah University medical sciences*, 13(5), 488–490.

Al-Worafi, Y.M., Patel, R.P., Zaidi, S.T.R., Alseragi, W.M., Almutairi, M.S., Alkhoshaiban, A.S., & Ming, L.C. (2018a). Completeness and legibility of handwritten prescriptions in Sana'a, Yemen. *Medical Principles and Practice*, 27, 290–292.

Al-Worafi, Y.M., Alseragi, W.M., Seng, L.K., Kassab, Y.W., Yeoh, S.F., Chiau, L., … & Husain, K. (2018b). Dispensing errors in community pharmacies: a prospective study in Sana'a, Yemen. *Arch Pharm Pract*, 9(4), 1–3.

Al-Worafi, Y.M., Alseragi, W.M., & Mahmoud, M.A. (2019). Competency of metered-dose inhaler use among community pharmacy dispensers in Ibb, Yemen: A simulation method study. *Latin American Journal of Pharmacy*, 38(3), 489–494.

Al-Worafi, Y.M. (Ed.). (2020a). *Drug Safety in Developing Countries: Achievements and Challenges.*

Al-Worafi, Y.M. (2020b). Medication errors. In *Drug Safety in Developing Countries* (pp. 105–117). Academic Press.

Al-Worafi, Y.M. (2020c). Adverse drug reactions. In *Drug Safety in Developing Countries* (pp. 39–57). Academic Press.

Al-Worafi, Y.M. (2020d). Medications registration and marketing: safety-related issues. In *Drug Safety in Developing Countries* (pp. 21–28). Academic Press.

Al-Worafi, Y.M. (2020e). Pharmacovigilance. In *Drug Safety in Developing Countries* (pp. 29–38). Academic Press.

Al-Worafi, Y.M. (2020f). Drug-related problems. In *Drug safety in developing countries* (pp. 59–71). Academic Press.

Al-Worafi, Y.M. (2020g). Medications safety-related terminology. In *Drug safety in developing countries* (pp. 7–19). Academic Press.

Al-Worafi, Y.M. (2020h). Self-medication. In *Drug Safety in Developing Countries* (pp. 73–86). Academic Press.

Al-Worafi, Y.M. (2020j). Antibiotics safety issues. In *Drug Safety in Developing Countries* (pp. 87–103). Academic Press.

Al-Worafi, Y.M. (2020k). Medications safety research issues. In *Drug Safety in Developing Countries* (pp. 213–227). Academic Press.

Al-Worafi, Y.M. (2020l). Counterfeit and substandard medications. In *Drug safety in developing countries* (pp. 119–126). Academic Press.

Al-Worafi, Y.M. (2020m). Medication abuse and misuse. In *Drug safety in developing countries* (pp. 127–135). Academic Press.

Al-Worafi, Y.M. (2020n). Storage and disposal of medications. In *Drug Safety in Developing Countries* (pp. 137–142). Academic Press.

Al-Worafi, Y.M. (2020o). Safety of medications in special population. In *Drug safety in developing countries* (pp. 143–162). Academic Press.

Al-Worafi, Y.M. (2020p). Herbal medicines safety issues. In *Drug Safety in developing countries* (pp. 163–178). Academic Press.

Al-Worafi, Y.M. (2020q). Medications safety pharmacoeconomics-related issues. In *Drug Safety in Developing Countries* (pp. 187–195). Academic Press.

Al-Worafi, Y.M. (2020r). Evidence-based medications safety practice. In *Drug Safety in Developing Countries* (pp. 197–201). Academic Press

Al-Worafi, Y.M. (2020s). Quality indicators for medications safety. In *Drug safety in developing countries* (pp. 229–242). Academic Press.

Al-Worafi, Y.M. (2020t). Drug safety in Yemen. In *Drug Safety in Developing Countries* (pp. 391–405). Academic Press.

Al-Worafi, Y.M. (2020u). Drug safety in Saudi Arabia. In *Drug Safety in Developing Countries* (pp. 407–417). Academic Press.

Al-Worafi, Y.M. (2020v). Drug safety in United Arab Emirates. In *Drug Safety in Developing Countries* (pp. 419–428). Academic Press.

Al-Worafi, Y.M. (2020w). Drug safety in Indonesia. In *Drug Safety in Developing Countries* (pp. 279–285). Academic Press.

Al-Worafi, Y.M. (2020x). Drug safety in Palestine. In *Drug Safety in Developing Countries* (pp. 471–480). Academic Press.

Al-Worafi, Y.M. (2020y). Drug safety: comparison between developing countries. In *Drug Safety in Developing Countries* (pp. 603–611). Academic Press.

Al-Worafi, Y.M. (2020z). Drug safety in developing versus developed countries. In *Drug Safety in Developing Countries* (pp. 613–615). Academic Press.

Al-Worafi, Y.M., Alseragi, W.M., Ming, L.C., & Alakhali, K.M. (2020a). Drug safety in China. In *Drug Safety in Developing Countries* (pp. 381–388). Academic Press.

Al-Worafi, Y.M., Alseragi, W.M., Alakhali, K.M., Ming, L.C., Othman, G., Halboup, A.M., … & Elkalmi, R.M. (2020b). Knowledge, beliefs and factors affecting the use of generic medicines among patients in Ibb, Yemen: a mixed-method study. *Journal of Pharmacy Practice and Community Medicine*, 6(4).

Al-Worafi, Y.M., Elkalmi, R.M., Ming, L.C., Othman, G., Halboup, A.M., Battah, M.M., ... & Mani, V. (2021a). *Dispensing errors in hospital pharmacies: A prospective study in Yemen.*

Al-Worafi, Y.M., Hasan, S., Hassan, N.M., & Gaili, A.A. (2021b). Knowledge, Attitude and Experience of Pharmacist in the UAE towards Pharmacovigilance. *Research Journal of Pharmacy and Technology*, 14(1), 265–269.

Al-Worafi, Y. (2022a). *A Guide to Online Pharmacy Education: Teaching Strategies and Assessment Methods*. CRC Press.

Al-Worafi, Y.M. (2022b). Patient care errors and related problems (part I): development and validation of the model. https://orcid.org/0000-0002-5752-2913

Al-Worafi, Y.M. (Ed.). (2023). *Clinical Case Studies on medication Safety*. Academic Press.

American Society of Health-System Pharmacists (ASHP) (1993). Guidelines on preventing medication errors in hospitals. *Am J Hosp Pharm*, 50, 305–314

Baig, M.R., Al-Worafi, Y.M., Alseragi, W.M., Ming, L.C., & Siddique, A. (2020). Drug safety in India. In *Drug Safety in Developing Countries* (pp. 327–334). Academic Press.

Billstein-Leber, M., Carrillo, C.J.D., Cassano, A.T., Moline, K., & Robertson, J.J. (2018). ASHP guidelines on preventing medication errors in hospitals. *American Journal of Health-System Pharmacy*, 75(19), 1493–1517.

Cowley, E., Williams, R., & Cousins, D. (2001). Medication errors in children: a descriptive summary of medication error reports submitted to the United States Pharmacopeia. *Current Therapeutic Research*, 62(9), 627–640.

Elkalmi, R.M., Al-Worafi, Y.M., Alseragi, W.M., Ming, L.C., & Siddique, A. (2020). Drug safety in Malaysia. In *Drug Safety in Developing Countries* (pp. 245–253). Academic Press.

Elsayed, T., & Al-Worafi, Y.M. (2020). Drug safety in Egypt. In *Drug Safety in Developing Countries* (pp. 511–523). Academic Press.

Hasan, S., Al-Omar, M.J., AlZubaidy, H., & Al-Worafi, Y.M. (2019). Use of medications in Arab Countries. *Handbook of Healthcare in the Arab World*. Cham: Springer, 42.

Hassan, Y., Abd Aziz, N., Kassab, Y.W., Elgasim, I., Shaharuddin, S., Al-Worafi, Y.M.A., ... & Ming, L.C. (2014). How to help patients to control their blood pressure? Blood pressure control and its predictor. *Archives of Pharmacy Practice*, 5(4).

Izahar, S., Lean, Q.Y., Hameed, M.A., Murugiah, M.K., Patel, R.P., Al-Worafi, Y.M., ... & Ming, L.C. (2017). Content analysis of mobile health applications on diabetes mellitus. *Frontiers in Endocrinology*, 8, 318.

Lee, K.S., Yee, S.M., Zaidi, S.T.R., Patel, R.P., Yang, Q., Al-Worafi, Y.M., & Ming, L.C., 2017. Combating sale of counterfeit and falsified medicines online: a losing battle. *Frontiers in pharmacology*, 8, p. 268.

Mahmoud, M.A., Wajid, S., Naqvi, A.A., Samreen, S., Althagfan, S.S., & Al-Worafi, Y. (2020). Self-medication with antibiotics: A cross-sectional community-based study. *Latin American Journal of Pharmacy*, 39(2), 348–353.

Manan, M.M., Rusli, R.A., Ang, W.C., Al-Worafi, Y.M., & Ming, L.C. (2014). Assessing the pharmaceutical care issues of antiepileptic drug therapy in hospitalised epileptic patients. *Journal of Pharmacy Practice and Research*, 44(3), 83–88.

Manan, M.M., Ibrahim, N.A., Aziz, N.A., Zulkifly, H.H., Al-Worafi, Y.M.A., & Long, C.M. (2016). Empirical use of antibiotic therapy in the prevention of early onset sepsis in neonates: a pilot study. *Archives of Medical Science*, 12(3), 603–613.

Ming, L.C., Hameed, M.A., Lee, D.D., Apidi, N.A., Lai, P.S.M., Hadi, M.A., Al-Worafi, Y.M.A., & Khan, T.M. (2016). Use of medical mobile applications among hospital pharmacists in Malaysia. *Therapeutic innovation & regulatory science*, 50(4), 419–426.

Ming, L.C., Untong, N., Aliudin, N.A., Osili, N., Kifli, N., Tan, C.S., ... & Goh, H.P. (2020). Mobile health apps on COVID-19 launched in the early days of the pandemic: content analysis and review. *JMIR mHealth and uHealth*, 8(9), e19796.

Othman, G., Ali, F., Ibrahim, M.I.M., Al-Worafi, Y.M., Ansari, M., & Halboup, A.M. (2020). Assessment of Anti-Diabetic Medications Adherence among Diabetic Patients in Sana'a City, Yemen: A Cross Sectional Study. *Journal of Pharmaceutical Research International*, 32(21), 114–122.

Reason, J. (1990). *Human error*. Cambridge university press.

Saeed, M.S., Alkhoshaiban, A.S., Al-Worafi, Y.M.A., & Long, C.M. (2014). Perception of self-medication among university students in Saudi Arabia. *Archives of Pharmacy Practice*, 5(4), 149.

15 Patient Care Errors and Related Problems

Dispensing and Administration Errors and Related Problems

15.1 BACKGROUND

Good dispensing has a good impact on patient's health as well as the healthcare system, it will help in achieving the best treating outcomes; decrease the admission rate to hospitals; decrease morbidity and mortality; decrease the cost of therapy, improve the quality of life and improve the patient satisfaction toward health care and decrease the burden on the hospitals. Dispensing quality indicators are very important and necessary in order to evaluate the dispensing practice, identify the problems as well as challenges, and develop and implement action plans to overcome the identified challenges and improve the practice (Al-Worafi, 2020a,b). Dispensing errors and related problems can be defined as any intentional or unintentional errors or problems that occur during the medication dispensing process. Administration errors and related problems can be defined as any intentional or unintentional errors or problems that occur during the administration process.

15.1.1 Dispensing Errors (For Dispensing Prescriptions and Orders)

Any error related to checking the appropriateness of the prescription for the prescribed medications such as dose, route of administration, frequency, duration, quantity, time of taking medications and instructions; monitoring for the efficacy and safety as well as disease; patient education and counseling related to adherence toward the management plan, self-management, potential adverse effects and reactions, possible interactions, cautions and precautions, contraindications and warning, proper storage and disposal of medications.

15.1.2 Dispensing Errors (For Patient's Self-medication, Prescribing and Dispensing Non-prescriptions Medications (OTC) Practice)

Any error related to gathering patients related information, medical and medications histories, allergies, chief complaints, history of present illness, assessment, management plan which includes objective and desired outcomes, non-pharmacological therapy and recommendations such as weight control, smoking cessation, appropriate and rational pharmacological therapy with dose, dosage form and route of administration, frequency, duration; time of taking medications and instructions; monitoring for the efficacy and safety as well as disease; patient education and counseling related to adherence toward the management plan, self-management, potential adverse effects and reactions, possible interactions, cautions and precautions, contraindications and warning, proper storage and disposal of medications; refer patients to physicians, clinics, hospitals.

15.2 POTENTIAL CAUSES AND FACTORS

The top 10 causes of medication errors identified by the United States Pharmacopoeia (USP) (Cowley et al, 2001; Al-Worafi, 2020a,b) are:

1. Performance deficit
2. Procedure or protocol not followed
3. Miscommunication
4. Inaccurate or omitted transcription
5. Improper documentation
6. Drug distribution system error
7. Knowledge deficit,
8. Calculation error
9. Computer entry errors and
10. Lack of system safeguards.

The Institute of Safe Medicine Practices (ISMP) identifies the following areas as potential causes of medication error (Reason, 1990):

DOI: 10.1201/9781003230465-17

- Failed communication

- Handwriting and oral communication

- Drugs with similar names

- Missing or misplaced zero and decimal points,

- Use of non-standard abbreviations

- Poor drug distribution practices

- Complex or poorly designed technology

- Access to drugs by no pharmacy personnel,

- Workplace environmental problems that lead to increased job stress

- Dose miscalculations

- Lack of patient information

- Lack of patient understanding of their therapy.

15.3 PREVENTION

Literature reported (ASHP, 1993; Billstein-Leber et al., 2018; Al-Worafi, 2020a,b) many recommendations in order to prevent medication errors as follows:

- Drug manufacturers and the Food and Drug Administration are urged to involve pharmacists, nurses, and physicians in decisions about drug names, labeling, and packaging.

- Look-alike or sound-alike trademarked names and generic names should be avoided.

- Organizational policies and procedures should be established to prevent medication errors. Development of the policies and procedures should involve multiple departments, including pharmacy, medicine, nursing, risk management, legal counsel, and organizational administration. The system should ensure adequate written and oral communications among personnel involved in the medication use process to optimize therapeutic appropriateness and to enable medications to be prescribed, dispensed, and administered in a timely fashion.

- To determine appropriate drug therapy, prescribers should stay abreast of the current state of knowledge through literature review, consultation with pharmacists, consultation with other physicians, participation in continuing professional education programs, and other means.

- Written drug or prescription orders (including signatures) should be legible. Prescribers with poor handwriting should print or type medication or prescription orders if direct order entry capabilities for computerized systems are unavailable. A handwritten order should be completely readable.

- Pharmacists should participate in drug therapy monitoring (including the following when indicated: The assessment of therapeutic appropriateness, medication administration appropriateness, and possible duplicate therapies; review for possible interactions; and evaluation of pertinent clinical and laboratory data) and Drug Use Evaluation (DUE) activities to help achieve a safe, effective, and rational use of drugs.

- To recommend and recognize appropriate drug therapy, pharmacists should stay abreast of the current state of knowledge through familiarity with literature, consultation with colleagues and other healthcare providers, participation in continuing professional education programs, and other means.

- Pharmacists should make themselves available to prescribers and nurses to offer information and advice about therapeutic drug regimens and the correct use of medications.

- Pharmacists should be familiar with the medication ordering system and drug distribution policies.

- Before dispensing medication in nonemergency situations, the pharmacist should review an original copy of the written medication order.

- When dispensing medications to patients, pharmacists should counsel patients or caregivers and verify that they understand why a medication was prescribed and dispensed, its intended use, any special precautions that might be observed, and other needed information. For inpatients, pharmacists should make their services available to counsel patients, families, or other caregivers when appropriate.

- Nurses should review patients' medications with respect to desired patient outcomes, therapeutic duplications, and possible drug interactions. Adequate drug information (including information on medication administration and product compatibilities) should be obtained from pharmacists, nurses, other healthcare providers, the literature, and other means when there are questions. There should be appropriate follow-up communication with the prescriber when this is indicated.

- All drug orders should be verified before medication administration. Nurses should carefully review original medication orders before administration of the first dose and compare them with medications dispensed.

- Patient identity should be verified before the administration of each prescribed dose. When appropriate, the patient should be observed after administration of the drug product to ensure that the doses were administered as prescribed and have the intended effect.

- All doses should be administered at scheduled times unless there are questions or problems to be resolved.

- Patients should inform appropriate direct healthcare providers (e.g., physicians, nurses, and pharmacists) about all known symptoms, allergies, sensitivities, and current medication use. Patients should communicate their actual self-medication practices, even if they differ from the prescribed directions.

- Patients should be educated and counseled about their medications.

15.4 CHALLENGES OF DISPENSING AND ADMINISTRATION ERRORS PREVENTION IN DEVELOPING COUNTRIES

Dispensing and administration errors are common in developing countries, however, there are many challenges which are as follows (Alshahrani et al., 2019a,b; Al-Qahtani et al., 2015; Alshahrani et al., 2020a,b; Al-Worafi, 2014; Al-Worafi, 2015; Al-Worafi, 2016; Al-Worafi et al., 2017; Al-Worafi, 2018a-d;Al-Worafi et al., 2018a-b; Al-Worafi et al., 2019; Al-Worafi, 2020a-z; Al-Worafi et al., 2020a-b; Al-Worafi et al., 2021a,b; Al-Worafi, 2022a,b; Al-Worafi, 2023; Baig et al., 2020; Elkalmi et al., 2020; Elsayed & Al-Worafi, 2020; Hasan et al., 2019; Hassan et al., 2014; Izhar et al., 2017; Lee et al., 2017; Mahmoud et al., 2020; Manan et al., 2014; Manan et al., 2016; Ming et al., 2016; Ming et al., 2020; Othman et al., 2020; Saeed et al., 2014).

15.4.1 Healthcare Systems

The quality of healthcare systems and healthcare services are the cornerstone in providing the most effective and safe patient care services; healthcare systems in many developing countries, especially low-income countries, are weak, with inadequate budgets and infrastructures, which affect patient safety in many ways. Therefore, strengthening the healthcare systems in developing countries is very important and highly recommended to improve patient care practice.

15.4.2 Financial Challenges

Patient care needs financial support in the public healthcare sectors as well as private healthcare sectors, which is missing in many developing countries, especially low-income countries. Therefore, increasing health expenditures and the public healthcare budget is very important and highly recommended. Increasing the contribution from the private and charity sectors is very important and highly recommended. Lack of financial support is the main challenge for medication errors reporting systems in developing countries. In order to run a comprehensive, effective, and high-quality system, and infrastructures—hiring highly qualified and trained healthcare professionals and staff is required, therefore, support from the policymakers, pharmaceutical industries and companies, and international organizations is highly recommended.

15.4.3 Workforce Challenges

The inadequate number of healthcare professionals throughout the public as well as private healthcare facilities is a major barrier affecting the quality of healthcare services throughout developing countries, especially low-income countries; therefore, hiring more healthcare professionals is very important and highly recommended. Lack of human resources and experts are major challenges for medication errors reporting systems in developing countries. In order to run a comprehensive, effective, and high-quality system, hiring highly qualified and trained healthcare professionals and staff is required, therefore, supports from the policymakers, pharmaceutical industries & companies, and international organizations are highly recommended.

15.4.4 Migration of Healthcare Professionals

Migration of healthcare professionals has increased during the last two decades from many developing countries, especially low- and middle-income countries, due to many reasons, such as the lack of jobs in healthcare facilities, low salaries, the attraction of jobs overseas, political and war issues, and others. Designing long-term plans and short-term plans to overcome this challenge is very important and highly recommended.

15.4.5 Reporting Challenges

Reporting patient care errors and related problems is very important to know the reasons and design the necessary interventions to overcome this challenge.

15.4.6 Research

There is little known about patient care errors and related problems in developing countries due to many reasons. Support from the Health Ministries, universities, pharmaceutical companies, organizations, and policymakers can overcome this challenge.

15.4.7 System Challenges

- Despite the efforts from the drug authorities in many developing countries toward the safety of medications by establishing pharmacovigilance systems in many developing countries but in general they are focusing on Adverse Drug reactions (ADRs) and ignoring medication errors, medication errors reporting systems either not available or very weak and centralized, all healthcare centers in general or a majority of them don't have medication errors reporting programs in developing countries. Therefore, establishing medication error reporting systems in all developing countries is highly recommended, and launching medication errors reporting programs in all developing countries is highly recommended.

15.4.8 Education and Training

Introducing the pharmacovigilance issues such as medication errors and their reporting to all medical and health sciences curriculums is highly recommended. Training the current healthcare professionals about pharmacovigilance issues is highly recommended. Launching postgraduate programs is recommended.

15.4.9 Knowledge and Attitude

Improving the knowledge and attitude of healthcare professionals and patients and public regarding the medication errors and their reporting is highly recommended and can be done through media, workshops, general lectures, brochures, and the distribution of educational material is needed to increase the awareness of healthcare professionals.

15.4.10 Reporting Challenges

Reporting medication errors and the absence of medication errors reporting is a major challenge in developing countries, and difficulties in reporting procedures are also another challenge. Therefore, designing the necessary interventions to overcome the barriers is very important and highly recommended. Mandatory reporting could help overcome this barrier.

15.4.11 Research

Lack of research about different issues of medication errors in the majority of developing countries due to lack of funds and other reasons. Support from the Health Ministries, universities, pharmaceutical companies, organizations, and policymakers can overcome this challenge. Collaborative research with researchers from developed countries could overcome this barrier.

15.4.12 International Collaboration

Collaborating with international organizations is highly recommended in order to share experiences, training, and research about medication errors and their reporting and various medication safety issues.

15.4.13 Quality and Accreditations of Pharmacovigilance Systems and Programs

This important concept should be implemented to measure the quality of the system in developing countries as well as in all healthcare settings in developing countries. Take the necessary actions toward it in order to improve the medication safety practice in all healthcare settings. Establishing a medication safety accreditation in developing countries and perhaps in the world is highly recommended in order to measure the safety of medication safety practice systems in the countries as well as in the healthcare settings, this could motivate the countries to improve their medications safety practice.

15.4.14 Technology Challenges

New technologies, applications, and social media could play an important role in the success of reporting, adapting such technologies could improve the pharmacovigilance practice.

15.4.15 Regulations and Guidelines Challenges

Developing and adapting regulations and guidelines related to medication safety issues such as mandatory reporting of medication errors is highly recommended in developing countries.

15.4.16 Documentation Challenges

Documenting the reporting and other activities is very important for the policymakers, healthcare professionals, researchers, and medical and health sciences students in order to develop the necessary interventions and improve the practice.

15.5 CONCLUSION

This chapter has discussed the dispensing and administration errors, causes, prevention, and recommendations for best practices in developing countries. Good dispensing and administration of the prescribed and recommended medications have a good impact on patient's health as well as the healthcare system and it will help in achieving the treating outcomes; decrease the admission rate to hospitals; decrease the morbidity and mortality; decrease the cost of therapy; improve the quality of life; improve the patient satisfaction toward healthcare; and decrease the burden on the hospitals.

REFERENCES

Al-Qahtani, I., Almoteb, T.M., & Al-Warafi, Y. (2015). Competency of metered-dose inhaler use among Saudi community pharmacists: A Simulation method study. *RRJPPS*, 4(2), 37–31.

Alshahrani, S.M., Alakhali, K.M., & Al-Worafi, Y.M. (2019a). Medication errors in a health care facility in southern Saudi Arabia. *Tropical Journal of Pharmaceutical Research*, 18(5), 1119–1122.

Alshahrani, S.M., Alavudeen, S.S., Alakhali, K.M., Al-Worafi, Y.M., Bahamdan, A.K., & Vigneshwaran, E. (2019b). Self-Medication Among King Khalid University Students, Saudi Arabia. *Risk Management and Healthcare Policy*, 12, 243–249.

Alshahrani, S.M., Alakhali, K.M., Al-Worafi, Y.M., & Alshahrani, N.Z. (2020a). Awareness and use of over the counter analgesic medication: A survey in the Aseer region population, Saudi Arabia. *International Journal of Advances in Applied Sciences*, 7(3), 130–134.

Alshahrani, S.M., Alzahran, M., Alakhali, K., Vigneshwaran, E., Iqbal, M.J., Khan, N.A., ... & Alavudeen, S.S. (2020b). Association Between Diabetes Consequences and Quality of Life Among Patients With Diabetes Mellitus in the Aseer Province of Saudi Arabia. *Open Access Macedonian Journal of Medical Sciences*, 8(E), 325–330.

Al-Worafi, Y.M. (2014). Prescription writing errors at a tertiary care hospital in Yemen: Prevalence, types, causes and recommendations. *American Journal of Pharmacy and Health Research*, 2, 134–140.

Al-Worafi, Y.M.A. (2015). Appropriateness of metered-dose inhaler use in the Yemeni community pharmacies. *Journal of Taibah University Medical Sciences*, 10(3), 353–358.

Al-Worafi, Y.M.A. (2016). Pharmacy practice in Yemen. In *Pharmacy Practice in Developing Countries* (pp. 267–287). Academic Press.

Al-Worafi, Y.M., Kassab, Y.W., Alseragi, W.M., Almutairi, M.S., Ahmed, A., Ming, L.C., Alkhoshaiban, A.S., & Hadi, M.A. (2017). Pharmacovigilance and adverse drg reaction reporting: A perspective of community pharmacists and pharmacy technicians in Sana'a, Yemen. *Therapeutics and Clinical Risk Management*, 13, 1175.

Al-Worafi, Y.M. (2018a). Knowledge, Attitude and Practice of Yemeni Physicians Toward Pharmacovigilance: A Mixed Method Study. *International Journal of Pharmacy and Pharmaceutical Sciences*, 10 (10), 74–77

Al-Worafi, Y. (2018b). Knowledge, attitude and practice of Yemeni physicians toward pharmacovigilance: A mixed method study. *International Journal of Pharmacy and Pharmaceutical Sciences*, 10, 74–77.

Al-Worafi, Y.M. (2018c). Dispensing errors observed by community pharmacy dispensers in IBB–YEMEN. *Asian Journal of Pharmaceutical and Clinical Research*, 11(11).

Al-Worafi, Y.M. (2018d). Evauation of inhaler technique among patients with asthma and COPD in Yemen. *Journal of Taibah University Medical Sciences*, 13(5), 488–490.

Al-Worafi, Y.M., Patel, R.P., Zaidi, S.T.R., Alseragi, W.M., Almutairi, M.S., Alkhoshaiban, A.S., & Ming, L.C. (2018a). Completeness and legibility of handwritten prescriptions in Sana'a, Yemen. *Medical Principles and Practice*, 27, 290–292.

Al-Worafi, Y.M., Alseragi, W.M., Seng, L.K., Kassab, Y.W., Yeoh, S.F., Chiau, L., … & Husain, K. (2018b). Dispensing errors in community pharmacies: A prospective study in Sana'a, Yemen. *Archives of Pharmacy Practice*, 9(4), 1–3.

Al-Worafi, Y.M., Alseragi, W.M., & Mahmoud, M.A. (2019). Competency of metered-dose inhaler use among community pharmacy dispensers in Ibb, Yemen: A simulation method study. *Latin American Journal of Pharmacy*, 38(3), 489–494.

Al-Worafi, Y.M. (Ed.). (2020a). *Drug Safety in Developing Countries: Achievements and Challenges*.

Al-Worafi, Y.M. (2020b). Medication errors. In *Drug Safety in Developing Countries* (pp. 105–117). Academic Press.

Al-Worafi, Y.M. (2020c). Adverse drug reactions. In *Drug Safety in Developing Countries* (pp. 39–57). Academic Press.

Al-Worafi, Y.M. (2020d). Medications registration and marketing: Safety-related issues. In *Drug Safety in Developing Countries* (pp. 21–28). Academic Press.

Al-Worafi, Y.M. (2020e). Pharmacovigilance. In *Drug Safety in Developing Countries* (pp. 29–38). Academic Press.

Al-Worafi, Y.M. (2020f). Drug-related problems. In *Drug Safety in Developing Countries* (pp. 59–71). Academic Press.

Al-Worafi, Y.M. (2020g). Medications safety-related terminology. In *Drug Safety in Developing Countries* (pp. 7–19). Academic Press.

Al-Worafi, Y.M. (2020h). Self-medication. In *Drug Safety in Developing Countries* (pp. 73–86). Academic Press.

Al-Worafi, Y.M. (2020j). Antibiotics safety issues. In *Drug Safety in Developing Countries* (pp. 87–103). Academic Press.

Al-Worafi, Y.M. (2020k). Medications safety research issues. In *Drug Safety in Developing Countries* (pp. 213–227). Academic Press.

Al-Worafi, Y.M. (2020l). Counterfeit and substandard medications. In *Drug Safety in Developing Countries* (pp. 119–126). Academic Press.

Al-Worafi, Y.M. (2020m). Medication abuse and misuse. In *Drug Safety in Developing Countries* (pp. 127–135). Academic Press.

Al-Worafi, Y.M. (2020n). Storage and disposal of medications. In *Drug Safety in Developing Countries* (pp. 137–142). Academic Press.

Al-Worafi, Y.M. (2020o). Safety of medications in special population. In *Drug Safety in Developing Countries* (pp. 143–162). Academic Press.

Al-Worafi, Y.M. (2020p). Herbal medicines safety issues. In *Drug Safety in Developing Countries* (pp. 163–178). Academic Press.

Al-Worafi, Y.M. (2020q). Medications safety pharmacoeconomics-related issues. In *Drug Safety in Developing Countries* (pp. 187–195). Academic Press.

Al-Worafi, Y.M. (2020r). Evidence-based medications safety practice. In *Drug Safety in Developing Countries* (pp. 197–201). Academic Press.

Al-Worafi, Y.M. (2020s). Quality indicators for medications safety. In *Drug Safety in Developing Countries* (pp. 229–242). Academic Press.

Al-Worafi, Y.M. (2020t). Drug safety in Yemen. In *Drug Safety in Developing Countries* (pp. 391–405). Academic Press.

Al-Worafi, Y.M. (2020u). Drug safety in Saudi Arabia. In *Drug Safety in Developing Countries* (pp. 407–417). Academic Press.

Al-Worafi, Y.M. (2020v). Drug safety in United Arab Emirates. In *Drug Safety in Developing Countries* (pp. 419–428). Academic Press.

Al-Worafi, Y.M. (2020w). Drug safety in Indonesia. In *Drug Safety in Developing Countries* (pp. 279–285). Academic Press.

Al-Worafi, Y.M. (2020x). Drug safety in Palestine. In *Drug Safety in Developing Countries* (pp. 471–480). Academic Press.

Al-Worafi, Y.M. (2020y). Drug safety: Comparison between developing countries. In *Drug Safety in Developing Countries* (pp. 603–611). Academic Press.

Al-Worafi, Y.M. (2020z). Drug safety in developing versus developed countries. In *Drug Safety in Developing Countries* (pp. 613–615). Academic Press.

Al-Worafi, Y.M., Alseragi, W.M., Ming, L.C., & Alakhali, K.M. (2020a). Drug safety in China. In *Drug Safety in Developing Countries* (pp. 381–388). Academic Press.

Al-Worafi, Y.M., Alseragi, W.M., Alakhali, K.M., Ming, L.C., Othman, G., Halboup, A.M., ... & Elkalmi, R.M. (2020b). Knowledge, beliefs and factors affecting the use of generic medicines among patients in Ibb, Yemen: A mixed-method study. *Journal of Pharmacy Practice and Community Medicine*, 6(4).

Al-Worafi, Y.M., Elkalmi, R.M., Ming, L.C., Othman, G., Halboup, A.M., Battah, M.M., ... & Mani, V. (2021a). *Dispensing Errors in Hospital Pharmacies: A Prospective Study in Yemen*.

Al-Worafi, Y.M., Hasan, S., Hassan, N.M., & Gaili, A.A. (2021b). Knowledge, Attitude and Experience of Pharmacist in the UAE towards Pharmacovigilance. *Research Journal of Pharmacy and Technology*, 14(1), 265–269.

Al-Worafi, Y. (2022a). *A Guide to Online Pharmacy Education: Teaching Strategies and Assessment Methods*. CRC Press.

Al-Worafi, Y.M. (2022b). Patient care errors and related problems (part I): Development and validation of the model. https://orcid.org/0000-0002-5752-2913

Al-Worafi, Y.M. (Ed.). (2023). *Clinical Case Studies on Medication Safety*. Academic Press.

American Society of Health-System Pharmacists (ASHP) (1993). guidelines on preventing medication errors in hospitals. *American Journal of Health-System Pharmacy*, 50, 305–314.

Baig, M.R., Al-Worafi, Y.M., Alseragi, W.M., Ming, L.C., & Siddique, A. (2020). Drug safety in India. In *Drug Safety in Developing Countries* (pp. 327–334). Academic Press.

Billstein-Leber, M., Carrillo, C.J.D., Cassano, A.T., Moline, K., & Robertson, J.J. (2018). ASHP guidelines on preventing medication errors in hospitals. *American Journal of Health-System Pharmacy*, 75(19), 1493–1517.

Cowley, E., Williams, R., & Cousins, D. (2001). Medication errors in children: A descriptive summary of medication error reports submitted to the United States Pharmacopeia. *Current Therapeutic Research*, 62(9), 627–640.

Elkalmi, R.M., Al-Worafi, Y.M., Alseragi, W.M., Ming, L.C., & Siddique, A. (2020). Drug safety in Malaysia. In *Drug Safety in Developing Countries* (pp. 245–253). Academic Press.

Elsayed, T., & Al-Worafi, Y.M. (2020). Drug safety in Egypt. In *Drug Safety in Developing Countries* (pp. 511–523). Academic Press.

Hasan, S., Al-Omar, M.J., AlZubaidy, H., & Al-Worafi, Y.M. (2019). Use of medications in Arab Countries. *Handbook of Healthcare in the Arab World*. Cham: Springer, 42.

Hassan, Y., Abd Aziz, N., Kassab, Y.W., Elgasim, I., Shaharuddin, S., Al-Worafi, Y.M.A., ... & Ming, L.C. (2014). How to help patients to control their blood pressure? Blood pressure control and its predictor. *Archives of Pharmacy Practice*, 5(4).

Izahar, S., Lean, Q.Y., Hameed, M.A., Murugiah, M.K., Patel, R.P., Al-Worafi, Y.M., ... & Ming, L.C. (2017). Content analysis of mobile health applications on diabetes mellitus. *Frontiers in Endocrinology*, 8, 318.

Lee, K.S., Yee, S.M., Zaidi, S.T.R., Patel, R.P., Yang, Q., Al-Worafi, Y.M., & Ming, L.C., 2017. Combating sale of counterfeit and falsified medicines online: A losing battle. *Frontiers in Pharmacology*, 8, p. 268.

Mahmoud, M.A., Wajid, S., Naqvi, A.A., Samreen, S., Althagfan, S.S., & Al-Worafi, Y. (2020). Self-medication with antibiotics: A cross-sectional community-based study. *Latin American Journal of Pharmacy*, 39(2), 348–353.

Manan, M.M., Rusli, R.A., Ang, W.C., Al-Worafi, Y.M., & Ming, L.C. (2014). Assessing the pharmaceutical care issues of antiepileptic drug therapy in hospitalised epileptic patients. *Journal of Pharmacy Practice and Research*, 44(3), 83–88.

Manan, M.M., Ibrahim, N.A., Aziz, N.A., Zulkifly, H.H., Al-Worafi, Y.M.A., & Long, C.M. (2016). Empirical use of antibiotic therapy in the prevention of early onset sepsis in neonates: A pilot study. *Archives of Medical Science*, 12(3), 603–613.

Ming, L.C., Hameed, M.A., Lee, D.D., Apidi, N.A., Lai, P.S.M., Hadi, M.A., Al-Worafi, Y.M.A., & Khan, T.M., (2016). Use of medical mobile applications among hospital pharmacists in Malaysia. *Therapeutic Innovation & Regulatory Science*, 50(4), 419–426.

Ming, L.C., Untong, N., Aliudin, N.A., Osili, N., Kifli, N., Tan, C.S., ... & Goh, H.P. (2020). Mobile health apps on COVID-19 launched in the early days of the pandemic: Content analysis and review. *JMIR mHealth and uHealth*, 8(9), e19796.

Othman, G., Ali, F., Ibrahim, M.I.M., Al-Worafi, Y.M., Ansari, M., & Halboup, A.M. (2020). Assessment of Anti-Diabetic Medications Adherence among Diabetic Patients in Sana'a City, Yemen: A Cross Sectional Study. *Journal of Pharmaceutical Research International*, 32(21), 114–122.

Reason, J. (1990). *Human Error*. Cambridge University Press.

Saeed, M.S., Alkhoshaiban, A.S., Al-Worafi, Y.M.A., & Long, C.M. (2014). Perception of self-medication among university students in Saudi Arabia. *Archives of Pharmacy Practice*, 5(4), 149.

16 Patient Care Errors and Related Problems

Monitoring Errors and Related Problems

16.1 BACKGROUND

Monitoring the efficacy and safety of medications is a very important part of the management of diseases and conditions, which help prescribers and healthcare professionals to provide the most effective patient care. Medication errors are responsible for more morbidity and mortality in developing countries and developed countries, it is associated with an increase in the admission rate to the emergency department, an increase in the length of hospitalization, an increase in the cost of illness, affecting patients' quality of life and lead to complications including life-threatening complications (Al-Worafi, 2020a-c). Evaluation of therapeutic outcomes and monitoring parameters are important aspects of patient care that help to assess the effectiveness and safety of a treatment.

This evaluation allows healthcare providers to adjust treatment plans to optimize patient outcomes and minimize adverse effects. Here are some important considerations for evaluating therapeutic outcomes and monitoring parameters:

1. Define the therapeutic outcome: Before initiating treatment, healthcare providers must define the desired therapeutic outcome based on the patient's condition and treatment goals. This definition will help guide the evaluation of treatment efficacy.

2. Choose appropriate monitoring parameters: To evaluate therapeutic outcomes, healthcare providers must choose appropriate monitoring parameters that will help assess treatment efficacy and safety. For example, monitoring blood pressure, blood glucose levels, or liver function tests may be necessary for certain treatments.

3. Establish a monitoring schedule: Healthcare providers must establish a monitoring schedule based on the patient's condition and treatment plan. This schedule may include periodic laboratory tests or regular follow-up appointments to assess treatment progress and identify any adverse effects.

4. Use validated assessment tools: Validated assessment tools can help healthcare providers to evaluate therapeutic outcomes objectively. For example, pain scales or quality-of-life question-naires may be used to assess the effectiveness of pain management or cancer treatments.

5. Document and communicate findings: Healthcare providers must document their findings and communicate them with the patient and other members of the healthcare team. This documentation allows for ongoing evaluation of treatment efficacy and safety and informs decision-making regarding changes to the treatment plan.

In summary, evaluating therapeutic outcomes and monitoring parameters are essential components of patient care. By defining therapeutic outcomes, choosing appropriate monitoring parameters, establishing a monitoring schedule, using validated assessment tools, and documenting findings, healthcare providers can optimize treatment plans to achieve the best possible outcomes for their patients.

16.2 TREATMENT EVALUATION AND MONITORING ERRORS AND RELATED PROBLEMS

Treatment evaluation and monitoring errors and related problems can be defined as any intentional or unintentional errors or problems that occur during the evaluation of therapy outcomes and monitoring parameters.

Monitoring parameters are the process of evaluating the therapeutic outcomes using different measurements and tools such as laboratory investigations to ensure the following:

The efficacy of medications (Is the prescribed medications effective?; Is the desired outcomes achieved?). This can be done by using the laboratory results, checking the improvement of the symptoms, patients report, and other criteria.

The safety of medications (Is the prescribed medications safe?). This can be done by patients' reports about side/adverse effects/reactions, evaluating the effects of the system on the patient's different systems such as renal, liver, etc, requesting laboratory tests, requesting Drug Therapy Monitoring (TDM), and others.

Adherence to the management plan (Al-Worafi, 2020a,b).

DOI: 10.1201/9781003230465-18

16.3 POTENTIAL CAUSES AND FACTORS

The top 10 causes of medication errors identified by the United States Pharmacopoeia (USP) (Al-Worafi, 2020a,b; Cowley et al, 2001) are:

1. Performance deficit

2. Procedure or protocol not followed

3. Miscommunication

4. Inaccurate or omitted transcription

5. Improper documentation

6. Drug distribution system error

7. Knowledge deficit,

8. Calculation error

9. Computer entry errors

10. Lack of system safeguards

The Institute of Safe Medicine Practices (ISMP) identifies the following areas as potential causes of medication error (Reason, 1990):

■ Failed communication

■ Handwriting and oral communication,

■ Drugs with similar names

■ Missing or misplaced zero and decimal points

■ Use of non-standard abbreviations

■ Poor drug distribution practices

■ Complex or poorly designed technology

■ Access to drugs by no pharmacy personnel

■ Workplace environmental problems that lead to increased job stress

■ Dose miscalculations

■ Lack of patient information

■ Lack of patient understanding of their therapy

There are several factors that can contribute to errors and problems with disease-therapy monitoring parameters:

1. Inaccurate or unreliable measurement tools: If the measurement tools used to monitor disease-therapy parameters are inaccurate or unreliable, the results may not reflect the true state of the patient's condition.

2. Interference from other medical conditions or medications: Other medical conditions or medications can interfere with the effectiveness of the therapy or the ability to monitor its effects accurately.

3. Patient factors: Patients may not adhere to the treatment plan, which can affect the accuracy of monitoring parameters. Additionally, patients may have factors outside of the treatment plan that affects their disease status, such as changes in lifestyle or exposure to environmental toxins.

4. Timing and frequency of monitoring: The timing and frequency of monitoring parameters can affect the accuracy of results. For example, if monitoring is not done frequently enough, changes in the patient's condition may be missed.

5. Variation in disease progression: The natural progression of the disease can vary from patient to patient, which can make it difficult to determine whether changes in monitoring parameters are due to the therapy or the natural course of the disease.

6. Inadequate training or experience of healthcare providers: Healthcare providers who are not adequately trained or experienced in monitoring disease-therapy parameters may not be able to accurately interpret the results.

7. Laboratory errors: Laboratory errors in sample collection or analysis can result in inaccurate monitoring parameter measurements. Laboratory testing can also be a source of errors, such as sample contamination, mishandling of specimens, or errors in test interpretation.

8. Environmental Factors: Environmental factors such as temperature, humidity, or atmospheric pressure can also affect monitoring parameters, especially in sensitive tests such as drug level monitoring.

9. Instrument Error: Monitoring instruments such as glucose meters or blood pressure monitors can malfunction, leading to inaccurate readings. It is important to regularly calibrate and maintain these instruments to ensure their accuracy.

10. Inappropriate outcome measures: If the outcome measures used in a study are not clinically meaningful or relevant to the target population, then the study results may not accurately reflect the impact of the treatment.

11. Short follow-up periods: If the follow-up period is too short, it may not be possible to assess the long-term impact of the treatment or the full extent of any side effects or adverse events.

12. Non-adherence: If participants do not adhere to the treatment protocol or do not complete the study as planned, then the study results may not accurately reflect the efficacy or safety of the treatment.

13. Lack of clear treatment goals: If there are no clear treatment goals established at the outset of therapy, it can be difficult to determine whether the therapy has been successful or not.

14. Limited assessment measures: If the assessment measures used to evaluate therapy are limited or not sensitive enough to capture changes in the patient's condition, it can be difficult to determine whether the therapy has been effective or not.

15. Inconsistent implementation of therapy: If therapy is not implemented consistently or if the therapist deviates from the established treatment plan, it can be difficult to evaluate the therapy's effectiveness.

16. Patient factors: Patients may not be fully committed to the therapy or may have personal issues that interfere with the therapy's effectiveness, making it difficult to evaluate the therapy's impact.

17. Therapist factors: Therapists may have biases or limitations that affect their ability to implement the therapy effectively or evaluate its effectiveness.

Overall, errors and problems with disease-therapy monitoring parameters can stem from a range of factors, including issues with the measurement tools, patient factors, timing and frequency of monitoring, natural variation in disease progression, healthcare provider factors, and laboratory errors.

16.4 PREVENTION

Treatment evaluation and monitoring errors and problems can have serious consequences on patient outcomes, so it's important to take steps to prevent them. Here are some strategies for preventing treatment evaluation and monitoring errors:

1. Standardize evaluation and monitoring protocols: Develop standardized protocols for evaluating and monitoring patients that are consistent across all providers. This can help reduce the likelihood of errors and inconsistencies in patient care.

2. Train providers on evaluation and monitoring protocols: Ensure that all providers are properly trained on the evaluation and monitoring protocols and that they understand the importance of adhering to them.

3. Use electronic health records: Electronic health records can help ensure that all patient data is accurately recorded and easily accessible to providers. This can help prevent errors that may occur when using paper records.

4. Conduct regular quality assurance checks: Conduct regular audits to ensure that evaluation and monitoring protocols are being followed correctly and that data is being accurately recorded.

5. Provide feedback and support to providers: Provide feedback to providers on their evaluation and monitoring practices, and offer support to help them improve their skills and knowledge.

6. Involve patients in the evaluation and monitoring process: Engage patients in their own care by involving them in the evaluation and monitoring process. This can help prevent errors and ensure that patients are actively involved in their own care.

7. Stay up-to-date with best practices: Stay informed about the latest best practices for evaluation and monitoring, and update protocols accordingly to ensure that patients receive the best possible care.

By implementing these strategies, providers can help prevent treatment evaluation and monitoring errors and problems and improve patient outcomes

16.5 CHALLENGES OF TREATMENT EVALUATION AND MONITORING ERRORS AND PROBLEMS IN DEVELOPING COUNTRIES

There are many challenges to treatment evaluation and monitoring in developing countries which are as follows (Alshahrani et al., 2019a,b; Al-Qahtani et al., 2015; Alshahrani et al., 2020a,b; Al-Worafi, 2014; Al-Worafi, 2015; Al-Worafi, 2016; Al-Worafi et al., 2017; Al-Worafi, 2018a-d; Al-Worafi et al., 2018a-b; Al-Worafi et al., 2019; Al-Worafi, 2020a-z; Al-Worafi et al., 2020a-b; Al-Worafi et al., 2021a,b; Al-Worafi, 2022a,b; Al-Worafi, 2023; Baig et al., 2020; Elkalmi et al., 2020; Elsayed & Al-Worafi, 2020; Hasan et al., 2019; Hassan et al., 2014; Izhar et al., 2017; Lee et al., 2017; Mahmoud et al., 2020; Manan et al., 2014; Manan et al., 2016; Ming et al., 2016; Ming et al., 2020; Othman et al., 2020; Saeed et al., 2014).

16.5.1 Healthcare Systems

The quality of healthcare systems and healthcare services are the cornerstone in providing the most effective and safe patient care services; healthcare systems in many developing countries, especially low-income countries, are weak, with inadequate budgets and infrastructures, which affect patient safety in many ways. Therefore, strengthening the healthcare systems in developing countries is very important and highly recommended to improve patient care practice.

16.5.2 Financial Challenges

Patient care needs financial support in the public healthcare sectors as well as private healthcare sectors, which is missing in many developing countries, especially low-income countries. Therefore, increasing health expenditures and the public healthcare budget is very important and highly recommended. Increasing the contribution from the private and charity sectors is very important and highly recommended. Lack of financial support is the main challenge for medication errors reporting systems in developing countries. In order to run a comprehensive, effective, and high-quality system with good infrastructures, hiring highly qualified and trained healthcare professionals and staff is required, therefore, support from the policymakers, pharmaceutical industries and companies, and international organizations is highly recommended.

16.5.3 Workforce Challenges

The inadequate number of healthcare professionals throughout the public as well as private healthcare facilities is a major barrier affecting the quality of healthcare services throughout developing countries, especially low-income countries; therefore, hiring more healthcare professionals is very important and highly recommended. Lack of human resources and experts are major challenges for medication errors reporting systems in developing countries. In order to run a comprehensive, effective, and high-quality system, hiring highly qualified and trained healthcare professionals and staff is required, therefore, support from the policymakers, pharmaceutical industries and companies, and international organizations is highly recommended.

16.5.4 Migration of Healthcare Professionals

Migration of healthcare professionals has increased during the last two decades from many developing countries, especially low and middle-income countries, due to many reasons, such as the lack of jobs in healthcare facilities, low salaries, the attraction of jobs overseas, political and war issues, and others. Designing long-term plans and short-term plans to overcome this challenge is very important and highly recommended.

16.5.5 Reporting Challenges

Reporting patient care errors and related problems is very important to know the reasons and design the necessary interventions to overcome this challenge.

16.5.6 Research

There is little known about patient care errors and related problems in developing countries due to many reasons. Support from the Health Ministries, universities, pharmaceutical companies, organizations, and policymakers can overcome this challenge.

16.5.7 System Challenges

■ Despite the efforts from the drug authorities in many developing countries toward the safety of medications by establishing pharmacovigilance systems in many developing countries but in general they are focusing on Adverse Drug reactions (ADRs) and ignoring medication errors, medication errors reporting systems either not available or very weak and centralized, all healthcare centers in general or a majority of them don't have medication errors reporting programs in developing countries. Therefore, establishing medication errors reporting systems and launching medication errors reporting programs in all developing countries is highly recommended.

16.5.8 Education and Training

Introducing the pharmacovigilance issues such as medication errors and their reporting to all medical and health sciences curriculums is highly recommended. Training the current healthcare professionals about pharmacovigilance issues is highly recommended. Launching postgraduate programs is also recommended.

16.5.9 Knowledge and Attitude

Improving the knowledge and attitude of healthcare professionals and patients and public regarding the medication errors and their reporting is highly recommended and can be done through media, workshops, general lectures, brochures, and distribution of educational material is needed to increase the awareness of healthcare professionals.

16.5.10 Reporting Challenges

Reporting medication errors and the absence of medication errors reporting is the major challenge in developing countries, difficulties in reporting procedures are also another challenge. Therefore, designing the necessary interventions to overcome the barriers is very important and highly recommended. Mandatory reporting could help overcome this barrier.

16.5.11 Research

Lack of research about different issues of medication errors in the majority of developing countries due to lack of funds and other reasons. Support from the Health Ministries, universities, pharmaceutical companies, organizations and policymakers can overcome this challenge. Collaborative research with researchers from developed countries could overcome this barrier.

16.5.12 International Collaboration

Collaborating with international organizations is highly recommended in order to share experiences, training, and research about medication errors and their reporting and various medication safety issues.

16.5.13 Quality and Accreditations of Pharmacovigilance Systems and Programs

This important concept should be implemented to measure the quality of the system in developing countries as well as in all healthcare settings in developing countries. Taking necessary actions toward it in order to improve the medication safety practice in all healthcare settings is crucial. Establishing a medication safety accreditation in developing countries and perhaps in the world is highly recommended in order to measure the safety of medication safety practice systems in the countries as well as in the healthcare settings, this could motivate the countries to improve their medication safety practice.

16.5.14 Technology Challenges

New technologies, applications, and social media could play an important role in the success of reporting, adapting such technologies could improve the pharmacovigilance practice.

16.5.15 Regulations and Guidelines Challenges

Developing and adapting regulations and guidelines related to medication safety issues such as mandatory reporting of medication errors is highly recommended in developing countries.

16.5.16 Documentation Challenges

Documenting the reporting and other activities is very important for the policymakers, healthcare professionals, researchers, and medical and health sciences students in order to develop the necessary interventions and improve the practice.

16.5.17 Limited Resources

Developing countries often have limited resources to invest in healthcare infrastructure, including access to medical equipment, medication, and trained healthcare professionals.

16.5.18 Inadequate Infrastructure

Lack of infrastructure, such as inadequate laboratory facilities, can limit the ability to conduct accurate diagnosis and monitoring of treatment.

16.5.19 Low Levels of Health Literacy

Patients in developing countries may have limited health literacy and may not understand the importance of adhering to treatment protocols, which can impact adherence to medication and monitoring of symptoms.

16.5.20 Socio-cultural Factors

Cultural beliefs and practices may impact the willingness of patients to seek medical care, adhere to treatment protocols, and participate in monitoring programs.

16.5.21 Geographical Barriers

In rural areas, patients may have limited access to medical facilities, which can impact their ability to receive treatment and access monitoring services.

16.5.22 Limited Data

Developing countries may lack reliable data on disease prevalence, treatment outcomes, and monitoring results, which can limit the ability to make informed decisions about treatment protocols.

16.6 CONCLUSION

This chapter has discussed the treatment evaluation and monitoring errors and problems, causes, prevention, and recommendations for the best practice in developing countries. Monitoring parameters are the process of evaluating the therapeutic outcomes using different measurements, and tools such as laboratory investigations to ensure the efficacy of medications, the safety of medications, and adherence to non-pharmacological and pharmacological therapies and interventions. Treatment evaluation and monitoring errors and related problems can be defined as any intentional or unintentional errors or problems that occur during the evaluation of therapy outcomes and monitoring parameters. Treatment evaluation and monitoring errors and problems can have serious consequences on patient outcomes, so it's important to take steps to prevent them.

REFERENCES

Al-Qahtani, I., Almoteb, T.M., & Al-Warafi, Y. (2015). Competency of metered-dose inhaler use among Saudi community pharmacists: A Simulation method study. *RRJPPS*, 4(2), 37–31.

Alshahrani, S.M., Alakhali, K.M., & Al-Worafi, Y.M. (2019a). Medication errors in a health care facility in southern Saudi Arabia. *Tropical Journal of Pharmaceutical Research*, 18(5), 1119–1122.

Alshahrani, S.M., Alavudeen, S.S., Alakhali, K.M., Al-Worafi, Y.M., Bahamdan, A.K., & Vigneshwaran, E. (2019b). Self-Medication Among King Khalid University Students, Saudi Arabia. *Risk Management and Healthcare Policy*, 12, 243–249.

Alshahrani, S.M., Alakhali, K.M., Al-Worafi, Y.M., & Alshahrani, N.Z. (2020a). Awareness and use of over the counter analgesic medication: A survey in the Aseer region population, Saudi Arabia. *International Journal of Advances in Applied Sciences*, 7(3), 130–134.

Alshahrani, S.M., Alzahran, M., Alakhali, K., Vigneshwaran, E., Iqbal, M.J., Khan, N.A., … & Alavudeen, S.S. (2020b). Association Between Diabetes Consequences and Quality of Life Among Patients With Diabetes Mellitus in the Aseer Province of Saudi Arabia. *Open Access Macedonian Journal of Medical Sciences*, 8(E), 325–330.

Al-Worafi, Y.M. (2014). Prescription writing errors at a tertiary care hospital in Yemen: Prevalence, types, causes and recommendations. *American Journal of Pharmacy and Health Research*, 2, 134–140.

Al-Worafi, Y.M.A. (2015). Appropriateness of metered-dose inhaler use in the Yemeni community pharmacies. *Journal of Taibah University Medical Sciences*, 10(3), 353–358.

Al-Worafi, Y.M.A. (2016). Pharmacy practice in Yemen. In *Pharmacy Practice in Developing Countries* (pp. 267–287). Academic Press.

Al-Worafi, Y.M., Kassab, Y.W., Alseragi, W.M., Almutairi, M.S., Ahmed, A., Ming, L.C., Alkhoshaiban, A.S., & Hadi, M.A. (2017). Pharmacovigilance and adverse drg reaction reporting: A perspective of community pharmacists and pharmacy technicians in Sana'a, Yemen. *Therapeutics and Clinical Risk Management*, 13, 1175.

Al-Worafi, Y.M. (2018a). Knowledge, Attitude and Practice of Yemeni Physicians Toward Pharmacovigilance: A Mixed Method Study. *International Journal of Pharmacy and Pharmaceutical Sciences*, 10 (10), 74–77.

Al-Worafi, Y. (2018b). Knowledge, attitude and practice of Yemeni physicians toward pharmacovigilance: A mixed method study. *International Journal of Pharmacy and Pharmaceutical Sciences*, 10, 74–77.

Al-Worafi, Y.M. (2018c). Dispensing errors observed by community pharmacy dispensers in IBB–YEMEN. *Asian Journal of Pharmaceutical and Clinical Research*, 11(11).

Al-Worafi, Y.M. (2018d). Evauation of inhaler technique among patients with asthma and COPD in Yemen. *Journal of Taibah University Medical Sciences*, 13(5), 488–490.

Al-Worafi, Y.M., Patel, R.P., Zaidi, S.T.R., Alseragi, W.M., Almutairi, M.S., Alkhoshaiban, A.S., & Ming, L.C. (2018a). Completeness and legibility of handwritten prescriptions in Sana'a, Yemen. *Medical Principles and Practice*, 27, 290–292.

Al-Worafi, Y.M., Alseragi, W.M., Seng, L.K., Kassab, Y.W., Yeoh, S.F., Chiau, L., … & Husain, K. (2018b). Dispensing errors in community pharmacies: A prospective study in Sana'a, Yemen. *Archives of Pharmacy Practice*, 9(4), 1–3.

Al-Worafi, Y.M., Alseragi, W.M., & Mahmoud, M.A. (2019). Competency of metered-dose inhaler use among community pharmacy dispensers in Ibb, Yemen: A simulation method study. *Latin American Journal of Pharmacy*, 38(3), 489–494.

Al-Worafi, Y.M. (Ed.). (2020a). *Drug Safety in Developing Countries: Achievements and Challenges.*

Al-Worafi, Y.M. (2020b). Medication errors. In *Drug Safety in Developing Countries* (pp. 105–117). Academic Press.

Al-Worafi, Y.M. (2020c). Adverse drug reactions. In *Drug Safety in Developing Countries* (pp. 39–57). Academic Press.

Al-Worafi, Y.M. (2020d). Medications registration and marketing: Safety-related issues. In *Drug Safety in Developing Countries* (pp. 21–28). Academic Press.

Al-Worafi, Y.M. (2020e). Pharmacovigilance. In *Drug Safety in Developing Countries* (pp. 29–38). Academic Press.

Al-Worafi, Y.M. (2020f). Drug-related problems. In *Drug Safety in Developing Countries* (pp. 59–71). Academic Press.

Al-Worafi, Y.M. (2020g). Medications safety-related terminology. In *Drug safety in Developing Countries* (pp. 7–19). Academic Press.

Al-Worafi, Y.M. (2020h). Self-medication. In *Drug Safety in Developing Countries* (pp. 73–86). Academic Press.

Al-Worafi, Y.M. (2020j). Antibiotics safety issues. In *Drug Safety in Developing Countries* (pp. 87–103). Academic Press.

Al-Worafi, Y.M. (2020k). Medications safety research issues. In *Drug Safety in Developing Countries* (pp. 213–227). Academic Press.

Al-Worafi, Y.M. (2020l). Counterfeit and substandard medications. In *Drug Safety in Developing Countries* (pp. 119–126). Academic Press.

Al-Worafi, Y.M. (2020m). Medication abuse and misuse. In *Drug Safety in Developing Countries* (pp. 127–135). Academic Press.

Al-Worafi, Y.M. (2020n). Storage and disposal of medications. In *Drug Safety in Developing Countries* (pp. 137–142). Academic Press.

Al-Worafi, Y.M. (2020o). Safety of medications in special population. In *Drug safety in Developing Countries* (pp. 143–162). Academic Press.

Al-Worafi, Y.M. (2020p). Herbal medicines safety issues. In *Drug Safety in Developing Countries* (pp. 163–178). Academic Press.

Al-Worafi, Y.M. (2020q). Medications safety pharmacoeconomics-related issues. In *Drug Safety in Developing Countries* (pp. 187–195). Academic Press.

Al-Worafi, Y.M. (2020r). Evidence-based medications safety practice. In *Drug Safety in Developing Countries* (pp. 197–201). Academic Press.

Al-Worafi, Y.M. (2020s). Quality indicators for medications safety. In *Drug Safety in Developing Countries* (pp. 229–242). Academic Press.

Al-Worafi, Y.M. (2020t). Drug safety in Yemen. In *Drug Safety in Developing Countries* (pp. 391–405). Academic Press.

Al-Worafi, Y.M. (2020u). Drug safety in Saudi Arabia. In *Drug Safety in Developing Countries* (pp. 407–417). Academic Press.

Al-Worafi, Y.M. (2020v). Drug safety in United Arab Emirates. In *Drug Safety in Developing Countries* (pp. 419–428). Academic Press.

Al-Worafi, Y.M. (2020w). Drug safety in Indonesia. In *Drug Safety in Developing Countries* (pp. 279–285). Academic Press.

Al-Worafi, Y.M. (2020x). Drug safety in Palestine. In *Drug Safety in Developing Countries* (pp. 471–480). Academic Press.

Al-Worafi, Y.M. (2020y). Drug safety: Comparison between developing countries. In *Drug Safety in Developing Countries* (pp. 603–611). Academic Press.

Al-Worafi, Y.M. (2020z). Drug safety in developing versus developed countries. In *Drug Safety in Developing Countries* (pp. 613–615). Academic Press.

Al-Worafi, Y.M., Alseragi, W.M., Ming, L.C., & Alakhali, K.M. (2020a). Drug safety in China. In *Drug Safety in Developing Countries* (pp. 381–388). Academic Press.

Al-Worafi, Y.M., Alseragi, W.M., Alakhali, K.M., Ming, L.C., Othman, G., Halboup, A.M., … & Elkalmi, R.M. (2020b). Knowledge, beliefs and factors affecting the use of generic medicines among patients in Ibb, Yemen: A mixed-method study. *Journal of Pharmacy Practice and Community Medicine*, 6(4).

Al-Worafi, Y.M., Elkalmi, R.M., Ming, L.C., Othman, G., Halboup, A.M., Battah, M.M., … & Mani, V. (2021a). Dispensing errors in hospital pharmacies: A prospective study in Yemen.

Al-Worafi, Y.M., Hasan, S., Hassan, N.M., & Gaili, A.A. (2021b). Knowledge, Attitude and Experience of Pharmacist in the UAE towards Pharmacovigilance. *Research Journal of Pharmacy and Technology*, 14(1), 265–269.

Al-Worafi, Y. (2022a). *A Guide to Online Pharmacy Education: Teaching Strategies and Assessment Methods*. CRC Press.

Al-Worafi, Y.M. (2022b). Patient care errors and related problems (part I): Development and validation of the model. https://orcid.org/0000-0002-5752-2913

Al-Worafi, Y.M. (Ed.). (2023). *Clinical Case Studies on Medication Safety*. Academic Press.

Baig, M.R., Al-Worafi, Y.M., Alseragi, W.M., Ming, L.C., & Siddique, A. (2020). Drug safety in India. In *Drug Safety in Developing Countries* (pp. 327–334). Academic Press.

Cowley, E., Williams, R., & Cousins, D. (2001). Medication errors in children: A descriptive summary of medication error reports submitted to the United States Pharmacopeia. *Current Therapeutic Research*, 62(9), 627–640.

Elkalmi, R.M., Al-Worafi, Y.M., Alseragi, W.M., Ming, L.C., & Siddique, A. (2020). Drug safety in Malaysia. In *Drug Safety in Developing Countries* (pp. 245–253). Academic Press.

Elsayed, T., & Al-Worafi, Y.M. (2020). Drug safety in Egypt. In *Drug Safety in Developing Countries* (pp. 511–523). Academic Press.

Hasan, S., Al-Omar, M.J., AlZubaidy, H., & Al-Worafi, Y.M. (2019). Use of medications in Arab Countries. *Handbook of Healthcare in the Arab World*. Cham: Springer, 42.

Hassan, Y., Abd Aziz, N., Kassab, Y.W., Elgasim, I., Shaharuddin, S., Al-Worafi, Y.M.A., ... & Ming, L.C. (2014). How to help patients to control their blood pressure? Blood pressure control and its predictor. *Archives of Pharmacy Practice*, 5(4).

Izahar, S., Lean, Q.Y., Hameed, M.A., Murugiah, M.K., Patel, R.P., Al-Worafi, Y.M., ... & Ming, L.C. (2017). Content analysis of mobile health applications on diabetes mellitus. *Frontiers in Endocrinology*, 8, 318.

Lee, K.S., Yee, S.M., Zaidi, S.T.R., Patel, R.P., Yang, Q., Al-Worafi, Y.M., & Ming, L.C., 2017. Combating sale of counterfeit and falsified medicines online: A losing battle. *Frontiers in Pharmacology*, 8, p.268.

Mahmoud, M.A., Wajid, S., Naqvi, A.A., Samreen, S., Althagfan, S.S., & Al-Worafi, Y. (2020). Self-medication with antibiotics: A cross-sectional community-based study. *Latin American Journal of Pharmacy*, 39(2), 348–353.

Manan, M.M., Rusli, R.A., Ang, W.C., Al-Worafi, Y.M., & Ming, L.C. (2014). Assessing the pharmaceutical care issues of antiepileptic drug therapy in hospitalised epileptic patients. *Journal of Pharmacy Practice and Research*, 44(3), 83–88.

Manan, M.M., Ibrahim, N.A., Aziz, N.A., Zulkifly, H.H., Al-Worafi, Y.M.A., & Long, C.M. (2016). Empirical use of antibiotic therapy in the prevention of early onset sepsis in neonates: A pilot study. *Archives of Medical Science*, 12(3), 603–613.

Ming, L.C., Hameed, M.A., Lee, D.D., Apidi, N.A., Lai, P.S.M., Hadi, M.A., Al-Worafi, Y.M.A., & Khan, T.M. (2016). Use of medical mobile applications among hospital pharmacists in Malaysia. *Therapeutic Innovation & Regulatory Science*, 50(4), 419–426.

Ming, L.C., Untong, N., Aliudin, N.A., Osili, N., Kifli, N., Tan, C.S., ... & Goh, H.P. (2020). Mobile health apps on COVID-19 launched in the early days of the pandemic: Content analysis and review. *JMIR mHealth and uHealth*, 8(9), e19796.

Othman, G., Ali, F., Ibrahim, M.I.M., Al-Worafi, Y.M., Ansari, M., & Halboup, A.M. (2020). Assessment of Anti-Diabetic Medications Adherence among Diabetic Patients in Sana'a City, Yemen: A Cross Sectional Study. *Journal of Pharmaceutical Research International*, 32(21), 114–122.

Reason, J. (1990). *Human Error*. Cambridge university press.

Saeed, M.S., Alkhoshaiban, A.S., Al-Worafi, Y.M.A., & Long, C.M. (2014). Perception of self-medication among university students in Saudi Arabia. *Archives of Pharmacy Practice*, 5(4), 149.

17 Patient Care Errors and Related Problems

Patient Education and Counseling Errors and Related Problems

17.1 BACKGROUND

Patient education and counseling is related to adherence towards the management plan, self-management, potential adverse effects and reactions, possible interactions, cautions and precautions, contraindications and warnings, and proper storage and disposal of medications. Patient education and counseling are essential components of healthcare. They involve providing patients with information about their condition, treatment options, and self-care strategies to help them manage their health effectively. The primary goal of patient education and counseling is to empower patients to make informed decisions about their health and to take an active role in their care. Patient education and counseling can take place in various settings, including hospitals, clinics, and community health centers. It can be delivered by various healthcare providers, such as physicians, nurses, pharmacists, and other allied health professionals.

Here are some key aspects of patient education and counseling:

1. Assessing patient needs: Healthcare providers should assess the patient's knowledge, understanding, and learning style to tailor the education and counseling to their individual needs.

2. Providing information: Healthcare providers should provide accurate and understandable information to patients about their condition, treatment options, and potential risks and benefits.

3. Addressing concerns and questions: Healthcare providers should encourage patients to ask questions and express their concerns. They should address any misconceptions and provide reassurance as needed.

4. Involving family members and caregivers: Healthcare providers should involve family members and caregivers in the education and counseling process to ensure that they have a clear understanding of the patient's condition and treatment plan.

5. Developing self-management skills: Healthcare providers should help patients develop the skills they need to manage their condition effectively, such as medication management, self-monitoring, and symptom recognition.

6. Follow-up: Healthcare providers should follow up with patients to assess their understanding and adherence to treatment plans and to address any ongoing concerns or questions.

In summary, patient education and counseling are critical components of healthcare that can help patients take an active role in their care, manage their condition effectively, and improve their overall health outcomes. Healthcare providers should assess patients' needs, provide accurate and understandable information, address concerns and questions, involve family members and caregivers, develop self-management skills, and follow up to ensure ongoing support and guidance.

17.2 PATIENT EDUCATION AND COUNSELING ERRORS AND RELATED PROBLEMS

Patient education and counseling errors and problems can occur at various stages of the healthcare process, and they can have serious consequences for patients. Here are some common errors that healthcare providers should try to avoid:

1. Lack of clear communication: Healthcare providers may use technical or medical jargon that patients may not understand. It is important to use plain language and check for understanding by asking patients to repeat what was discussed.

2. Insufficient time: Providers may not allocate enough time to provide comprehensive patient education or counseling. This can lead to incomplete or rushed discussions, which may result in patients not fully understanding their condition or treatment options.

3. Cultural differences: Providers may not be aware of or sensitive to cultural differences that can affect communication and understanding. It is important to acknowledge and respect cultural differences to facilitate effective communication. Cultural differences can also impact patient education and counseling. Healthcare providers may not be aware of cultural norms and values that may impact a patient's understanding of their health condition.

DOI: 10.1201/9781003230465-19

4. Assumptions about patient knowledge: Providers may assume that patients have prior knowledge or experience with their condition, which can lead to gaps in understanding. It is important to assess patients' knowledge and address any gaps.

5. Inadequate documentation: Providers may not document important information discussed during patient education or counseling, which can lead to confusion or misunderstandings later on.

6. Lack of follow-up: Providers may not follow up with patients to ensure that they have understood and implemented the information provided during education and counseling sessions. This can result in patients not adhering to treatment plans or experiencing adverse outcomes.

7. Health literacy: Low health literacy can make it difficult for patients to understand medical terminology and follow treatment plans. Healthcare providers should use plain language and provide written materials that are easy to understand.

8. Lack of patient engagement: Patients may not be engaged in their own care, which can lead to poor adherence to treatment plans and poor health outcomes. Healthcare providers should involve patients in the decision-making process and encourage them to ask questions.

9. Inadequate training: Healthcare providers may not have received adequate training in patient education and counseling. This can lead to ineffective communication and poor health outcomes.

10. Overreliance on technology: While technology can be helpful in patient education and counseling, healthcare providers should not rely solely on technology. Personal interaction and face-to-face communication are important for building trust and rapport with patients.

17.3 POTENTIAL CAUSES AND FACTORS

Patient education is an essential aspect of healthcare, as it helps patients to understand their condition, treatment options, and how to manage their health effectively. However, errors and problems can occur during patient education, which can lead to misunderstandings and negative health outcomes. Some of the causes of patient education errors and problems include:

1. Limited health literacy: Many patients may have limited health literacy, which means they may have difficulty understanding health-related information. This can lead to misunderstandings and incorrect self-management.

2. Cultural and language barriers: Patients who come from different cultural and linguistic backgrounds may face difficulties in understanding health-related information. This can lead to misunderstandings and incorrect self-management.

3. Lack of communication skills: Healthcare providers may not have adequate communication skills to explain complex health-related information to patients. This can lead to misunderstandings and incorrect self-management.

4. Limited time: Healthcare providers may have limited time to explain health-related information to patients, leading to incomplete or inadequate patient education.

5. Inadequate patient assessment: Healthcare providers may not assess the patient's level of understanding, learning style, or preferred method of communication, leading to inadequate patient education.

6. Use of medical jargon: Healthcare providers may use medical jargon that patients may not understand, leading to misunderstandings and incorrect self-management.

7. Lack of patient engagement: Patients may not be engaged in the patient education process, leading to limited understanding and incorrect self-management.

8. Health literacy: Patients with low health literacy may struggle to understand medical information and instructions, leading to errors.

9. Cultural differences: Cultural differences can lead to misunderstandings in communication and different expectations regarding medical care, which can result in patient education errors.

10. Time constraints: Healthcare providers may have limited time to explain complex medical information to patients, which can result in incomplete or inaccurate patient education.

11. Technology: Healthcare providers may rely on technology to provide patient education, but if the technology is not accessible or user-friendly, it can lead to errors.

12. Health system issues: Issues within the healthcare system, such as inadequate training or staffing shortages, can result in errors in patient education.

It is essential to address these causes of patient education errors and problems to improve patient outcomes and ensure effective patient education. Healthcare providers should adopt clear communication strategies, assess patients' understanding, use plain language, and engage patients in the education process.

The top 10 causes of medication errors identified by the United States Pharmacopoeia (USP) (Al-Worafi, 2020a,b; Cowley et al., 2001) are:

1. Performance deficit

2. Procedure or protocol not followed

3. Miscommunication

4. Inaccurate or omitted transcription

5. Improper documentation

6. Drug distribution system error

7. Knowledge deficit

8. Calculation error

9. Computer entry error

10. Lack of system safeguards

The Institute of Safe Medicine Practices (ISMP) identifies the following areas as potential causes of medication error (Reason, 1990):

- Failed communication

- Hand writing and oral communication,

- Drugs with similar names

- Missing or misplaced zero and decimal points

- Use of non-standard abbreviations,

- Poor drug distribution practices

- Complex or poorly designed technology

- Access to drugs by no pharmacy personnel

- Work place environmental problem that lead to increased job stress

- Dose miscalculations

- Lack of patient information

- Lack of patient understanding of their therapy.

17.4 PREVENTION

Here are some strategies to prevent errors and problems during patient education and counseling:

1. Assess patient literacy: Assessing patient literacy is important to identify patients who may have difficulty understanding health information. Health literacy assessments can be done using simple questionnaires or tools. Health professionals can then adjust their communication style and use simpler language to improve patient understanding.

2. Use plain language: Using plain language is important in patient education and counseling. Avoid medical jargon and complex terminology that patients may not understand. Explain terms in simple language and use visual aids to enhance understanding.

3. Tailor education to patient needs: Patients have different levels of understanding and learning styles. Health professionals should tailor education and counseling to the patient's individual needs, preferences, and cultural background.

4. Confirm patient understanding: Confirming patient understanding is crucial to prevent errors and misunderstandings. Health professionals can use the teach-back method, where patients are asked to explain what they have learned in their own words. This allows health professionals to identify areas where patients may need further education or clarification.

5. Provide written materials: Providing written materials such as pamphlets, brochures, or handouts can reinforce patient education and serve as a reference for patients. Ensure that written materials are in plain language and easily understandable.

6. Address barriers to adherence: Patients may face barriers to adhering to treatment plans, such as financial constraints or transportation issues. Health professionals should address these barriers during patient education and counseling and provide resources to overcome them.

7. Continually assess and evaluate patient education: Continual assessment and evaluation of patient education and counseling is important to identify areas for improvement. Feedback from patients can help health professionals tailor education to better meet patient needs and improve health outcomes.

8. Prioritize patient education: Healthcare providers should make patient education and counseling a priority and allocate adequate time to each patient.

9. Involve patients in the decision-making process: Healthcare providers should involve patients in the decision-making process and encourage them to ask questions and express their concerns.

10. Be aware of cultural differences: Healthcare providers should be aware of cultural differences that may impact patient education and counseling and tailor their communication accordingly.

11. Receive training: Healthcare providers should receive training in patient education and counseling to improve their communication skills and reduce the likelihood of errors and problems.

12. Use a multidisciplinary approach: Healthcare providers should consider using a multi-disciplinary approach to patient education and counseling, involving other healthcare professionals such as nurses, pharmacists, and social workers.

By taking these steps, healthcare providers can help ensure that patient education and counseling are effective and contribute to better health outcomes and patient satisfaction.

17.5 CHALLENGES OF PATIENT EDUCATION AND COUNSELING IN DEVELOPING COUNTRIES

There are many challenges for the patient education and counseling in developing countries which are as follows (Alshahrani et al., 2019a,b; Al-Qahtani et al., 2015; Alshahrani et al., 2020a,b; Al-Worafi, 2014; Al-Worafi, 2015; Al-Worafi, 2016; Al-Worafi et al., 2017; Al-Worafi, 2018a-d;Al-Worafi et al., 2018a-b; Al-Worafi et al., 2019; Al-Worafi, 2020a-z; Al-Worafi et al., 2020a-b; Al-Worafi et al., 2021a,b; Al-Worafi, 2022a,b; Al-Worafi, 2023; Baig et al., 2020; Elkalmi et al., 2020; Elsayed & Al-Worafi, 2020; Hasan et al., 2019; Hassan et al., 2014; Izhar et al., 2017; Lee et al., 2017; Mahmoud et al., 2020; Manan et al., 2014; Manan et al., 2016; Ming et al., 2016; Ming et al., 2020; Othman et al., 2020; Saeed et al., 2014).

17.5.1 Healthcare Systems

The quality of healthcare systems and healthcare services are the cornerstone in providing the most effective and safe patient care services; healthcare systems in many developing countries, especially low-income countries, are weak, with inadequate budgets and infrastructures, which affect patient safety in many ways. Therefore, strengthening the healthcare systems in developing countries is very important and highly recommended to improve patient care practice.

17.5.2 Financial Challenges

Patient care need financial support in the public healthcare sectors as well as private healthcare sectors, which is missing in many developing countries, especially low-income countries. Therefore, increasing the health expenditure and the public healthcare budget is very important and highly recommended. Increasing the contribution from the private and charity sectors is very important and highly recommended.

17.5.3 Workforce Challenges

The inadequate number of healthcare professionals throughout the public as well as private healthcare facilities is a major barrier affecting the quality of healthcare services throughout developing countries, especially low-income countries; therefore, hiring more healthcare professionals is very important and highly recommended.

17.5.4 Migration of Healthcare Professionals

Migration of healthcare professionals has increased during the last two decades from many developing countries, especially low and middle-income countries, due to many reasons, such as the lack of jobs in healthcare facilities, low salaries, the attraction of jobs overseas, political and war issues and others. Designing long-term plans and short-term plans to overcome this challenge is very important and highly recommended.

17.5.5 Reporting Challenges

Reporting patient care errors and related problems is very important to know the reasons and design the necessary interventions to overcome this challenge.

17.5.6 Research

There is little known about patient care errors and related problems in developing countries due to many reasons. Support from the Health Ministries, universities, pharmaceutical companies, organizations, and policymakers can overcome this challenge.

17.5.7 Technology Challenges

New technologies, applications, and social media can play an important role in patient process.
   Low health literacy: Many patients in developing countries have low health literacy, which refers to their ability to understand and act upon health information. This can make it challenging for healthcare providers to convey health information effectively and ensure that patients understand it.

17.5.8 Cultural Barriers

Cultural beliefs and practices can sometimes conflict with recommended healthcare practices, making it difficult to provide effective patient education and counseling. For example, in some cultures, herbal remedies are preferred over conventional medicines, which can complicate treatment and adherence to prescribed medication.

17.5.9 Language Barriers

In many developing countries, both patients and healthcare providers may not speak the same language. This can lead to miscommunication and misunderstandings, making it challenging to provide effective patient education and counseling.
   In conclusion, patient education and counseling are essential components of healthcare delivery, and overcoming the challenges that hinder them in developing countries is critical to improving health outcomes. Healthcare providers, policymakers, and other stakeholders must work together to address these challenges and ensure that patients receive effective patient education, and counseling.

17.6 CONCLUSION

This chapter has discussed the patient education and counseling errors and problems, causes, prevention, and recommendations for the best practice in the developing countries. Patient education and counseling is related to adherence toward the management plan, self-management, potential adverse effects and reactions, possible interactions, cautions and precautions, contra-indications and warnings, and proper storage and disposal of medications. Patient education and counseling errors and problems can occur at various stages of the healthcare process, and they can have serious consequences for patients. patient education and counseling are essential components of healthcare delivery, and overcoming the challenges that hinder them in developing countries is critical to improving health outcomes. Healthcare providers, policymakers, and other stakeholders must work together to address these challenges and ensure that patients receive effective patient education and counseling.

REFERENCES

Al-Qahtani, I., Almoteb, T.M., & Al-Warafi, Y. (2015). Competency of metered-dose inhaler use among Saudi community pharmacists: A Simulation method study. *RRJPPS*, 4(2), 37–31.

Alshahrani, S.M., Alakhali, K.M., & Al-Worafi, Y.M. (2019a). Medication errors in a health care facility in southern Saudi Arabia. *Tropical Journal of Pharmaceutical Research*, 18(5), 1119–1122.

Alshahrani, S.M., Alavudeen, S.S., Alakhali, K.M., Al-Worafi, Y.M., Bahamdan, A.K., & Vigneshwaran, E. (2019b). Self-Medication Among King Khalid University Students, Saudi Arabia. *Risk Management and Healthcare Policy*, 12, 243–249.

Alshahrani, S.M., Alakhali, K.M., Al-Worafi, Y.M., & Alshahrani, N.Z. (2020a). Awareness and use of over the counter analgesic medication: A survey in the Aseer region population, Saudi Arabia. *International Journal of Advances in Applied Sciences*, 7(3), 130–134.

Alshahrani, S.M., Alzahran, M., Alakhali, K., Vigneshwaran, E., Iqbal, M.J., Khan, N.A., ... & Alavudeen, S.S. (2020b). Association Between Diabetes Consequences and Quality of Life Among Patients With Diabetes Mellitus in the Aseer Province of Saudi Arabia. *Open Access Macedonian Journal of Medical Sciences*, 8(E), 325–330.

Al-Worafi, Y.M. (2014). Prescription writing errors at a tertiary care hospital in Yemen: Prevalence, types, causes and recommendations. *American Journal of Pharmacy and Health Research*, 2, 134–140.

Al-Worafi, Y.M.A. (2015). Appropriateness of metered-dose inhaler use in the Yemeni community pharmacies. *Journal of Taibah University Medical Sciences*, 10(3), 353–358.

Al-Worafi, Y.M.A. (2016). Pharmacy practice in Yemen. In *Pharmacy Practice in Developing Countries* (pp. 267–287). Academic Press.

Al-Worafi, Y.M., Kassab, Y.W., Alseragi, W.M., Almutairi, M.S., Ahmed, A., Ming, L.C., Alkhoshaiban, A.S., & Hadi, M.A., (2017). Pharmacovigilance and adverse drg reaction reporting: A perspective of community pharmacists and pharmacy technicians in Sana'a, Yemen. *Therapeutics and Clinical Risk Management*, 13, 1175.

Al-Worafi, Y.M. (2018a). Knowledge, Attitude and Practice of Yemeni Physicians Toward Pharmacovigilance: A Mixed Method Study. *International Journal of Pharmacy and Pharmaceutical Sciences*, 10 (10), 74–77

Al-Worafi, Y. (2018b). Knowledge, attitude and practice of Yemeni physicians toward pharmacovigilance: A mixed method study. *International Journal of Pharmacy and Pharmaceutical Sciences*, 10, 74–77.

Al-Worafi, Y.M. (2018c). Dispensing errors observed by community pharmacy dispensers in IBB–YEMEN. *Asian Journal of Pharmaceutical and Clinical Research*, 11(11).

Al-Worafi, Y.M. (2018d). Evauation of inhaler technique among patients with asthma and COPD in Yemen. *Journal of Taibah University Medical Sciences*, 13(5), 488–490.

Al-Worafi, Y.M., Patel, R.P., Zaidi, S.T.R., Alseragi, W.M., Almutairi, M.S., Alkhoshaiban, A.S., & Ming, L.C. (2018a). Completeness and legibility of handwritten prescriptions in Sana'a, Yemen. *Medical Principles and Practice*, 27, 290–292.

Al-Worafi, Y.M., Alseragi, W.M., Seng, L.K., Kassab, Y.W., Yeoh, S.F., Chiau, L., ... & Husain, K. (2018b). Dispensing errors in community pharmacies: a prospective study in Sana'a, Yemen. *Archives of Pharmacy Practice*, 9(4), 1–3.

Al-Worafi, Y.M., Alseragi, W.M., & Mahmoud, M.A. (2019). Competency of metered-dose inhaler use among community pharmacy dispensers in Ibb, Yemen: A simulation method study. *Latin American Journal of Pharmacy*, 38(3), 489–494.

Al-Worafi, Y.M. (Ed.). (2020a). *Drug Safety in Developing Countries: Achievements and Challenges.*

Al-Worafi, Y.M. (2020b). Medication errors. In *Drug Safety in Developing Countries* (pp. 105–117). Academic Press.

Al-Worafi, Y.M. (2020c). Adverse drug reactions. In *Drug Safety in Developing Countries* (pp. 39–57). Academic Press.

Al-Worafi, Y.M. (2020d). Medications registration and marketing: Safety-related issues. In *Drug Safety in Developing Countries* (pp. 21–28). Academic Press.

Al-Worafi, Y.M. (2020e). Pharmacovigilance. In *Drug Safety in Developing Countries* (pp. 29–38). Academic Press.

Al-Worafi, Y.M. (2020f). Drug-related problems. In *Drug Safety in Developing Countries* (pp. 59–71). Academic Press.

Al-Worafi, Y.M. (2020g). Medications safety-related terminology. In *Drug Safety in Developing Countries* (pp. 7–19). Academic Press.

Al-Worafi, Y.M. (2020h). Self-medication. In *Drug Safety in Developing Countries* (pp. 73–86). Academic Press.

Al-Worafi, Y.M. (2020j). Antibiotics safety issues. In *Drug Safety in Developing Countries* (pp. 87–103). Academic Press.

Al-Worafi, Y.M. (2020k). Medications safety research issues. In *Drug Safety in Developing Countries* (pp. 213–227). Academic Press.

Al-Worafi, Y.M. (2020l). Counterfeit and substandard medications. In *Drug Safety in Developing Countries* (pp. 119–126). Academic Press.

Al-Worafi, Y.M. (2020m). Medication abuse and misuse. In *Drug Safety in Developing Countries* (pp. 127–135). Academic Press.

Al-Worafi, Y.M. (2020n). Storage and disposal of medications. In *Drug Safety in Developing Countries* (pp. 137–142). Academic Press.

Al-Worafi, Y.M. (2020o). Safety of medications in special population. In *Drug Safety in Developing Countries* (pp. 143–162). Academic Press.

Al-Worafi, Y.M. (2020p). Herbal medicines safety issues. In *Drug Safety in Developing Countries* (pp. 163–178). Academic Press.

Al-Worafi, Y.M. (2020q). Medications safety pharmacoeconomics-related issues. In *Drug Safety in Developing Countries* (pp. 187–195). Academic Press.

Al-Worafi, Y.M. (2020r). Evidence-based medications safety practice. In *Drug Safety in Developing Countries* (pp. 197–201). Academic Press.

Al-Worafi, Y.M. (2020s). Quality indicators for medications safety. In *Drug Safety in Developing Countries* (pp. 229–242). Academic Press.

Al-Worafi, Y.M. (2020t). Drug safety in Yemen. In *Drug Safety in Developing Countries* (pp. 391–405). Academic Press.

Al-Worafi, Y.M. (2020u). Drug safety in Saudi Arabia. In *Drug Safety in Developing Countries* (pp. 407–417). Academic Press.

Al-Worafi, Y.M. (2020v). Drug safety in United Arab Emirates. In *Drug Safety in Developing Countries* (pp. 419–428). Academic Press.

Al-Worafi, Y.M. (2020w). Drug safety in Indonesia. In *Drug Safety in Developing Countries* (pp. 279–285). Academic Press.

Al-Worafi, Y.M. (2020x). Drug safety in Palestine. In *Drug Safety in Developing Countries* (pp. 471–480). Academic Press.

Al-Worafi, Y.M. (2020y). Drug safety: Comparison between developing countries. In *Drug Safety in Developing Countries* (pp. 603–611). Academic Press.

Al-Worafi, Y.M. (2020z). Drug safety in developing versus developed countries. In *Drug Safety in Developing Countries* (pp. 613–615). Academic Press.

Al-Worafi, Y.M., Alseragi, W.M., Ming, L.C., & Alakhali, K.M. (2020a). Drug safety in China. In *Drug Safety in Developing Countries* (pp. 381–388). Academic Press.

Al-Worafi, Y.M., Alseragi, W.M., Alakhali, K.M., Ming, L.C., Othman, G., Halboup, A.M., … & Elkalmi, R.M. (2020b). Knowledge, beliefs and factors affecting the use of generic medicines among patients in Ibb, Yemen: A mixed-method study. *Journal of Pharmacy Practice and Community Medicine*, 6(4).

Al-Worafi, Y.M., Elkalmi, R.M., Ming, L.C., Othman, G., Halboup, A.M., Battah, M.M., … & Mani, V. (2021a). *Dispensing Errors in Hospital Pharmacies: A Prospective Study in Yemen*.

Al-Worafi, Y.M., Hasan, S., Hassan, N.M., & Gaili, A.A. (2021b). Knowledge, Attitude and Experience of Pharmacist in the UAE towards Pharmacovigilance. *Research Journal of Pharmacy and Technology*, 14(1), 265–269.

Al-Worafi, Y. (2022a). *A Guide to Online Pharmacy Education: Teaching Strategies and Assessment Methods*. CRC Press.

Al-Worafi, Y.M. (2022b). Patient care errors and related problems (part I): Development and validation of the model. https://orcid.org/0000-0002-5752-2913

Al-Worafi, Y.M. (Ed.). (2023). *Clinical Case Studies on Medication Safety*. Academic Press.

Baig, M.R., Al-Worafi, Y.M., Alseragi, W.M., Ming, L.C., & Siddique, A. (2020). Drug safety in India. In *Drug Safety in Developing Countries* (pp. 327–334). Academic Press.

Cowley, E., Williams, R., & Cousins, D. (2001). Medication errors in children: A descriptive summary of medication error reports submitted to the United States Pharmacopeia. *Current Therapeutic Research*, 62(9), 627–640.

Elkalmi, R.M., Al-Worafi, Y.M., Alseragi, W.M., Ming, L.C., & Siddique, A. (2020). Drug safety in Malaysia. In *Drug Safety in Developing Countries* (pp. 245–253). Academic Press.

Elsayed, T., & Al-Worafi, Y.M. (2020). Drug safety in Egypt. In *Drug Safety in Developing Countries* (pp. 511–523). Academic Press.

Hasan, S., Al-Omar, M.J., AlZubaidy, H., & Al-Worafi, Y.M. (2019). Use of medications in Arab Countries. *Handbook of Healthcare in the Arab World*. Cham: Springer, 42.

Hassan, Y., Abd Aziz, N., Kassab, Y.W., Elgasim, I., Shaharuddin, S., Al-Worafi, Y.M.A., ... & Ming, L.C. (2014). How to help patients to control their blood pressure? Blood pressure control and its predictor. *Archives of Pharmacy Practice*, 5(4).

Izahar, S., Lean, Q.Y., Hameed, M.A., Murugiah, M.K., Patel, R.P., Al-Worafi, Y.M., ... & Ming, L.C. (2017). Content analysis of mobile health applications on diabetes mellitus. *Frontiers in Endocrinology*, 8, 318.

Lee, K.S., Yee, S.M., Zaidi, S.T.R., Patel, R.P., Yang, Q., Al-Worafi, Y.M., & Ming, L.C., 2017. Combating sale of counterfeit and falsified medicines online: A losing battle. *Frontiers in Pharmacology*, 8, 268.

Mahmoud, M.A., Wajid, S., Naqvi, A.A., Samreen, S., Althagfan, S.S., & Al-Worafi, Y. (2020). Self-medication with antibiotics: A cross-sectional community-based study. *Latin American Journal of Pharmacy*, 39(2), 348–353.

Manan, M.M., Rusli, R.A., Ang, W.C., Al-Worafi, Y.M., & Ming, L.C. (2014). Assessing the pharmaceutical care issues of antiepileptic drug therapy in hospitalised epileptic patients. *Journal of Pharmacy Practice and Research*, 44(3), 83–88.

Manan, M.M., Ibrahim, N.A., Aziz, N.A., Zulkifly, H.H., Al-Worafi, Y.M.A., & Long, C.M. (2016). Empirical use of antibiotic therapy in the prevention of early onset sepsis in neonates: A pilot study. *Archives of Medical Science*, 12(3), 603–613.

Ming, L.C., Hameed, M.A., Lee, D.D., Apidi, N.A., Lai, P.S.M., Hadi, M.A., Al-Worafi, Y.M.A., & Khan, T.M. (2016). Use of medical mobile applications among hospital pharmacists in Malaysia. *Therapeutic Innovation & Regulatory Science*, 50(4), 419–426.

Ming, L.C., Untong, N., Aliudin, N.A., Osili, N., Kifli, N., Tan, C.S., ... & Goh, H.P. (2020). Mobile health apps on COVID-19 launched in the early days of the pandemic: Content analysis and review. *JMIR mHealth and uHealth*, 8(9), e19796.

Othman, G., Ali, F., Ibrahim, M.I.M., Al-Worafi, Y.M., Ansari, M., & Halboup, A.M. (2020). Assessment of Anti-Diabetic Medications Adherence among Diabetic Patients in Sana'a City, Yemen: A Cross Sectional Study. *Journal of Pharmaceutical Research International*, 32(21), 114–122.

Reason, J. (1990). *Human Error*. Cambridge university press.

Saeed, M.S., Alkhoshaiban, A.S., Al-Worafi, Y.M.A., & Long, C.M. (2014). Perception of self-medication among university students in Saudi Arabia. *Archives of Pharmacy Practice*, 5(4), 149.

18 Patient Safety-Related Issues

Other Medication Safety Issues

18.1 BACKGROUND

Medication safety issues such as adverse Drug Reactions (ADRs), medication errors, Drug-Related Problems (DRPs), drug abuse and misuse, and inappropriate use of antibiotics are examples of medication safety issues, which are affecting patients, families, and ministries of health worldwide. They lead to failure in the treatment outcomes, increase in the length of hospitalization, increase in morbidity and mortality, reduction in the quality of life, and increase in the cost of illness and health expenditure. Healthcare professionals are the cornerstone in improving medication safety practices in developed countries and developing countries. There are many medication safety issues in developing countries which are as follows (Alshahrani et al., 2019a,b; Al-Qahtani et al., 2015; Alshahrani et al., 2020a,b; Al-Worafi, 2014; Al-Worafi, 2015; Al-Worafi, 2016; Al-Worafi et al., 2017; Al-Worafi, 2018a-d; Al-Worafi et al., 2018a-b; Al-Worafi et al., 2019; Al-Worafi, 2020a-z; Al-Worafi et al., 2020a-b; Al-Worafi et al., 2021a,b; Al-Worafi, 2022a,b; Al-Worafi, 2023; Baig et al., 2020; Elkalmi et al., 2020; Elsayed & Al-Worafi, 2020; Hasan et al., 2019; Hassan et al., 2014; Izhar et al., 2017; Lee et al., 2017; Mahmoud et al., 2020; Manan et al., 2014; Manan et al., 2016; Ming et al., 2016; Ming et al., 2020; Othman et al., 2020; Saeed et al., 2014).

18.2 PHARMACOVIGILANCE IN DEVELOPING COUNTRIES

Pharmacovigilance is the science and activities related to the detection, assessment, understanding, and prevention of adverse effects or any other drug-related problem. Pharmacovigilance is an essential part of ensuring drug safety and is critical to promoting public health. Developing countries often face significant challenges in implementing and maintaining effective pharmacovigilance systems. These challenges can include a lack of resources, infrastructure, trained personnel, and regulatory frameworks. However, pharmacovigilance is crucial in developing countries because of the high burden of disease, limited healthcare resources, and increased risk of adverse drug reactions due to the use of substandard or falsified medicines.

Several initiatives have been undertaken to strengthen pharmacovigilance in developing countries. The World Health Organization (WHO) has developed guidelines and training materials to help countries establish pharmacovigilance systems. The WHO also supports the development of pharmacovigilance networks in regions and countries to share information and promote collaboration. Several developing countries have established pharmacovigilance systems that comply with international standards. For example, in India, the Central Drugs Standard Control Organization (CDSCO) has established a nationwide pharmacovigilance program to monitor the safety of medicines. Similarly, in South Africa, the Medicines Control Council (MCC) has implemented a pharmacovigilance system that meets international standards. In conclusion, pharmacovigilance is a critical component of drug safety and public health, and developing countries must establish and maintain effective pharmacovigilance systems. While significant challenges exist, several initiatives have been undertaken to strengthen pharmacovigilance in developing countries, and many countries have established pharmacovigilance systems that comply with international standards.

18.3 ADVERSE DRUG REACTIONS AND MEDICATION ERRORS REPORTING IN DEVELOPING COUNTRIES

Adverse drug reactions (ADRs) and medication errors are significant public health concerns worldwide. However, reporting of ADRs and medication errors is often inadequate in developing countries due to various factors such as lack of awareness, insufficient infrastructure, and underdeveloped pharmacovigilance systems. Inadequate reporting of ADRs and medication errors in developing countries can lead to a delay in detecting safety signals, preventing harm to patients, and reducing the burden on healthcare systems. Therefore, it is crucial to improve reporting mechanisms in developing countries to ensure better patient safety. To improve reporting of ADRs and medication errors, several initiatives have been undertaken. The World Health Organization (WHO) has developed guidelines and tools to support developing countries in establishing pharmacovigilance systems and improving ADR reporting. The WHO also supports the establishment of national pharmacovigilance centers in developing countries. Many developing countries have also implemented ADR reporting systems. For example, in India, the Pharmacovigilance Program of India (PvPI) was established in 2010 to improve ADR reporting and

DOI: 10.1201/9781003230465-20

monitoring. The PvPI has created a network of ADR monitoring centers across the country and has also implemented an online reporting system to increase the efficiency of ADR reporting. In addition, healthcare providers in developing countries need to be educated on the importance of ADR reporting and medication safety. Healthcare providers need to be trained on how to identify and report ADRs and medication errors to ensure that accurate and timely information is captured.

In conclusion, improving ADR and medication error reporting in developing countries is critical to improving patient safety and reducing the burden on healthcare systems. Initiatives such as the establishment of pharmacovigilance centers and the education of healthcare providers can help improve reporting mechanisms in developing countries. It is essential that the global community continues to support developing countries in improving their pharmacovigilance systems and reporting mechanisms.

18.4 SELF-CARE AND SELF-MEDICATIONS IN DEVELOPING COUNTRIES

Self-care and self-medication are common practices in many developing countries, where access to healthcare services may be limited or expensive. While self-care practices can be beneficial in promoting health and preventing disease, self-medication can also be risky if not done properly.

Self-medication refers to the use of over-the-counter (OTC) medications, herbal remedies, or traditional medicines to treat symptoms of illness without consulting a healthcare provider. In many developing countries, self-medication is widespread due to the high cost of healthcare services and limited access to healthcare providers. Self-medication can be beneficial if done correctly, but it can also be harmful if the wrong medication or dose is taken, leading to adverse reactions or drug interactions. In developing countries, where medications may be of questionable quality or counterfeit, self-medication can pose an even greater risk. To promote safe self-medication practices, healthcare providers in developing countries need to educate the public on the risks and benefits of self-medication. Healthcare providers can also provide guidance on how to select and use OTC medications safely and appropriately. In addition, regulatory bodies need to ensure that OTC medications are safe, effective, and of good quality. This can be challenging in developing countries, where regulatory systems may be weak or non-existent. However, efforts are being made to strengthen regulatory systems in many developing countries to ensure that medications are safe and effective. In conclusion, self-care and self-medication are common practices in many developing countries. While self-care practices can promote health and prevent disease, self-medication can be risky if not done properly. Education and guidance on safe self-medication practices, as well as the regulation of OTC medications, are essential to promote safe self-medication practices in developing countries.

18.5 SELF-MEDICATIONS WITH ANTIMICROBIALS IN DEVELOPING COUNTRIES

Self-medication with antimicrobials is a significant problem in many developing countries. In these countries, antimicrobials are often readily available without a prescription, and individuals may self-medicate to treat common infections such as respiratory tract infections, diarrhea, and urinary tract infections. The inappropriate use of antimicrobials can lead to the development of antimicrobial resistance (AMR), which is a global public health threat. AMR can lead to the emergence of superbugs, which are difficult to treat with existing antimicrobial agents, resulting in increased morbidity, mortality, and healthcare costs. Several factors contribute to the high prevalence of self-medication with antimicrobials in developing countries. These factors include lack of access to healthcare services, high cost of healthcare, limited availability of quality healthcare services, and inadequate regulation of antimicrobial use. To address the problem of self-medication with antimicrobials in developing countries, several initiatives have been undertaken. These include the development of policies and guidelines for the appropriate use of antimicrobials, improving access to quality healthcare services, and strengthening regulatory systems to ensure the appropriate use of antimicrobials. Education and awareness campaigns targeted at the general public and healthcare providers are also essential to promote the appropriate use of antimicrobials. These campaigns can include information on the risks of self-medication with antimicrobials, the importance of completing a full course of treatment, and the need to seek healthcare services for serious infections. In conclusion, self-medication with antimicrobials is a significant problem in many developing countries, contributing to the development of AMR. Addressing this issue requires a multifaceted approach that includes improving access to quality healthcare services, developing policies and guidelines for the appropriate use of antimicrobials, and educating the public and healthcare providers on the risks of self-medication with antimicrobials.

18.6 COUNTERFEIT AND SUBSTANDARD MEDICATIONS IN DEVELOPING COUNTRIES

Counterfeit and substandard medications are a significant problem in many developing countries. These medications may be produced without proper quality control measures, may contain incorrect or inactive ingredients, or may be packaged to look like a genuine medication. Counterfeit and substandard medications can be found in both prescription and over-the-counter medications. The problem of counterfeit and substandard medications in developing countries is driven by several factors, including weak regulatory systems, limited resources for drug quality monitoring, and inadequate enforcement of existing regulations. In addition, the high cost of genuine medications may lead individuals to purchase cheaper, counterfeit medications. The use of counterfeit and substandard medications can have serious consequences, including treatment failure, development of drug resistance, and adverse drug reactions. It can also undermine public confidence in the healthcare system and result in the loss of resources and lives.

Several initiatives have been undertaken to address the problem of counterfeit and substandard medications in developing countries. These initiatives include strengthening regulatory systems, increasing the capacity for drug quality monitoring, and improving enforcement of existing regulations. Other initiatives include the use of technology such as barcoding and serialization to track medications and prevent counterfeit products from entering the supply chain. Education and awareness campaigns targeted at the general public and healthcare providers are also essential to promote the use of genuine medications and to raise awareness of the risks associated with counterfeit and substandard medications. In conclusion, counterfeit and substandard medications are a significant problem in many developing countries, driven by weak regulatory systems and inadequate enforcement of existing regulations. Addressing this problem requires a multifaceted approach that includes strengthening regulatory systems, increasing capacity for drug quality monitoring, and improving public awareness of the risks associated with counterfeit and substandard medications.

18.7 MEDICATIONS ABUSE AND MISUSE IN DEVELOPING COUNTRIES

Medication abuse and misuse are significant problems in many developing countries. Medication abuse refers to the intentional use of medications for non-medical purposes, while medication misuse refers to the inappropriate use of medications, such as taking incorrect doses or using medications for an extended period. The problem of medication abuse and misuse in developing countries is driven by several factors, including lack of access to healthcare services, limited availability of quality healthcare services, poverty, and cultural beliefs. In some cases, individuals may also use medications as a coping mechanism for social or emotional problems. The misuse and abuse of medications can have serious consequences, including addiction, dependence, overdose, and death. It can also result in the development of drug resistance, making it more difficult to treat infectious diseases. Several initiatives have been undertaken to address the problem of medication abuse and misuse in developing countries. These initiatives include improving access to quality healthcare services, increasing awareness of the risks associated with medication abuse and misuse, and developing policies and guidelines for the appropriate use of medications. Other initiatives include the implementation of drug monitoring systems to track the use of medications and identify cases of abuse and misuse. Education and awareness campaigns targeted at the general public and healthcare providers are also essential to promote the appropriate use of medications and to raise awareness of the risks associated with medication abuse and misuse. In conclusion, medication abuse and misuse are significant problems in many developing countries, driven by a lack of access to healthcare services, poverty, and cultural beliefs. Addressing this problem requires a multi-faceted approach that includes improving access to quality healthcare services, increasing awareness of the risks associated with medication abuse and misuse, and developing policies and guidelines for the appropriate use of medications.

18.8 SUBSTANCE ABUSE IN DEVELOPING COUNTRIES

Substance abuse is a significant public health concern in developing countries. Substance abuse can lead to addiction, health problems, and social issues, including poverty, unemployment, and crime.

Several factors contribute to the high rates of substance abuse in developing countries, including:

1. Poverty and social inequality: Poverty and social inequality can lead to increased stress and mental health issues, which may lead to substance abuse as a coping mechanism.

2. Lack of education and awareness: Many people in developing countries may not be aware of the risks and dangers associated with substance abuse, and education about substance abuse prevention and treatment may be limited.

3. Limited access to healthcare: Many people in developing countries do not have easy access to healthcare services, including addiction treatment and mental health services.

4. Availability of illicit substances: Illicit substances may be more readily available in developing countries, making them easier to access and abuse.

To address the problem of substance abuse in developing countries, it is important to prioritize public education and awareness campaigns about the risks and dangers of substance abuse, as well as promoting the availability of addiction treatment and mental health services. Additionally, regulations on the production, sale, and distribution of illicit substances can help to reduce their availability and prevent substance abuse. Community-based programs, such as support groups and peer counseling, can also be effective in addressing substance abuse in developing countries.

18.9 STORAGE AND DISPOSAL OF MEDICINES

Proper storage and disposal of medicines is important to ensure their effectiveness and prevent harm to individuals and the environment. However, in developing countries, there are often challenges in maintaining adequate storage conditions and implementing safe disposal practices due to factors such as limited resources, inadequate infrastructure, and lack of awareness.

Storage of medicines:

- Store medicines in a cool, dry place, away from direct sunlight and moisture.

- Avoid storing medicines in places where temperature and humidity fluctuations are common, such as near windows or in bathrooms.

- Keep medicines out of reach of children and pets.

- Follow any specific storage instructions provided with the medicine, such as storing in the refrigerator or at room temperature.

- Ensure medicines are stored in their original packaging and not mixed with other medications.

Disposal of medicines:

- Follow any specific disposal instructions provided with the medicine, such as flushing down the toilet or placing in a hazardous waste bin.

- If there are no specific instructions, do not flush medicines down the toilet or drain, as this can contaminate water sources.

- Check with local authorities to determine the proper method of disposal for unused or expired medications.

- If possible, return unused or expired medications to a pharmacy or healthcare provider for proper disposal.

- Do not share medications with others, as this can be dangerous and contribute to the development of drug-resistant infections.

In developing countries, there may be additional challenges in implementing safe storage and disposal practices due to factors such as limited resources, inadequate infrastructure, and lack of awareness. Strategies to address these challenges may include:

- Providing education and training on proper storage and disposal practices for healthcare providers and the general public.

- Improving access to proper storage facilities, such as refrigerators and secure cabinets.

- Implementing community-based collection and disposal programs for unused and expired medications.

- Developing and enforcing regulations and policies for the safe disposal of medications.

■ Encouraging manufacturers to design and package medications in a way that minimizes waste and environmental impact.

Overall, proper storage and disposal of medications is important to ensure their effectiveness and prevent harm to individuals and the environment. In developing countries, efforts are needed to address the unique challenges that may impact safe storage and disposal practices. In general, inappropriate storage and disposal of medications is common practice in the majority of developing countries, so an increase in the awareness of people and healthcare professionals about the safe and appropriate storage and disposal of medications is very important and highly recommended; Drug Take Back Programs is very important and highly recommended; conduct research about storage and disposal of medications challenges, interventions and impact of interventions is very important and highly recommended; monitor and supervise the disposal of medications by the drug authorities is very important and highly recommended. Patient education and counseling at pharmacies is the key for the best practice.

18.10 HERBAL MEDICINES

Herbal medicines are commonly used in developing countries for their therapeutic benefits. However, there are safety issues associated with the use of herbal medicines in these regions due to various factors such as lack of regulation, poor quality control, and inadequate knowledge about their potential risks. Here are some of the safety issues associated with herbal medicines in developing countries:

1. Lack of regulation: In many developing countries, there is little or no regulation of herbal medicines, which means that there are no standards for quality control, safety, or efficacy. This can lead to the production and sale of herbal medicines that are contaminated, adulterated, or mislabeled, which can pose a serious health risk to consumers.

2. Poor quality control: Due to the lack of regulation, there may be poor quality control in the production of herbal medicines. This can result in variations in the potency and purity of herbal medicines, which can affect their safety and efficacy.

3. Adverse effects: Herbal medicines can cause adverse effects, just like any other medication. However, in developing countries, there may be inadequate reporting and monitoring of adverse effects associated with herbal medicines, which can make it difficult to identify potential safety issues.

4. Interactions with conventional medicines: Herbal medicines can interact with conventional medicines, which can lead to adverse effects. However, in developing countries, there may be a lack of awareness and knowledge about potential interactions, which can increase the risk of adverse effects.

5. Contamination with heavy metals: Herbal medicines can be contaminated with heavy metals such as lead, arsenic, and mercury, which can be harmful to human health. This can occur due to environmental pollution, poor quality control, or improper harvesting and processing of the herbs.

6. Lack of knowledge and education: In developing countries, there may be a lack of knowledge and education about the safe and effective use of herbal medicines. This can lead to inappropriate use, such as self-medication and the use of herbal medicines without consulting a healthcare professional, which can increase the risk of adverse effects.

To address these safety issues, it is important to implement regulations for the production, quality control, and sale of herbal medicines. Healthcare professionals and consumers should be educated about the safe and effective use of herbal medicines, and efforts should be made to improve reporting and monitoring of adverse effects associated with herbal medicines. Additionally, there should be increased awareness about potential interactions between herbal medicines and conventional medicines, and efforts should be made to reduce environmental pollution to prevent contamination of herbal medicines with heavy metals.

18.11 NUTRACEUTICALS SAFETY ISSUES IN DEVELOPING COUNTRIES

Nutraceuticals, which are dietary supplements or functional foods that provide health benefits beyond basic nutrition, are gaining popularity in developing countries due to their perceived health benefits and affordability. However, there are several safety issues associated with nutraceuticals in developing countries.

1. Lack of Regulation: In many developing countries, there is a lack of regulation or inadequate regulation of nutraceuticals. This makes it difficult to ensure the safety and efficacy of these products.

2. Quality Control Issues: The quality of nutraceuticals can vary widely due to inadequate quality control measures. This can result in products that are contaminated with harmful substances or do not contain the claimed ingredients in the proper amounts.

3. Adulteration: Adulteration of nutraceuticals with unapproved or harmful substances is a common problem in developing countries. This can lead to serious health consequences for consumers.

4. Lack of Information: Consumers in developing countries may not have access to accurate and reliable information about nutraceuticals, including their potential risks and benefits. This can lead to uninformed decisions about their use.

5. Interactions with Conventional Medicines: Nutraceuticals may interact with prescription medications, leading to adverse effects. Consumers in developing countries may not be aware of these potential interactions or may not disclose their use of nutraceuticals to healthcare providers.

6. Overdose: Overdosing on nutraceuticals can lead to serious health consequences, including liver damage and kidney failure. Consumers in developing countries may not be aware of the appropriate dosages or may not have access to products with accurate labeling.

Overall, nutraceutical safety issues in developing countries highlight the need for better regulation and quality control measures, as well as increased education and awareness among consumers and healthcare providers.

18.12 RECOMMENDATIONS FOR THE BEST MEDICATION SAFETY PRACTICE IN DEVELOPING COUNTRIES

There are many challenges in developing countries to overcome it and there are many suggested recommendations (Alshahrani et al., 2019a,b; Al-Qahtani et al., 2015; Alshahrani et al., 2020a,b; Al-Worafi, 2014; Al-Worafi, 2015; Al-Worafi, 2016; Al-Worafi et al., 2017; Al-Worafi, 2018a-d;Al-Worafi et al., 2018a-b; Al-Worafi et al., 2019; Al-Worafi, 2020a-z; Al-Worafi et al., 2020a-b; Al-Worafi et al., 2021a,b; Al-Worafi, 2022a,b; Al-Worafi, 2023a; Baig et al., 2020; Elkalmi et al., 2020; Elsayed & Al-Worafi, 2020; Hasan et al., 2019; Hassan et al., 2014; Izhar et al., 2017; Lee et al., 2017; Mahmoud et al., 2020; Manan et al., 2014; Manan et al., 2016; Ming et al., 2016; Ming et al., 2020; Othman et al., 2020; Saeed et al., 2014) which are discussed below:

1. Increase public awareness: Educate the public on the safe use of medications, including how to read labels, store and dispose of medications, and recognize potential side effects. This can be done through public health campaigns, patient education materials, and community outreach programs.

2. Improve healthcare provider training: Healthcare providers in developing countries may not have access to the same level of training and resources as those in developed countries. Providing regular training on medication safety practices can help reduce medication errors and improve patient outcomes.

3. Implement medication reconciliation: Medication reconciliation is a process of comparing a patient's current medication regimen to what is prescribed. This helps prevent medication errors due to miscommunication or duplication of medications. Developing countries can implement medication reconciliation in their healthcare systems to improve medication safety.

4. Establish a medication safety committee: Developing countries can create a committee focused on medication safety. This committee can develop and implement medication safety protocols, conduct regular medication safety audits, and provide recommendations for improving medication safety practices.

5. Strengthen drug regulatory systems: Developing countries should strengthen their drug regulatory systems to ensure that medications are safe, effective, and of high quality. This

includes regulating the import and distribution of medications, monitoring adverse drug reactions, and conducting regular inspections of drug manufacturing facilities.

6. Enhance patient monitoring: Developing countries can enhance patient monitoring by implementing electronic health records systems and improving medication dispensing and tracking systems. This can help healthcare providers identify potential medication errors or adverse drug reactions.

7. Improve medication access: Access to essential medicines is essential for ensuring medication safety. Developing countries should prioritize improving access to essential medicines by addressing issues such as availability, affordability, and distribution.

8. Strengthen regulatory systems: Developing countries should establish and strengthen regulatory systems for medicines to ensure that they are safe, effective, and of good quality. Regulatory systems should include procedures for registration, licensing, inspection, and post-marketing surveillance.

9. Increase awareness and education: Healthcare professionals and patients in developing countries should be educated about medication safety, including the proper use, storage, and disposal of medications. Education should also include information on potential medication interactions, side effects, and adverse events.

10. Develop medication guidelines: Developing countries should establish medication guidelines that outline the appropriate use of medications based on evidence-based practices. These guidelines should be regularly updated to reflect new evidence and changes in medication safety practices.

11. Enhance medication labeling: Medication labeling should be improved to include clear and concise information on the name of the medication, dosage, instructions for use, and potential side effects. Labeling should be available in local languages and should be easy to understand.

12. Encourage reporting of adverse events: Healthcare professionals and patients should be encouraged to report adverse events associated with medications to relevant regulatory bodies. Reporting can help identify potential medication safety issues and inform regulatory decisions.

13. Improve medication storage and disposal: Developing countries should establish guidelines for the proper storage and disposal of medications to prevent contamination and ensure their effectiveness. Storage should be in a cool, dry place, and disposal should follow local regulations to prevent environmental harm.

14. Support research and development: Developing countries should support research and development in medication safety, including the development of new medications, improved medication delivery systems, and the identification of new medication safety issues.

18.13 CONCLUSION

This chapter has discussed medication safety practices in developing countries, improving access to essential medicines, strengthening regulatory systems, increasing awareness and education, developing medication guidelines, enhancing medication labeling, encouraging reporting of adverse events, improving medication storage and disposal, and supporting research and development. These recommendations can help improve medication safety and improve health outcomes in developing countries.

REFERENCES

Al-Qahtani, I., Almoteb, T.M., & Al-Warafi, Y. (2015). Competency of metered-dose inhaler use among Saudi community pharmacists: A Simulation method study. *RRJPPS*, 4(2), 37–31.

Alshahrani, S.M., Alakhali, K.M., & Al-Worafi, Y.M. (2019a). Medication errors in a health care facility in southern Saudi Arabia. *Tropical Journal of Pharmaceutical Research*, 18(5), 1119–1122.

Alshahrani, S.M., Alavudeen, S.S., Alakhali, K.M., Al-Worafi, Y.M., Bahamdan, A.K., & Vigneshwaran, E. (2019b). Self-Medication Among King Khalid University Students, Saudi Arabia. *Risk Management and Healthcare Policy*, 12, 243–249.

Alshahrani, S.M., Alakhali, K.M., Al-Worafi, Y.M., & Alshahrani, N.Z. (2020a). Awareness and use of over the counter analgesic medication: a survey in the Aseer region population, Saudi Arabia. *International Journal of Advances in Applied Sciences*, 7(3), 130–134.

Alshahrani, S.M., Alzahran, M., Alakhali, K., Vigneshwaran, E., Iqbal, M.J., Khan, N.A., ... & Alavudeen, S.S. (2020b). Association Between Diabetes Consequences and Quality of Life Among Patients With Diabetes Mellitus in the Aseer Province of Saudi Arabia. *Open Access Macedonian Journal of Medical Sciences*, 8(E), 325–330.

Al-Worafi, Y.M. (2014). Prescription writing errors at a tertiary care hospital in Yemen: prevalence, types, causes and recommendations. *American Journal of Pharmacy and Health Research*, 2, 134–140.

Al-Worafi, Y.M.A. (2015). Appropriateness of metered-dose inhaler use in the Yemeni community pharmacies. *Journal of Taibah University Medical Sciences*, 10(3), 353–358.

Al-Worafi, Y.M.A. (2016). Pharmacy practice in Yemen. In *Pharmacy Practice in Developing Countries* (pp. 267–287). Academic Press.

Al-Worafi, Y.M., Kassab, Y.W., Alseragi, W.M., Almutairi, M.S., Ahmed, A., Ming, L.C., Alkhoshaiban, A.S., & Hadi, M.A. (2017). Pharmacovigilance and adverse drg reaction reporting: a perspective of community pharmacists and pharmacy technicians in Sana'a, Yemen. *Ther. Clin. Risk. Manag.*, 13, 1175.

Al-Worafi, Y.M. (2018a). Knowledge, Attitude and Practice of Yemeni Physicians Toward Pharmacovigilance: A Mixed Method Study. *International Journal of Pharmacy and Pharmaceutical Sciences*, 10 (10), 74–77.

Al-Worafi, Y. (2018b). Knowledge, attitude and practice of Yemeni physicians toward pharmacovigilance: A mixed method study. *International Journal of Pharmacy and Pharmaceutical Sciences*, 10, 74–77.

Al-Worafi, Y.M. (2018c). Dispensing errors observed by community pharmacy dispensers in IBB–YEMEN. *Asian Journal of Pharmaceutical and Clinical Research*, 11(11).

Al-Worafi, Y.M. (2018d). Evauation of inhaler technique among patients with asthma and COPD in Yemen. *Journal of Taibah University Medical Sciences*, 13(5), 488–490.

Al-Worafi, Y.M., Patel, R.P., Zaidi, S.T.R., Alseragi, W.M., Almutairi, M.S., Alkhoshaiban, A.S., & Ming, L.C. (2018a). Completeness and legibility of handwritten prescriptions in Sana'a, Yemen. *Medical Principles and Practice*, 27, 290–292.

Al-Worafi, Y.M., Alseragi, W.M., Seng, L.K., Kassab, Y.W., Yeoh, S.F., Chiau, L., ... & Husain, K. (2018b). Dispensing errors in community pharmacies: A prospective study in Sana'a, Yemen. *Arch Pharm Pract*, 9(4), 1–3.

Al-Worafi, Y.M., Alseragi, W.M., & Mahmoud, M.A. (2019). Competency of metered-dose inhaler use among community pharmacy dispensers in Ibb, Yemen: A simulation method study. *Latin American Journal of Pharmacy*, 38(3), 489–494.

Al-Worafi, Y.M. (Ed.). (2020a). *Drug Safety in Developing Countries: Achievements and Challenges*.

Al-Worafi, Y.M. (2020b). Medication errors. In *Drug Safety in Developing Countries* (pp. 105–117). Academic Press.

Al-Worafi, Y.M. (2020c). Adverse drug reactions. In *Drug Safety in Developing Countries* (pp. 39–57). Academic Press.

Al-Worafi, Y.M. (2020d). Medications registration and marketing: safety-related issues. In *Drug Safety in Developing Countries* (pp. 21–28). Academic Press.

Al-Worafi, Y.M. (2020e). Pharmacovigilance. In *Drug Safety in Developing Countries* (pp. 29–38). Academic Press.

Al-Worafi, Y.M. (2020f). Drug-related problems. In *Drug Safety In Developing Countries* (pp. 59–71). Academic Press.

Al-Worafi, Y.M. (2020g). Medications safety-related terminology. In *Drug safety in Developing Countries* (pp. 7–19). Academic Press.

Al-Worafi, Y.M. (2020h). Self-medication. In *Drug Safety in Developing Countries* (pp. 73–86). Academic Press.

Al-Worafi, Y.M. (2020j). Antibiotics safety issues. In *Drug Safety in Developing Countries* (pp. 87–103). Academic Press.

Al-Worafi, Y.M. (2020k). Medications safety research issues. In *Drug Safety in Developing Countries* (pp. 213–227). Academic Press.

Al-Worafi, Y.M. (2020l). Counterfeit and substandard medications. In *Drug Safety in Developing Countries* (pp. 119–126). Academic Press.

Al-Worafi, Y.M. (2020m). Medication abuse and misuse. In *Drug Safety in Developing Countries* (pp. 127–135). Academic Press.

Al-Worafi, Y.M. (2020n). Storage and disposal of medications. In *Drug Safety in Developing Countries* (pp. 137–142). Academic Press.

Al-Worafi, Y.M. (2020o). Safety of medications in special population. In *Drug Safety in Developing Countries* (pp. 143–162). Academic Press.

Al-Worafi, Y.M. (2020p). Herbal medicines safety issues. In *Drug Safety in Developing Countries* (pp. 163–178). Academic Press.

Al-Worafi, Y.M. (2020q). Medications safety pharmacoeconomics-related issues. In *Drug Safety in Developing Countries* (pp. 187–195). Academic Press.

Al-Worafi, Y.M. (2020r). Evidence-based medications safety practice. In *Drug Safety in Developing Countries* (pp. 197–201). Academic Press.

Al-Worafi, Y.M. (2020s). Quality indicators for medications safety. In *Drug Safety in Developing Countries* (pp. 229–242). Academic Press.

Al-Worafi, Y.M. (2020t). Drug safety in Yemen. In *Drug Safety in Developing Countries* (pp. 391–405). Academic Press.

Al-Worafi, Y.M. (2020u). Drug safety in Saudi Arabia. In *Drug Safety in Developing Countries* (pp. 407–417). Academic Press.

Al-Worafi, Y.M. (2020v). Drug safety in United Arab Emirates. In *Drug Safety in Developing Countries* (pp. 419–428). Academic Press.

Al-Worafi, Y.M. (2020w). Drug safety in Indonesia. In *Drug Safety in Developing Countries* (pp. 279–285). Academic Press.

Al-Worafi, Y.M. (2020x). Drug safety in Palestine. In *Drug Safety in Developing Countries* (pp. 471–480). Academic Press.

Al-Worafi, Y.M. (2020y). Drug safety: comparison between developing countries. In *Drug Safety in Developing Countries* (pp. 603–611). Academic Press.

Al-Worafi, Y.M. (2020z). Drug safety in developing versus developed countries. In *Drug Safety in Developing Countries* (pp. 613–615). Academic Press.

Al-Worafi, Y.M., Alseragi, W.M., Ming, L.C., & Alakhali, K.M. (2020a). Drug safety in China. In *Drug Safety in Developing Countries* (pp. 381–388). Academic Press.

Al-Worafi, Y.M., Alseragi, W.M., Alakhali, K.M., Ming, L.C., Othman, G., Halboup, A.M., … & Elkalmi, R.M. (2020b). Knowledge, beliefs and factors affecting the use of generic medicines among patients in Ibb, Yemen: A mixed-method study. *Journal of Pharmacy Practice and Community Medicine*, 6(4).

Al-Worafi, Y.M., Elkalmi, R.M., Ming, L.C., Othman, G., Halboup, A.M., Battah, M.M., … & Mani, V. (2021a). Dispensing errors in hospital pharmacies: A prospective study in Yemen.

Al-Worafi, Y.M., Hasan, S., Hassan, N.M., & Gaili, A.A. (2021b). Knowledge, Attitude and Experience of Pharmacist in the UAE towards Pharmacovigilance. *Research Journal of Pharmacy and Technology*, 14(1), 265–269.

Al-Worafi, Y. (2022a). *A Guide to Online Pharmacy Education: Teaching Strategies and Assessment Methods*. CRC Press.

Al-Worafi, Y.M. (2022b). Patient care errors and related problems (part I): development and validation of the model. https://orcid.org/0000-0002-5752-2913

Al-Worafi, Y.M. (Ed.). (2023). *Clinical Case Studies on Medication Safety*. Academic Press.

Baig, M.R., Al-Worafi, Y.M., Alseragi, W.M., Ming, L.C., & Siddique, A. (2020). Drug safety in India. In *Drug Safety in Developing Countries* (pp. 327–334). Academic Press.

Elkalmi, R.M., Al-Worafi, Y.M., Alseragi, W.M., Ming, L.C., & Siddique, A. (2020). Drug safety in Malaysia. In *Drug Safety in Developing Countries* (pp. 245–253). Academic Press.

Elsayed, T., & Al-Worafi, Y.M. (2020). Drug safety in Egypt. In *Drug Safety in Developing Countries* (pp. 511–523). Academic Press.

Hasan, S., Al-Omar, M.J., AlZubaidy, H., & Al-Worafi, Y.M. (2019). Use of medications in Arab Countries. *Handbook of Healthcare in the Arab World*. Cham: Springer, 42.

Hassan, Y., Abd Aziz, N., Kassab, Y.W., Elgasim, I., Shaharuddin, S., Al-Worafi, Y.M.A., … & Ming, L.C. (2014). How to help patients to control their blood pressure? Blood pressure control and its predictor. *Archives of Pharmacy Practice*, 5(4).

Izahar, S., Lean, Q.Y., Hameed, M.A., Murugiah, M.K., Patel, R.P., Al-Worafi, Y.M., … & Ming, L.C. (2017). Content analysis of mobile health applications on diabetes mellitus. *Frontiers in Endocrinology*, 8, 318.

Lee, K.S., Yee, S.M., Zaidi, S.T.R., Patel, R.P., Yang, Q., Al-Worafi, Y.M., & Ming, L.C., 2017. Combating sale of counterfeit and falsified medicines online: a losing battle. *Frontiers in Pharmacology*, 8, 268.

Mahmoud, M.A., Wajid, S., Naqvi, A.A., Samreen, S., Althagfan, S.S., & Al-Worafi, Y. (2020). Self-medication with antibiotics: A cross-sectional community-based study. *Latin American Journal of Pharmacy*, 39(2), 348–353.

Manan, M.M., Rusli, R.A., Ang, W.C., Al-Worafi, Y.M., & Ming, L.C. (2014). Assessing the pharmaceutical care issues of antiepileptic drug therapy in hospitalised epileptic patients. *Journal of Pharmacy Practice and Research*, 44(3), 83–88.

Manan, M.M., Ibrahim, N.A., Aziz, N.A., Zulkifly, H.H., Al-Worafi, Y.M.A., & Long, C.M. (2016). Empirical use of antibiotic therapy in the prevention of early onset sepsis in neonates: a pilot study. *Archives of Medical Science*, 12(3), 603–613.

Ming, L.C., Hameed, M.A., Lee, D.D., Apidi, N.A., Lai, P.S.M., Hadi, M.A., Al-Worafi, Y.M.A. and Khan, T.M., (2016). Use of medical mobile applications among hospital pharmacists in Malaysia. *Therapeutic Innovation & Regulatory Science*, 50(4), pp. 419–426.

Ming, L.C., Untong, N., Aliudin, N.A., Osili, N., Kifli, N., Tan, C.S., ... & Goh, H.P. (2020). Mobile health apps on COVID-19 launched in the early days of the pandemic: content analysis and review. *JMIR mHealth and uHealth*, 8(9), e19796.

Othman, G., Ali, F., Ibrahim, M.I.M., Al-Worafi, Y.M., Ansari, M., & Halboup, A.M. (2020). Assessment of Anti-Diabetic Medications Adherence among Diabetic Patients in Sana'a City, Yemen: A Cross Sectional Study. *Journal of Pharmaceutical Research International*, 32(21), 114–122.

Saeed, M.S., Alkhoshaiban, A.S., Al-Worafi, Y.M.A., & Long, C.M. (2014). Perception of self-medication among university students in Saudi Arabia. *Archives of Pharmacy Practice*, 5(4), 149.

19 Patient Safety Culture

19.1 BACKGROUND

Patient safety culture refers to the attitudes, beliefs, values, and practices that shape the way healthcare providers and organizations approach patient safety. It encompasses the entire healthcare system, from individual providers to hospitals and other healthcare organizations, and encompasses a range of activities designed to reduce the risk of harm to patients. Patient safety culture is focused on the aspects of organizational culture that relate to patient safety. It is defined as a pattern of individual and organizational behavior, based upon shared beliefs and values that continuously seek to minimize patient harm, which may result from the process of care delivery. A positive patient safety culture is one in which all stakeholders are committed to promoting safety, and where there is a shared understanding of the importance of patient safety. This includes a willingness to report errors, near-misses, and adverse events, and a commitment to learning from these incidents and making improvements to prevent them from happening in the future. Positive patient safety cultures have strong leadership that drives and prioritizes safety. Commitment from leaders and managers is key, their actions and attitudes influence the perceptions, attitudes, and behaviors of the wider workforce. Key elements of a positive patient safety culture include effective communication, leadership commitment, continuous improvement, transparency, and a focus on learning and education. By fostering a positive patient safety culture, healthcare organizations can improve patient outcomes, reduce the risk of adverse events, and enhance the overall quality of care they provide (Kristensen & Bartels, 2010; Reynard et al., 2009; Salas & Frush, 2012; Vincent, 2011).

Other important aspects of positive patient safety culture include:

- Shared perceptions of the importance of safety

- Constructive communication

- Mutual trust

- A workforce that is engaged and always aware that things can go wrong

- Acknowledgment at all levels that mistakes occur

- Ability to recognize, respond to, give feedback about, and learn from, adverse events.

Patient safety inquiries provide insights into the potentially catastrophic impact of dysfunctional workplace cultures on patient care.

A review of inquiries identified the following common deficits4:

- Limitations in the Standard of clinical governance

- An absence of monitoring important metrics in relation to patient outcomes

- A preference to focus on financial targets rather than healthcare process and outcome targets

- Pressure on staff

- An organizational culture that is considered unhealthy and fails to place the patient at the center of all activities

19.2 THE FIELD OF PATIENT SAFETY CULTURE

The field of patient safety culture focuses on promoting a culture of safety in healthcare organizations. It is concerned with identifying and addressing factors that can contribute to medical errors, adverse events, and harm to patients. Patient safety culture is defined as the collective beliefs, values, attitudes, and behaviors that determine how safety is prioritized and operationalized within an organization. A positive patient safety culture is one in which there is a shared commitment to safety, open communication, active learning, and continuous improvement. Efforts to improve patient safety culture may involve implementing evidence-based practices, such as team training, communication skills training, and error reporting systems. It may also involve addressing organizational factors, such as staffing levels, leadership support, and work environment Kristensen & Bartels,2010; Reynard et al., 2009; Salas & Frush, 2012; Vincent, 2011).

19.3 PATIENT SAFETY CULTURE DIMENSIONS

There are several dimensions that are typically used to assess patient safety culture. These dimensions include:

1. Leadership support for patient safety: This dimension assesses the extent to which leaders within the organization prioritize patient safety and provide support for initiatives to improve patient safety.

2. Teamwork: This dimension assesses the level of collaboration and communication among healthcare providers within the organization, as well as the extent to which providers work together to promote patient safety.

3. Communication openness: This dimension assesses the extent to which healthcare providers feel comfortable reporting errors, near-misses, and other safety concerns, and the organization's response to these reports.

4. Feedback and communication about errors: This dimension assesses the extent to which healthcare providers receive feedback and information about errors and near-misses, and how this feedback is used to improve patient safety.

5. Staffing: This dimension assesses the adequacy of staffing levels and the impact of staffing on patient safety.

6. Non-punitive response to error: This dimension assesses the extent to which healthcare providers feel comfortable reporting errors without fear of punishment or retribution.

7. Organizational learning and continuous improvement: This dimension assesses the organization's commitment to learning from errors and near-misses and implementing changes to improve patient safety.

8. Patient-centered care: This dimension assesses the extent to which the organization prioritizes the needs and preferences of patients and involves patients in their care.

9. Handoffs and transitions: This dimension assesses the communication and collaboration between healthcare providers during handoffs and transitions in care.

By assessing these dimensions of patient safety culture, healthcare organizations can identify areas for improvement and develop strategies to enhance patient safety and reduce the risk of harm to patients.

19.4 RATIONALITY OF PATIENT SAFETY CULTURE

The goal of improving patient safety culture is to create a healthcare system in which patients receive safe, high-quality care. By focusing on patient safety culture, healthcare organizations can reduce medical errors, improve patient outcomes, and enhance patient and staff satisfaction. The rationality of patient safety culture lies in the fact that it promotes the delivery of safe, effective, and high-quality healthcare to patients. Patient safety culture recognizes that errors and adverse events can occur in any healthcare setting, but by establishing a culture of safety, organizations can minimize the likelihood of such events and improve patient outcomes Kristensen & Bartels, 2010; Reynard et al., 2009; Salas & Frush, 2012; Vincent, 2011). A positive patient safety culture can lead to a number of benefits, including:

1. Improved patient outcomes: A culture of safety can reduce medical errors, adverse events, and harm to patients, ultimately leading to better patient outcomes.

2. Increased staff engagement and satisfaction: Staff who work in a culture of safety are more engaged and satisfied with their work, leading to improved staff retention and recruitment.

3. Enhanced organizational reputation: Organizations with a strong patient safety culture are viewed positively by patients, their families, and the community, leading to enhanced organizational reputation.

4. Reduced healthcare costs: A culture of safety can reduce healthcare costs associated with medical errors, adverse events, and lawsuits.

Overall, the rationality of patient safety culture is clear: it is essential for healthcare organizations to prioritize patient safety in order to improve patient outcomes, reduce healthcare costs, and enhance organizational reputation.

19.5 IMPORTANCE OF PATIENT SAFETY CULTURE

Patient safety culture is critical to the delivery of safe, high-quality healthcare. A patient safety culture is a set of values, beliefs, and behaviors that shape the attitudes and practices of healthcare professionals and organizations toward patient safety.

Here are some of the reasons why patient safety culture is important:

1. Reduces errors and adverse events: A strong patient safety culture can reduce errors and adverse events that can harm patients. It encourages healthcare professionals to be vigilant, identify risks, and take corrective actions before harm occurs.

2. Improves quality of care: A patient safety culture supports the delivery of high-quality care by promoting a focus on patient-centeredness, teamwork, and continuous improvement.

3. Enhances patient satisfaction: When patients feel safe and confident in the care they receive, they are more satisfied with their healthcare experience.

4. Increases trust: Patient safety culture increases trust between patients and healthcare providers, which is essential for building strong and effective relationships.

5. Reduces healthcare costs: Improving patient safety culture can help reduce healthcare costs associated with medical errors, adverse events, and malpractice claims.

In summary, a patient safety culture is essential for improving patient outcomes, enhancing the quality of care, increasing patient satisfaction, building trust, and reducing healthcare costs

19.6 MEASURING PATIENT SAFETY CULTURE

Measurement of patient safety culture enables the identification of strengths and areas for improvement. This information can be used to develop appropriate interventions. Patient safety culture measures can also be used to evaluate new safety programs by comparing results before and after implementation. Patient safety culture can be measured through surveys of hospital staff, qualitative measurement (focus groups, interviews), ethnographic investigation, or a combination of these. Surveys of hospital staff are the most common way of measuring patient safety culture. Patient safety culture forms one component of a comprehensive measurement and improvement system; it should be measured alongside other indicators of safety and quality, such as complications acquired while in the hospital, accreditation outcomes, mortality, patient-reported measures, and serious in-hospital incidents.

Patient safety culture assessment is a process of evaluating the safety culture of healthcare organizations to identify areas for improvement and implement strategies to enhance patient safety. It involves collecting and analyzing data on various aspects of an organization's safety culture, such as its policies and procedures, leadership, communication, and teamwork. There are several methods for conducting patient safety culture assessments, including surveys, interviews, and focus groups. Surveys are the most common methods and typically involve asking healthcare providers to rate their perceptions of various aspects of patient safety culture on a Likert scale. The Agency for Healthcare Research and Quality (AHRQ) has developed a widely used patient safety culture survey, the Hospital Survey on Patient Safety Culture, which consists of 42 items that assess 12 dimensions of patient safety culture. Other organizations may use different surveys or customize the AHRQ survey to meet their specific needs. In addition to surveys, interviews and focus groups can provide valuable qualitative data about the strengths and weaknesses of an organization's safety culture. These methods allow for a more in-depth exploration of the attitudes and behaviors of healthcare providers and can uncover issues that may not be apparent in survey data.

Once the data has been collected, it is analyzed to identify areas for improvement and develop strategies to enhance patient safety culture. This may involve developing new policies and procedures, providing additional training and education to healthcare providers, improving communication and teamwork, or making changes to the physical environment.

Patient safety culture assessment is an important tool for improving patient safety and reducing the risk of harm to patients. By regularly assessing and monitoring their safety culture, healthcare organizations can identify and address potential risks and continuously improve the quality of care they provide.

19.7 FACTORS AFFECTING PATIENT SAFETY CULTURE

Several factors can affect patient safety culture in healthcare organizations, including:

1. Leadership: The leadership style and actions of senior management can have a significant impact on the patient safety culture within an organization. Effective leadership should prioritize patient safety, communicate this priority to staff, and model safe behaviors.

2. Communication: Open and transparent communication is essential for a positive patient safety culture. Healthcare organizations should establish channels for staff to report errors and near misses, and encourage a culture of learning from mistakes.

3. Staffing levels: Adequate staffing levels are critical for ensuring patient safety. When staffing levels are insufficient, staff may feel pressured to rush through tasks and may be more likely to make errors.

4. Training and education: Providing staff with regular training and education on patient safety practices and procedures can help to create a culture of safety. This includes training on communication skills, teamwork, and error prevention strategies.

5. Work environment: The physical and emotional work environment can have a significant impact on patient safety culture. A safe and supportive work environment can promote staff engagement and reduce the likelihood of errors.

6. Regulatory requirements: Compliance with regulatory requirements, such as those from accreditation bodies and government agencies, can also affect patient safety culture. Organizations that prioritize compliance may be more likely to prioritize patient safety.

By addressing these factors, healthcare organizations can work to promote a culture of safety and improve patient outcomes.

19.8 PERCEPTIONS AND ATTITUDES OF HEALTHCARE PROVIDERS AND PROFESSIONALS TOWARD PATIENT SAFETY CULTURE

The perceptions and attitudes of healthcare providers and professionals towards patient safety culture can have a significant impact on the delivery of safe and effective healthcare. Here are some common perceptions and attitudes of healthcare providers toward patient safety culture:

- Importance of patient safety: Many healthcare providers recognize the importance of patient safety and the need for a strong patient safety culture to prevent medical errors and adverse events.

- Resistance to change: Some healthcare providers may resist changes in practice or procedures that are designed to improve patient safety, either due to a lack of understanding or a perceived burden on their workload.

- Fear of blame and punishment: Healthcare providers may be hesitant to report errors or adverse events due to fear of blame, punishment, or legal consequences.

- Lack of teamwork and communication: Poor communication and teamwork can lead to breakdowns in patient safety and contribute to errors and adverse events.

- Prioritization of other goals: Some healthcare providers may prioritize other goals, such as cost savings or productivity, over patient safety.

- Emphasis on individual responsibility: While individual accountability is important, healthcare providers may view patient safety as solely their responsibility rather than a collective responsibility shared by the entire healthcare team.

- Safety culture is important: Most healthcare providers recognize the importance of safety culture in promoting patient safety and quality of care.

- Safety culture is everyone's responsibility: Healthcare providers understand that promoting safety culture is not the sole responsibility of any one individual or department, but rather a shared responsibility among all healthcare professionals.

- Time constraints and workload: Healthcare providers may feel overwhelmed by their workload and may prioritize completing tasks over safety concerns, leading to potential safety incidents.

- Lack of resources and support: Healthcare providers may not have adequate resources and support to implement safety measures effectively, such as staffing, training, and equipment.

- Communication breakdown: Communication breakdown between healthcare providers can contribute to safety incidents, particularly when information is not shared effectively or when there is a lack of collaboration among team members.

To promote a positive patient safety culture, healthcare organizations should prioritize the promotion of open communication, encourage reporting of safety incidents without fear of blame or punishment, provide resources and support to staff, and implement effective training programs. It is essential to recognize that creating and maintaining a positive safety culture requires a sustained effort and a commitment to continuous improvement.

9.9 RECOMMENDATIONS FOR THE BEST PATIENT CULTURE SAFETY PRACTICE IN DEVELOPING COUNTRIES

Despite the progress in research about patient care and safety in developing countries, there is little research about the patient safety culture in the majority of developing countries (Alshahrani et al., 2019a,b; Al-Qahtani et al., 2015; Alshahrani et al., 2020a,b; Al-Worafi, 2014; Al-Worafi, 2015; Al-W1orafi, 2016; Al-Worafi et al., 2017; Al-Worafi, 2018a-d; Al-Worafi et al., 2018a-b; Al-Worafi et al., 2019; Al-Worafi, 2020a-z; Al-Worafi et al., 2020a-b; Al-Worafi et al., 2021a,b; Al-Worafi, 2022a,b; Al-Worafi, 2023; Baig et al., 2020; Elkalmi et al., 2020; Elsayed & Al-Worafi, 2020; Hasan et al., 2019; Hassan et al., 2014; Izhar et al., 2017; Lee et al., 2017; Mahmoud et al., 2020; Manan et al., 2014; Manan et al., 2016; Ming et al., 2016; Ming et al., 2020; Othman et al., 2020; Saeed et al., 2014). Improving patient safety culture is a complex and ongoing process that requires the commitment of all healthcare providers and stakeholders. However, there are several recommendations that can be implemented in developing countries to enhance patient safety culture. Here are some of them:

1. Develop a safety culture program: Developing a comprehensive safety culture program that includes policies, procedures, and training programs can help promote a culture of safety within healthcare organizations.

2. Encourage open communication: Encouraging open communication among healthcare providers and patients can help identify and address potential safety issues before they become serious.

3. Use of checklists: The use of checklists in clinical practice has been shown to improve patient safety and reduce errors. Developing and implementing checklists can be particularly beneficial in developing countries where resources may be limited.

4. Improve infection control: Infection control is a critical component of patient safety culture. Implementing effective infection control measures such as hand hygiene, sterilization of equipment, and appropriate use of personal protective equipment can help reduce the risk of healthcare-associated infections.

5. Increase access to information: Providing patients with access to information about their healthcare and treatment options can help them make informed decisions and participate more fully in their care.

6. Implement patient safety reporting systems: Developing a patient safety reporting system can help healthcare providers identify and address safety concerns in real time.

7. Invest in healthcare workforce training: Investing in training programs for healthcare providers can help improve their knowledge and skills and promote a culture of safety within healthcare organizations.

Overall, developing a patient safety culture requires a sustained effort and a commitment to continuous improvement. These recommendations can help provide a framework for promoting patient safety culture in developing countries.

19.10 CONCLUSION

This chapter has discussed and described patient safety culture-related issues, and also described the recommendations for the best practice in developing countries. Patient safety culture refers to the attitudes, beliefs, values, and practices that shape the way healthcare providers and organizations approach patient safety. It encompasses the entire healthcare system, from individual providers to hospitals and other healthcare organizations, and encompasses a range of activities designed to reduce the risk of harm to patients. Patient safety culture is focused on the aspects of organizational culture that relate to patient safety.

REFERENCES

Al-Qahtani, I., Almoteb, T.M., & Al-Warafi, Y. (2015). Competency of metered-dose inhaler use among Saudi community pharmacists: A Simulation method study. *RRJPPS*, 4(2), 37–31.

Alshahrani, S.M., Alakhali, K.M., & Al-Worafi, Y.M. (2019a). Medication errors in a health care facility in southern Saudi Arabia. *Tropical Journal of Pharmaceutical Research*, 18(5), 1119–1122.

Alshahrani, S.M., Alavudeen, S.S., Alakhali, K.M., Al-Worafi, Y.M., Bahamdan, A.K., & Vigneshwaran, E. (2019b). Self-Medication Among King Khalid University Students, *Saudi Arabia. Risk Management and Healthcare Policy*, 12, 243–249.

Alshahrani, S.M., Alakhali, K.M., Al-Worafi, Y.M., & Alshahrani, N.Z. (2020a). Awareness and use of over the counter analgesic medication: a survey in the Aseer region population, Saudi Arabia. *International Journal of Advances in Applied Sciences*, 7(3), 130–134.

Alshahrani, S.M., Alzahran, M., Alakhali, K., Vigneshwaran, E., Iqbal, M.J., Khan, N.A., … & Alavudeen, S.S. (2020b). Association Between Diabetes Consequences and Quality of Life Among Patients With Diabetes Mellitus in the Aseer Province of Saudi Arabia. *Open Access Macedonian Journal of Medical Sciences*, 8(E), 325–330.

Al-Worafi, Y.M. (2014). Prescription writing errors at a tertiary care hospital in Yemen: prevalence, types, causes and recommendations. *American Journal of Pharmacy and Health Research*, 2, 134–140.

Al-Worafi, Y.M.A. (2015). Appropriateness of metered-dose inhaler use in the Yemeni community pharmacies. *Journal of Taibah University Medical Sciences*, 10(3), 353–358.

Al-Worafi, Y.M.A. (2016). Pharmacy practice in Yemen. In *Pharmacy Practice in Developing Countries* (pp. 267–287). Academic Press.

Al-Worafi, Y.M., Kassab, Y.W., Alseragi, W.M., Almutairi, M.S., Ahmed, A., Ming, L.C., Alkhoshaiban, A.S., & Hadi, M.A. (2017). Pharmacovigilance and adverse drg reaction reporting: a perspective of community pharmacists and pharmacy technicians in Sana'a, Yemen. *Therapeutics and Clinical Risk Management*, 13, 1175.

Al-Worafi, Y.M. (2018a). Knowledge, Attitude and Practice of Yemeni Physicians Toward Pharmacovigilance: A Mixed Method Study. *International Journal of Pharmacy and Pharmaceutical Sciences*, 10 (10), 74–77.

Al-Worafi, Y. (2018b). Knowledge, attitude and practice of Yemeni physicians toward pharmacovigilance: A mixed method study. *International Journal of Pharmacy and Pharmaceutical Sciences*, 10, 74–77.

Al-Worafi, Y.M. (2018c). Dispensing errors observed by community pharmacy dispensers in IBB–YEMEN. *Asian Journal of Pharmaceutical and Clinical Research*, 11(11).

Al-Worafi, Y.M. (2018d). Evauation of inhaler technique among patients with asthma and COPD in Yemen. *Journal of Taibah University Medical Sciences*, 13(5), 488–490.

Al-Worafi, Y.M., Patel, R.P., Zaidi, S.T.R., Alseragi, W.M., Almutairi, M.S., Alkhoshaiban, A.S., & Ming, L.C. (2018a). Completeness and legibility of handwritten prescriptions in Sana'a, Yemen. *Medical Principles and Practice*, 27, 290–292.

Al-Worafi, Y.M., Alseragi, W.M., Seng, L.K., Kassab, Y.W., Yeoh, S.F., Chiau, L., … & Husain, K. (2018b). Dispensing errors in community pharmacies: a prospective study in Sana'a, Yemen. *Archives of Pharmacy Practice*, 9(4), 1–3.

Al-Worafi, Y.M., Alseragi, W.M., & Mahmoud, M.A. (2019). Competency of metered-dose inhaler use among community pharmacy dispensers in Ibb, Yemen: A simulation method study. *Latin American Journal of Pharmacy*, 38(3), 489–494.

Al-Worafi, Y.M. (Ed.). (2020a). *Drug Safety in Developing Countries: Achievements and Challenges.*

Al-Worafi, Y.M. (2020b). Medication errors. In *Drug Safety in Developing Countries* (pp. 105–117). Academic Press.

Al-Worafi, Y.M. (2020c). Adverse drug reactions. In *Drug Safety in Developing Countries* (pp. 39–57). Academic Press.

Al-Worafi, Y.M. (2020d). Medications registration and marketing: safety-related issues. In *Drug Safety in Developing Countries* (pp. 21–28). Academic Press.

Al-Worafi, Y.M. (2020e). Pharmacovigilance. In *Drug Safety in Developing Countries* (pp. 29–38). Academic Press.

Al-Worafi, Y.M. (2020f). Drug-related problems. In *Drug Safety in Developing Countries* (pp. 59–71). Academic Press.

Al-Worafi, Y.M. (2020g). Medications safety-related terminology. In *Drug Safety in Developing Countries* (pp. 7–19). Academic Press.

Al-Worafi, Y.M. (2020h). Self-medication. In *Drug Safety in Developing Countries* (pp. 73–86). Academic Press.

Al-Worafi, Y.M. (2020j). Antibiotics safety issues. In *Drug Safety in Developing Countries* (pp. 87–103). Academic Press.

Al-Worafi, Y.M. (2020k). Medications safety research issues. In *Drug Safety in Developing Countries* (pp. 213–227). Academic Press.

Al-Worafi, Y.M. (2020l). Counterfeit and substandard medications. In *Drug Safety in Developing Countries* (pp. 119–126). Academic Press.

Al-Worafi, Y.M. (2020m). Medication abuse and misuse. In *Drug Safety in Developing Countries* (pp. 127–135). Academic Press.

Al-Worafi, Y.M. (2020n). Storage and disposal of medications. In *Drug Safety in Developing Countries* (pp. 137–142). Academic Press.

Al-Worafi, Y.M. (2020o). Safety of medications in special population. In *Drug safety in Developing Countries* (pp. 143–162). Academic Press.

Al-Worafi, Y.M. (2020p). Herbal medicines safety issues. In *Drug Safety in Developing Countries* (pp. 163–178). Academic Press.

Al-Worafi, Y.M. (2020q). Medications safety pharmacoeconomics-related issues. In *Drug Safety in Developing Countries* (pp. 187–195). Academic Press.

Al-Worafi, Y.M. (2020r). Evidence-based medications safety practice. In *Drug Safety in Developing Countries* (pp. 197–201). Academic Press.

Al-Worafi, Y.M. (2020s). Quality indicators for medications safety. In *Drug Safety in Developing Countries* (pp. 229–242). Academic Press.

Al-Worafi, Y.M. (2020t). Drug safety in Yemen. In *Drug Safety in Developing Countries* (pp. 391–405). Academic Press.

Al-Worafi, Y.M. (2020u). Drug safety in Saudi Arabia. In *Drug Safety in Developing Countries* (pp. 407–417). Academic Press.

Al-Worafi, Y.M. (2020v). Drug safety in United Arab Emirates. In *Drug Safety in Developing Countries* (pp. 419–428). Academic Press.

Al-Worafi, Y.M. (2020w). Drug safety in Indonesia. In *Drug Safety in Developing Countries* (pp. 279–285). Academic Press.

Al-Worafi, Y.M. (2020x). Drug safety in Palestine. In *Drug Safety in Developing Countries* (pp. 471–480). Academic Press.

Al-Worafi, Y.M. (2020y). Drug safety: comparison between developing countries. In *Drug Safety in Developing Countries* (pp. 603–611). Academic Press.

Al-Worafi, Y.M. (2020z). Drug safety in developing versus developed countries. In *Drug Safety in Developing Countries* (pp. 613–615). Academic Press.

Al-Worafi, Y.M., Alseragi, W.M., Ming, L.C., & Alakhali, K.M. (2020a). Drug safety in China. In *Drug Safety in Developing Countries* (pp. 381–388). Academic Press.

Al-Worafi, Y.M., Alseragi, W.M., Alakhali, K.M., Ming, L.C., Othman, G., Halboup, A.M., ... & Elkalmi, R.M. (2020b). Knowledge, beliefs and factors affecting the use of generic medicines among patients in Ibb, Yemen: a mixed-method study. *Journal of Pharmacy Practice and Community Medicine*, 6(4).

Al-Worafi, Y.M., Elkalmi, R.M., Ming, L.C., Othman, G., Halboup, A.M., Battah, M.M., ... & Mani, V. (2021a). *Dispensing Errors in Hospital Pharmacies: A Prospective Study in Yemen*.

Al-Worafi, Y.M., Hasan, S., Hassan, N.M., & Gaili, A.A. (2021b). Knowledge, Attitude and Experience of Pharmacist in the UAE towards Pharmacovigilance. *Research Journal of Pharmacy and Technology*, 14(1), 265–269.

Al-Worafi, Y. (2022a). *A Guide to Online Pharmacy Education: Teaching Strategies and Assessment Methods*. CRC Press.

Al-Worafi, Y.M. (2022b). Patient care errors and related problems (part I): development and validation of the model. https://orcid.org/0000-0002-5752-2913

Al-Worafi, Y.M. (Ed.). (2023). *Clinical Case Studies on Medication Safety*. Academic Press.

Baig, M.R., Al-Worafi, Y.M., Alseragi, W.M., Ming, L.C., & Siddique, A. (2020). Drug safety in India. In *Drug Safety in Developing Countries* (pp. 327–334). Academic Press.

Elkalmi, R.M., Al-Worafi, Y.M., Alseragi, W.M., Ming, L.C., & Siddique, A. (2020). Drug safety in Malaysia. In *Drug Safety in Developing Countries* (pp. 245–253). Academic Press.

Elsayed, T., & Al-Worafi, Y.M. (2020). Drug safety in Egypt. In *Drug Safety in Developing Countries* (pp. 511–523). Academic Press.

Hasan, S., Al-Omar, M.J., AlZubaidy, H., & Al-Worafi, Y.M. (2019). Use of medications in Arab Countries. *Handbook of Healthcare in the Arab World*. Cham: Springer, 42.

Hassan, Y., Abd Aziz, N., Kassab, Y.W., Elgasim, I., Shaharuddin, S., Al-Worafi, Y.M.A., ... & Ming, L.C. (2014). How to help patients to control their blood pressure? Blood pressure control and its predictor. *Archives of Pharmacy Practice*, 5(4).

Izahar, S., Lean, Q.Y., Hameed, M.A., Murugiah, M.K., Patel, R.P., Al-Worafi, Y.M., ... & Ming, L.C. (2017). Content analysis of mobile health applications on diabetes mellitus. *Frontiers in Endocrinology*, 8, 318.

Kristensen, S., & Bartels, P. (2010). Use of patient safety culture instruments and recommendations. *Aarhus, Denmark, European Society for Quality in HealthCare-Office for Quality Indicators*, 113.

Lee, K.S., Yee, S.M., Zaidi, S.T.R., Patel, R.P., Yang, Q., Al-Worafi, Y.M., & Ming, L.C., 2017. Combating sale of counterfeit and falsified medicines online: a losing battle. *Frontiers in Pharmacology*, 8, 268.

Mahmoud, M.A., Wajid, S., Naqvi, A.A., Samreen, S., Althagfan, S.S., & Al-Worafi, Y. (2020). Self-medication with antibiotics: A cross-sectional community-based study. *Latin American Journal of Pharmacy*, 39(2), 348–353.

Manan, M.M., Rusli, R.A., Ang, W.C., Al-Worafi, Y.M., & Ming, L.C. (2014). Assessing the pharmaceutical care issues of antiepileptic drug therapy in hospitalised epileptic patients. *Journal of Pharmacy Practice and Research*, 44(3), 83–88.

Manan, M.M., Ibrahim, N.A., Aziz, N.A., Zulkifly, H.H., Al-Worafi, Y.M.A., & Long, C.M. (2016). Empirical use of antibiotic therapy in the prevention of early onset sepsis in neonates: a pilot study. *Archives of Medical Science*, 12(3), 603–613.

Ming, L.C., Hameed, M.A., Lee, D.D., Apidi, N.A., Lai, P.S.M., Hadi, M.A., Al-Worafi, Y.M.A., & Khan, T.M. (2016). Use of medical mobile applications among hospital pharmacists in Malaysia. *Therapeutic Innovation & Regulatory Science*, 50(4), 419–426.

Ming, L.C., Untong, N., Aliudin, N.A., Osili, N., Kifli, N., Tan, C.S., ... & Goh, H.P. (2020). Mobile health apps on COVID-19 launched in the early days of the pandemic: content analysis and review. *JMIR mHealth and uHealth*, 8(9), e19796.

Othman, G., Ali, F., Ibrahim, M.I.M., Al-Worafi, Y.M., Ansari, M., & Halboup, A.M. (2020). Assessment of Anti-Diabetic Medications Adherence among Diabetic Patients in Sana'a City, Yemen: A Cross Sectional Study. *Journal of Pharmaceutical Research International*, 32(21), 114–122.

Reynard, J., Reynolds, J., & Stevenson, P. (2009). *Practical Patient Safety*. OUP Oxford.

Saeed, M.S., Alkhoshaiban, A.S., Al-Worafi, Y.M.A., & Long, C.M. (2014). Perception of self-medication among university students in Saudi Arabia. *Archives of Pharmacy Practice*, 5(4), 149.

Salas, E., & Frush, K. (2012). *Improving Patient Safety through Teamwork and Team Training*. Oxford University Press.

Vincent, C. (2011). *Patient Safety*. John Wiley & Sons.

20 Nosocomial Infections in Developing Countries

20.1 BACKGROUND

Nosocomial, or hospital-acquired, infections are infections that are acquired while in a hospital or other healthcare setting. They are caused by a variety of factors, including poor hygiene, improper handling of medical equipment, and contact with infectious agents. The most common nosocomial infections include urinary tract infections, surgical site infections, and bloodstream infections. While many nosocomial infections are preventable, they are still a leading cause of healthcare-associated morbidity and mortality worldwide. Good hygiene practices, careful use of antibiotics, and the proper handling of equipment can help reduce the occurrence and spread of nosocomial infections. The most common types of nosocomial infections include urinary tract infections, surgical site infections, and bloodstream infections. Urinary tract infections are the most prevalent nosocomial infection and can be caused by bacteria, fungi, or viruses. Surgical site infections are infections that occur in or near the surgical incision site and can be caused by bacteria, fungi, or viruses. Bloodstream infections, also called sepsis, are caused by bacteria entering the body through the bloodstream and can be fatal if not treated quickly. Other types of nosocomial infections include pneumonia, skin and soft tissue infections, and eye infections (Allegranzi et al., 2011).

20.2 EPIDEMIOLOGY, BURDEN, AND COST OF TREATMENT

The global burden of nosocomial infections is significant and has a significant impact on healthcare costs. The World Health Organization (WHO) estimates that up to 10% of all hospitalized patients acquire a nosocomial infection and that between 5% and 15% of all hospital deaths are attributable to nosocomial infections. The cost of treating nosocomial infections is estimated to be about 7.7 billion US dollars annually. The costs relate to medications, additional doctor visits, and extended hospital stays. The financial burden of nosocomial infections can be reduced by better infection control practices and improved use of antibiotics. Nosocomial infections are a major public health issue in developing countries, where the prevalence and burden of nosocomial infections is higher than in developed countries. This is primarily due to the lack of adequate infection control measures and access to proper healthcare. The WHO estimates that the incidence of nosocomial infections in developing countries is three to four times higher than in developed countries. The financial burden of nosocomial infections in developing countries is even higher due to the limited access to healthcare and limited resources. As such, the economic impact of nosocomial infections is greater in developing countries than in developed countries. The prevalence of nosocomial infections in developing countries is significantly higher than in developed countries. The World Health Organization estimates that the incidence of nosocomial infections in developing countries is three to four times higher than in developed countries. This is due to the lack of adequate infection control measures, limited access to healthcare, and the use of substandard drugs and medical supplies. The prevalence of nosocomial infections is particularly high in poorer countries and in areas with limited access to health care. In addition, overcrowding and lack of hygiene in many medical facilities can further increase the risk of nosocomial infections. The cost of treating nosocomial infections in developing countries is significantly higher than in developed countries, due to the limited access to healthcare and resources. The occurrence of infection was associated with significantly higher treatment costs. It is estimated that, on average, treatment of a patient with HAI would cost the hospital $1400 more than a control case. Therefore, it is essential that hospitals in developing countries focus on the prevention and control of nosocomial infections in order to reduce the economic burden associated with them (Allegranzi et al., 2011).

20.3 CAUSES AND RISK FACTORS

The causes and risk factors of nosocomial infections vary from country to country and from healthcare setting to setting. Generally, the main risk factors for nosocomial infections include overcrowding in healthcare facilities, lack of adequate infection control measures, lack of adequate staff training, inappropriate use of antibiotics and other medical supplies, and poor hygiene. In addition, contact with infected patients, contact with contaminated equipment and surfaces, and contact with contaminated medical personnel are also risk factors for nosocomial infections. Poor sanitation and inadequate cleaning of healthcare facilities, inadequate hand hygiene practices, and lack of availability of antiseptic solutions are also associated with higher rates of nosocomial infections. Causes and risk factors of nosocomial infections in developing countries are often similar

DOI: 10.1201/9781003230465-22

to those in developed countries. However, in developing countries, the lack of access to resources and inadequate infection control measures are key drivers of nosocomial infections. In addition, overcrowding in healthcare facilities, inadequate staff training, inappropriate use of antibiotics and other medical supplies, and poor hygiene are all risk factors for nosocomial infections in developing countries. Inadequate sanitation and cleaning of healthcare facilities, lack of availability of antiseptic solutions, and poor hand hygiene practices are also associated with higher rates of nosocomial infections in developing countries.

20.4 PREVENTION OF NOSOCOMIAL INFECTIONS

Prevention of nosocomial infections requires multiple strategies and measures, both at the individual and the healthcare system level. At the individual level, healthcare workers should practice hand hygiene, use personal protective equipment, follow proper techniques for managing medical supplies and equipment, and properly dispose of hazardous materials. Patients and their families should also be educated about proper hand hygiene, the appropriate use of antibiotics, and other infection control practices. At the healthcare system level, adequate staffing, resources, and training should be ensured. Proper sanitation and cleaning of healthcare facilities is also essential, along with the availability of antiseptic solutions and other preventive measures. Regular staff training and audits should also be conducted to ensure that infection control practices are being properly implemented. Finally, surveillance systems should be developed to monitor the incidence of nosocomial infections and the effectiveness of prevention efforts.

20.5 NOSOCOMIAL INFECTIONS IN DEVELOPING COUNTRIES: Challenges and Recommendations

The WHO reports that, in spite of significant improvements in healthcare infrastructure, nosocomial infections remain a leading cause of morbidity and mortality in developing countries. Challenges such as overcrowding, inadequate medical staff, inadequate medical equipment, and poor sanitation all contribute to the prevalence of nosocomial infections. The most effective way to prevent and contain nosocomial infections is to adhere to the WHO's guidelines on infection prevention and control. These guidelines include proper hand washing, proper cleaning of medical equipment, and proper waste management. Furthermore, it is important to ensure that medical staff and patients receive the necessary training on the proper methods of infection control, as well as understanding the signs and symptoms of nosocomial infections. In addition to following these guidelines, it is important to invest in improving the overall healthcare infrastructure in developing countries. This includes improving access to medical supplies and proper medical equipment, as well as training staff in the latest infection prevention and control techniques. Furthermore, increased public education on the proper hygiene protocols and the dangers of nosocomial infections is essential. Ultimately, nosocomial infections are a significant public health challenge in developing countries, but with proper guidelines, improved infrastructure, and increased public awareness, these infections can be reduced and better managed. It is also important to ensure that healthcare facilities are regularly monitored and inspected to ensure that they are adhering to the necessary guidelines and protocols. Additionally, it is essential to ensure that the necessary resources are available to healthcare facilities in order to adequately treat nosocomial infections. For example, there should be access to antibiotics, antifungals, and antiviral medications to ensure effective treatment of nosocomial infections. Another important factor is to establish a system of surveillance and reporting of nosocomial infections in order to track the prevalence of nosocomial infections over time. This would allow health authorities to better identify and isolate outbreaks and implement the necessary control measures. Furthermore, it would enable healthcare providers to identify areas for improvement and implement better infection control protocols. It is important to ensure that healthcare workers receive the necessary support and training in order to properly handle and treat nosocomial infections. This includes providing proper protective gear and educating healthcare workers on the proper protocols and techniques for preventing and managing nosocomial infections. Despite the progress in research about patient care and safety in developing countries, there is little research about the nosocomial infections culture in the majority of developing countries (Alshahrani et al., 2019a,b; Al-Qahtani et al., 2015; Alshahrani et al., 2020a,b; Al-Worafi, 2014; Al-Worafi, 2015; Al-Worafi, 2016; Al-Worafi et al., 2017; Al-Worafi, 2018a-d; Al-Worafi et al., 2018a-b; Al-Worafi et al., 2019; Al-Worafi, 2020a-z; Al-Worafi et al., 2020a-b; Al-Worafi et al., 2021a,b; Al-Worafi, 2022a,b; Al-Worafi, 2023; Baig et al., 2020; Elkalmi et al., 2020; Elsayed & Al-Worafi, 2020; Hasan et al., 2019; Hassan et al., 2014; Izhar et al., 2017; Lee et al., 2017; Mahmoud

et al., 2020; Manan et al., 2014; Manan et al., 2016; Ming et al., 2016; Ming et al., 2020; Othman et al., 2020; Saeed et al., 2014). Challenges and recommendations can be summarized as follows.
  Challenges

1. Limited resources: Developing countries often have limited resources to invest in infection control measures, such as personal protective equipment, disinfectants, and staff training.

2. Poor infrastructure: Many healthcare facilities in developing countries lack basic infrastructure such as reliable water supply, electricity, and waste management systems. This can contribute to the spread of infection.

3. High patient volumes: Developing countries often have high patient volumes and overcrowded healthcare facilities, which can increase the risk of infection transmission.

4. Limited surveillance systems: Surveillance systems for HAIs are often lacking or poorly implemented in developing countries, which makes it difficult to identify outbreaks and monitor the effectiveness of infection control measures.

Recommendations

1. Improve basic infrastructure: Healthcare facilities in developing countries need basic infrastructure such as reliable water supply, electricity, and waste management systems. These are essential for infection control measures to be effective.

2. Increase resources for infection control: Adequate resources should be provided for infection control measures, including personal protective equipment, disinfectants, and staff training. This will help to prevent the spread of infection and protect healthcare workers.

3. Implement surveillance systems: Surveillance systems for HAIs should be implemented and strengthened in developing countries. This will help to identify outbreaks, monitor trends, and evaluate the effectiveness of infection control measures.

4. Promote hand hygiene: Hand hygiene is the most effective way to prevent the spread of infection. Hand hygiene education should be provided to healthcare workers and patients in developing countries.

5. Improve antibiotic stewardship: Overuse and misuse of antibiotics contribute to the development of antibiotic-resistant bacteria. Antibiotic stewardship programs should be implemented in healthcare facilities in developing countries to promote appropriate antibiotic use.

6. Implement infection prevention and control measures: Healthcare facilities in developing countries should implement infection prevention and control measures, such as isolation precautions, environmental cleaning, and sterilization of medical equipment.

20.6 CONCLUSION

This chapter has discussed the patent safety issues related to nosocomial infections in developing countries. Nosocomial, or hospital-acquired, infections are infections that are acquired while in a hospital or other healthcare setting. They are caused by a variety of factors, including poor hygiene, improper handling of medical equipment, and contact with infectious agents. The most common nosocomial infections include urinary tract infections, surgical site infections, and bloodstream infections. While many nosocomial infections are preventable, they are still a leading cause of healthcare-associated morbidity and mortality worldwide. Good hygiene practices, careful use of antibiotics, and the proper handling of equipment can help reduce the occurrence and spread of nosocomial infections. nosocomial infections are a significant problem in developing countries, and the challenges are numerous. Improving basic infrastructure, increasing resources for infection control, implementing surveillance systems, promoting hand hygiene, improving antibiotic stewardship, and implementing infection prevention and control measures are all essential to reduce the burden of HAIs in developing countries.

REFERENCES
Allegranzi, B., Nejad, S.B., Combescure, C., Graafmans, W., Attar, H., Donaldson, L., & Pittet, D. (2011). Burden of endemic health-care-associated infection in developing countries: systematic review and meta-analysis. *The Lancet*, 377(9761), 228–241.

Al-Qahtani, I., Almoteb, T.M., & Al-Warafi, Y. (2015). Competency of metered-dose inhaler use among Saudi community pharmacists: A Simulation method study. *RRJPPS*, 4(2), 37-31.

Alshahrani, S.M., Alakhali, K.M., & Al-Worafi, Y.M. (2019a). Medication errors in a health care facility in southern Saudi Arabia. *Tropical Journal of Pharmaceutical Research*, 18(5), 1119–1122.

Alshahrani, S.M., Alavudeen, S.S., Alakhali, K.M., Al-Worafi, Y.M., Bahamdan, A.K., & Vigneshwaran, E. (2019b). Self-Medication Among King Khalid University Students, Saudi Arabia. *Risk Management and Healthcare Policy*, 12, 243–249.

Alshahrani, S.M., Alakhali, K.M., Al-Worafi, Y.M., & Alshahrani, N.Z. (2020a). Awareness and use of over the counter analgesic medication: a survey in the Aseer region population, Saudi Arabia. *Int J Advan Appl Sci*, 7(3), 130–134.

Alshahrani, S.M., Alzahran, M., Alakhali, K., Vigneshwaran, E., Iqbal, M.J., Khan, N.A.,... ... & Alavudeen, S.S. (2020b). Association Between Diabetes Consequences and Quality of Life Among Patients With Diabetes Mellitus in the Aseer Province of Saudi Arabia. *Open Access Macedonian Journal of Medical Sciences*, 8(E), 325–330.

Al-Worafi, Y.M. (2014). Prescription writing errors at a tertiary care hospital in Yemen: prevalence, types, causes and recommendations. *Am J Pharm Health Res*, 2, 134–140.

Al-Worafi, Y.M.A. (2015). Appropriateness of metered-dose inhaler use in the Yemeni community pharmacies. *Journal of Taibah University Medical Sciences*, 10(3), 353–358.

Al-Worafi, Y.M.A. (2016). Pharmacy practice in Yemen. In *Pharmacy Practice in Developing Countries* (pp. 267–287). Academic Press.

Al-Worafi, Y.M., Kassab, Y.W., Alseragi, W.M., Almutairi, M.S., Ahmed, A., Ming, L.C., Alkhoshaiban, A.S., & Hadi, M.A. (2017). Pharmacovigilance and adverse drg reaction reporting: a perspective of community pharmacists and pharmacy technicians in Sana'a, Yemen. *Therapeutics and clinical risk management*, 13, 1175.

Al-Worafi, Y.M. (2018a). Knowledge, Attitude and Practice of Yemeni Physicians Toward Pharmacovigilance: A Mixed Method Study. *International Journal of Pharmacy and Pharmaceutical Sciences*, 10 (10), 74–77.

Al-Worafi, Y. (2018b). Knowledge, attitude and practice of Yemeni physicians toward pharmacovigilance: A mixed method study. *Int. J. Pharm. Pharm. Sci*, 10, 74–77.

Al-Worafi, Y.M. (2018c). Dispensing errors observed by community pharmacy dispensers in IBB–YEMEN. *Asian J. Pharm. Clin. Res*, 11(11).

Al-Worafi, Y.M. (2018d). Evauation of inhaler technique among patients with asthma and COPD in Yemen. *Journal of Taibah University medical sciences*, 13(5), 488–490.

Al-Worafi, Y.M., Patel, R.P., Zaidi, S.T.R., Alseragi, W.M., Almutairi, M.S., Alkhoshaiban, A.S., & Ming, L.C. (2018a). Completeness and legibility of handwritten prescriptions in Sana'a, Yemen. *Medical Principles and Practice*, 27, 290–292.

Al-Worafi, Y.M., Alseragi, W.M., Seng, L.K., Kassab, Y.W., Yeoh, S.F., Chiau, L., … & Husain, K. (2018b). Dispensing errors in community pharmacies: a prospective study in Sana'a, Yemen. *Arch Pharm Pract*, 9(4), 1–3.

Al-Worafi, Y.M., Alseragi, W.M., & Mahmoud, M.A. (2019). Competency of metered-dose inhaler use among community pharmacy dispensers in Ibb, Yemen: A simulation method study. *Latin American Journal of Pharmacy*, 38(3), 489–494.

Al-Worafi, Y.M. (Ed.). (2020a). *Drug Safety in Developing Countries: Achievements and Challenges.*

Al-Worafi, Y.M. (2020b). Medication errors. In *Drug Safety in Developing Countries* (pp. 105–117). Academic Press.

Al-Worafi, Y.M. (2020c). Adverse drug reactions. In *Drug Safety in Developing Countries* (pp. 39–57). Academic Press.

Al-Worafi, Y.M. (2020d). Medications registration and marketing: safety-related issues. In *Drug Safety in Developing Countries* (pp. 21–28). Academic Press.

Al-Worafi, Y.M. (2020e). Pharmacovigilance. In *Drug Safety in Developing Countries* (pp. 29–38). Academic Press.

Al-Worafi, Y.M. (2020f). Drug-related problems. In *Drug safety in developing countries* (pp. 59–71). Academic Press.

Al-Worafi, Y.M. (2020g). Medications safety-related terminology. In *Drug safety in developing countries* (pp. 7–19). Academic Press.

Al-Worafi, Y.M. (2020h). Self-medication. In *Drug Safety in Developing Countries* (pp. 73–86). Academic Press.

Al-Worafi, Y.M. (2020j). Antibiotics safety issues. In *Drug Safety in Developing Countries* (pp. 87–103). Academic Press.

Al-Worafi, Y.M. (2020k). Medications safety research issues. In *Drug Safety in Developing Countries* (pp. 213–227). Academic Press.

Al-Worafi, Y.M. (2020l). Counterfeit and substandard medications. In *Drug safety in developing countries* (pp. 119–126). Academic Press.

Al-Worafi, Y.M. (2020m). Medication abuse and misuse. In *Drug safety in developing countries* (pp. 127–135). Academic Press.

Al-Worafi, Y.M. (2020n). Storage and disposal of medications. In *Drug Safety in Developing Countries* (pp. 137–142). Academic Press.

Al-Worafi, Y.M. (2020o). Safety of medications in special population. In *Drug safety in developing countries* (pp. 143–162). Academic Press.

Al-Worafi, Y.M. (2020p). Herbal medicines safety issues. In *Drug Safety in developing countries* (pp. 163–178). Academic Press.

Al-Worafi, Y.M. (2020q). Medications safety pharmacoeconomics-related issues. In *Drug Safety in Developing Countries* (pp. 187–195). Academic Press.

Al-Worafi, Y.M. (2020r). Evidence-based medications safety practice. In *Drug Safety in Developing Countries* (pp. 197–201). Academic Press.

Al-Worafi, Y.M. (2020s). Quality indicators for medications safety. In *Drug safety in developing countries* (pp. 229–242). Academic Press.

Al-Worafi, Y.M. (2020t). Drug safety in Yemen. In *Drug Safety in Developing Countries* (pp. 391–405). Academic Press.

Al-Worafi, Y.M. (2020u). Drug safety in Saudi Arabia. In *Drug Safety in Developing Countries* (pp. 407–417). Academic Press.

Al-Worafi, Y.M. (2020v). Drug safety in United Arab Emirates. In *Drug Safety in Developing Countries* (pp. 419–428). Academic Press.

Al-Worafi, Y.M. (2020w). Drug safety in Indonesia. In *Drug Safety in Developing Countries* (pp. 279–285). Academic Press.

Al-Worafi, Y.M. (2020x). Drug safety in Palestine. In *Drug Safety in Developing Countries* (pp. 471–480). Academic Press.

Al-Worafi, Y.M. (2020y). Drug safety: comparison between developing countries. In *Drug Safety in Developing Countries* (pp. 603–611). Academic Press.

Al-Worafi, Y.M. (2020z). Drug safety in developing versus developed countries. In *Drug Safety in Developing Countries* (pp. 613–615). Academic Press.

Al-Worafi, Y.M., Alseragi, W.M., Ming, L.C., & Alakhali, K.M. (2020a). Drug safety in China. In *Drug Safety in Developing Countries* (pp. 381–388). Academic Press.

Al-Worafi, Y.M., Alseragi, W.M., Alakhali, K.M., Ming, L.C., Othman, G., Halboup, A.M., … & Elkalmi, R.M. (2020b). Knowledge, beliefs and factors affecting the use of generic medicines among patients in Ibb, Yemen: a mixed-method study. *Journal of Pharmacy Practice and Community Medicine*, 6(4).

Al-Worafi, Y.M., Elkalmi, R.M., Ming, L.C., Othman, G., Halboup, A.M., Battah, M.M., … & Mani, V. (2021a). *Dispensing errors in hospital pharmacies: A prospective study in Yemen*.

Al-Worafi, Y.M., Hasan, S., Hassan, N.M., & Gaili, A.A. (2021b). Knowledge, Attitude and Experience of Pharmacist in the UAE towards Pharmacovigilance. *Research Journal of Pharmacy and Technology*, 14(1), 265–269.

Al-Worafi, Y. (2022a). *A Guide to Online Pharmacy Education: Teaching Strategies and Assessment Methods*. CRC Press.

Al-Worafi, Y.M. (2022b). Patient care errors and related problems (part I): development and validation of the model. https://orcid.org/0000-0002-5752-2913

Al-Worafi, Y.M. (Ed.). (2023). *Clinical Case Studies on medication Safety*. Academic Press.

Baig, M.R., Al-Worafi, Y.M., Alseragi, W.M., Ming, L.C., & Siddique, A. (2020). Drug safety in India. In *Drug Safety in Developing Countries* (pp. 327–334). Academic Press.

Elkalmi, R.M., Al-Worafi, Y.M., Alseragi, W.M., Ming, L.C., & Siddique, A. (2020). Drug safety in Malaysia. In *Drug Safety in Developing Countries* (pp. 245–253). Academic Press.

Elsayed, T., & Al-Worafi, Y.M. (2020). Drug safety in Egypt. In *Drug Safety in Developing Countries* (pp. 511–523). Academic Press.

Hasan, S., Al-Omar, M.J., AlZubaidy, H., & Al-Worafi, Y.M. (2019). Use of medications in Arab Countries. *Handbook of Healthcare in the Arab World*. Cham: Springer, 42.

Hassan, Y., Abd Aziz, N., Kassab, Y.W., Elgasim, I., Shaharuddin, S., Al-Worafi, Y.M.A., … & Ming, L.C. (2014). How to help patients to control their blood pressure? Blood pressure control and its predictor. *Archives of Pharmacy Practice*, 5(4).

Izahar, S., Lean, Q.Y., Hameed, M.A., Murugiah, M.K., Patel, R.P., Al-Worafi, Y.M., ... & Ming, L.C. (2017). Content analysis of mobile health applications on diabetes mellitus. *Frontiers in Endocrinology*, 8, 318.

Lee, K.S., Yee, S.M., Zaidi, S.T.R., Patel, R.P., Yang, Q., Al-Worafi, Y.M., & Ming, L.C., 2017. Combating sale of counterfeit and falsified medicines online: a losing battle. *Frontiers in pharmacology*, 8, p. 268.

Mahmoud, M.A., Wajid, S., Naqvi, A.A., Samreen, S., Althagfan, S.S., & Al-Worafi, Y. (2020). Self-medication with antibiotics: A cross-sectional community-based study. *Latin American Journal of Pharmacy*, 39(2), 348–353.

Manan, M.M., Rusli, R.A., Ang, W.C., Al-Worafi, Y.M., & Ming, L.C. (2014). Assessing the pharmaceutical care issues of antiepileptic drug therapy in hospitalised epileptic patients. *Journal of Pharmacy Practice and Research*, 44(3), 83–88.

Manan, M.M., Ibrahim, N.A., Aziz, N.A., Zulkifly, H.H., Al-Worafi, Y.M.A., & Long, C.M. (2016). Empirical use of antibiotic therapy in the prevention of early onset sepsis in neonates: a pilot study. *Archives of Medical Science*, 12(3), 603–613.

Ming, L.C., Hameed, M.A., Lee, D.D., Apidi, N.A., Lai, P.S.M., Hadi, M.A., Al-Worafi, Y.M.A., & Khan, T.M. (2016). Use of medical mobile applications among hospital pharmacists in Malaysia. *Therapeutic innovation & regulatory science*, 50(4), 419–426.

Ming, L.C., Untong, N., Aliudin, N.A., Osili, N., Kifli, N., Tan, C.S., ... & Goh, H.P. (2020). Mobile health apps on COVID-19 launched in the early days of the pandemic: content analysis and review. *JMIR mHealth and uHealth*, 8(9), e19796.

Othman, G., Ali, F., Ibrahim, M.I.M., Al-Worafi, Y.M., Ansari, M., & Halboup, A.M. (2020). Assessment of Anti-Diabetic Medications Adherence among Diabetic Patients in Sana'a City, Yemen: A Cross Sectional Study. *Journal of Pharmaceutical Research International*, 32(21), 114–122.

Saeed, M.S., Alkhoshaiban, A.S., Al-Worafi, Y.M.A., & Long, C.M. (2014). Perception of self-medication among university students in Saudi Arabia. *Archives of Pharmacy Practice*, 5(4), 149.

21 Patient Safety in Laboratory Medicine

21.1 BACKGROUND

Laboratory medicine, also known as clinical pathology or clinical laboratory science, is a medical specialty that involves the analysis of body fluids, tissues, and other specimens to diagnose and monitor diseases. Laboratory medicine encompasses a wide range of laboratory tests, including blood tests, urine tests, and microbiological cultures, among others. Laboratory medicine plays a critical role in the diagnosis and treatment of disease. Laboratory tests are used to identify the presence of pathogens, monitor the effectiveness of treatments, and detect changes in a patient's health status. Laboratory professionals work closely with healthcare providers to provide accurate and timely laboratory results that are essential for making medical decisions. Laboratory medicine also involves the use of advanced technologies, such as molecular diagnostic techniques and mass spectrometry, to provide more precise and accurate results. These technologies have greatly improved the ability to diagnose and treat diseases. Laboratory professionals who specialize in laboratory medicine include medical laboratory scientists, medical technologists, pathologists, and laboratory technicians. These professionals are highly trained and educated in laboratory science and work in a variety of settings, including hospitals, clinical laboratories, research institutions, and public health laboratories. Laboratory medicine professionals use a variety of tools and techniques to interpret and analyze data, such as microscopy, cell culture, and molecular testing. Furthermore, laboratory medicine professionals must be knowledgeable about the latest technology and instruments available, as well as the proper protocols and procedures for collecting and handling specimens. Laboratory medicine professionals must also be aware of the ethical and regulatory issues associated with laboratory testing, as well as the potential for errors in laboratory testing. Additionally, laboratory medicine requires a team-based approach, as it involves multiple healthcare professionals working together to ensure accurate results. In conclusion, laboratory medicine is an important component of healthcare that involves the use of a variety of tools and techniques to help diagnose and manage diseases. It is a team-based approach that involves multiple healthcare professionals and requires knowledge of the latest technology and instruments, as well as a deep understanding of the ethical and regulatory issues associated with laboratory testing (Kristensen & Bartels, 2010; McClatchey, 2002; Reynard et al., 2009; Salas & Frush, 2012; Vincent, 2011).

21.2 LABORATORY MEDICINES ERRORS AND RELATED PROBLEMS

Errors in laboratory medicine can lead to serious consequences, including misdiagnosis and mistreatment of diseases. Errors can occur at different stages of laboratory testing, such as pre-analytical errors (e.g., incorrect patient identification, improper specimen collection), analytical errors (e.g., wrong test ordered, wrong reagent used), and post-analytical errors (e.g., incorrect interpretation of results, wrong reporting of results). To reduce errors in laboratory medicine, healthcare professionals must ensure that proper protocols and procedures are followed. This includes ensuring that patient identification and specimen collection are accurate, that the right test is ordered, and the correct reagents are used. Furthermore, healthcare professionals must be aware of the potential for errors in laboratory testing and develop systems to detect and correct errors. It is also important that laboratory personnel receive adequate training on laboratory techniques and protocols, as well as quality assurance and quality control measures. Additionally, laboratory personnel must be aware of the potential sources of error and how to prevent them. Laboratory medicine is a critical component of healthcare, and errors in laboratory testing can have serious consequences for patients. Some of the common laboratory medicine errors and related problems include:

1. Sample collection errors: Errors in sample collection can lead to inaccurate test results. Examples of sample collection errors include incorrect labeling of samples, insufficient quantity of samples, and inappropriate storage conditions.

2. Pre-analytical errors: Pre-analytical errors occur during the process of preparing samples for testing. These errors can include problems with sample transport, handling, and processing, which can result in inaccurate test results.

3. Analytical errors: Analytical errors can occur during the actual testing process. These errors can include problems with instrumentation, calibration, or reagent quality, which can lead to inaccurate test results.

4. Post-analytical errors: Post-analytical errors occur after testing is complete, during the process of reporting and interpreting test results. These errors can include problems with data entry, report generation, and communication of results to clinicians.

5. Misinterpretation of results: Misinterpretation of laboratory test results can lead to inappropriate treatment decisions or delayed diagnosis, which can harm patients.

To mitigate these errors and related problems, laboratories must have robust quality control and quality assurance programs in place, and laboratory professionals must adhere to established protocols and best practices. It is also important for clinicians to understand the limitations of laboratory testing and to collaborate closely with laboratory professionals to ensure the accuracy and reliability of laboratory results.

21.3 CAUSES OF LABORATORY MEDICINES ERRORS AND RELATED PROBLEMS

There are a variety of causes of errors in laboratory medicine, such as pre-analytical errors, analytical errors, and post-analytical errors. Pre-analytical errors include incorrect patient identification, improper specimen collection, and incorrect labeling of specimens. Analytical errors include wrong test ordered, wrong reagents used, and incorrect interpretation of results. Post-analytical errors include wrong reporting of results, delays in reporting results, and failure to follow up on abnormal results. Other causes of errors in laboratory medicine include human errors, such as fatigue and negligence, as well as technical errors, such as instrument malfunction or failure. Additionally, errors can occur due to environmental factors, such as improper storage conditions. Additionally, errors can occur due to environmental factors, such as improper storage conditions. Laboratory medicine errors and related problems can be summarized as:

Human error: Laboratory medicine involves several steps, including sample collection, transport, processing, testing, and reporting. Any of these steps can be prone to errors if laboratory professionals are not properly trained, or if they are fatigued, distracted, or under stress.

Equipment failure: Laboratory testing relies on sophisticated instrumentation and equipment, and any malfunction or failure can lead to inaccurate test results.

Improper sample collection and handling: Sample collection and handling errors, such as incorrect labeling, insufficient quantity, or inappropriate storage conditions, can lead to inaccurate test results.

Lack of standardization: Laboratory testing involves a complex array of assays and tests, and variations in testing protocols, instrumentation, or reagents can lead to inconsistent and unreliable results.

Communication breakdowns: Communication breakdowns between laboratory professionals and clinicians can lead to misunderstandings, inappropriate test orders, and delays in diagnosis or treatment.

Quality control and quality assurance deficiencies: Laboratories must have robust quality control and quality assurance programs in place to ensure the accuracy and reliability of test results. Deficiencies in these programs can lead to errors and related problems.

To address these causes, laboratories must implement effective training and quality control programs, adhere to established testing protocols and maintain open communication with clinicians to ensure the accuracy and reliability of laboratory results. It is also important to establish a culture of safety and continuous improvement within the laboratory to reduce the risk of errors and related problems.

21.4 PREVENTION OF LABORATORY MEDICINES ERRORS AND RELATED PROBLEMS

Errors in laboratory medicine can be prevented through proper protocols and procedures, adequate training, and quality assurance and control measures. To ensure proper protocols and procedures are followed, healthcare professionals should ensure that patient identification and specimen collection are accurate, that the right test is ordered, and that the correct reagents are used.

Additionally, healthcare professionals should be aware of the potential sources of errors and how to prevent them. Furthermore, laboratory personnel should receive adequate training on laboratory techniques and protocols, as well as quality assurance and quality control measures. This will provide them with the knowledge and skills needed to identify and address errors. Quality assurance and quality control measures should be implemented to detect and correct errors. This could include regular audits, reviews of results, and corrective action plans. In conclusion, laboratory medicine errors can occur at any stage of the laboratory process, including sample collection, transportation, processing, analysis, and interpretation. These errors can result in misdiagnosis, delayed treatment, and even patient harm. Therefore, it is essential to take preventive measures to minimize the risk of laboratory medicine errors. Here are some strategies to prevent laboratory medicine errors and related problems:

1. Standardize laboratory procedures and protocols: Developing standardized procedures and protocols can minimize the likelihood of errors. This includes standardizing sample collection procedures, test methods, and equipment maintenance protocols.

2. Implement quality control measures: Quality control measures should be implemented throughout the laboratory process. This includes regular calibration and maintenance of equipment, ensuring that laboratory staff is properly trained, and following established procedures for reporting and addressing errors.

3. Use barcode technology: Barcoding technology can be used to ensure accurate sample identification and tracking throughout the laboratory process.

4. Develop a system for reporting and addressing errors: Establishing a system for reporting and addressing errors can help identify potential errors before they result in harm to patients. This includes encouraging staff to report errors, investigating reported errors, and developing corrective actions to prevent similar errors from occurring in the future.

5. Ensure clear communication between healthcare providers: Effective communication between healthcare providers can help prevent errors. This includes providing clear and concise instructions for sample collection and test ordering and ensuring that results are reported in a timely and accurate manner.

6. Continuously monitor and evaluate laboratory processes: Regular monitoring and evaluation of laboratory processes can identify areas for improvement and help prevent errors from occurring in the future. This includes tracking error rates, implementing corrective actions, and continuously improving laboratory procedures.

21.5 LABORATORY MEDICINES SAFETY CULTURE

A laboratory medicine safety culture is an environment in which laboratory personnel are aware of potential errors and sources of errors, and strive to continuously improve safety, quality, and performance. It is based on a shared commitment to patient safety and includes communication, teamwork, and collaboration between lab personnel, healthcare providers, and other stakeholders. Safety culture in a laboratory medicine setting is achieved through a combination of policies, procedures, training, and education. Policies should be established to ensure that patient safety is a priority and that lab personnel are aware of the potential sources of errors. Procedures should be in place to ensure accuracy and quality of results, and training should be provided to laboratory personnel on laboratory techniques and protocols, as well as quality assurance and control measures. Finally, education should be provided to healthcare providers on the importance of laboratory results, and how they can use them to make informed decisions. A laboratory medicine safety culture is an environment in which laboratory personnel are aware of potential errors and sources of errors, and strive to continuously improve safety, quality, and performance. It is based on a shared commitment to patient safety and includes communication, teamwork, and collaboration between lab personnel, healthcare providers, and other stakeholders. To ensure a safe environment, policies should be established to ensure that patient safety is a priority and that lab personnel are aware of the potential sources of errors. Procedures should be in place to ensure accuracy and quality of results, and training should be provided to laboratory personnel on laboratory techniques and protocols, as well as quality assurance and control measures. Additionally, education should be provided to healthcare providers on the importance of laboratory results, and how they can use them to make informed decisions. It is important to emphasize the importance of reporting errors, near-misses, and adverse events so that lessons can be learned and mistakes avoided in the future. Creating a safety culture is essential to ensure that laboratory professionals are aware of the potential risks associated with laboratory testing and take the necessary steps to prevent errors Some of the key components of a laboratory safety culture include:

1. Leadership commitment: Laboratory leadership should prioritize safety and demonstrate their commitment to safety through actions and communication.

2. Open communication: Laboratory staff should feel comfortable reporting safety concerns, incidents, and near-misses without fear of retribution.

3. Education and training: Laboratory staff should receive regular training on safety procedures and policies.

4. Risk assessment: Laboratory management should conduct regular risk assessments to identify and mitigate potential hazards in laboratory operations.

5. Continuous improvement: The laboratory should have a process for continuous improvement, where safety incidents are analyzed, and corrective actions are taken to prevent reoccurrence.

6. Standardization: Standardized procedures, policies, and protocols should be in place to ensure consistency and minimize errors.

7. Collaboration: Laboratory staff should work collaboratively with other stakeholders to promote safety and share best practices.

Overall, a laboratory safety culture is essential for ensuring the accuracy and reliability of laboratory results while protecting the safety of laboratory staff, patients, and the public.

21.6 LABORATORY MEDICINES ERRORS AND RELATED PROBLEMS IN DEVELOPING COUNTRIES: Challenges and Recommendations

Laboratory medicine errors and related problems are a significant concern in developing countries, where healthcare systems may be under-resourced and underdeveloped. These problems can have serious consequences, including misdiagnosis, incorrect treatment, and even patient harm or death. Here are some challenges and recommendations to address laboratory medicine errors and related problems in developing countries:

Challenges:

1. Limited resources: Developing countries often lack the necessary resources to invest in laboratory infrastructure, equipment, and personnel, leading to inadequate testing capacity and a higher risk of errors.

2. Inadequate training: Laboratory technicians and other healthcare professionals may not receive sufficient training in laboratory medicine, leading to a lack of knowledge and skills in testing procedures, equipment use, and quality assurance.

3. Poor quality control: Quality control measures may not be adequately implemented, leading to inaccurate or unreliable test results.

4. Limited access to quality assurance programs: Developing countries may not have access to external quality assurance programs or proficiency testing, which are essential for ensuring the accuracy and reliability of laboratory results.

Recommendations:

1. Investment in laboratory infrastructure and resources: Governments and healthcare organizations should prioritize investment in laboratory infrastructure, including equipment, supplies, and personnel.

2. Improved training and education: Healthcare professionals working in laboratory medicine should receive regular training and education to improve their knowledge and skills in testing procedures, equipment use, and quality assurance.

3. Implementation of quality control measures: Laboratories should implement quality control measures, such as internal and external quality control programs, to ensure the accuracy and reliability of test results.

4. Access to quality assurance programs: Developing countries should have access to external quality assurance programs and proficiency testing, which can help to identify and address errors and improve the quality of laboratory testing.

5. Collaboration and partnerships: Collaboration and partnerships between healthcare organizations and governments, as well as with international organizations, can help to improve laboratory medicine practices and address issues related to errors and quality control.

6. Despite the progress in research about patient care and safety in developing countries, there is little research about patient safety related to laboratory medicines in majority of developing countries, therefore, conduct research is very important and highly recommended (Alshahrani et al., 2019a,b; Al-Qahtani et al., 2015; Alshahrani et al., 2020a,b; Al-Worafi, 2014; Al-Worafi, 2015; Al-Worafi, 2016; Al-Worafi et al., 2017; Al-Worafi, 2018a–d; Al-Worafi et al., 2018a,b; Al-Worafi et al., 2019; Al-Worafi, 2020a–z; Al-Worafi et al., 2020a,b; Al-Worafi et al., 2021a,b; Al-Worafi, 2022a,b; Al-Worafi, 2023; Baig et al., 2020; Elkalmi et al., 2020; Elsayed & Al-Worafi, 2020; Hasan et al., 2019; Hassan et al., 2014; Izhar et al., 2017; Lee et al., 2017; Mahmoud et al., 2020; Manan et al., 2014; Manan et al., 2016; Ming et al., 2016; Ming et al., 2020; Othman et al., 2020; Saeed et al., 2014).

21.7 CONCLUSION

In conclusion, addressing laboratory medicine errors and related problems in developing countries requires a multifaceted approach that addresses challenges related to resources, training, quality control, and access to quality assurance programs. Through collaboration and investment in laboratory medicine infrastructure and practices, healthcare organizations and governments can help to improve the quality and safety of laboratory testing and enhance patient outcomes.

REFERENCES

Al-Qahtani, I., Almoteb, T.M., & Al-Warafi, Y. (2015). Competency of metered-dose inhaler use among Saudi community pharmacists: A Simulation method study. *RRJPPS*, 4(2), 37–31.

Alshahrani, S.M., Alakhali, K.M., & Al-Worafi, Y.M. (2019a). Medication errors in a health care facility in southern Saudi Arabia. *Tropical Journal of Pharmaceutical Research*, 18(5), pp. 1119–1122.

Alshahrani, S.M., Alavudeen, S.S., Alakhali, K.M., Al-Worafi, Y.M., Bahamdan, A.K., & Vigneshwaran, E. (2019b). Self-Medication Among King Khalid University Students, Saudi Arabia. *Risk Management and Healthcare Policy*, 12, pp. 243–249.

Alshahrani, S.M., Alakhali, K.M., Al-Worafi, Y.M., & Alshahrani, N.Z. (2020b). Awareness and use of over the counter analgesic medication: a survey in the Aseer region population, Saudi Arabia. *Int J Advan Appl Sci*, 7(3), 130–134.

Alshahrani, S.M., Alzahran, M., Alakhali, K., Vigneshwaran, E., Iqbal, M.J., Khan, N.A., … & Alavudeen, S.S. (2020b). Association Between Diabetes Consequences and Quality of Life Among Patients With Diabetes Mellitus in the Aseer Province of Saudi Arabia. *Open Access Macedonian Journal of Medical Sciences*, 8(E), 325–330.

Al-Worafi, Y.M. (2014). Prescription writing errors at a tertiary care hospital in Yemen: prevalence, types, causes and recommendations. *Am J Pharm Health Res*, 2, 134–140.

Al-Worafi, Y.M.A. (2015). Appropriateness of metered-dose inhaler use in the Yemeni community pharmacies. *Journal of Taibah University Medical Sciences*, 10(3), 353–358.

Al-Worafi, Y.M.A. (2016). Pharmacy practice in Yemen. In *Pharmacy Practice in Developing Countries* (pp. 267–287). Academic Press.

Al-Worafi, Y.M., Kassab, Y.W., Alseragi, W.M., Almutairi, M.S., Ahmed, A., Ming, L.C., Alkhoshaiban, A.S., & Hadi, M.A. (2017). Pharmacovigilance and adverse drg reaction reporting: a perspective of community pharmacists and pharmacy technicians in Sana'a, Yemen. *Therapeutics and clinical risk management*, 13, p. 1175.

Al-Worafi, Y.M. (2018a). Knowledge, Attitude and Practice of Yemeni Physicians Toward Pharmacovigilance: A Mixed Method Study. *International Journal of Pharmacy and Pharmaceutical Sciences*, 10(10), 74–77.

Al-Worafi, Y. (2018b). Knowledge, attitude and practice of Yemeni physicians toward pharmacovigilance: A mixed method study. *Int. J. Pharm. Pharm. Sci*, 10, 74–77.

Al-Worafi, Y.M. (2018c). Dispensing errors observed by community pharmacy dispensers in IBB–YEMEN. *Asian J. Pharm. Clin. Res*, 11(11).

Al-Worafi, Y.M. (2018d). Evauation of inhaler technique among patients with asthma and COPD in Yemen. *Journal of Taibah University medical sciences*, 13(5), 488–490.

Al-Worafi, Y.M., Patel, R.P., Zaidi, S.T.R., Alseragi, W.M., Almutairi, M.S., Alkhoshaiban, A.S., & Ming, L.C. (2018a). Completeness and legibility of handwritten prescriptions in Sana'a, Yemen. *Medical Principles and Practice*, 27, 290–292.

Al-Worafi, Y.M., Alseragi, W.M., Seng, L.K., Kassab, Y.W., Yeoh, S.F., Chiau, L., … & Husain, K. (2018b). Dispensing errors in community pharmacies: a prospective study in Sana'a, Yemen. *Arch Pharm Pract*, 9(4), 1–3.

Al-Worafi, Y.M., Alseragi, W.M., & Mahmoud, M.A. (2019). Competency of metered-dose inhaler use among community pharmacy dispensers in Ibb, Yemen: A simulation method study. *Latin American Journal of Pharmacy*, 38(3), 489–494.

Al-Worafi, Y.M. (Ed.). (2020a). *Drug Safety in Developing Countries: Achievements and Challenges.*

Al-Worafi, Y.M. (2020b). Medication errors. In *Drug Safety in Developing Countries* (pp. 105–117). Academic Press.

Al-Worafi, Y.M. (2020c). Adverse drug reactions. In *Drug Safety in Developing Countries* (pp. 39–57). Academic Press.

Al-Worafi, Y.M. (2020d). Medications registration and marketing: safety-related issues. In *Drug Safety in Developing Countries* (pp. 21–28). Academic Press.

Al-Worafi, Y.M. (2020e). Pharmacovigilance. In *Drug Safety in Developing Countries* (pp. 29–38). Academic Press.

Al-Worafi, Y.M. (2020f). Drug-related problems. In *Drug safety in developing countries* (pp. 59–71). Academic Press.

Al-Worafi, Y.M. (2020g). Medications safety-related terminology. In *Drug safety in developing countries* (pp. 7–19). Academic Press.

Al-Worafi, Y.M. (2020h). Self-medication. In *Drug Safety in Developing Countries* (pp. 73–86). Academic Press.

Al-Worafi, Y.M. (2020j). Antibiotics safety issues. In *Drug Safety in Developing Countries* (pp. 87–103). Academic Press.

Al-Worafi, Y.M. (2020k). Medications safety research issues. In *Drug Safety in Developing Countries* (pp. 213–227). Academic Press.

Al-Worafi, Y.M. (2020l). Counterfeit and substandard medications. In *Drug safety in developing countries* (pp. 119–126). Academic Press.

Al-Worafi, Y.M. (2020m). Medication abuse and misuse. In *Drug safety in developing countries* (pp. 127–135). Academic Press.

Al-Worafi, Y.M. (2020n). Storage and disposal of medications. In *Drug Safety in Developing Countries* (pp. 137–142). Academic Press.

Al-Worafi, Y.M. (2020o). Safety of medications in special population. In *Drug safety in developing countries* (pp. 143–162). Academic Press.

Al-Worafi, Y.M. (2020p). Herbal medicines safety issues. In *Drug Safety in developing countries* (pp. 163–178). Academic Press.

Al-Worafi, Y.M. (2020q). Medications safety pharmacoeconomics-related issues. In *Drug Safety in Developing Countries* (pp. 187–195). Academic Press.

Al-Worafi, Y.M. (2020r). Evidence-based medications safety practice. In *Drug Safety in Developing Countries* (pp. 197–201). Academic Press.

Al-Worafi, Y.M. (2020s). Quality indicators for medications safety. In *Drug safety in developing countries* (pp. 229–242). Academic Press.

Al-Worafi, Y.M. (2020t). Drug safety in Yemen. In *Drug Safety in Developing Countries* (pp. 391–405). Academic Press.

Al-Worafi, Y.M. (2020u). Drug safety in Saudi Arabia. In *Drug Safety in Developing Countries* (pp. 407–417). Academic Press.

Al-Worafi, Y.M. (2020v). Drug safety in United Arab Emirates. In *Drug Safety in Developing Countries* (pp. 419–428). Academic Press.

Al-Worafi, Y.M. (2020w). Drug safety in Indonesia. In *Drug Safety in Developing Countries* (pp. 279–285). Academic Press.

Al-Worafi, Y.M. (2020x). Drug safety in Palestine. In *Drug Safety in Developing Countries* (pp. 471–480). Academic Press.

Al-Worafi, Y.M. (2020y). Drug safety: comparison between developing countries. In *Drug Safety in Developing Countries* (pp. 603–611). Academic Press.

Al-Worafi, Y.M. (2020z). Drug safety in developing versus developed countries. In *Drug Safety in Developing Countries* (pp. 613–615). Academic Press.

Al-Worafi, Y.M., Alseragi, W.M., Ming, L.C., & Alakhali, K.M. (2020a). Drug safety in China. In *Drug Safety in Developing Countries* (pp. 381–388). Academic Press.

Al-Worafi, Y.M., Alseragi, W.M., Alakhali, K.M., Ming, L.C., Othman, G., Halboup, A.M., … & Elkalmi, R.M. (2020b). Knowledge, beliefs and factors affecting the use of generic medicines among patients in Ibb, Yemen: a mixed-method study. *Journal of Pharmacy Practice and Community Medicine*, 6(4).

Al-Worafi, Y.M., Elkalmi, R.M., Ming, L.C., Othman, G., Halboup, A.M., Battah, M.M., ... & Mani, V. (2021a). *Dispensing errors in hospital pharmacies: A prospective study in Yemen.*

Al-Worafi, Y.M., Hasan, S., Hassan, N.M., & Gaili, A.A. (2021b). Knowledge, Attitude and Experience of Pharmacist in the UAE towards Pharmacovigilance. *Research Journal of Pharmacy and Technology,* 14(1), 265–269.

Al-Worafi, Y. (2022a). *A Guide to Online Pharmacy Education: Teaching Strategies and Assessment Methods.* CRC Press.

Al-Worafi, Y.M. (2022b). Patient care errors and related problems (part I): development and validation of the model. 0000-0002-5752-2913

Al-Worafi, Y.M. (Ed.). (2023). *Clinical Case Studies on medication Safety.* Academic Press.

Baig, M.R., Al-Worafi, Y.M., Alseragi, W.M., Ming, L.C., & Siddique, A. (2020). Drug safety in India. In *Drug Safety in Developing Countries* (pp. 327–334). Academic Press.

Elkalmi, R.M., Al-Worafi, Y.M., Alseragi, W.M., Ming, L.C., & Siddique, A. (2020). Drug safety in Malaysia. In *Drug Safety in Developing Countries* (pp. 245–253). Academic Press.

Elsayed, T., & Al-Worafi, Y.M. (2020). Drug safety in Egypt. In *Drug Safety in Developing Countries* (pp. 511–523). Academic Press.

Hasan, S., Al-Omar, M.J., AlZubaidy, H., & Al-Worafi, Y.M. (2019). Use of medications in Arab Countries. *Handbook of Healthcare in the Arab World.* Cham: Springer, 42.

Hassan, Y., Abd Aziz, N., Kassab, Y.W., Elgasim, I., Shaharuddin, S., Al-Worafi, Y.M.A., ... & Ming, L.C. (2014). How to help patients to control their blood pressure? Blood pressure control and its predictor. *Archives of Pharmacy Practice,* 5(4).

Izahar, S., Lean, Q.Y., Hameed, M.A., Murugiah, M.K., Patel, R.P., Al-Worafi, Y.M., ... & Ming, L.C. (2017). Content analysis of mobile health applications on diabetes mellitus. *Frontiers in Endocrinology,* 8, 318.

Kristensen, S., & Bartels, P. (2010). Use of patient safety culture instruments and recommendations. *Aarhus, Denmark, European Society for Quality in HealthCare-Office for Quality Indicators,* 113.

Lee, K.S., Yee, S.M., Zaidi, S.T.R., Patel, R.P., Yang, Q., Al-Worafi, Y.M., & Ming, L.C., 2017. Combating sale of counterfeit and falsified medicines online: a losing battle. *Frontiers in pharmacology,* 8, p. 268.

McClatchey, K.D. (Ed.). (2002). *Clinical laboratory medicine.* Lippincott Williams & Wilkins.

Mahmoud, M.A., Wajid, S., Naqvi, A.A., Samreen, S., Althagfan, S.S., & Al-Worafi, Y. (2020). Self-medication with antibiotics: A cross-sectional community-based study. *Latin american journal of pharmacy,* 39(2), 348–353.

Manan, M.M., Rusli, R.A., Ang, W.C., Al-Worafi, Y.M., & Ming, L.C. (2014). Assessing the pharmaceutical care issues of antiepileptic drug therapy in hospitalised epileptic patients. *Journal of Pharmacy Practice and Research,* 44(3), 83–88.

Manan, M.M., Ibrahim, N.A., Aziz, N.A., Zulkifly, H.H., Al-Worafi, Y.M.A., & Long, C.M. (2016). Empirical use of antibiotic therapy in the prevention of early onset sepsis in neonates: a pilot study. *Archives of Medical Science,* 12(3), 603–613.

Ming, L.C., Hameed, M.A., Lee, D.D., Apidi, N.A., Lai, P.S.M., Hadi, M.A., Al-Worafi, Y.M.A., & Khan, T.M. (2016). Use of medical mobile applications among hospital pharmacists in Malaysia. *Therapeutic innovation & regulatory science*, 50(4), pp. 419–426.

Ming, L.C., Untong, N., Aliudin, N.A., Osili, N., Kifli, N., Tan, C.S., ... & Goh, H.P. (2020). Mobile health apps on COVID-19 launched in the early days of the pandemic: content analysis and review. *JMIR mHealth and uHealth*, 8(9), e19796.

Othman, G., Ali, F., Ibrahim, M.I.M., Al-Worafi, Y.M., Ansari, M., & Halboup, A.M. (2020). Assessment of Anti-Diabetic Medications Adherence among Diabetic Patients in Sana'a City, Yemen: A Cross Sectional Study. *Journal of Pharmaceutical Research International*, 32(21), 114–122.

Reynard, J., Reynolds, J., & Stevenson, P. (2009). *Practical patient safety*. OUP Oxford.

Saeed, M.S., Alkhoshaiban, A.S., Al-Worafi, Y.M.A., & Long, C.M., (2014). Perception of self-medication among university students in Saudi Arabia. *Archives of Pharmacy Practice*, 5(4), p. 149.

Salas, E., & Frush, K. (2012). *Improving patient safety through teamwork and team training*. Oxford University Press.

Vincent, C. (2011). *Patient safety*. John Wiley & Sons.

22 Patient Safety in Radiology

22.1 BACKGROUND

Radiology is a branch of medicine that uses imaging techniques, such as X-rays, CT scans, MRI, and ultrasound, to diagnose and treat diseases and injuries. Radiology is used in various medical fields, including oncology, cardiology, neurology, orthopedics, and others. Radiology plays a critical role in patient care, as it helps physicians diagnose and treat a wide range of medical conditions. Imaging tests such as X-rays, CT scans, and MRI scans provide detailed images of the body that can help identify injuries, tumors, and other abnormalities. This information is essential for physicians to make accurate diagnoses and develop effective treatment plans. Radiology also plays a critical role in patient safety by minimizing the need for invasive procedures. Imaging tests can often provide the same information as invasive procedures without the added risks and complications associated with surgery. Additionally, radiologists use specialized equipment and techniques to minimize radiation exposure and ensure that imaging tests are performed safely. To ensure patient safety, radiologists work closely with other healthcare providers to coordinate care and ensure that patients receive the appropriate imaging tests. This involves communicating effectively with physicians, nurses, and other healthcare providers to ensure that imaging tests are performed at the appropriate time and that patients receive the care they need. Radiology involves the use of medical imaging techniques such as X-rays, CT scans, MRI, and ultrasound to diagnose and treat various medical conditions. Below are some ways in which radiology contributes to patient care and safety:

1. Diagnosis: Radiology is an important tool for diagnosing medical conditions. Medical imaging techniques can help physicians identify and locate abnormalities or injuries within the body that may be difficult to detect through physical examination. Early detection of medical conditions can lead to better patient outcomes.

2. Treatment: Radiology can also be used to treat medical conditions. For example, radiation therapy can be used to destroy cancerous cells. Other minimally invasive procedures, such as image-guided biopsies or vascular interventions, can be performed using radiologic techniques.

3. Patient safety: Radiology plays a vital role in ensuring patient safety. Radiology professionals follow strict safety protocols to minimize patient exposure to ionizing radiation, which can be harmful in large amounts. Radiology also uses advanced technology, such as dose monitoring software, to ensure that patients receive the lowest possible dose of radiation during imaging procedures.

4. Communication: Radiology professionals often serve as key communicators between different medical specialties. They work closely with referring physicians and other healthcare professionals to ensure that patients receive the appropriate imaging studies and that imaging findings are communicated effectively.

Overall, radiology plays a crucial role in patient care and safety. Medical imaging techniques can help diagnose and treat medical conditions, while also ensuring that patients are exposed to the lowest possible levels of radiation during imaging procedures. Radiology professionals work closely with other healthcare professionals to ensure that patients receive the best possible care (Kristensen & Bartels, 2010; Reynard et al., 2009; Salas & Frush, 2012; Vincent, 2011).

22.2 RADIOLOGY ERRORS AND RELATED PROBLEMS

Despite the significant role radiology plays in patient care and safety, errors in radiology can occur, which can lead to patient harm or even death. Some of the common radiology errors and related problems are:

1. Interpretation errors: One of the most common radiology errors is interpretation errors, where a radiologist misinterprets an image or fails to detect a significant abnormality. These errors can lead to missed or delayed diagnoses, resulting in patient harm or even death.

2. Technical errors: Technical errors can occur during the imaging process, such as equipment malfunction or improper positioning of the patient, leading to inaccurate or unusable images.

3. Communication errors: Communication errors can occur when radiology professionals fail to communicate imaging results effectively to referring physicians or other healthcare providers, leading to delayed or inappropriate treatment.

DOI: 10.1201/9781003230465-24

4. Overuse of imaging: Overuse of imaging, such as ordering unnecessary imaging tests, can lead to increased radiation exposure and unnecessary costs.

5. Lack of standardization: There is a lack of standardization in radiology practices, which can lead to variations in image interpretation and reporting, leading to potential errors.

6. Workflow issues: Workflow issues, such as delays in image acquisition or interpretation, can result in delayed diagnoses or treatment, affecting patient outcomes.

To address these problems, radiology professionals and healthcare organizations can implement various strategies, such as improving communication and collaboration among healthcare providers, developing standardized protocols and guidelines, implementing quality control measures, and providing ongoing education and training to radiology professionals. These efforts can help reduce the occurrence of radiology errors and improve patient outcomes.

22.3 CAUSES OF RADIOLOGY ERRORS AND RELATED PROBLEMS

Radiology errors can occur for various reasons, including technical errors, interpretation errors, communication errors, and system errors. Some of the common causes of radiology errors and problems are:

1. Technical errors: These errors can occur due to equipment malfunction, incorrect positioning of the patient, and inadequate quality control.

2. Interpretation errors: Interpretation errors can occur when radiologists misinterpret the images, fail to detect abnormalities or misdiagnose a condition. This can be due to various factors such as lack of experience, fatigue, distraction, or poor image quality.

3. Communication errors: Communication errors can occur between the radiologist and the referring physician, between the radiologist and the patient, or within the radiology department. Examples of communication errors include failure to convey critical findings, incorrect or incomplete information in the medical record, and failure to follow up on abnormal results.

4. System errors: System errors can occur due to a breakdown in the workflow, inadequate staffing, lack of standardization, or failure to use technology effectively.

5. Cognitive biases: Cognitive biases can lead to errors in radiology interpretation. For example, confirmation bias can lead radiologists to look for evidence that confirms their initial diagnosis and ignore contradictory evidence.

6. Inadequate training: Inadequate training of radiologists and technologists can also contribute to errors in radiology. New technologies and procedures require continuous training to ensure that radiologists and technologists are up-to-date on the latest techniques and procedures.

7. Time pressures: Radiologists often face time pressures due to the high volume of cases they need to review. This can lead to errors, as radiologists may not have enough time to carefully review the images and make an accurate diagnosis.

8. Lack of access to patient information: Radiologists may not have access to all of the patient's medical information, which can lead to errors in diagnosis and treatment.

9. Inadequate training and experience: Radiologists require extensive training and experience to accurately interpret images and make diagnoses. Inexperienced radiologists or those with inadequate training may misinterpret images or miss important findings.

10. Workload and time pressures: Radiologists are often required to interpret a large volume of images in a short period of time. This can lead to errors and oversights, as radiologists may not have enough time to thoroughly review images.

11. Technical issues with imaging equipment: Technical problems with imaging equipment, such as malfunctioning machines or poor image quality, can lead to misinterpretation of images and inaccurate diagnoses.

12. Communication breakdowns: Poor communication between radiologists and other healthcare providers can lead to misunderstandings and errors in diagnosis and treatment. Radiology errors can also be caused by human factors, such as fatigue, stress, and distraction.

Overall, radiology errors and related problems are complex and multifactorial, and addressing them requires a multifaceted approach that addresses the various underlying causes.

22.4 PREVENTION OF RADIOLOGY ERRORS AND RELATED PROBLEMS

Preventing radiology errors and related problems requires a multi-pronged approach that addresses the various causes of errors. Some strategies that can help prevent radiology errors include:

1. Quality control: Ensuring proper quality control of equipment and procedures can help prevent technical errors and improve the quality of images.

2. Standardization: Standardizing procedures and protocols across the radiology department can help reduce the risk of errors due to inconsistent practices.

3. Continuous education and training: Continuous education and training can help keep radiologists and technologists up-to-date on the latest techniques and procedures, reducing the risk of errors due to inadequate training.

4. Decision support tools: The use of decision support tools, such as computer-aided detection and diagnosis, can help improve accuracy and reduce errors in interpretation.

5. Double reading: Implementing a system of double reading, where two radiologists independently review the same images, can help reduce errors in interpretation.

6. Improved communication: Ensuring clear and effective communication between radiologists, referring physicians, and patients can help reduce communication errors and ensure timely and appropriate follow-up.

7. Workflow optimization: Optimizing workflow can help reduce time pressures and prevent errors due to fatigue or distraction.

8. Patient-centered care: Ensuring that patient-centered care is a priority can help improve patient safety and reduce the risk of errors due to inadequate patient information or patient involvement.

Overall, preventing radiology errors requires a culture of safety that values continuous improvement and prioritizes patient safety. By implementing these strategies, radiology departments can work toward reducing the risk of errors and improving the quality of care they provide to their patients.

22.5 RADIOLOGY SAFETY CULTURE

Radiology safety culture refers to the values, beliefs, and attitudes of individuals and organizations that prioritize patient safety in radiology. A strong safety culture is critical for minimizing the risks associated with radiology procedures and ensuring that imaging tests are performed safely and effectively. To promote a culture of safety in radiology, healthcare organizations should prioritize patient safety and make it a core value. This includes providing ongoing training and education for radiologists and other healthcare providers, implementing quality control measures to ensure accurate interpretation of images, and encouraging open communication and collaboration among team members. Organizations should also establish policies and procedures to promote safety, such as protocols for reducing radiation exposure and guidelines for patient positioning and use of protective equipment. Additionally, healthcare organizations should encourage a culture of reporting and learning from errors, so that mistakes can be identified and prevented in the future. Radiology safety culture refers to the values, attitudes, and behaviors of individuals and organizations within the radiology community that prioritize safety and aim to prevent errors and improve patient outcomes. A strong safety culture in radiology is essential for ensuring patient safety, reducing errors, and improving the quality of care.

Here are some characteristics of a strong radiology safety culture:

1. Open communication: A culture of open communication encourages team members to report errors, near misses, and safety concerns without fear of retribution. This can help identify and address safety issues before they cause harm.

2. Learning from errors: A culture of continuous improvement requires learning from errors and near misses to identify ways to prevent similar incidents in the future.

3. Accountability: A culture of accountability ensures that individuals and organizations take responsibility for their actions and are held accountable for ensuring patient safety.

4. Standardization: A culture of standardization promotes the use of standardized procedures and protocols to reduce the risk of errors due to inconsistent practices.

5. Continuous education and training: A culture of continuous education and training ensures that radiologists and technologists are up-to-date on the latest techniques and procedures and are equipped to provide the best possible care to their patients.

6. Patient-centered care: A culture of patient-centered care places the patient at the center of the care process and ensures that their safety and well-being are a top priority.

7. Leadership support: A strong safety culture requires support from leadership at all levels, from the radiology department to the hospital or healthcare organization.

Overall, a strong safety culture in radiology is essential for ensuring patient safety, reducing errors, and improving the quality of care. By prioritizing safety and promoting a culture of continuous improvement, radiology departments can work toward improving patient outcomes and reducing the risk of harm. In conclusion, promoting a culture of safety in radiology requires a comprehensive approach that involves prioritizing patient safety, ongoing training and education, quality control measures, open communication and collaboration, policies and procedures to promote safety, and a culture of reporting and learning from errors. By implementing these strategies, healthcare organizations can create a culture of safety in radiology and improve patient outcomes.

22.6 RADIOLOGY ERRORS AND RELATED PROBLEMS IN DEVELOPING COUNTRIES: Challenges and Recommendations

Radiology errors and related problems are a global issue, but they are particularly challenging in developing countries. Here are some challenges and recommendations for addressing these issues:
  Challenges:

1. Limited access to technology and equipment: Many developing countries have limited access to advanced imaging technology and equipment, which can lead to errors due to inadequate image quality and interpretation.

2. Lack of trained personnel: Developing countries may have a shortage of trained radiologists and technologists, leading to errors due to inadequate training and experience.

3. Language barriers: In countries where there are multiple languages spoken, communication between radiologists and patients can be challenging, leading to errors in interpretation and diagnosis.

4. Financial constraints: Many developing countries have limited financial resources, which can make it challenging to invest in advanced imaging technology and equipment, as well as training and continuing education for radiologists and technologists.

Recommendations:

  To address these challenges, there are several recommendations that can be implemented:

1. Increased investment in imaging equipment and infrastructure: Developing countries should prioritize investment in imaging equipment and infrastructure to improve access to imaging tests and support accurate diagnoses.

2. Training and education: Developing countries should prioritize training and education for radiologists and other healthcare providers to improve skills and knowledge.

3. Quality control measures: Developing countries should implement quality control measures to ensure accurate interpretation of images and timely communication of results.

4. Partnerships and collaborations: Developing countries can benefit from partnerships and collaborations with organizations in developed countries to share knowledge, expertise, and resources.

5. Despite the progress in research about patient care and safety in developing countries, there is little research about patient safety related to the radiology in the majority of developing

countries, therefore, conduct research is very important and highly recommended (Alshahrani et al., 2019a,b; Al-Qahtani et al., 2015; Alshahrani et al., 2020a,b; Al-Worafi, 2014; Al-Worafi, 2015; Al-Worafi, 2016; Al-Worafi et al., 2017; Al-Worafi, 2018a–d; Al-Worafi et al., 2018a–b; Al-Worafi et al., 2019; Al-Worafi, 2020a–z; Al-Worafi et al., 2020a–b; Al-Worafi et al., 2021a,b; Al-Worafi, 2022a,b; Al-Worafi, 2023; Baig et al., 2020; Elkalmi et al., 2020; Elsayed & Al-Worafi, 2020; Hasan et al., 2019; Hassan et al., 2014; Izhar et al., 2017; Lee et al., 2017; Mahmoud et al., 2020; Manan et al., 2014; Manan et al., 2016; Ming et al., 2016; Ming et al., 2020; Othman et al., 2020; Saeed et al., 2014).

In conclusion, radiology errors and related problems are significant issues in developing countries, but there are steps that can be taken to address these challenges. By implementing recommendations such as increased investment in equipment and infrastructure, training and education, quality control measures, and partnerships and collaborations, healthcare organizations in developing countries can improve patient outcomes and promote a culture of safety in radiology.

22.7 CONCLUSION

This chapter has discussed the radiology safety issues in developing countries. Despite the significant role radiology plays in patient care and safety, errors in radiology can occur, which can lead to patient harm or even death. Radiology errors can occur for various reasons, including technical errors, interpretation errors, communication errors, and system errors. Radiology errors and related problems are significant issues in developing countries, but there are steps that can be taken to address these challenges. With increased investment in equipment and infrastructure, training and education, quality control measures, and partnerships and collaborations, healthcare organizations in developing countries can improve patient outcomes and promote a culture of safety in radiology.

REFERENCES

Al-Qahtani, I., Almoteb, T.M., & Al-Warafi, Y. (2015). Competency of metered-dose inhaler use among Saudi community pharmacists: A Simulation method study. *RRJPPS*, 4(2), pp. 27–31.

Alshahrani, S.M., Alakhali, K.M., & Al-Worafi, Y.M., (2019a). Medication errors in a health care facility in southern Saudi Arabia. *Tropical Journal of Pharmaceutical Research*, 18(5), pp. 1119–1122.

Alshahrani, S.M., Alavudeen, S.S., Alakhali, K.M., Al-Worafi, Y.M., Bahamdan, A.K., & Vigneshwaran, E., (2019b). Self-Medication Among King Khalid University Students, Saudi Arabia. *Risk Management and Healthcare Policy*, 12, pp. 243–249.

Alshahrani, S.M., Alakhali, K.M., Al-Worafi, Y.M., & Alshahrani, N.Z. (2020a). Awareness and use of over the counter analgesic medication: A survey in the Aseer region population, Saudi Arabia. *International Journal of Advances in Applied Sciences*, 7(3), pp. 130–134.

Alshahrani, S.M., Alzahran, M., Alakhali, K., Vigneshwaran, E., Iqbal, M.J., Khan, N.A., … & Alavudeen, S.S. (2020b). Association between diabetes consequences and quality of life among patients with diabetes mellitus in the Aseer Province of Saudi Arabia. *Open Access Macedonian Journal of Medical Sciences*, 8(E), pp. 325–330.

Al-Worafi, Y.M. (2014). Prescription writing errors at a tertiary care hospital in Yemen: Prevalence, types, causes and recommendations. *American Journal of Pharmacy and Health Research*, 2, pp. 134–140.

Al-Worafi, Y.M.A. (2015). Appropriateness of metered-dose inhaler use in the Yemeni community pharmacies. *Journal of Taibah University Medical Sciences*, 10(3), pp. 353–358.

Al-Worafi, Y.M.A., (2016). Pharmacy practice in Yemen. In *Pharmacy Practice in Developing Countries* (pp. 267–287). Academic Press.

Al-Worafi, Y.M., Kassab, Y.W., Alseragi, W.M., Almutairi, M.S., Ahmed, A., Ming, L.C., Alkhoshaiban, A.S., & Hadi, M.A., (2017). Pharmacovigilance and adverse drg reaction reporting: A perspective of community pharmacists and pharmacy technicians in Sana'a, Yemen. *Therapeutics and Clinical Risk Management*, 13, p. 1175.

Al-Worafi, Y.M. (2018a). Knowledge, attitude and practice of Yemeni physicians toward pharmacovigilance: A mixed method study. *International Journal of Pharmacy and Pharmaceutical Sciences*, 10(10), pp. 74–77.

Al-Worafi, Y. (2018b). Knowledge, attitude and practice of Yemeni physicians toward pharmacovigilance: A mixed method study. *International Journal of Pharmacy and Pharmaceutical Sciences*, 10, pp. 74–77.

Al-Worafi, Y.M. (2018c). Dispensing errors observed by community pharmacy dispensers in IBB–YEMEN. *Asian Journal of Pharmaceutical and Clinical Research*, 11(11) 478.481.

Al-Worafi, Y.M. (2018d). Evauation of inhaler technique among patients with asthma and COPD in Yemen. *Journal of Taibah University Medical Sciences*, 13(5), pp. 488–490.

Al-Worafi, Y.M., Patel, R.P., Zaidi, S.T.R., Alseragi, W.M., Almutairi, M.S., Alkhoshaiban, A.S., & Ming, L.C. (2018a). Completeness and legibility of handwritten prescriptions in Sana'a, Yemen. *Medical Principles and Practice*, 27, pp. 290–292.

Al-Worafi, Y.M., Alseragi, W.M., Seng, L.K., Kassab, Y.W., Yeoh, S.F., Chiau, L., ... & Husain, K. (2018b). Dispensing errors in community pharmacies: A prospective study in Sana'a, Yemen. *Archives of Pharmacy Practice*, 9(4), pp. 1–3.

Al-Worafi, Y.M., Alseragi, W.M., & Mahmoud, M.A. (2019). Competency of metered-dose inhaler use among community pharmacy dispensers in Ibb, Yemen: A simulation method study. *Latin American Journal of Pharmacy*, 38(3), pp. 489–494.

Al-Worafi, Y.M. (Ed.). (2020a). *Drug Safety in Developing Countries: Achievements and Challenges.*

Al-Worafi, Y.M. (2020b). Medication errors. In *Drug Safety in Developing Countries* (pp. 105–117). Academic Press.

Al-Worafi, Y.M. (2020c). Adverse drug reactions. In *Drug Safety in Developing Countries* (pp. 39–57). Academic Press.

Al-Worafi, Y.M. (2020d). Medications registration and marketing: Safety-related issues. In *Drug Safety in Developing Countries* (pp. 21–28). Academic Press.

Al-Worafi, Y.M. (2020e). Pharmacovigilance. In *Drug Safety in Developing Countries* (pp. 29–38). Academic Press.

Al-Worafi, Y.M. (2020f). Drug-related problems. In *Drug Safety in Developing Countries* (pp. 59–71). Academic Press.

Al-Worafi, Y.M. (2020g). Medications safety-related terminology. In *Drug Safety in Developing Countries* (pp. 7–19). Academic Press.

Al-Worafi, Y.M. (2020h). Self-medication. In *Drug Safety in Developing Countries* (pp. 73–86). Academic Press.

Al-Worafi, Y.M. (2020j). Antibiotics safety issues. In *Drug Safety in Developing Countries* (pp. 87–103). Academic Press.

Al-Worafi, Y.M. (2020k). Medications safety research issues. In *Drug Safety in Developing Countries* (pp. 213–227). Academic Press.

Al-Worafi, Y.M. (2020l). Counterfeit and substandard medications. In *Drug Safety in Developing Countries* (pp. 119–126). Academic Press.

Al-Worafi, Y.M. (2020m). Medication abuse and misuse. In *Drug Safety in Developing Countries* (pp. 127–135). Academic Press.

Al-Worafi, Y.M. (2020n). Storage and disposal of medications. In *Drug Safety in Developing Countries* (pp. 137–142). Academic Press.

Al-Worafi, Y.M. (2020o). Safety of medications in special population. In *Drug Safety in Developing Countries* (pp. 143–162). Academic Press.

Al-Worafi, Y.M. (2020p). Herbal medicines safety issues. In *Drug Safety in Developing Countries* (pp. 163–178). Academic Press.

Al-Worafi, Y.M. (2020q). Medications safety pharmacoeconomics-related issues. In *Drug Safety in Developing Countries* (pp. 187–195). Academic Press.

Al-Worafi, Y.M. (2020r). Evidence-based medications safety practice. In *Drug Safety in Developing Countries* (pp. 197–201). Academic Press.

Al-Worafi, Y.M. (2020s). Quality indicators for medications safety. In *Drug Safety in Developing Countries* (pp. 229–242). Academic Press.

Al-Worafi, Y.M. (2020t). Drug safety in Yemen. In *Drug Safety in Developing Countries* (pp. 391–405). Academic Press.

Al-Worafi, Y.M. (2020u). Drug safety in Saudi Arabia. In *Drug Safety in Developing Countries* (pp. 407–417). Academic Press.

Al-Worafi, Y.M. (2020v). Drug safety in United Arab Emirates. In *Drug Safety in Developing Countries* (pp. 419–428). Academic Press.

Al-Worafi, Y.M. (2020w). Drug safety in Indonesia. In *Drug Safety in Developing Countries* (pp. 279–285). Academic Press.

Al-Worafi, Y.M. (2020x). Drug safety in Palestine. In *Drug Safety in Developing Countries* (pp. 471–480). Academic Press.

Al-Worafi, Y.M. (2020y). Drug safety: Comparison between developing countries. In *Drug Safety in Developing Countries* (pp. 603–611). Academic Press.

Al-Worafi, Y.M. (2020z). Drug safety in developing versus developed countries. In *Drug Safety in Developing Countries* (pp. 613–615). Academic Press.

Al-Worafi, Y.M., Alseragi, W.M., Ming, L.C., & Alakhali, K.M. (2020a). Drug safety in China. In *Drug Safety in Developing Countries* (pp. 381–388). Academic Press.

Al-Worafi, Y.M., Alseragi, W.M., Alakhali, K.M., Ming, L.C., Othman, G., Halboup, A.M., … & Elkalmi, R.M. (2020b). Knowledge, beliefs and factors affecting the use of generic medicines among patients in Ibb, Yemen: A mixed-method study. *Journal of Pharmacy Practice and Community Medicine*, 6(4). 53–56

Al-Worafi, Y.M., Elkalmi, R.M., Ming, L.C., Othman, G., Halboup, A.M., Battah, M.M., … & Mani, V. (2021a). Dispensing errors in hospital pharmacies: A prospective study in Yemen.AlQalam Journal of Medical and Applied Sciences, 4(2), 13–17.

Al-Worafi, Y.M., Hasan, S., Hassan, N.M., & Gaili, A.A. (2021b). Knowledge, attitude and experience of pharmacist in the UAE towards pharmacovigilance. *Research Journal of Pharmacy and Technology*, 14(1), pp. 265–269.

Al-Worafi, Y. (2022a). *A Guide to Online Pharmacy Education: Teaching Strategies and Assessment Methods*. CRC Press.

Al-Worafi, Y.M. (2022b). Patient care errors and related problems (part I): Development and validation of the model. 0000-0002-5752-2913

Al-Worafi, Y.M. (Ed.). (2023). *Clinical Case Studies on Medication Safety*. Academic Press.

Baig, M.R., Al-Worafi, Y.M., Alseragi, W.M., Ming, L.C., & Siddique, A. (2020). Drug safety in India. In *Drug Safety in Developing Countries* (pp. 327–334). Academic Press.

Elkalmi, R.M., Al-Worafi, Y.M., Alseragi, W.M., Ming, L.C., & Siddique, A. (2020). Drug safety in Malaysia. In *Drug Safety in Developing Countries* (pp. 245–253). Academic Press.

Elsayed, T., & Al-Worafi, Y.M. (2020). Drug safety in Egypt. In *Drug Safety in Developing Countries* (pp. 511–523). Academic Press.

Hasan, S., Al-Omar, M.J., AlZubaidy, H., & Al-Worafi, Y.M. (2019). Use of medications in Arab Countries. *Handbook of Healthcare in the Arab World*(pp 1–42), Springer, 42.

Hassan, Y., Abd Aziz, N., Kassab, Y.W., Elgasim, I., Shaharuddin, S., Al-Worafi, Y.M.A., … & Ming, L.C. (2014). How to help patients to control their blood pressure? Blood pressure control and its predictor. *Archives of Pharmacy Practice*, 5(4)153–161.

Izahar, S., Lean, Q.Y., Hameed, M.A., Murugiah, M.K., Patel, R.P., Al-Worafi, Y.M., … & Ming, L.C. (2017). Content analysis of mobile health applications on diabetes mellitus. *Frontiers in Endocrinology*, 8, p. 318.

Kristensen, S., & Bartels, P. (2010). Use of patient safety culture instruments and recommendations. *Aarhus, Denmark, European Society for Quality in HealthCare-Office for Quality Indicators*, 113. 1–35.

Lee, K.S., Yee, S.M., Zaidi, S.T.R., Patel, R.P., Yang, Q., Al-Worafi, Y.M., & Ming, L.C., 2017. Combating sale of counterfeit and falsified medicines online: A losing battle. *Frontiers in Pharmacology*, 8, p. 268.

McClatchey, K.D. (Ed.). (2002). *Clinical Laboratory Medicine*. Lippincott Williams & Wilkins.

Mahmoud, M.A., Wajid, S., Naqvi, A.A., Samreen, S., Althagfan, S.S., & Al-Worafi, Y. (2020). Self-medication with antibiotics: A cross-sectional community-based study. *Latin American Journal of Pharmacy*, 39(2), pp. 348–353.

Manan, M.M., Rusli, R.A., Ang, W.C., Al-Worafi, Y.M., & Ming, L.C. (2014). Assessing the pharmaceutical care issues of antiepileptic drug therapy in hospitalised epileptic patients. *Journal of Pharmacy Practice and Research*, 44(3), pp. 83–88.

Manan, M.M., Ibrahim, N.A., Aziz, N.A., Zulkifly, H.H., Al-Worafi, Y.M.A., & Long, C.M. (2016). Empirical use of antibiotic therapy in the prevention of early onset sepsis in neonates: A pilot study. *Archives of Medical Science*, 12(3), pp. 603–613.

Ming, L.C., Hameed, M.A., Lee, D.D., Apidi, N.A., Lai, P.S.M., Hadi, M.A., Al-Worafi, Y.M.A., & Khan, T.M., (2016). Use of medical mobile applications among hospital pharmacists in Malaysia. *Therapeutic Innovation & Regulatory Science*, 50(4), pp. 419–426.

Ming, L.C., Untong, N., Aliudin, N.A., Osili, N., Kifli, N., Tan, C.S., … & Goh, H.P. (2020). Mobile health apps on COVID-19 launched in the early days of the pandemic: Content analysis and review. *JMIR mHealth and uHealth*, 8(9), p. e19796.

Othman, G., Ali, F., Ibrahim, M.I.M., Al-Worafi, Y.M., Ansari, M., & Halboup, A.M. (2020). Assessment of anti-diabetic medications adherence among diabetic patients in Sana'a City, Yemen: A cross sectional study. *Journal of Pharmaceutical Research International*, 32(21), pp. 114–122.

Reynard, J., Reynolds, J., & Stevenson, P. (2009). *Practical patient safety*. OUP Oxford.

Saeed, M.S., Alkhoshaiban, A.S., Al-Worafi, Y.M.A., & Long, C.M., (2014). Perception of self-medication among university students in Saudi Arabia. *Archives of Pharmacy Practice*, 5(4), p. 149.

Salas, E., & Frush, K. (2012). *Improving Patient Safety Through Teamwork and Team Training*. Oxford University Press.

Vincent, C. (2011). *Patient Safety*. John Wiley & Sons.

23 Patient Safety in the Emergency Department (ED)

23.1 BACKGROUND

The emergency department (ED) plays a crucial role in patient care and patient safety by providing immediate medical care to patients with acute illnesses or injuries. The ED is equipped with advanced medical technology and resources to diagnose and treat patients quickly and effectively, often in life-threatening situations. The ED also plays a critical role in coordinating care for patients after they leave the hospital. This includes follow-up care, referrals to specialists, and assistance with accessing community resources. This coordination of care helps to ensure that patients receive appropriate care and are less likely to experience complications or readmissions. In terms of patient safety, the ED has a responsibility to identify and address potential safety risks for patients. This includes ensuring that patients receive the correct medication and treatment, preventing infections and falls, and identifying and responding to medical emergencies. To improve patient safety in the ED, healthcare organizations are implementing strategies such as patient safety checklists, electronic medical records, and standardized protocols for care. These strategies help to ensure that patients receive the highest quality of care and minimize the risk of errors or complications. EDs are the gateway to the healthcare system for patients who are experiencing acute illnesses or injuries, and they are often the first point of contact for patients seeking medical attention. EDs are staffed by a team of healthcare professionals, including physicians, nurses, and other support staff who work together to provide timely and effective care. One of the primary roles of EDs is to triage patients based on the severity of their condition. Patients who are critically ill or injured are given priority for care, while patients with less urgent conditions may have to wait longer to be seen. Triage helps ensure that the most critical patients receive care quickly, which can be life-saving in some cases. EDs also play a critical role in patient safety. The ED team must ensure that patients receive the correct diagnosis and treatment, which requires a thorough assessment of the patient's condition and medical history. This assessment may include diagnostic tests, such as blood tests, imaging studies, or electrocardiograms, to help identify the cause of the patient's symptoms. EDs also have protocols in place to manage patients with infectious diseases or other communicable illnesses. These protocols help prevent the spread of disease and protect both patients and healthcare workers from exposure. EDs are often called upon to manage patients with behavioral health issues, such as anxiety, depression, or substance abuse. The ED team must provide a safe and supportive environment for these patients and ensure that they receive appropriate care and follow-up. In conclusion, EDs play a critical role in patient care and patient safety. They are often the first point of contact for patients seeking medical attention and are staffed by a team of healthcare professionals who work together to provide timely and effective care. By triaging patients based on the severity of their condition, ensuring accurate diagnosis and treatment, managing infectious diseases, and addressing behavioral health issues, EDs help ensure that patients receive the care they need and stay safe (Croskerry et al., 2009; Kristensen & Bartels, 2010; Reynard et al., 2009; Salas & Frush, 2012; Vincent, 2011; Wyatt et al., 2020).

23.2 EMERGENCY DEPARTMENT ERRORS AND RELATED PROBLEMS

The ED is a fast-paced and high-stress environment where errors can occur. Some of the common errors and related problems in the ED include:

1. Misdiagnosis: Misdiagnosis is a significant problem in the ED, and it can result in delayed or inappropriate treatment, patient harm, and even death.

2. Medication errors: Medication errors, such as administering the wrong medication or dosage, can cause harm to patients and result in adverse drug reactions.

3. Communication breakdowns: Communication breakdowns between healthcare providers can result in missed diagnoses, delayed treatment, and other errors.

4. Overcrowding: Overcrowding in the ED can lead to long wait times, delayed treatment, and patient dissatisfaction.

5. Lack of resources: The ED may face shortages of staff, equipment, and supplies, which can lead to errors and delays in care.

Despite the critical role that EDs play in patient care, there are several challenges and issues that can lead to errors and related problems. Some of the most common ED errors and related problems include the following:

1. Misdiagnosis: EDs are fast-paced and high-pressure environments, and misdiagnosis is a common error that can occur due to various factors such as inadequate assessment, limited diagnostic capabilities, and cognitive biases.

2. Medication errors: EDs often use high-risk medications, and medication errors such as incorrect dosage or administration can occur due to factors such as inadequate communication, misreading of prescription orders, and patient-related factors such as allergies or non-disclosure of medication history.

3. Delayed treatment: EDs may experience overcrowding, staffing shortages, or delays in diagnostic testing, which can lead to delayed treatment and poorer outcomes for patients.

4. Communication breakdowns: EDs involve several healthcare professionals, and communication breakdowns between team members, or with the patient or their family, can lead to errors such as misdiagnosis or medication errors.

5. Violence and aggression: EDs may be exposed to high levels of violence and aggression, which can create an unsafe work environment for healthcare professionals and affect the quality of care provided to patients.

To address these problems, healthcare organizations are implementing strategies such as improved communication and collaboration among healthcare providers, increased staffing and resources, and the use of technology to support accurate diagnosis and treatment. Additionally, healthcare organizations are investing in training and education for ED staff to improve their skills and knowledge and promote a culture of safety. In conclusion, errors and related problems in the ED can have significant consequences for patients and healthcare organizations. By implementing strategies to address these issues, healthcare organizations can improve patient outcomes and promote a culture of safety in the ED.

23.3 CAUSES OF EMERGENCY DEPARTMENT ERRORS AND RELATED PROBLEMS

There are several causes of ED errors and related problems, including:

1. High patient volume: The high volume of patients in the ED can create a stressful and fast-paced environment, which can contribute to errors and delays in care.

2. Complexity of cases: Patients who come to the ED often have complex medical conditions that require urgent and specialized care, which can increase the risk of errors.

3. Communication breakdowns: Communication breakdowns between healthcare providers can result in missed diagnoses, delayed treatment, and other errors.

4. Overcrowding: Overcrowding in the ED can lead to long wait times, delayed treatment, and patient dissatisfaction.

5. Lack of resources: The ED may face shortages of staff, equipment, and supplies, which can lead to errors and delays in care.

By identifying and addressing these causes, healthcare organizations can implement strategies to improve the quality and safety of care in the ED. These strategies may include increased staffing and resources, improved communication and collaboration among healthcare providers, and the use of technology to support accurate diagnosis and treatment. Additionally, healthcare organizations can invest in training and education for ED staff to improve their skills and knowledge and promote a culture of safety.

23.4 PREVENTION OF EMERGENCY DEPARTMENT ERRORS AND RELATED PROBLEMS

Preventing errors and related problems in the ED involves a multi-faceted approach that includes:

1. Staff education and training: Healthcare organizations should invest in ongoing education and training for ED staff to improve their skills and knowledge, promote a culture of safety, and reduce the risk of errors.

2. Process improvements: Healthcare organizations should implement process improvements to streamline care delivery, reduce wait times, and improve patient flow in the ED.

3. Use of technology: Healthcare organizations should leverage technology to support accurate diagnosis and treatment, such as electronic medical records, decision support tools, and telemedicine.

4. Standardization of care: Healthcare organizations should standardize care delivery through the use of evidence-based protocols, checklists, and guidelines to reduce the risk of errors and improve patient outcomes.

5. Patient engagement: Healthcare organizations should engage patients in their care by providing clear communication, involving them in decision-making, and providing education and resources to support self-management.

6. Improving communication: Clear and effective communication is key to preventing errors in the ED. Healthcare professionals should communicate important information clearly and ensure that it is understood by all team members.

7. Standardizing processes: Standardizing processes such as triage, documentation, and medication administration can help to prevent errors by ensuring that all patients receive consistent and high-quality care.

8. Using technology: Implementing technology such as electronic health records, barcode scanning, and decision support systems can help to reduce errors by improving accuracy and efficiency.

9. Providing education and training: Healthcare professionals should receive regular education and training on topics such as patient safety, communication, and team dynamics to help them provide safe and effective care in the ED.

10. Improving staffing levels: Adequate staffing levels can help to prevent errors by reducing the workload on individual healthcare professionals and ensuring that patients receive timely and appropriate care.

11. Encouraging a culture of safety: Healthcare organizations should promote a culture of safety by encouraging staff to report errors and near-misses, analyzing the root causes of errors, and implementing strategies to prevent similar errors from occurring in the future.

By implementing these strategies, healthcare organizations can help to prevent ED errors and related problems, ultimately improving patient safety and outcomes.

23.5 EMERGENCY DEPARTMENT SAFETY CULTURE

ED safety culture refers to the attitudes, beliefs, and values of healthcare professionals and organizations toward patient safety in the ED. A positive safety culture is characterized by a shared commitment to patient safety, open communication, and a willingness to learn from errors and near-misses. Here are some key components of a positive safety culture in the ED:

1. Leadership commitment: Leaders in the ED must prioritize patient safety and create a culture that supports it. This includes providing resources for staff training and education, encouraging open communication, and actively supporting staff in their efforts to improve patient safety.

2. Open communication: Effective communication is essential to a positive safety culture. Healthcare professionals must be able to communicate openly and honestly about errors and near-misses, without fear of retribution. This includes reporting errors and near-misses, providing feedback to colleagues, and sharing information about patient care.

3. Learning from errors: A positive safety culture involves learning from errors and near-misses, rather than blaming individuals for mistakes. Healthcare organizations should establish systems to analyze errors and near-misses, identify root causes, and implement strategies to prevent similar errors from occurring in the future.

4. Teamwork: Effective teamwork is essential to a positive safety culture in the ED. Healthcare professionals must work collaboratively, communicate effectively, and support one another in their efforts to provide safe and effective care.

5. Continuous improvement: A positive safety culture involves a commitment to continuous improvement. Healthcare organizations must regularly assess their processes and systems, identify areas for improvement, and implement strategies to enhance patient safety.

By promoting a positive safety culture in the ED, healthcare organizations can improve patient safety, reduce the risk of errors and adverse events, and enhance the overall quality of care.

23.6 EMERGENCY DEPARTMENT ERRORS AND RELATED PROBLEMS IN DEVELOPING COUNTRIES: Challenges and Recommendations

ED errors and related problems in developing countries can be particularly challenging due to a variety of factors, including limited resources, inadequate infrastructure, and workforce shortages. Here are some challenges and recommendations for improving ED safety in developing countries.
  Challenges:

1. Limited resources: Many developing countries have limited resources for healthcare, including emergency services. This can result in overcrowded EDs, inadequate staffing, and insufficient medical supplies and equipment.

2. Inadequate infrastructure: In many developing countries, EDs lack adequate infrastructure, including appropriate triage systems, patient monitoring equipment, and diagnostic tools.

3. Workforce shortages: Developing countries may face workforce shortages in the healthcare sector, including emergency medicine specialists, nurses, and other healthcare professionals. This can result in overworked staff, poor quality care, and higher rates of errors and adverse events.

Recommendations:

1. Strengthen emergency services: Developing countries should prioritize strengthening their emergency services by increasing resources and investing in infrastructure. This can include expanding ED capacity, improving triage systems, and increasing the availability of medical supplies and equipment.

2. Workforce development: Developing countries should prioritize workforce development by investing in training and education for emergency medicine specialists, nurses, and other healthcare professionals. This can help to improve the quality of care and reduce the risk of errors and adverse events.

3. Technology adoption: Developing countries can leverage technology to improve ED safety, including the use of electronic health records, decision support systems, and telemedicine. These technologies can help to improve accuracy, efficiency, and communication among healthcare professionals.

4. Quality improvement: Developing countries should prioritize quality improvement initiatives in their EDs. This can include establishing systems for error reporting, analyzing root causes of errors, and implementing strategies to prevent similar errors from occurring in the future.

5. Collaboration and partnerships: Developing countries can benefit from collaboration and partnerships with international organizations, academic institutions, and other healthcare stakeholders. These collaborations can provide resources, expertise, and support for improving ED safety in developing countries.

6. Despite the progress in research about patient care and safety in developing countries, there is little research about patient safety related to the ED in the majority of developing countries, therefore, conducting research is very important and highly recommended (Alshahrani et al., 2019a,b; Al-Qahtani et al., 2015; Alshahrani et al., 2020a,b; Al-Worafi, 2014; Al-Worafi, 2015; Al-Worafi, 2016; Al-Worafi et al., 2017; Al-Worafi, 2018a–d; Al-Worafi et al., 2018a–b; Al-Worafi et al., 2019; Al-Worafi, 2020a–z; Al-Worafi et al., 2020a–b; Al-Worafi et al., 2021a,b; Al-Worafi, 2022a,b; Al-Worafi, 2023; Baig et al., 2020; Elkalmi et al., 2020; Elsayed & Al-Worafi, 2020; Hasan et al., 2019; Hassan et al., 2014; Izhar et al., 2017; Lee et al., 2017; Mahmoud et al., 2020; Manan et al., 2014; Manan et al., 2016; Ming et al., 2016; Ming et al., 2020; Othman et al., 2020; Saeed et al., 2014).

Improving ED safety in developing countries will require a multifaceted approach that addresses the challenges unique to these settings. By investing in resources, workforce development, technology, quality improvement, and collaboration, developing countries can improve ED safety, ultimately improving patient outcomes and saving lives.

23.7 CONCLUSION

This chapter has discussed ED safety issues, prevention, challenges, and recommendations for achieving the best practice in developing countries. Improving ED safety in developing countries will require a multifaceted approach that addresses the challenges unique to these settings. By investing in resources, workforce development, technology, quality improvement, and collaboration, developing countries can improve ED safety, ultimately improving patient outcomes and saving lives.

REFERENCES

Al-Qahtani, I., Almoteb, T.M., & Al-Warafi, Y. (2015). Competency of metered-dose inhaler use among Saudi community pharmacists: A Simulation method study. *RRJPPS*, 4(2), pp. 27–31.

Alshahrani, S.M., Alakhali, K.M., & Al-Worafi, Y.M., (2019a). Medication errors in a health care facility in southern Saudi Arabia. *Tropical Journal of Pharmaceutical Research*, 18(5), pp. 1119–1122.

Alshahrani, S.M., Alavudeen, S.S., Alakhali, K.M., Al-Worafi, Y.M., Bahamdan, A.K., & Vigneshwaran, E., (2019b). Self-medication among King Khalid University students, Saudi Arabia. *Risk Management and Healthcare Policy*, 12, pp. 243–249.

Alshahrani, S.M., Alakhali, K.M., Al-Worafi, Y.M., & Alshahrani, N.Z. (2020a). Awareness and use of over the counter analgesic medication: A survey in the Aseer region population, Saudi Arabia. *International Journal of Advances in Applied Sciences*, 7(3), pp. 130–134.

Alshahrani, S.M., Alzahran, M., Alakhali, K., Vigneshwaran, E., Iqbal, M.J., Khan, N.A., … & Alavudeen, S.S. (2020b). Association between diabetes consequences and quality of life among patients with diabetes mellitus in the Aseer Province of Saudi Arabia. *Open Access Macedonian Journal of Medical Sciences*, 8(E), pp. 325–330.

Al-Worafi, Y.M. (2014). Prescription writing errors at a tertiary care hospital in Yemen: Prevalence, types, causes and recommendations. *American Journal of Pharmacy and Health Research*, 2, pp. 134–140.

Al-Worafi, Y.M.A. (2015). Appropriateness of metered-dose inhaler use in the Yemeni community pharmacies. *Journal of Taibah University Medical Sciences*, 10(3), pp. 353–358.

Al-Worafi, Y.M.A., (2016). Pharmacy practice in Yemen. In *Pharmacy Practice in Developing Countries* (pp. 267–287). Academic Press.

Al-Worafi, Y.M., Kassab, Y.W., Alseragi, W.M., Almutairi, M.S., Ahmed, A., Ming, L.C., Alkhoshaiban, A.S., & Hadi, M.A., (2017). Pharmacovigilance and adverse drg reaction reporting: A perspective of community pharmacists and pharmacy technicians in Sana'a, Yemen. *Therapeutics and Clinical Risk Management*, 13, p. 1175.

Al-Worafi, Y.M., (2018a). Knowledge, attitude and practice of Yemeni physicians toward pharmacovigilance: A mixed method study. *International Journal of Pharmacy and Pharmaceutical Sciences*, 10(10), pp. 74–77.

Al-Worafi, Y. (2018b). Knowledge, attitude and practice of Yemeni physicians toward pharmacovigilance: A mixed method study. *International Journal of Pharmacy and Pharmaceutical Sciences*, 10, pp. 74–77.

Al-worafi, Y.M. (2018c). Dispensing errors observed by community pharmacy dispensers in IBB–YEMEN. *Asian Journal of Pharmaceutical and Clinical Research*, 11(11)478.481.

Al-Worafi, Y.M. (2018d). Evauation of inhaler technique among patients with asthma and COPD in Yemen. *Journal of Taibah University Medical Sciences*, 13(5), pp. 488–490.

Al-Worafi, Y.M., Patel, R.P., Zaidi, S.T.R., Alseragi, W.M., Almutairi, M.S., Alkhoshaiban, A.S., & Ming, L.C. (2018a). Completeness and legibility of handwritten prescriptions in Sana'a, Yemen. *Medical Principles and Practice*, 27, pp. 290–292.

Al-Worafi, Y.M., Alseragi, W.M., Seng, L.K., Kassab, Y.W., Yeoh, S.F., Chiau, L., ... & Husain, K. (2018b). Dispensing errors in community pharmacies: A prospective study in Sana'a, Yemen. *Archives of Pharmacy Practice*, 9(4), pp. 1–3.

Al-Worafi, Y.M., Alseragi, W.M., & Mahmoud, M.A. (2019). Competency of metered-dose inhaler use among community pharmacy dispensers in Ibb, Yemen: A simulation method study. *Latin American Journal of Pharmacy*, 38(3), pp. 489–494.

Al-Worafi, Y.M. (Ed.). (2020a). *Drug Safety in Developing Countries: Achievements and Challenges*.

Al-Worafi, Y.M. (2020b). Medication errors. In *Drug Safety in Developing Countries* (pp. 105–117). Academic Press.

Al-Worafi, Y.M. (2020c). Adverse drug reactions. In *Drug Safety in Developing Countries* (pp. 39–57). Academic Press.

Al-Worafi, Y.M. (2020d). Medications registration and marketing: Safety-related issues. In *Drug Safety in Developing Countries* (pp. 21–28). Academic Press.

Al-Worafi, Y.M. (2020e). Pharmacovigilance. In *Drug Safety in Developing Countries* (pp. 29–38). Academic Press.

Al-Worafi, Y.M. (2020f). Drug-related problems. In *Drug Safety in Developing Countries* (pp. 59–71). Academic Press.

Al-Worafi, Y.M. (2020g). Medications safety-related terminology. In *Drug Safety in Developing Countries* (pp. 7–19). Academic Press.

Al-Worafi, Y.M. (2020h). Self-medication. In *Drug Safety in Developing Countries* (pp. 73–86). Academic Press.

Al-Worafi, Y.M. (2020j). Antibiotics safety issues. In *Drug Safety in Developing Countries* (pp. 87–103). Academic Press.

Al-Worafi, Y.M. (2020k). Medications safety research issues. In *Drug Safety in Developing Countries* (pp. 213–227). Academic Press.

Al-Worafi, Y.M. (2020l). Counterfeit and substandard medications. In *Drug Safety in Developing Countries* (pp. 119–126). Academic Press.

Al-Worafi, Y.M. (2020m). Medication abuse and misuse. In *Drug Safety in Developing Countries* (pp. 127–135). Academic Press.

Al-Worafi, Y.M. (2020n). Storage and disposal of medications. In *Drug Safety in Developing Countries* (pp. 137–142). Academic Press.

Al-Worafi, Y.M. (2020o). Safety of medications in special population. In *Drug Safety in Developing Countries* (pp. 143–162). Academic Press.

Al-Worafi, Y.M. (2020p). Herbal medicines safety issues. In *Drug Safety in Developing Countries* (pp. 163–178). Academic Press.

Al-Worafi, Y.M. (2020q). Medications safety pharmacoeconomics-related issues. In *Drug Safety in Developing Countries* (pp. 187–195). Academic Press.

Al-Worafi, Y.M. (2020r). Evidence-based medications safety practice. In *Drug Safety in Developing Countries* (pp. 197–201). Academic Press.

Al-Worafi, Y.M. (2020s). Quality indicators for medications safety. In *Drug Safety in Developing Countries* (pp. 229–242). Academic Press.

Al-Worafi, Y.M. (2020t). Drug safety in Yemen. In *Drug Safety in Developing Countries* (pp. 391–405). Academic Press.

Al-Worafi, Y.M. (2020u). Drug safety in Saudi Arabia. In *Drug Safety in Developing Countries* (pp. 407–417). Academic Press.

Al-Worafi, Y.M. (2020v). Drug safety in United Arab Emirates. In *Drug Safety in Developing Countries* (pp. 419–428). Academic Press.

Al-Worafi, Y.M. (2020w). Drug safety in Indonesia. In *Drug Safety in Developing Countries* (pp. 279–285). Academic Press.

Al-Worafi, Y.M. (2020x). Drug safety in Palestine. In *Drug Safety in Developing Countries* (pp. 471–480). Academic Press.

Al-Worafi, Y.M. (2020y). Drug safety: comparison between developing countries. In *Drug Safety in Developing Countries* (pp. 603–611). Academic Press.

Al-Worafi, Y.M. (2020z). Drug safety in developing versus developed countries. In *Drug Safety in Developing Countries* (pp. 613–615). Academic Press.

Al-Worafi, Y.M., Alseragi, W.M., Ming, L.C., & Alakhali, K.M. (2020a). Drug safety in China. In *Drug Safety in Developing Countries* (pp. 381–388). Academic Press.

Al-Worafi, Y.M., Alseragi, W.M., Alakhali, K.M., Ming, L.C., Othman, G., Halboup, A.M., … & Elkalmi, R.M. (2020b). Knowledge, beliefs and factors affecting the use of generic medicines among patients in Ibb, Yemen: A mixed-method study. *Journal of Pharmacy Practice and Community Medicine*, 6(4) 53–56.

Al-Worafi, Y.M., Elkalmi, R.M., Ming, L.C., Othman, G., Halboup, A.M., Battah, M.M., … & Mani, V. (2021a). Dispensing errors in hospital pharmacies: A prospective study in Yemen.AlQalam Journal of Medical and Applied Sciences, 4(2), 13–17.

Al-Worafi, Y.M., Hasan, S., Hassan, N.M., & Gaili, A.A. (2021b). Knowledge, Attitude and Experience of Pharmacist in the UAE towards Pharmacovigilance. *Research Journal of Pharmacy and Technology*, 14(1), pp. 265–269.

Al-Worafi, Y. (2022a). *A Guide to Online Pharmacy Education: Teaching Strategies and Assessment Methods*. CRC Press.

Al-Worafi, Y.M. (2022b). Patient care errors and related problems (part I): Development and validation of the model. 0000-0002-5752-2913

Al-Worafi, Y.M. (Ed.). (2023). *Clinical Case Studies on Medication Safety*. Academic Press.

Baig, M.R., Al-Worafi, Y.M., Alseragi, W.M., Ming, L.C., & Siddique, A. (2020). Drug safety in India. In *Drug Safety in Developing Countries* (pp. 327–334). Academic Press.

Croskerry, P., Cosby, K.S., Schenkel, S.M., & Wears, R.L. (2009). *Patient Safety in Emergency Medicine* (pp. 219–227). Philadelphia, PA: Wolters Kluwer Health/Lippincott Williams & Wilkins.

Elkalmi, R.M., Al-Worafi, Y.M., Alseragi, W.M., Ming, L.C., & Siddique, A. (2020). Drug safety in Malaysia. In *Drug Safety in Developing Countries* (pp. 245–253). Academic Press.

Elsayed, T., & Al-Worafi, Y.M. (2020). Drug safety in Egypt. In *Drug Safety in Developing Countries* (pp. 511–523). Academic Press.

Hasan, S., Al-Omar, M.J., AlZubaidy, H., & Al-Worafi, Y.M. (2019). Use of medications in Arab Countries. *Handbook of Healthcare in the Arab World*, Springer,

Hassan, Y., Abd Aziz, N., Kassab, Y.W., Elgasim, I., Shaharuddin, S., Al-Worafi, Y.M.A., ... & Ming, L.C. (2014). How to help patients to control their blood pressure? Blood pressure control and its predictor. *Archives of Pharmacy Practice*, 5(4), pp. 153–161.

Izahar, S., Lean, Q.Y., Hameed, M.A., Murugiah, M.K., Patel, R.P., Al-Worafi, Y.M., ... & Ming, L.C. (2017). Content analysis of mobile health applications on diabetes mellitus. *Frontiers in Endocrinology*, 8, p. 318.

Kristensen, S., & Bartels, P. (2010). Use of patient safety culture instruments and recommendations. *Aarhus, Denmark, European Society for Quality in HealthCare-Office for Quality Indicators*, 113. 1–35.

Lee, K.S., Yee, S.M., Zaidi, S.T.R., Patel, R.P., Yang, Q., Al-Worafi, Y.M., & Ming, L.C., 2017. Combating sale of counterfeit and falsified medicines online: A losing battle. *Frontiers in Pharmacology*, 8, p. 268.

Mahmoud, M.A., Wajid, S., Naqvi, A.A., Samreen, S., Althagfan, S.S., & Al-Worafi, Y. (2020). Self-medication with antibiotics: A cross-sectional community-based study. *Latin American Journal of Pharmacy*, 39(2), pp. 348–353.

Manan, M.M., Rusli, R.A., Ang, W.C., Al-Worafi, Y.M., & Ming, L.C. (2014). Assessing the pharmaceutical care issues of antiepileptic drug therapy in hospitalised epileptic patients. *Journal of Pharmacy Practice and Research*, 44(3), pp. 83–88.

Manan, M.M., Ibrahim, N.A., Aziz, N.A., Zulkifly, H.H., Al-Worafi, Y.M.A., & Long, C.M. (2016). Empirical use of antibiotic therapy in the prevention of early onset sepsis in neonates: A pilot study. *Archives of Medical Science*, 12(3), pp. 603–613.

Ming, L.C., Hameed, M.A., Lee, D.D., Apidi, N.A., Lai, P.S.M., Hadi, M.A., Al-Worafi, Y.M.A., & Khan, T.M., (2016). Use of medical mobile applications among hospital pharmacists in Malaysia. *Therapeutic Innovation & Regulatory Science*, 50(4), pp. 419–426.

Ming, L.C., Untong, N., Aliudin, N.A., Osili, N., Kifli, N., Tan, C.S., ... & Goh, H.P. (2020). Mobile health apps on COVID-19 launched in the early days of the pandemic: Content analysis and review. *JMIR mHealth and uHealth*, 8(9), p. e19796.

Othman, G., Ali, F., Ibrahim, M.I.M., Al-Worafi, Y.M., Ansari, M., & Halboup, A.M. (2020). Assessment of anti-diabetic medications adherence among diabetic patients in Sana'a City, Yemen: A cross sectional study. *Journal of Pharmaceutical Research International*, 32(21), pp. 114–122.

Reynard, J., Reynolds, J., & Stevenson, P. (2009). *Practical Patient Safety*. OUP Oxford.

Saeed, M.S., Alkhoshaiban, A.S., Al-Worafi, Y.M.A., & Long, C.M., (2014). Perception of self-medication among university students in Saudi Arabia. *Archives of Pharmacy Practice*, 5(4), p. 149.

Salas, E., & Frush, K. (2012). *Improving Patient Safety Through Teamwork and Team Training*. Oxford University Press.

Vincent, C. (2011). *Patient Safety*. John Wiley & Sons.

Wyatt, J.P., Taylor, R.G., de Wit, K., & Hotton, E.J. (2020). *Oxford Handbook of Emergency Medicine*. Oxford University Press, USA.

24 Patient Safety in Intensive Care Unit (ICU)

24.1 BACKGROUND

The intensive care unit (ICU) is a specialized unit within a hospital that provides care for critically ill patients. The ICU plays a critical role in patient care and patient safety by providing close monitoring, specialized treatment, and a multidisciplinary team approach to care delivery. Patient care in the ICU involves a comprehensive approach to addressing the unique needs of critically ill patients. This includes close monitoring of vital signs, medication management, and specialized treatments such as mechanical ventilation and renal replacement therapy. The ICU team works together to provide coordinated care and ensure that patients receive appropriate interventions to optimize their recovery. Patient safety in the ICU is a top priority, given the high acuity of patients and the potential for adverse events. To promote patient safety, healthcare organizations implement strategies such as standardized protocols, checklists, and electronic medical records to support accurate diagnosis and treatment. In addition, the ICU team works closely to identify and address potential safety risks for patients, such as infections, falls, and medication errors. To improve patient care and patient safety in the ICU, healthcare organizations are investing in training and education for ICU staff, implementing evidence-based practices, and leveraging technology to support accurate diagnosis and treatment. By providing high-quality care and promoting a culture of safety in the ICU, healthcare organizations can improve patient outcomes and reduce the risk of adverse events (Kristensen & Bartels, 2010; Reynard et al., 2009; Salas & Frush, 2012; Vincent, 2011; Webb et al., 2016).

24.2 INTENSIVE CARE UNIT (ICU) ERRORS AND RELATED PROBLEMS

ICUs are specialized hospital departments that provide critical care to patients with life-threatening illnesses or injuries. Despite the best efforts of healthcare providers, ICU errors and related problems can occur. Here are some examples:

1. Medication errors: These can include giving the wrong medication, the wrong dose, or administering medications at the wrong time. These errors can have serious consequences, especially in critically ill patients who may be more susceptible to medication-related complications.

2. Infections: ICU patients are at a higher risk of developing infections due to their weakened immune systems, invasive procedures, and prolonged hospital stays. Infections acquired in the ICU can lead to sepsis, organ failure, and even death.

3. Ventilator-associated complications: Patients on mechanical ventilators are at risk of complications such as pneumonia, ventilator-associated lung injury, and ventilator-associated pneumonia.

4. Delayed diagnosis and treatment: ICU patients often have complex medical conditions that require prompt and accurate diagnosis and treatment. Delayed or missed diagnoses can lead to serious complications or even death.

5. Communication breakdowns: The fast-paced, high-pressure environment of the ICU can lead to communication breakdowns between healthcare providers. These breakdowns can result in missed information, misunderstandings, and errors in care.

6. Equipment malfunction: The ICU relies on a variety of specialized equipment, such as ventilators, monitors, and infusion pumps. Equipment malfunctions can lead to serious complications, such as delayed treatment or medication errors.

7. Staffing shortages: Staffing shortages in the ICU can lead to increased workload, fatigue, and burnout among healthcare providers. This can increase the risk of errors and compromise patient safety.

Reducing ICU errors and related problems requires a multifaceted approach, including ongoing education and training for healthcare providers, improvements in communication and teamwork, and the implementation of best practices and safety protocols.

24.3 CAUSES OF INTENSIVE CARE UNIT (ICU) ERRORS AND RELATED PROBLEMS

There are several potential causes of ICU errors and related problems, including:

1. Human error: Healthcare providers, like anyone else, are fallible and can make mistakes. These mistakes may be due to factors such as fatigue, stress, distraction, or lack of experience or training.

DOI: 10.1201/9781003230465-26

2. Systemic issues: In some cases, ICU errors may be caused by systemic issues within the healthcare system, such as inadequate staffing, poor communication between healthcare providers, or a lack of resources or equipment.

3. Patient factors: Patients who are critically ill or have complex medical conditions may be at a higher risk of experiencing complications or errors in care. This may be due to factors such as their underlying medical conditions, their level of consciousness or ability to communicate, or their medication regimen.

4. Medication-related factors: Medication-related errors in the ICU may be caused by a variety of factors, including inadequate medication reconciliation, confusion between similarly named medications, or improper dosing or administration.

5. Technical problems: Equipment malfunctions, power outages, or other technical issues may also contribute to ICU errors and complications.

6. Communication breakdowns: Communication breakdowns between healthcare providers can lead to missed information, misunderstandings, and errors in care. This may be due to factors such as language barriers, poor documentation, or conflicting priorities.

7. Organizational factors: Organizational factors, such as a lack of support for healthcare providers, inadequate resources or training, or a culture of blame or shame, may also contribute to ICU errors and related problems.

It's important to note that ICU errors and complications often have multiple contributing factors, and addressing them may require a multi-pronged approach.

24.4 PREVENTION OF INTENSIVE CARE UNIT (ICU) ERRORS AND RELATED PROBLEMS

Prevention of ICU errors and related problems is critical to ensuring patient safety and improving outcomes. Strategies for preventing errors and related problems in the ICU include:

1. Standardized protocols and checklists: Standardized protocols and checklists can help to ensure that all ICU staff follow consistent procedures and take the necessary steps to prevent errors and complications.

2. Monitoring and surveillance: Continuous monitoring of vital signs, medication administration, and other aspects of care can help to identify potential problems before they become serious concerns.

3. Communication and teamwork: Effective communication and teamwork among ICU staff can help to prevent errors and related problems by ensuring that everyone is aware of the patient's condition and needs.

4. Staff education and training: Ongoing education and training for ICU staff can help to ensure that they are up-to-date on the latest techniques and best practices for preventing errors and complications.

5. Technology and automation: The use of technology and automation, such as electronic medical records and smart infusion pumps, can help to reduce the risk of errors and improve the accuracy of care.

By implementing these strategies and prioritizing patient safety, healthcare organizations can reduce the risk of errors and related problems in the ICU and improve patient

24.5 INTENSIVE CARE UNIT (ICU) SAFETY CULTURE

To promote a strong ICU safety culture, healthcare organizations should prioritize patient safety and create an environment that supports open communication and collaboration among healthcare providers. ICU staff should be engaged in the development of safety policies, procedures, and protocols to ensure that they are relevant and effective in the ICU setting. Education and training on patient safety, error prevention, and best practices for care delivery in the ICU are essential to promoting a safety culture. In addition, healthcare organizations should encourage reporting of errors and near-misses, and conduct a thorough analysis to identify areas for improvement and implement changes to prevent future errors. By promoting a safety culture in the ICU, healthcare organizations can improve the quality and safety of care, reduce the risk of errors and adverse events, and improve patient outcomes. It is important for healthcare providers in the ICU to prioritize patient safety and work together to identify and address potential safety risks for patients.

24.6 INTENSIVE CARE UNIT (ICU) ERRORS AND RELATED PROBLEMS IN DEVELOPING COUNTRIES: Challenges and Recommendations

ICU errors and related problems can have a significant impact on patient outcomes in developing countries, where healthcare resources may be limited and healthcare systems may be less well-established. Here are some of the challenges and recommendations related to ICU errors in developing countries:

Challenges:

1. Limited Resources: Developing countries may have limited resources, including equipment, medications, and trained healthcare professionals, which can contribute to errors in ICU care.

2. Poor Infrastructure: Inadequate infrastructure, including outdated facilities and unreliable electricity and water supply, can further exacerbate challenges in providing quality care in ICU settings.

3. Lack of Training: Healthcare professionals in developing countries may not receive adequate training in critical care, including ICU-specific protocols and procedures, which can contribute to errors.

4. Communication Barriers: Communication barriers, including language and cultural differences, can make it challenging for healthcare professionals to provide effective care and collaborate effectively.

Recommendations:

1. Strengthen Healthcare Infrastructure: Developing countries should invest in improving their healthcare infrastructure, including updating facilities, ensuring reliable utilities, and providing essential equipment.

2. Increase Education and Training: Healthcare professionals in developing countries should receive comprehensive training in critical care, including ICU-specific protocols and procedures, to reduce errors and improve patient outcomes.

3. Develop Standardized Protocols: Developing standardized protocols and procedures for ICU care can help healthcare professionals provide consistent, high-quality care, regardless of location or resources.

4. Encourage Collaboration: Encouraging collaboration between healthcare professionals, including through regular team meetings and interprofessional education, can improve communication and reduce errors.

5. Emphasize Patient and Family Engagement: Including patients and their families in the care process can help healthcare professionals better understand patients' needs and improve communication, ultimately leading to better outcomes.

6. Establish Quality Improvement Programs: Developing countries should establish quality improvement programs to identify areas of weakness in ICU care and implement changes to improve patient outcomes.

7. Despite the progress in research about patient care and safety in developing countries, there is little research about patient safety related to the ICU in the majority of developing countries, therefore, conducting research is very important and highly recommended (Alshahrani et al., 2019a,b; Al-Qahtani et al., 2015; Alshahrani et al., 2020a,b; Al-Worafi, 2014; Al-Worafi, 2015; Al-Worafi, 2016; Al-Worafi et al., 2017; Al-Worafi, 2018a–d; Al-Worafi et al., 2018a–b; Al-Worafi et al., 2019; Al-Worafi, 2020a–z; Al-Worafi et al., 2020a–b; Al-Worafi et al., 2021a,b; Al-Worafi, 2022a,b; Al-Worafi, 2023; Baig et al., 2020; Elkalmi et al., 2020; Elsayed & Al-Worafi, 2020; Hasan et al., 2019; Hassan et al., 2014; Izhar et al., 2017; Lee et al., 2017; Mahmoud et al., 2020; Manan et al., 2014; Manan et al., 2016; Ming et al., 2016; Ming et al., 2020; Othman et al., 2020; Saeed et al., 2014).

24.7 CONCLUSION

This chapter has discussed ICU safety issues, prevention, challenges, and recommendations for achieving the best practice in developing countries. ICU is a specialized unit within a hospital that provides care for critically ill patients, it plays a critical role in patient care and patient safety by providing close monitoring, specialized treatment, and a multidisciplinary team approach to care delivery. Patient care in the ICU involves a comprehensive approach to addressing the unique needs of critically ill patients. Reducing ICU errors and related problems requires a multifaceted approach, including ongoing education and training for healthcare providers, improvements in communication and teamwork, and the implementation of best practices and safety protocols.

REFERENCES

Al-Qahtani, I., Almoteb, T.M., & Al-Warafi, Y. (2015). Competency of metered-dose inhaler use among Saudi community pharmacists: A Simulation method study. *RRJPPS*, 4(2), 27–31.

Alshahrani, S.M., Alakhali, K.M., & Al-Worafi, Y.M., (2019a). Medication errors in a health care facility in southern Saudi Arabia. *Tropical Journal of Pharmaceutical Research*, 18(5), pp. 1119–1122.

Alshahrani, S.M., Alavudeen, S.S., Alakhali, K.M., Al-Worafi, Y.M., Bahamdan, A.K., & Vigneshwaran, E., (2019b). Self-Medication Among King Khalid University Students, Saudi Arabia. *Risk Management and Healthcare Policy*, 12, pp. 243–249.

Alshahrani, S.M., Alakhali, K.M., Al-Worafi, Y.M., & Alshahrani, N.Z. (2020a). Awareness and use of over the counter analgesic medication: A survey in the Aseer region population, Saudi Arabia. *International Journal of Advances in Applied Sciences*, 7(3), pp. 130–134.

Alshahrani, S.M., Alzahran, M., Alakhali, K., Vigneshwaran, E., Iqbal, M.J., Khan, N.A., ... & Alavudeen, S.S. (2020b). Association between diabetes consequences and quality of life among patients with diabetes mellitus in the Aseer Province of Saudi Arabia. *Open Access Macedonian Journal of Medical Sciences*, 8(E), pp. 325–330.

Al-Worafi, Y.M. (2014). Prescription writing errors at a tertiary care hospital in Yemen: Prevalence, types, causes and recommendations. *American Journal of Pharmacy and Health Research*, 2, pp. 134–140.

Al-Worafi, Y.M.A. (2015). Appropriateness of metered-dose inhaler use in the Yemeni community pharmacies. *Journal of Taibah University Medical Sciences*, 10(3), pp. 353–358.

Al-Worafi, Y.M.A., (2016). Pharmacy practice in Yemen. In *Pharmacy Practice in Developing Countries* (pp. 267–287). Academic Press.

Al-Worafi, Y.M., Kassab, Y.W., Alseragi, W.M., Almutairi, M.S., Ahmed, A., Ming, L.C., Alkhoshaiban, A.S., & Hadi, M.A., (2017). Pharmacovigilance and adverse drg reaction reporting: A perspective of community pharmacists and pharmacy technicians in Sana'a, Yemen. *Therapeutics and Clinical Risk Management*, 13, p. 1175.

Al-Worafi, Y.M. (2018a). Knowledge, attitude and practice of Yemeni physicians toward pharmacovigilance: A mixed method study. *International Journal of Pharmacy and Pharmaceutical Sciences*, 10(10), pp. 74–77.

Al-Worafi, Y. (2018b). Knowledge, attitude and practice of Yemeni physicians toward pharmacovigilance: A mixed method study. *International Journal of Pharmacy and Pharmaceutical Sciences*, 10, pp. 74–77.

Al-Worafi, Y.M. (2018c). Dispensing errors observed by community pharmacy dispensers in IBB–YEMEN. *Asian Journal of Pharmaceutical and Clinical Research*, 11(11).478.481.

Al-Worafi, Y.M. (2018d). Evauation of inhaler technique among patients with asthma and COPD in Yemen. *Journal of Taibah University Medical Sciences*, 13(5), pp. 488–490.

Al-Worafi, Y.M., Patel, R.P., Zaidi, S.T.R., Alseragi, W.M., Almutairi, M.S., Alkhoshaiban, A.S., & Ming, L.C. (2018a). Completeness and legibility of handwritten prescriptions in Sana'a, Yemen. *Medical Principles and Practice*, 27, pp. 290–292.

Al-Worafi, Y.M., Alseragi, W.M., Seng, L.K., Kassab, Y.W., Yeoh, S.F., Chiau, L., ... & Husain, K. (2018b). Dispensing errors in community pharmacies: A prospective study in Sana'a, Yemen. *Archives of Pharmacy Practice*, 9(4), pp. 1–3.

Al-Worafi, Y.M., Alseragi, W.M., & Mahmoud, M.A. (2019). Competency of metered-dose inhaler use among community pharmacy dispensers in Ibb, Yemen: A simulation method study. *Latin American Journal of Pharmacy*, 38(3), pp. 489–494.

Al-Worafi, Y.M. (Ed.). (2020a). *Drug Safety in Developing Countries: Achievements and Challenges*.

Al-Worafi, Y.M. (2020b). Medication errors. In *Drug Safety in Developing Countries* (pp. 105–117). Academic Press.

Al-Worafi, Y.M. (2020c). Adverse drug reactions. In *Drug Safety in Developing Countries* (pp. 39–57). Academic Press.

Al-Worafi, Y.M. (2020d). Medications registration and marketing: Safety-related issues. In *Drug Safety in Developing Countries* (pp. 21–28). Academic Press.

Al-Worafi, Y.M. (2020e). Pharmacovigilance. In *Drug Safety in Developing Countries* (pp. 29–38). Academic Press.

Al-Worafi, Y.M. (2020f). Drug-related problems. In *Drug Safety in Developing Countries* (pp. 59–71). Academic Press.

Al-Worafi, Y.M. (2020g). Medications safety-related terminology. In *Drug Safety in Developing Countries* (pp. 7–19). Academic Press.

Al-Worafi, Y.M. (2020h). Self-medication. In *Drug Safety in Developing Countries* (pp. 73–86). Academic Press.

Al-Worafi, Y.M. (2020j). Antibiotics safety issues. In *Drug Safety in Developing Countries* (pp. 87–103). Academic Press.

Al-Worafi, Y.M. (2020k). Medications safety research issues. In *Drug Safety in Developing Countries* (pp. 213–227). Academic Press.

Al-Worafi, Y.M. (2020l). Counterfeit and substandard medications. In *Drug Safety in Developing Countries* (pp. 119–126). Academic Press.

Al-Worafi, Y.M. (2020m). Medication abuse and misuse. In *Drug Safety in Developing Countries* (pp. 127–135). Academic Press.

Al-Worafi, Y.M. (2020n). Storage and disposal of medications. In *Drug Safety in Developing Countries* (pp. 137–142). Academic Press.

Al-Worafi, Y.M. (2020o). Safety of medications in special population. In *Drug Safety in Developing Countries* (pp. 143–162). Academic Press.

Al-Worafi, Y.M. (2020p). Herbal medicines safety issues. In *Drug Safety in Developing Countries* (pp. 163–178). Academic Press.

Al-Worafi, Y.M. (2020q). Medications safety pharmacoeconomics-related issues. In *Drug Safety in Developing Countries* (pp. 187–195). Academic Press.

Al-Worafi, Y.M. (2020r). Evidence-based medications safety practice. In *Drug Safety in Developing Countries* (pp. 197–201). Academic Press.

Al-Worafi, Y.M. (2020s). Quality indicators for medications safety. In *Drug Safety in Developing Countries* (pp. 229–242). Academic Press.

Al-Worafi, Y.M. (2020t). Drug safety in Yemen. In *Drug Safety in Developing Countries* (pp. 391–405). Academic Press.

Al-Worafi, Y.M. (2020u). Drug safety in Saudi Arabia. In *Drug Safety in Developing Countries* (pp. 407–417). Academic Press.

Al-Worafi, Y.M. (2020v). Drug safety in United Arab Emirates. In *Drug Safety in Developing Countries* (pp. 419–428). Academic Press.

Al-Worafi, Y.M. (2020w). Drug safety in Indonesia. In *Drug Safety in Developing Countries* (pp. 279–285). Academic Press.

Al-Worafi, Y.M. (2020x). Drug safety in Palestine. In *Drug Safety in Developing Countries* (pp. 471–480). Academic Press.

Al-Worafi, Y.M. (2020y). Drug safety: Comparison between developing countries. In *Drug Safety in Developing Countries* (pp. 603–611). Academic Press.

Al-Worafi, Y.M. (2020z). Drug safety in developing versus developed countries. In *Drug Safety in Developing Countries* (pp. 613–615). Academic Press.

Al-Worafi, Y.M., Alseragi, W.M., Ming, L.C., & Alakhali, K.M. (2020a). Drug safety in China. In *Drug Safety in Developing Countries* (pp. 381–388). Academic Press.

Al-Worafi, Y.M., Alseragi, W.M., Alakhali, K.M., Ming, L.C., Othman, G., Halboup, A.M., … & Elkalmi, R.M. (2020b). Knowledge, beliefs and factors affecting the use of generic medicines among patients in Ibb, Yemen: A mixed-method study. *Journal of Pharmacy Practice and Community Medicine*, 6(4)53-56.

Al-Worafi, Y.M., Elkalmi, R.M., Ming, L.C., Othman, G., Halboup, A.M., Battah, M.M., … & Mani, V. (2021a). *Dispensing errors in hospital pharmacies: A prospective study in Yemen.*AlQalam Journal of Medical and Applied Sciences, 4(2), 13–17.

Al-Worafi, Y.M., Hasan, S., Hassan, N.M., & Gaili, A.A. (2021b). Knowledge, attitude and experience of pharmacist in the UAE towards pharmacovigilance. *Research Journal of Pharmacy and Technology*, 14(1), pp. 265–269.

Al-Worafi, Y. (2022a). *A Guide to Online Pharmacy Education: Teaching Strategies and Assessment Methods*. CRC Press.

Al-Worafi, Y.M. (2022b). Patient care errors and related problems (part I): Development and validation of the model. 0000-0002-5752-2913

Al-Worafi, Y.M. (Ed.). (2023). *Clinical Case Studies on Medication Safety*. Academic Press.

Baig, M.R., Al-Worafi, Y.M., Alseragi, W.M., Ming, L.C., & Siddique, A. (2020). Drug safety in India. In *Drug Safety in Developing Countries* (pp. 327–334). Academic Press.

Elkalmi, R.M., Al-Worafi, Y.M., Alseragi, W.M., Ming, L.C., & Siddique, A. (2020). Drug safety in Malaysia. In *Drug Safety in Developing Countries* (pp. 245–253). Academic Press.

Elsayed, T., & Al-Worafi, Y.M. (2020). Drug safety in Egypt. In *Drug Safety in Developing Countries* (pp. 511–523). Academic Press.

Hasan, S., Al-Omar, M.J., AlZubaidy, H., & Al-Worafi, Y.M. (2019). Use of medications in Arab Countries. *Handbook of Healthcare in the Arab World*, Springer, 42.

Hassan, Y., Abd Aziz, N., Kassab, Y.W., Elgasim, I., Shaharuddin, S., Al-Worafi, Y.M.A., ... & Ming, L.C. (2014). How to help patients to control their blood pressure? Blood pressure control and its predictor. *Archives of Pharmacy Practice*, 5(4), 153–161.

Izahar, S., Lean, Q.Y., Hameed, M.A., Murugiah, M.K., Patel, R.P., Al-Worafi, Y.M., ... & Ming, L.C. (2017). Content analysis of mobile health applications on diabetes mellitus. *Frontiers in Endocrinology*, 8, p. 318.

Kristensen, S., & Bartels, P. (2010). Use of patient safety culture instruments and recommendations. *Aarhus, Denmark, European Society for Quality in HealthCare-Office for Quality Indicators*, 113, 1–35.

Lee, K.S., Yee, S.M., Zaidi, S.T.R., Patel, R.P., Yang, Q., Al-Worafi, Y.M., & Ming, L.C., 2017. Combating sale of counterfeit and falsified medicines online: A losing battle. *Frontiers in Pharmacology*, 8, p. 268.

Mahmoud, M.A., Wajid, S., Naqvi, A.A., Samreen, S., Althagfan, S.S., & Al-Worafi, Y. (2020). Self-medication with antibiotics: A cross-sectional community-based study. *Latin American Journal of Pharmacy*, 39(2), pp. 348–353.

Manan, M.M., Rusli, R.A., Ang, W.C., Al-Worafi, Y.M., & Ming, L.C. (2014). Assessing the pharmaceutical care issues of antiepileptic drug therapy in hospitalised epileptic patients. *Journal of Pharmacy Practice and Research*, 44(3), pp. 83–88.

Manan, M.M., Ibrahim, N.A., Aziz, N.A., Zulkifly, H.H., Al-Worafi, Y.M.A., & Long, C.M. (2016). Empirical use of antibiotic therapy in the prevention of early onset sepsis in neonates: A pilot study. *Archives of Medical Science*, 12(3), pp. 603–613.

Ming, L.C., Hameed, M.A., Lee, D.D., Apidi, N.A., Lai, P.S.M., Hadi, M.A., Al-Worafi, Y.M.A., & Khan, T.M., (2016). Use of medical mobile applications among hospital pharmacists in Malaysia. *Therapeutic Innovation & Regulatory Science*, 50(4), pp. 419–426.

Ming, L.C., Untong, N., Aliudin, N.A., Osili, N., Kifli, N., Tan, C.S., ... & Goh, H.P. (2020). Mobile health apps on COVID-19 launched in the early days of the pandemic: Content analysis and review. *JMIR mHealth and uHealth*, 8(9), p. e19796.

Othman, G., Ali, F., Ibrahim, M.I.M., Al-Worafi, Y.M., Ansari, M., & Halboup, A.M. (2020). Assessment of anti-diabetic medications adherence among diabetic patients in Sana'a City, Yemen: A cross sectional study. *Journal of Pharmaceutical Research International*, 32(21), 114–122.

Reynard, J., Reynolds, J., & Stevenson, P. (2009). *Practical Patient Safety*. OUP Oxford.

Saeed, M.S., Alkhoshaiban, A.S., Al-Worafi, Y.M.A., & Long, C.M., (2014). Perception of self-medication among university students in Saudi Arabia. *Archives of Pharmacy Practice*, 5(4), p. 149.

Salas, E., & Frush, K. (2012). *Improving Patient Safety Through Teamwork and Team Training*. Oxford University Press.

Vincent, C. (2011). *Patient Safety*. John Wiley & Sons.

Webb, A., Angus, D., Finfer, S., Gattioni, L., & Singer, M. (2016). *Oxford Textbook of Critical Care*. Oxford University Press.

25 Patient Safety in Surgery

25.1 BACKGROUND

Surgery is a medical specialty that involves using invasive procedures to diagnose, treat, and manage a wide range of conditions and injuries. Surgeries can be performed on different parts of the body, including organs, tissues, bones, and joints. Surgeries can be categorized into different types based on the purpose and method of the procedure. Some common types of surgeries include:

1. Diagnostic surgery: This type of surgery is performed to determine the cause of a medical problem, such as a biopsy to diagnose cancer.

2. Therapeutic surgery: This type of surgery is performed to treat or cure a medical problem, such as removing a tumor or repairing a broken bone.

3. Elective surgery: This type of surgery is planned in advance and is not considered to be an emergency, such as cosmetic surgery.

4. Emergency surgery: This type of surgery is performed urgently to address a life-threatening situation, such as an appendectomy for acute appendicitis.

5. Minimally invasive surgery: This type of surgery involves using small incisions and specialized tools to minimize damage to surrounding tissues and speed up recovery time.

6. Open surgery: This type of surgery involves making a larger incision to access the affected area, and may be necessary for more complex procedures.

Before undergoing surgery, patients will typically undergo a comprehensive evaluation to determine their overall health status and any potential risks associated with the procedure. During the surgery itself, patients may be given anesthesia to prevent pain and discomfort. After the surgery, patients will typically receive postoperative care and follow-up to ensure a successful recovery. Patient care and safety are critical aspects of surgery, as surgical procedures can potentially cause harm or even death. To ensure patient safety and the best possible outcomes, there are several important considerations that should be taken into account during surgery:

1. Patient selection: Patients should be carefully selected for surgical procedures, taking into account their medical history, current health status, and any other risk factors that could increase the likelihood of complications.

2. Preoperative evaluation and preparation: Patients should be thoroughly evaluated before surgery to ensure that they are medically stable and prepared for the procedure. This may involve diagnostic tests, such as blood tests and imaging scans, as well as optimization of any underlying medical conditions.

3. Informed consent: Patients should be fully informed about the risks and benefits of the surgical procedure and provide informed consent before the procedure.

4. Use of standardized surgical protocols: The use of standardized protocols and checklists can help to ensure that surgical procedures are performed consistently and safely, reducing the risk of errors and complications.

5. Proper surgical technique: Surgeons should adhere to proper surgical technique, including sterile preparation and the use of appropriate instruments and equipment.

6. Continuous monitoring during surgery: Patients should be continuously monitored during surgery, including vital signs and anesthesia administration, to detect and address any potential complications.

7. Postoperative care: Adequate postoperative care is essential to ensure a safe and successful recovery. This may involve pain management, monitoring for complications, and appropriate follow-up care.

By prioritizing patient care and safety in surgery through careful patient selection, preoperative evaluation, informed consent, standardized protocols, proper surgical technique, continuous monitoring, and postoperative care, surgeons can help to ensure the best possible outcomes for their patients (Kristensen & Bartels, 2010; Reynard et al., 2009; Salas & Frush, 2012; Vincent, 2011).

DOI: 10.1201/9781003230465-27

25.2 SURGERY ERRORS AND RELATED PROBLEMS

Surgery errors and related problems are unfortunately common and can have serious consequences for patients. Some common surgery errors and related problems include:

1. Wrong site surgery: This occurs when surgery is performed on the wrong part of the body, such as performing surgery on the left leg instead of the right.

2. Anesthesia errors: Anesthesia errors can include giving too much or too little anesthesia, failing to monitor the patient's vital signs during the procedure, or failing to take into account the patient's medical history and any potential risks.

3. Infections: Surgical procedures can increase the risk of infection, and if proper infection control procedures are not followed, patients may develop serious infections that can lead to complications or even death.

4. Bleeding: Surgical procedures can sometimes cause excessive bleeding, which can lead to complications and even death if not promptly addressed.

5. Nerve damage: Surgery can sometimes result in nerve damage, which can lead to numbness, weakness, or other neurological symptoms.

6. Postoperative complications: Patients may experience a range of postoperative complications, such as pain, nausea, vomiting, or difficulty breathing.

To minimize the risk of surgery errors and related problems, it is important for surgeons and surgical teams to follow established protocols and checklists, maintain clear communication with patients and other healthcare providers, and prioritize patient safety and well-being throughout the surgical process. If surgery errors or related problems do occur, it is important for patients to speak up and report any concerns to their healthcare providers.

25.3 CAUSES OF SURGERY ERRORS AND RELATED PROBLEMS

There are many factors that can contribute to surgery errors and related problems, including:

1. Communication breakdowns: Poor communication between members of the surgical team, or between the surgical team and the patient, can lead to misunderstandings or miscommunications that can result in errors.

2. Lack of training or experience: Surgeons or other members of the surgical team who are not properly trained or experienced in a particular procedure may be more likely to make mistakes.

3. Fatigue or burnout: Surgical team members who are fatigued or experiencing burnout may be more prone to errors or oversights.

4. Distractions or interruptions: Distractions or interruptions during surgery, such as phone calls or alarms, can disrupt concentration and increase the risk of errors.

5. Inadequate preparation or planning: Inadequate preparation or planning, such as failing to properly review the patient's medical history or plan for potential complications, can increase the risk of errors.

6. Time pressure: Surgeons or other members of the surgical team may feel pressure to complete the procedure quickly, which can increase the risk of errors.

7. Equipment failure: Malfunctioning or improperly maintained equipment can contribute to errors and complications during surgery.

To minimize the risk of surgery errors and related problems, it is important for surgical teams to address these potential contributing factors through effective communication, adequate training and experience, appropriate staffing levels, careful preparation and planning, and appropriate use of equipment and technology. Additionally, healthcare providers and organizations can implement policies and procedures to identify and address errors and near-misses and provide ongoing training and education to improve patient safety and quality of care.

25.4 PREVENTION OF SURGERY ERRORS AND RELATED PROBLEMS

Preventing surgery errors and related problems requires a multi-faceted approach that involves the entire surgical team, including the surgeon, anesthesiologist, nurses, and other healthcare providers. Some key strategies for preventing surgery errors and related problems include:

1. Effective communication: Clear and effective communication between all members of the surgical team, as well as with the patient and their family, is essential to preventing errors. This can include using standardized communication protocols, such as "read-back" or "time-out" procedures, to confirm critical information.

2. Standardized protocols and checklists: Standardized protocols and checklists can help to ensure that all steps of the surgical process are performed consistently and safely, reducing the risk of errors and complications.

3. Proper training and experience: All members of the surgical team should be properly trained and experienced in their roles, and should undergo regular training and education to maintain their skills and knowledge.

4. Adequate staffing levels: Ensuring that there are enough staff members present to properly monitor the patient and perform the procedure can help to reduce the risk of errors.

5. Careful preparation and planning: Thorough preparation and planning, including reviewing the patient's medical history and planning for potential complications, can help to prevent errors.

6. Use of technology and equipment: Proper use of technology and equipment, including maintenance and calibration, can help to prevent errors and complications.

7. Ongoing quality improvement: Regular review of surgical outcomes and processes, and ongoing quality improvement initiatives, can help to identify and address potential areas for improvement in patient safety.

By prioritizing effective communication, standardized protocols and checklists, proper training and experience, adequate staffing levels, careful preparation and planning, appropriate use of technology and equipment, and ongoing quality improvement, surgical teams can help to prevent errors and related problems and ensure the best possible outcomes for their patients.

25.5 SURGERY SAFETY CULTURE

Surgery safety culture refers to the shared values, beliefs, attitudes, and practices that prioritize patient safety and well-being within the surgical setting. A strong safety culture in surgery is essential to preventing errors and complications and ensuring high-quality, patient-centered care. Some key elements of a strong surgery safety culture include:

1. Open and honest communication: Members of the surgical team should feel comfortable speaking up about concerns or errors, without fear of retribution or blame. This can help to identify potential areas for improvement and prevent errors from occurring.

2. Teamwork and collaboration: Effective teamwork and collaboration between members of the surgical team, as well as with the patient and their family, can help to ensure that all aspects of the surgical process are performed safely and consistently.

3. Continuous learning and improvement: Regular education and training, as well as ongoing quality improvement initiatives, can help to promote a culture of learning and continuous improvement in surgical care.

4. Patient-centered care: Prioritizing the patient's safety, preferences, and well-being throughout the surgical process can help to ensure that care is patient-centered and responsive to individual needs.

5. Leadership commitment: Strong leadership commitment to patient safety and a culture of safety is essential to promoting and maintaining a safety culture in surgery.

Creating and maintaining a strong safety culture in surgery requires a commitment from all members of the surgical team, as well as from healthcare organizations and leaders. By prioritizing open and honest communication, effective teamwork and collaboration, continuous learning and improvement, patient-centered care, and strong leadership commitment, surgical teams can help to prevent errors and complications and ensure the best possible outcomes for their patients.

25.6 SURGERY ERRORS AND RELATED PROBLEMS IN DEVELOPING COUNTRIES: Challenges and Recommendations

Surgery errors and related problems in developing countries are a significant challenge that affects millions of people every year. These issues arise due to several factors, including limited resources, inadequate training, and a lack of regulations and oversight. In this response, we will discuss the challenges and recommendations for improving surgical care in developing countries.

Challenges:

1. Limited resources: Developing countries have limited resources, including personnel, medical equipment, and medications. These shortages can lead to delayed or inadequate surgical care, which increases the risk of complications and errors.

2. Inadequate training: Many healthcare professionals in developing countries receive limited training in surgical procedures, leading to a lack of technical skills and knowledge. This situation can result in poor surgical outcomes and increased patient morbidity and mortality.

3. Lack of regulations and oversight: Developing countries often have inadequate regulations and oversight mechanisms for surgical care. This situation can lead to poor quality control, lack of standardization, and limited accountability for surgical errors and malpractice.

Recommendations:

1. Increase funding and resources: Governments and international organizations should increase funding and resources for surgical care in developing countries. This step will help to improve infrastructure, increase the availability of medical equipment and medications, and provide more training opportunities for healthcare professionals.

2. Develop training programs: Developing countries should invest in training programs to improve the technical skills and knowledge of healthcare professionals. This step will help to ensure that surgeries are conducted safely and effectively, reducing the risk of errors and complications.

3. Strengthen regulations and oversight: Developing countries should develop and enforce regulations and oversight mechanisms for surgical care. This step will help to improve quality control, standardization, and accountability for surgical errors and malpractice.

4. Promote collaboration: International organizations, governments, and healthcare professionals should collaborate to promote best practices in surgical care. This step will help to share knowledge and expertise, improve patient outcomes, and reduce the risk of errors and complications.

5. Implement technology: Developing countries should implement technological solutions, such as telemedicine and electronic medical records, to improve surgical care. These solutions can help to increase access to specialized care and reduce the risk of errors and complications.

6. Despite the progress in research about patient care and safety in developing countries, there is little research about patient safety related to surgery in the majority of developing countries, therefore, conducting research is very important and highly recommended (Alshahrani et al., 2019a,b; Al-Qahtani et al., 2015; Alshahrani et al., 2020a,b; Al-Worafi, 2014; Al-Worafi, 2015; Al-Worafi, 2016; Al-Worafi et al., 2017; Al-Worafi, 2018a-d; Al-Worafi et al., 2018a-b; Al-Worafi et al., 2019; Al-Worafi, 2020a-z; Al-Worafi et al., 2020a-b; Al-Worafi et al., 2021a,b; Al-Worafi, 2022a,b; Al-Worafi, 2023; Baig et al., 2020; Elkalmi et al., 2020; Elsayed & Al-Worafi, 2020; Hasan et al., 2019; Hassan et al., 2014; Izhar et al., 2017; Lee et al., 2017; Mahmoud et al., 2020; Manan et al., 2014; Manan et al., 2016; Ming et al., 2016; Ming et al., 2020; Othman et al., 2020; Saeed et al., 2014).

In conclusion, improving surgical care in developing countries is a complex and multifaceted challenge. By increasing funding and resources, developing training programs, strengthening regulations and oversight, promoting collaboration, and implementing technology, we can make progress toward reducing surgical errors and improving patient outcomes.

25.7 CONCLUSION

This chapter has discussed the surgery safety issues, prevention, challenges, and recommendations for achieving the best practice in developing countries. Surgery errors and related problems in developing countries are a significant challenge that affects millions of people every year. These issues arise due to several factors, including limited resources, inadequate training, and a lack of regulations and oversight. improving surgical care in developing countries is a complex and multifaceted challenge. By increasing funding and resources, developing training programs, strengthening regulations and oversight, promoting collaboration, and implementing technology, we can make progress toward reducing surgical errors and improving patient outcomes.

REFERENCES

Al-Qahtani, I., Almoteb, T.M., & Al-Warafi, Y. (2015). Competency of metered-dose inhaler use among Saudi community pharmacists: A simulation method study. *RRJPPS*, 4(2), 27–31.

Alshahrani, S.M., Alakhali, K.M., & Al-Worafi, Y.M., (2019a). Medication errors in a health care facility in southern Saudi Arabia. *Tropical Journal of Pharmaceutical Research*, 18(5), pp. 1119–1122.

Alshahrani, S.M., Alavudeen, S.S., Alakhali, K.M., Al-Worafi, Y.M., Bahamdan, A.K., & Vigneshwaran, E., (2019b). Self-Medication Among King Khalid University Students, Saudi Arabia. *Risk Management and Healthcare Policy*, 12, pp. 243–249.

Alshahrani, S.M., Alakhali, K.M., Al-Worafi, Y.M., & Alshahrani, N.Z. (2020b). Awareness and use of over the counter analgesic medication: A survey in the Aseer region population, Saudi Arabia. *International Journal of Advances in Applied Sciences*, 7(3), pp. 130–134.

Alshahrani, S.M., Alzahran, M., Alakhali, K., Vigneshwaran, E., Iqbal, M.J., Khan, N.A.,... ... & Alavudeen, S.S. (2020b). Association between diabetes consequences and quality of life among patients with diabetes mellitus in the Aseer Province of Saudi Arabia. *Open Access Macedonian Journal of Medical Sciences*, 8(E), pp. 325–330.

Al-Worafi, Y.M. (2014). Prescription writing errors at a tertiary care hospital in Yemen: Prevalence, types, causes and recommendations. *American Journal of Pharmacy and Health Research*, 2, pp. 134–140.

Al-Worafi, Y.M.A. (2015). Appropriateness of metered-dose inhaler use in the Yemeni community pharmacies. *Journal of Taibah University Medical Sciences*, 10(3), pp. 353–358.

Al-Worafi, Y.M.A., (2016). Pharmacy practice in Yemen. In *Pharmacy Practice in Developing Countries* (pp. 267–287). Academic Press.

Al-Worafi, Y.M., Kassab, Y.W., Alseragi, W.M., Almutairi, M.S., Ahmed, A., Ming, L.C., Alkhoshaiban, A.S., & Hadi, M.A., (2017). Pharmacovigilance and adverse drg reaction reporting: A perspective of community pharmacists and pharmacy technicians in Sana'a, Yemen. *Therapeutics and Clinical Risk Management*, 13, p. 1175.

Al-Worafi, Y.M., (2018a). Knowledge, attitude and practice of Yemeni physicians toward pharmacovigilance: A mixed method study. *International Journal of Pharmacy and Pharmaceutical Sciences*, 10(10), pp. 74–77.

Al-Worafi, Y. (2018b). Knowledge, attitude and practice of Yemeni physicians toward pharmacovigilance: A mixed method study. *International Journal of Pharmacy and Pharmaceutical Sciences*, 10, pp. 74–77.

Al-Worafi, Y.M. (2018c). Dispensing errors observed by community pharmacy dispensers in IBB–YEMEN. *Asian Journal of Pharmaceutical and Clinical Research*, 11(11), 478.481.

Al-Worafi, Y.M. (2018d). Evauation of inhaler technique among patients with asthma and COPD in Yemen. *Journal of Taibah University Medical Sciences*, 13(5), pp. 488–490.

Al-Worafi, Y.M., Patel, R.P., Zaidi, S.T.R., Alseragi, W.M., Almutairi, M.S., Alkhoshaiban, A.S., & Ming, L.C. (2018a). Completeness and legibility of handwritten prescriptions in Sana'a, Yemen. *Medical Principles and Practice*, 27, pp. 290–292.

Al-Worafi, Y.M., Alseragi, W.M., Seng, L.K., Kassab, Y.W., Yeoh, S.F., Chiau, L.,... ... & Husain, K. (2018b). Dispensing errors in community pharmacies: A prospective study in Sana'a, Yemen. *Archives of Pharmacy Practice*, 9(4), pp. 1–3.

Al-Worafi, Y.M., Alseragi, W.M., & Mahmoud, M.A. (2019). Competency of metered-dose inhaler use among community pharmacy dispensers in Ibb, Yemen: A simulation method study. *Latin American Journal of Pharmacy*, 38(3), pp. 489–494.

Al-Worafi, Y.M. (Ed.). (2020a). *Drug Safety in Developing Countries: Achievements and Challenges*.

Al-Worafi, Y.M. (2020b). Medication errors. In *Drug Safety in Developing Countries* (pp. 105–117). Academic Press.

Al-Worafi, Y.M. (2020c). Adverse drug reactions. In *Drug Safety in Developing Countries* (pp. 39–57). Academic Press.

Al-Worafi, Y.M. (2020d). Medications registration and marketing: Safety-related issues. In *Drug Safety in Developing Countries* (pp. 21–28). Academic Press.

Al-Worafi, Y.M. (2020e). Pharmacovigilance. In *Drug Safety in Developing Countries* (pp. 29–38). Academic Press.

Al-Worafi, Y.M. (2020f). Drug-related problems. In *Drug Safety in Developing Countries* (pp. 59–71). Academic Press.

Al-Worafi, Y.M. (2020g). Medications safety-related terminology. In *Drug Safety in Developing Countries* (pp. 7–19). Academic Press.

Al-Worafi, Y.M. (2020h). Self-medication. In *Drug Safety in Developing Countries* (pp. 73–86). Academic Press.

Al-Worafi, Y.M. (2020j). Antibiotics safety issues. In *Drug Safety in Developing Countries* (pp. 87–103). Academic Press.

Al-Worafi, Y.M. (2020k). Medications safety research issues. In *Drug Safety in Developing Countries* (pp. 213–227). Academic Press.

Al-Worafi, Y.M. (2020l). Counterfeit and substandard medications. In *Drug safety in developing countries* (pp. 119–126). Academic Press.

Al-Worafi, Y.M. (2020m). Medication abuse and misuse. In *Drug safety in developing countries* (pp. 127–135). Academic Press.

Al-Worafi, Y.M. (2020n). Storage and disposal of medications. In *Drug Safety in Developing Countries* (pp. 137–142). Academic Press.

Al-Worafi, Y.M. (2020o). Safety of medications in special population. In *Drug Safety in Developing Countries* (pp. 143–162). Academic Press.

Al-Worafi, Y.M. (2020p). Herbal medicines safety issues. In *Drug Safety in Developing Countries* (pp. 163–178). Academic Press.

Al-Worafi, Y.M. (2020q). Medications safety pharmacoeconomics-related issues. In *Drug Safety in Developing Countries* (pp. 187–195). Academic Press.

Al-Worafi, Y.M. (2020r). Evidence-based medications safety practice. In *Drug Safety in Developing Countries* (pp. 197–201). Academic Press.

Al-Worafi, Y.M. (2020s). Quality indicators for medications safety. In *Drug Safety in Developing Countries* (pp. 229–242). Academic Press.

Al-Worafi, Y.M. (2020t). Drug safety in Yemen. In *Drug Safety in Developing Countries* (pp. 391–405). Academic Press.

Al-Worafi, Y.M. (2020u). Drug safety in Saudi Arabia. In *Drug Safety in Developing Countries* (pp. 407–417). Academic Press.

Al-Worafi, Y.M. (2020v). Drug safety in United Arab Emirates. In *Drug Safety in Developing Countries* (pp. 419–428). Academic Press.

Al-Worafi, Y.M. (2020w). Drug safety in Indonesia. In *Drug Safety in Developing Countries* (pp. 279–285). Academic Press.

Al-Worafi, Y.M. (2020x). Drug safety in Palestine. In *Drug Safety in Developing Countries* (pp. 471–480). Academic Press.

Al-Worafi, Y.M. (2020y). Drug safety: Comparison between developing countries. In *Drug Safety in Developing Countries* (pp. 603–611). Academic Press.

Al-Worafi, Y.M. (2020z). Drug safety in developing versus developed countries. In *Drug Safety in Developing Countries* (pp. 613–615). Academic Press.

Al-Worafi, Y.M., Alseragi, W.M., Ming, L.C., & Alakhali, K.M. (2020a). Drug safety in China. In *Drug Safety in Developing Countries* (pp. 381–388). Academic Press.

Al-Worafi, Y.M., Alseragi, W.M., Alakhali, K.M., Ming, L.C., Othman, G., Halboup, A.M., … & Elkalmi, R.M. (2020b). Knowledge, beliefs and factors affecting the use of generic medicines among patients in Ibb, Yemen: A mixed-method study. *Journal of Pharmacy Practice and Community Medicine*, 6(4), 53–56

Al-Worafi, Y.M., Elkalmi, R.M., Ming, L.C., Othman, G., Halboup, A.M., Battah, M.M., … & Mani, V. (2021a). Dispensing errors in hospital pharmacies: A prospective study in Yemen.AlQalam Journal of Medical and Applied Sciences, 4(2), 13–17.

Al-Worafi, Y.M., Hasan, S., Hassan, N.M., & Gaili, A.A. (2021b). Knowledge, Attitude and Experience of Pharmacist in the UAE towards Pharmacovigilance. *Research Journal of Pharmacy and Technology*, 14(1), pp. 265–269.

Al-Worafi, Y. (2022a). *A Guide to Online Pharmacy Education: Teaching Strategies and Assessment Methods*. CRC Press.

Al-Worafi, Y.M. (2022b). Patient care errors and related problems (part I): Development and validation of the model. 0000-0002-5752-2913

Al-Worafi, Y.M. (Ed.). (2023). *Clinical Case Studies on Medication Safety*. Academic Press.

Baig, M.R., Al-Worafi, Y.M., Alseragi, W.M., Ming, L.C., & Siddique, A. (2020). Drug safety in India. In *Drug Safety in Developing Countries* (pp. 327–334). Academic Press.

Elkalmi, R.M., Al-Worafi, Y.M., Alseragi, W.M., Ming, L.C., & Siddique, A. (2020). Drug safety in Malaysia. In *Drug Safety in Developing Countries* (pp. 245–253). Academic Press.

Elsayed, T., & Al-Worafi, Y.M. (2020). Drug safety in Egypt. In *Drug Safety in Developing Countries* (pp. 511–523). Academic Press.

Hasan, S., Al-Omar, M.J., AlZubaidy, H., & Al-Worafi, Y.M. (2019). Use of medications in Arab Countries. In *Handbook of Healthcare in the Arab World*. Springer, 42.

Hassan, Y., Abd Aziz, N., Kassab, Y.W., Elgasim, I., Shaharuddin, S., Al-Worafi, Y.M.A., ... & Ming, L.C. (2014). How to help patients to control their blood pressure? Blood pressure control and its predictor. *Archives of Pharmacy Practice*, 5(4). 153–161.

Izahar, S., Lean, Q.Y., Hameed, M.A., Murugiah, M.K., Patel, R.P., Al-Worafi, Y.M., ... & Ming, L.C. (2017). Content analysis of mobile health applications on diabetes mellitus. *Frontiers in Endocrinology*, 8, p. 318.

Kristensen, S., & Bartels, P. (2010). Use of patient safety culture instruments and recommendations. *Aarhus, Denmark, European Society for Quality in HealthCare-Office for Quality Indicators*, 113, 1–35.

Lee, K.S., Yee, S.M., Zaidi, S.T.R., Patel, R.P., Yang, Q., Al-Worafi, Y.M., & Ming, L.C., 2017. Combating sale of counterfeit and falsified medicines online: A losing battle. *Frontiers in Pharmacology*, 8, p. 268.

Mahmoud, M.A., Wajid, S., Naqvi, A.A., Samreen, S., Althagfan, S.S., & Al-Worafi, Y. (2020). Self-medication with antibiotics: A cross-sectional community-based study. *Latin American Journal of Pharmacy*, 39(2), 348–353.

Manan, M.M., Rusli, R.A., Ang, W.C., Al-Worafi, Y.M., & Ming, L.C. (2014). Assessing the pharmaceutical care issues of antiepileptic drug therapy in hospitalised epileptic patients. *Journal of Pharmacy Practice and Research*, 44(3), pp. 83–88.

Manan, M.M., Ibrahim, N.A., Aziz, N.A., Zulkifly, H.H., Al-Worafi, Y.M.A., & Long, C.M. (2016). Empirical use of antibiotic therapy in the prevention of early onset sepsis in neonates: A pilot study. *Archives of Medical Science*, 12(3), pp. 603–613.

Ming, L.C., Hameed, M.A., Lee, D.D., Apidi, N.A., Lai, P.S.M., Hadi, M.A., Al-Worafi, Y.M.A., & Khan, T.M., (2016). Use of medical mobile applications among hospital pharmacists in Malaysia. *Therapeutic Innovation & Regulatory Science*, 50(4), pp. 419–426.

Ming, L.C., Untong, N., Aliudin, N.A., Osili, N., Kifli, N., Tan, C.S., ... & Goh, H.P. (2020). Mobile health apps on COVID-19 launched in the early days of the pandemic: Content analysis and review. *JMIR mHealth and uHealth*, 8(9), p. e19796.

Othman, G., Ali, F., Ibrahim, M.I.M., Al-Worafi, Y.M., Ansari, M., & Halboup, A.M. (2020). Assessment of anti-diabetic medications adherence among diabetic patients in Sana'a City, Yemen: A cross sectional study. *Journal of Pharmaceutical Research International*, 32(21), pp. 114–122.

Reynard, J., Reynolds, J., & Stevenson, P. (2009). *Practical Patient Safety*. OUP Oxford.

Saeed, M.S., Alkhoshaiban, A.S., Al-Worafi, Y.M.A., & Long, C.M., (2014). Perception of self-medication among university students in Saudi Arabia. *Archives of Pharmacy Practice*, 5(4), p. 149.

Salas, E., & Frush, K. (2012). *Improving Patient Safety Through Teamwork and Team Training*. Oxford University Press.

Vincent, C. (2011). *Patient Safety*. John Wiley & Sons.

26 Patient Safety in Internal Medicine (IM)

26.1 BACKGROUND

Internal medicine (IM) is a medical specialty that focuses on the prevention, diagnosis, and treatment of adult diseases. Physicians who specialize in IM are called internists, or sometimes simply "doctors." Internists provide comprehensive care for patients with a wide range of health conditions, including chronic diseases such as diabetes, hypertension, and heart disease, as well as acute illnesses and infections. They often serve as primary care physicians, but may also work in hospitals or specialized clinics. In addition to diagnosing and treating medical conditions, internists also provide preventive care and health education to help patients maintain their health and well-being. They may also coordinate care with other healthcare providers and specialists to ensure that patients receive the most appropriate and effective treatment. IM is a medical specialty that places a high emphasis on patient care and patient safety. Internists are trained to provide comprehensive, patient-centered care that takes into account not only a patient's medical condition but also their overall health, lifestyle, and other factors that may impact their health and well-being. To ensure patient safety, internists are trained in a variety of techniques and best practices, such as proper hand hygiene, infection control, and medication safety. They also work closely with other healthcare providers to ensure that patients receive the appropriate care and treatment at all stages of their illness. Internists may use a variety of tools and technologies to monitor patients and ensure their safety. For example, they may use electronic health records (EHRs) to track patients' medical history, medications, and allergies, and to communicate with other healthcare providers involved in their care. They may also use technology such as telemedicine to provide remote consultations and monitor patients who are receiving care at home. In addition to providing medical care, internists also place a high priority on patient education and empowerment. They work with patients to help them understand their medical conditions, treatment options, and ways to manage their health and well-being. By providing patients with the knowledge and tools they need to take control of their health, internists can help improve patient outcomes and reduce the risk of adverse events (Kristensen & Bartels, 2010; Reynard et al., 2009; Salas & Frush, 2012; Vincent, 2011).

26.2 INTERNAL MEDICINE ERRORS AND RELATED PROBLEMS

As with any medical specialty, IM is not immune to errors and related problems. Some common errors and problems that can occur in IM include:

1. Medication errors: This can include prescribing the wrong medication or dose, failing to check for drug interactions or allergies, or administering medication incorrectly.

2. Diagnostic errors: This can include misinterpreting test results, failing to order necessary tests, or misdiagnosing a condition.

3. Communication errors: This can include miscommunications between healthcare providers, failure to communicate important information to patients or their families, or failure to document important information in a patient's medical record.

4. System errors: This can include issues with the healthcare system itself, such as lack of resources or staffing, inadequate training or supervision, or problems with equipment or technology.

These errors and problems can lead to adverse events such as medication reactions, complications from misdiagnosis or delayed treatment, or even death in some cases. They can also lead to decreased patient satisfaction, increased healthcare costs, and increased liability for healthcare providers. To address these issues, internists and other healthcare providers must take steps to improve patient safety and reduce the risk of errors. This can include implementing protocols and best practices for medication safety, improving communication and collaboration among healthcare providers, implementing systems for tracking and reporting errors and adverse events, and investing in training and education for healthcare providers. Additionally, patients can play a role in reducing the risk of errors by being proactive about their healthcare and advocating for their own safety and well-being.

26.3 CAUSES OF INTERNAL MEDICINE ERRORS AND RELATED PROBLEMS

The causes of IM errors and related problems can be complex and multifactorial, involving a variety of factors related to the patient, the healthcare provider, and the healthcare system as a whole. Some common causes of IM errors and related problems include:

DOI: 10.1201/9781003230465-28

1. Communication breakdowns: Miscommunications between healthcare providers, between providers and patients, or between different departments within a healthcare system can lead to errors and adverse events.

2. Inadequate training or supervision: Lack of training, inadequate supervision, or insufficient staffing can lead to errors and adverse events, particularly in high-stress situations.

3. Systemic problems: Issues with the healthcare system itself, such as inadequate resources, lack of standardization, or inconsistent policies and procedures, can contribute to errors and adverse events.

4. Patient factors: Patients with complex medical histories, multiple chronic conditions, or cognitive or physical impairments may be at increased risk of errors and adverse events.

5. Medication errors: Errors related to medication can occur due to factors such as incorrect dosing, incorrect administration, or failure to check for drug interactions or allergies.

6. Diagnostic errors: Misdiagnosis, delayed diagnosis, or failure to order necessary tests can lead to errors and adverse events.

7. Human error: Healthcare providers are human and may make mistakes due to factors such as fatigue, stress, or distraction.

8. Lack of follow-up: Failure to follow up on test results or communicate important information to patients or other healthcare providers can contribute to errors and adverse events.

By understanding the complex causes of IM errors and related problems, healthcare providers and systems can take steps to address these issues and improve patient safety. This may include implementing protocols and best practices for communication, training and education for healthcare providers, investing in technology and equipment, and engaging patients as partners in their own care.

26.4 PREVENTION OF INTERNAL MEDICINE ERRORS AND RELATED PROBLEMS

Prevention refers to actions taken to prevent or reduce the occurrence of disease, injury, or other adverse health events. There are three levels of prevention: primary prevention, secondary prevention, and tertiary prevention.

1. Primary prevention: This level of prevention involves measures taken to prevent the onset of disease or injury before it occurs. Examples of primary prevention include vaccination, health education and promotion, and lifestyle modifications such as healthy eating, regular exercise, and not smoking.

2. Secondary prevention: This level of prevention involves early detection and treatment of disease or injury before it becomes symptomatic or progresses. Examples of secondary prevention include screening tests such as mammograms, colonoscopies, and blood pressure checks.

3. Tertiary prevention: This level of prevention involves interventions aimed at preventing further complications or disability in individuals with established disease or injury. Examples of tertiary prevention include rehabilitation, physical therapy, and disease management programs.

Prevention is an important aspect of healthcare because it can help reduce the incidence and burden of disease, improve overall health outcomes, and reduce healthcare costs. By focusing on prevention, individuals can take an active role in maintaining their health and well-being, while healthcare providers can work to identify and manage risk factors and implement interventions to prevent or mitigate the impact of disease or injury. Additionally, public health efforts aimed at prevention can help promote healthy behaviors and environments, reduce health disparities, and improve the overall health of populations.

Preventing IM errors and related problems is an important aspect of ensuring patient safety and improving healthcare outcomes. Some strategies for preventing these errors and problems include:

1. Improve communication: Effective communication is critical in preventing errors and adverse events. Healthcare providers should use clear and concise language when communicating with patients and other providers, verify and clarify information, and document important information in the patient's medical record.

2. Implement medication safety measures: To prevent medication errors, healthcare providers should follow best practices for prescribing, dispensing, and administering medication. This may include using electronic prescribing systems, double-checking medication orders and dosages, and educating patients on how to properly take their medications.

3. Use technology: Technology can be a valuable tool in preventing errors and improving patient safety. Healthcare providers can use electronic health records (EHRs) to track patient information and medication orders, use barcode scanning systems to ensure the right medication is given to the right patient, and implement decision support systems to help providers make informed decisions about patient care.

4. Engage patients: Patients can play an important role in preventing errors and adverse events by actively participating in their own care. Providers should educate patients about their conditions, treatment options, and medications, encourage patients to ask questions and provide resources for patients to learn more about their health.

5. Implement quality improvement initiatives: Healthcare providers and systems should engage in ongoing quality improvement initiatives to identify and address potential areas for improvement in patient care. This may include conducting root cause analyses to identify the causes of errors and adverse events, implementing process improvements to prevent errors from occurring, and monitoring and measuring the effectiveness of these interventions over time.

By implementing these strategies and working collaboratively to improve patient safety, healthcare providers and systems can help prevent IM errors and related problems and ensure the best possible outcomes for their patients.

26.5 INTERNAL MEDICINE SAFETY CULTURE

IM safety culture refers to the attitudes, values, and behaviors of healthcare providers and organizations that prioritize patient safety and quality of care. A strong safety culture in IM can help prevent errors, adverse events, and other patient safety problems.

Safety culture in IM is characterized by:

1. Open communication: A culture that encourages open communication allows healthcare providers to share information about patient care and safety concerns without fear of retribution or punishment. This includes communication between different healthcare providers and departments, as well as between providers and patients.

2. Learning from mistakes: In a strong safety culture, mistakes are viewed as opportunities for learning and improvement, rather than blame or punishment. Healthcare providers are encouraged to report errors and adverse events, and organizations use these reports to identify areas for improvement and implement changes to prevent future incidents.

3. Collaboration and teamwork: Collaboration and teamwork are essential components of a strong safety culture in IM. Providers work together to ensure the best possible outcomes for their patients and support one another in identifying and addressing potential patient safety risks.

4. Commitment to quality improvement: A strong safety culture includes a commitment to ongoing quality improvement initiatives that focus on improving patient safety and the overall quality of care. These initiatives may include regular safety training, ongoing process improvement, and ongoing monitoring and evaluation of patient safety measures.

5. Patient-centered care: A strong safety culture in IM is centered around the needs and preferences of patients. Healthcare providers work collaboratively with patients to ensure that their care is personalized, coordinated, and effective.

Overall, a strong safety culture in IM is essential to ensuring patient safety and improving healthcare outcomes. By prioritizing communication, learning, collaboration, quality improvement, and patient-centered care, healthcare providers and organizations can create a culture of safety that supports the best possible outcomes for patients.

26.6 INTERNAL MEDICINE ERRORS AND RELATED PROBLEMS IN DEVELOPING COUNTRIES: Challenges and Recommendations

Internal medicine errors and related problems in developing countries pose unique challenges due to the limited resources, infrastructure, and healthcare workforce available. Some of the challenges faced by developing countries in preventing and addressing IM errors and related problems include:

1. Limited resources: Developing countries often have limited resources, including access to medications, diagnostic tests, and medical equipment, which can lead to errors in diagnosis and treatment.

2. Lack of training and education: Healthcare providers in developing countries may have limited access to ongoing training and education, which can impact their ability to provide high-quality care and prevent errors.

3. Fragmented healthcare systems: Healthcare systems in developing countries may be fragmented and lack coordination, making it difficult to provide comprehensive and coordinated care for patients.

4. Cultural and language barriers: In some developing countries, cultural and language barriers can make it difficult to effectively communicate with patients and provide appropriate care.

To address these challenges and prevent IM errors and related problems in developing countries, some recommendations include:

1. Increase access to resources: Efforts should be made to increase access to medications, diagnostic tests, and medical equipment to improve the accuracy of diagnosis and treatment.

2. Provide ongoing training and education: Healthcare providers in developing countries should have access to ongoing training and education to improve their knowledge and skills and reduce the risk of errors.

3. Strengthen healthcare systems: Healthcare systems in developing countries should be strengthened and coordinated to provide comprehensive and coordinated care for patients.

4. Address cultural and language barriers: Efforts should be made to address cultural and language barriers by providing training and resources to healthcare providers and improving communication with patients.

5. Emphasize patient-centered care: Patient-centered care should be emphasized, with a focus on understanding and addressing the unique needs and preferences of patients.

6. Despite the progress in research about patient care and safety in developing countries, there is little research about patient safety related to IM in the majority of developing countries, therefore, conducting research is very important and highly recommended (Alshahrani et al., 2019a,b; Al-Qahtani et al., 2015; Alshahrani et al., 2020a,b; Al-Worafi, 2014; Al-Worafi, 2015; Al-Worafi, 2016; Al-Worafi et al., 2017; Al-Worafi, 2018a-d; Al-Worafi et al., 2018a-b; Al-Worafi et al., 2019; Al-Worafi, 2020a-z; Al-Worafi et al., 2020a-b; Al-Worafi et al., 2021a,b; Al-Worafi, 2022a,b; Al-Worafi, 2023; Baig et al., 2020; Elkalmi et al., 2020; Elsayed & Al-Worafi, 2020; Hasan et al., 2019; Hassan et al., 2014; Izahar et al., 2017; Lee et al., 2017; Mahmoud et al., 2020; Manan et al., 2014; Manan et al., 2016; Ming et al., 2016; Ming et al., 2020; Othman et al., 2020; Saeed et al., 2014).

By implementing these recommendations and working collaboratively to address the unique challenges faced by developing countries, healthcare providers and organizations can help prevent IM errors and related problems and improve patient outcomes.

26.7 CONCLUSION

This chapter has discussed and described the IM safety issues, prevention, challenges, and recommendations for achieving the best practice in developing countries. IM is a medical specialty that focuses on the prevention, diagnosis, and treatment of adult diseases. Physicians who specialize in IM are called internists, or sometimes simply "doctors." Internists provide comprehensive care for patients with a wide range of health conditions, including chronic diseases such as diabetes, hypertension, and heart disease, as well as acute illnesses and infections. Preventing IM errors and related problems is an important aspect of ensuring patient safety and improving healthcare outcomes.

REFERENCES

Al-Qahtani, I., Almoteb, T.M., & Al-Warafi, Y. (2015). Competency of metered-dose inhaler use among Saudi community pharmacists: A Simulation method study. *RRJPPS*, 4(2), 37– 31.

Alshahrani, S.M., Alakhali, K.M., & Al-Worafi, Y.M., (2019a). Medication errors in a health care facility in southern Saudi Arabia. *Tropical Journal of Pharmaceutical Research*, 18(5), pp. 1119–1122.

Alshahrani, S.M., Alavudeen, S.S., Alakhali, K.M., Al-Worafi, Y.M., Bahamdan, A.K., & Vigneshwaran, E., (2019b). Self-Medication Among King Khalid University Students, Saudi Arabia. *Risk Management and Healthcare Policy*, 12, pp. 243–249.

Alshahrani, S.M., Alakhali, K.M., Al-Worafi, Y.M., & Alshahrani, N.Z. (2020b). Awareness and use of over the counter analgesic medication: a survey in the Aseer region population, Saudi Arabia. *Int J Advan Appl Sci*, 7(3), 130–134.

Alshahrani, S.M., Alzahran, M., Alakhali, K., Vigneshwaran, E., Iqbal, M.J., Khan, N.A., … & Alavudeen, S.S. (2020b). Association Between Diabetes Consequences and Quality of Life Among Patients With Diabetes Mellitus in the Aseer Province of Saudi Arabia. *Open Access Macedonian Journal of Medical Sciences*, 8(E), 325–330.

Al-Worafi, Y.M. (2014). Prescription writing errors at a tertiary care hospital in Yemen: prevalence, types, causes and recommendations. *Am J Pharm Health Res*, 2, 134–140.

Al-Worafi, Y.M.A. (2015). Appropriateness of metered-dose inhaler use in the Yemeni community pharmacies. *Journal of Taibah University Medical Sciences*, 10(3), 353–358.

Al-Worafi, Y.M.A., (2016). Pharmacy practice in Yemen. In *Pharmacy Practice in Developing Countries* (pp. 267–287). Academic Press.

Al-Worafi, Y.M., Kassab, Y.W., Alseragi, W.M., Almutairi, M.S., Ahmed, A., Ming, L.C., Alkhoshaiban, A.S., & Hadi, M.A., (2017). Pharmacovigilance and adverse drg reaction reporting: a perspective of community pharmacists and pharmacy technicians in Sana'a, Yemen. *Therapeutics and clinical risk management*, 13, p. 1175.

Al-Worafi, Y.M., (2018a). Knowledge, Attitude and Practice of Yemeni Physicians Toward Pharmacovigilance: A Mixed Method Study. *International Journal of Pharmacy and Pharmaceutical Sciences*, 10(10), 74–77.

Al-Worafi, Y. (2018b). Knowledge, attitude and practice of Yemeni physicians toward pharmacovigilance: A mixed method study. *Int. J. Pharm. Pharm. Sci*, 10, 74–77.

Al-Worafi, Y.M. (2018c). Dispensing errors observed by community pharmacy dispensers in IBB–YEMEN. *Asian J. Pharm. Clin. Res*, 11(11).

Al-Worafi, Y.M. (2018d). Evauation of inhaler technique among patients with asthma and COPD in Yemen. *Journal of Taibah University medical sciences*, 13(5), 488–490.

Al-Worafi, Y.M., Patel, R.P., Zaidi, S.T.R., Alseragi, W.M., Almutairi, M.S., Alkhoshaiban, A.S., & Ming, L.C. (2018a). Completeness and legibility of handwritten prescriptions in Sana'a, Yemen. *Medical Principles and Practice*, 27, 290–292.

Al-Worafi, Y.M., Alseragi, W.M., Seng, L.K., Kassab, Y.W., Yeoh, S.F., Chiau, L., … & Husain, K. (2018b). Dispensing errors in community pharmacies: a prospective study in Sana'a, Yemen. *Arch Pharm Pract*, 9(4), 1–3.

Al-Worafi, Y.M., Alseragi, W.M., & Mahmoud, M.A. (2019). Competency of metered-dose inhaler use among community pharmacy dispensers in Ibb, Yemen: A simulation method study. *Latin American Journal of Pharmacy*, 38(3), 489–494.

Al-Worafi, Y.M. (Ed.). (2020a). *Drug Safety in Developing Countries: Achievements and Challenges.*

Al-Worafi, Y.M. (2020b). Medication errors. In *Drug Safety in Developing Countries* (pp. 105–117). Academic Press.

Al-Worafi, Y.M. (2020c). Adverse drug reactions. In *Drug Safety in Developing Countries* (pp. 39–57). Academic Press.

Al-Worafi, Y.M. (2020d). Medications registration and marketing: safety-related issues. In *Drug Safety in Developing Countries* (pp. 21–28). Academic Press.

Al-Worafi, Y.M. (2020e). Pharmacovigilance. In *Drug Safety in Developing Countries* (pp. 29–38). Academic Press.

Al-Worafi, Y.M. (2020f). Drug-related problems. In *Drug safety in developing countries* (pp. 59–71). Academic Press.

Al-Worafi, Y.M. (2020g). Medications safety-related terminology. In *Drug safety in developing countries* (pp. 7–19). Academic Press.

Al-Worafi, Y.M. (2020h). Self-medication. In *Drug Safety in Developing Countries* (pp. 73–86). Academic Press.

Al-Worafi, Y.M. (2020j). Antibiotics safety issues. In *Drug Safety in Developing Countries* (pp. 87–103). Academic Press.

Al-Worafi, Y.M. (2020k). Medications safety research issues. In *Drug Safety in Developing Countries* (pp. 213–227). Academic Press.

Al-Worafi, Y.M. (2020l). Counterfeit and substandard medications. In *Drug safety in developing countries* (pp. 119–126). Academic Press.

Al-Worafi, Y.M. (2020m). Medication abuse and misuse. In *Drug safety in developing countries* (pp. 127–135). Academic Press.

Al-Worafi, Y.M. (2020n). Storage and disposal of medications. In *Drug Safety in Developing Countries* (pp. 137–142). Academic Press.

Al-Worafi, Y.M. (2020o). Safety of medications in special population. In *Drug safety in developing countries* (pp. 143–162). Academic Press.

Al-Worafi, Y.M. (2020p). Herbal medicines safety issues. In *Drug Safety in developing countries* (pp. 163–178). Academic Press.

Al-Worafi, Y.M. (2020q). Medications safety pharmacoeconomics-related issues. In *Drug Safety in Developing Countries* (pp. 187–195). Academic Press.

Al-Worafi, Y.M. (2020r). Evidence-based medications safety practice. In *Drug Safety in Developing Countries* (pp. 197–201). Academic Press.

Al-Worafi, Y.M. (2020s). Quality indicators for medications safety. In *Drug safety in developing countries* (pp. 229–242). Academic Press.

Al-Worafi, Y.M. (2020t). Drug safety in Yemen. In *Drug Safety in Developing Countries* (pp. 391–405). Academic Press.

Al-Worafi, Y.M. (2020u). Drug safety in Saudi Arabia. In *Drug Safety in Developing Countries* (pp. 407–417). Academic Press.

Al-Worafi, Y.M. (2020v). Drug safety in United Arab Emirates. In *Drug Safety in Developing Countries* (pp. 419–428). Academic Press.

Al-Worafi, Y.M. (2020w). Drug safety in Indonesia. In *Drug Safety in Developing Countries* (pp. 279–285). Academic Press.

Al-Worafi, Y.M. (2020x). Drug safety in Palestine. In *Drug Safety in Developing Countries* (pp. 471–480). Academic Press.

Al-Worafi, Y.M. (2020y). Drug safety: comparison between developing countries. In *Drug Safety in Developing Countries* (pp. 603–611). Academic Press.

Al-Worafi, Y.M. (2020z). Drug safety in developing versus developed countries. In *Drug Safety in Developing Countries* (pp. 613–615). Academic Press.

Al-Worafi, Y.M., Alseragi, W.M., Ming, L.C., & Alakhali, K.M. (2020a). Drug safety in China. In *Drug Safety in Developing Countries* (pp. 381–388). Academic Press.

Al-Worafi, Y.M., Alseragi, W.M., Alakhali, K.M., Ming, L.C., Othman, G., Halboup, A.M., … & Elkalmi, R.M. (2020b). Knowledge, beliefs and factors affecting the use of generic medicines among patients in Ibb, Yemen: a mixed-method study. *Journal of Pharmacy Practice and Community Medicine*, 6(4).

Al-Worafi, Y.M., Elkalmi, R.M., Ming, L.C., Othman, G., Halboup, A.M., Battah, M.M., … & Mani, V. (2021a). Dispensing errors in hospital pharmacies: A prospective study in Yemen.

Al-Worafi, Y.M., Hasan, S., Hassan, N.M., & Gaili, A.A. (2021b). Knowledge, Attitude and Experience of Pharmacist in the UAE towards Pharmacovigilance. *Research Journal of Pharmacy and Technology*, 14(1), 265–269.

Al-Worafi, Y. (2022a). *A Guide to Online Pharmacy Education: Teaching Strategies and Assessment Methods*. CRC Press.

Al-Worafi, Y.M. (2022b). Patient care errors and related problems (part I): development and validation of the model. 0000-0002-5752-2913

Al-Worafi, Y.M. (Ed.). (2023). *Clinical Case Studies on medication Safety*. Academic Press.

Baig, M.R., Al-Worafi, Y.M., Alseragi, W.M., Ming, L.C., & Siddique, A. (2020). Drug safety in India. In *Drug Safety in Developing Countries* (pp. 327–334). Academic Press.

Elkalmi, R.M., Al-Worafi, Y.M., Alseragi, W.M., Ming, L.C., & Siddique, A. (2020). Drug safety in Malaysia. In *Drug Safety in Developing Countries* (pp. 245–253). Academic Press.

Elsayed, T., & Al-Worafi, Y.M. (2020). Drug safety in Egypt. In *Drug Safety in Developing Countries* (pp. 511–523). Academic Press.

Hasan, S., Al-Omar, M.J., AlZubaidy, H., & Al-Worafi, Y.M. (2019). Use of medications in Arab Countries. *Handbook of Healthcare in the Arab World*. Cham: Springer, 42.

Hassan, Y., Abd Aziz, N., Kassab, Y.W., Elgasim, I., Shaharuddin, S., Al-Worafi, Y.M.A., ... & Ming, L.C. (2014). How to help patients to control their blood pressure? Blood pressure control and its predictor. *Archives of Pharmacy Practice*, 5(4).

Izahar, S., Lean, Q.Y., Hameed, M.A., Murugiah, M.K., Patel, R.P., Al-Worafi, Y.M., ... & Ming, L.C. (2017). Content analysis of mobile health applications on diabetes mellitus. *Frontiers in Endocrinology*, 8, 318.

Kristensen, S., & Bartels, P. (2010). Use of patient safety culture instruments and recommendations. *Aarhus, Denmark, European Society for Quality in HealthCare-Office for Quality Indicators*, 113.

Lee, K.S., Yee, S.M., Zaidi, S.T.R., Patel, R.P., Yang, Q., Al-Worafi, Y.M., & Ming, L.C., 2017. Combating sale of counterfeit and falsified medicines online: a losing battle. *Frontiers in pharmacology*, 8, p. 268.

Mahmoud, M.A., Wajid, S., Naqvi, A.A., Samreen, S., Althagfan, S.S., & Al-Worafi, Y. (2020). Self-medication with antibiotics: A cross-sectional community-based study. *Latin american journal of pharmacy*, 39(2), 348–353.

Manan, M.M., Rusli, R.A., Ang, W.C., Al-Worafi, Y.M., & Ming, L.C. (2014). Assessing the pharmaceutical care issues of antiepileptic drug therapy in hospitalised epileptic patients. *Journal of Pharmacy Practice and Research*, 44(3), 83–88.

Manan, M.M., Ibrahim, N.A., Aziz, N.A., Zulkifly, H.H., Al-Worafi, Y.M.A., & Long, C.M. (2016). Empirical use of antibiotic therapy in the prevention of early onset sepsis in neonates: a pilot study. *Archives of Medical Science*, 12(3), 603–613.

Ming, L.C., Hameed, M.A., Lee, D.D., Apidi, N.A., Lai, P.S.M., Hadi, M.A., Al-Worafi, Y.M.A., & Khan, T.M., (2016). Use of medical mobile applications among hospital pharmacists in Malaysia. *Therapeutic innovation & regulatory science*, 50(4), pp. 419–426.

Ming, L.C., Untong, N., Aliudin, N.A., Osili, N., Kifli, N., Tan, C.S., ... & Goh, H.P. (2020). Mobile health apps on COVID-19 launched in the early days of the pandemic: content analysis and review. *JMIR mHealth and uHealth*, 8(9), e19796.

Othman, G., Ali, F., Ibrahim, M.I.M., Al-Worafi, Y.M., Ansari, M., & Halboup, A.M. (2020). Assessment of Anti-Diabetic Medications Adherence among Diabetic Patients in Sana'a City, Yemen: A Cross Sectional Study. *Journal of Pharmaceutical Research International*, 32(21), 114–122.

Reynard, J., Reynolds, J., & Stevenson, P. (2009). *Practical patient safety*. OUP Oxford.

Saeed, M.S., Alkhoshaiban, A.S., Al-Worafi, Y.M.A., & Long, C.M., (2014). Perception of self-medication among university students in Saudi Arabia. *Archives of Pharmacy Practice*, 5(4), p. 149.

Salas, E., & Frush, K. (2012). *Improving patient safety through teamwork and team training*. Oxford University Press.

Vincent, C. (2011). *Patient safety*. John Wiley & Sons.

215

27 Patient safety in oncology

27.1 BACKGROUND

Oncology is the branch of medicine that deals with the prevention, diagnosis, and treatment of cancer. It involves the study and treatment of tumors, which are abnormal growths of cells that can occur in any part of the body. There are several different types of cancer, each with its own unique characteristics and treatment options. Some of the most common types of cancer include breast cancer, lung cancer, prostate cancer, and colon cancer. Oncologists are medical professionals who specialize in the diagnosis and treatment of cancer. They may work in hospitals, cancer centers, or private practices, and may be involved in a variety of different types of cancer treatments, including chemotherapy, radiation therapy, and surgery. The field of oncology is constantly evolving, as new treatments and technologies are developed to improve outcomes for cancer patients. Ongoing research is focused on understanding the underlying causes of cancer, as well as developing more effective treatments and prevention strategies. Patient care and safety are critical aspects of oncology, as patients with cancer are often undergoing complex and intensive treatments that require careful monitoring and management. Here are some key considerations for patient care and safety in oncology:

1. Patient education: Oncology patients need to be educated about their diagnosis, treatment options, and potential side effects. They should also receive information on how to manage their symptoms, how to take their medications, and when to seek medical help.

2. Pain management: Pain is a common symptom of cancer and its treatment. Effective pain management is crucial to improving patient comfort and quality of life.

3. Infection control: Cancer patients are at increased risk of infection due to their weakened immune systems. Healthcare providers should take extra precautions to prevent the spread of infection.

4. Chemotherapy safety: Chemotherapy is a potent treatment for cancer, but it can also have serious side effects. Patients receiving chemotherapy should be closely monitored for side effects and given clear instructions on how to manage them.

5. Nutritional support: Good nutrition is essential for cancer patients, as it helps to maintain strength and support the immune system. Patients may require special diets or nutritional supplements to support their treatment.

6. Psychosocial support: Cancer can be emotionally challenging, and patients may require additional support to manage their mental health. Oncology patients should have access to counseling services or support groups.

7. End-of-life care: For patients with advanced cancer, end-of-life care is a critical consideration. Healthcare providers should work with patients and their families to ensure that end-of-life care is appropriate and in line with the patient's wishes.

In conclusion, patient care and safety in oncology require a multi-disciplinary approach, involving a range of healthcare providers, including physicians, nurses, nutritionists, and mental health professionals. By taking a holistic approach to patient care, healthcare providers can help to improve patient outcomes and quality of life (Kristensen & Bartels, 2010; Reynard et al., 2009; Salas & Frush, 2012; Vincent, 2011).

27.2 ONCOLOGY ERRORS AND RELATED PROBLEMS

Oncology errors and related problems can have serious consequences for patients, including delayed diagnosis, inappropriate treatment, and even death. Here are some common oncology errors and problems:

1. Diagnostic errors: Oncology diagnostic errors can occur when healthcare providers fail to correctly identify a patient's cancer or misinterpret test results. This can result in delays in treatment or inappropriate treatment.

2. Treatment errors: Treatment errors can occur when patients receive the wrong medication, incorrect dosage, or when treatment is not administered properly. These errors can lead to severe side effects or complications.

DOI: 10.1201/9781003230465-29

3. Communication errors: Communication errors can occur between healthcare providers or between providers and patients. This can result in confusion, misinterpretation of information, or missed appointments.

4. Adverse drug reactions: Adverse drug reactions can occur when patients have an unexpected or dangerous reaction to a medication. This can result in severe side effects, hospitalization, or even death.

5. Medical device malfunctions: Medical device malfunctions can occur during cancer treatment, such as radiation therapy or chemotherapy. Malfunctions can result in underdosing or overdosing of treatment or other harmful effects.

6. Infection control breaches: Infection control breaches can occur when healthcare providers fail to follow proper protocols for preventing the spread of infection. This can result in serious infections, hospitalization, or even death.

7. Inadequate follow-up: Inadequate follow-up can occur when patients do not receive appropriate monitoring or care after their cancer treatment. This can lead to complications or disease recurrence.

In conclusion, oncology errors and related problems can have serious consequences for patients. Healthcare providers must take steps to prevent these errors by improving communication, following proper protocols, and monitoring patients closely. Patients can also help to reduce the risk of errors by being informed and engaged in their care.

27.3 CAUSES OF ONCOLOGY ERRORS AND RELATED PROBLEMS

There are many causes of oncology errors and related problems, including:

1. Human error: Mistakes can be made by healthcare providers at any stage of the care process, from diagnosis to treatment and follow-up. Human error can occur due to fatigue, stress, distraction, or lack of training.

2. Communication breakdowns: Communication breakdowns can occur between healthcare providers or between providers and patients. This can lead to confusion, misinterpretation of information, or missed appointments.

3. Systemic issues: Systemic issues within healthcare systems can contribute to oncology errors and problems. This can include inadequate staffing, poor coordination between departments, or outdated technology.

4. Inadequate training: Healthcare providers may lack the necessary training or experience to effectively diagnose, treat, or manage cancer patients.

5. Medication errors: Medication errors can occur when patients receive the wrong medication, incorrect dosage, or when treatment is not administered properly. This can be due to mistakes in prescribing, dispensing, or administration.

6. Infection control breaches: Infection control breaches can occur when healthcare providers fail to follow proper protocols for preventing the spread of infection. This can be due to inadequate training, lack of resources, or failure to adhere to best practices.

7. Patient-related factors: Patient-related factors, such as non-adherence to treatment regimens or failure to communicate symptoms to healthcare providers, can contribute to oncology errors and problems.

In conclusion, there are many factors that can contribute to oncology errors and related problems. Healthcare providers must take steps to identify and address these issues in order to improve patient care and safety. This can involve improving communication, providing adequate training, and implementing best practices for infection control and medication management. Patients can also play a role in reducing the risk of errors by being informed and engaged in their care.

27.4 PREVENTION OF ONCOLOGY ERRORS AND RELATED PROBLEMS

Preventing oncology errors and related problems is critical to ensuring the safety and well-being of cancer patients. Here are some strategies that healthcare providers can use to prevent these errors:

1. Implement standardized protocols: Standardized protocols can help to ensure that healthcare providers follow consistent and effective practices for diagnosing, treating, and managing cancer patients. These protocols can be developed based on best practices and evidence-based guidelines.

2. Improve communication: Effective communication is essential to preventing errors in oncology care. This can involve using electronic health records, providing clear and concise instructions to patients, and encouraging patients to ask questions and provide feedback.

3. Provide training and education: Healthcare providers should receive ongoing training and education on best practices for oncology care. This can include training in communication skills, infection control, medication management, and other critical aspects of care.

4. Use technology: Technology can play a key role in preventing oncology errors and related problems. For example, electronic prescribing systems can reduce the risk of medication errors, while electronic health records can improve communication and coordination between healthcare providers.

5. Involve patients in their care: Patients can play a critical role in preventing errors by being informed and engaged in their care. Healthcare providers should encourage patients to ask questions, report symptoms, and provide feedback on their care.

6. Conduct regular quality assessments: Regular quality assessments can help to identify areas for improvement in oncology care. Healthcare providers should conduct audits of their practices and outcomes to identify and address potential areas for improvement.

In conclusion, preventing oncology errors and related problems requires a multi-faceted approach that involves improving communication, providing training and education, using technology, involving patients in their care, and conducting regular quality assessments. By taking these steps, healthcare providers can improve patient outcomes and ensure the safety and well-being of cancer patients.

27.5 ONCOLOGY SAFETY CULTURE

Oncology safety culture refers to the values, attitudes, and behaviors that shape the safety of oncology care. A strong safety culture in oncology is characterized by a commitment to patient safety, open communication, continuous learning, and a willingness to report errors and near misses. Here are some key elements of a strong oncology safety culture:

1. Leadership commitment: Strong leadership is essential to creating a culture of safety in oncology care. Leaders must communicate a clear commitment to patient safety, allocate resources to support safety initiatives and empower staff to report errors and near misses.

2. Communication and teamwork: Effective communication and teamwork are critical to ensuring safe and effective oncology care. This includes open and transparent communication between healthcare providers and patients, as well as between different departments and disciplines.

3. Learning and continuous improvement: A strong safety culture in oncology also involves a commitment to learning and continuous improvement. This includes ongoing education and training for healthcare providers, regular assessments of safety practices and outcomes, and a willingness to learn from errors and near misses.

4. Reporting and analysis of errors: Healthcare providers must be encouraged to report errors and near misses without fear of retribution. This includes implementing reporting systems and processes that allow for anonymous reporting and analysis of errors to identify opportunities for improvement.

5. Patient engagement: Patients should be involved in their care and treated as partners in the safety process. This includes educating patients about their care and treatment options, encouraging them to ask questions and report symptoms, and involving them in the development of care plans.

In conclusion, a strong oncology safety culture is critical to ensuring safe and effective cancer care. This involves a commitment to leadership, communication and teamwork, learning and continuous improvement, reporting and analysis of errors, and patient engagement. By prioritizing these elements, healthcare providers can create a culture of safety that supports the best possible outcomes for cancer patients.

27.6 ONCOLOGY ERRORS AND RELATED PROBLEMS IN DEVELOPING COUNTRIES: Challenges and recommendations

Oncology errors and related problems are a significant challenge in developing countries, where healthcare resources may be limited and oncology care may be less accessible. Here are some of the challenges that contribute to oncology errors in developing countries, as well as some recommendations for addressing these challenges:

Challenges:

1. Limited resources: Developing countries often have limited resources to allocate to healthcare, including oncology care. This can lead to a lack of equipment, supplies, and trained personnel, which can contribute to errors and poor outcomes.

2. Inadequate infrastructure: Developing countries may have inadequate infrastructure to support effective oncology care. This includes insufficient facilities, poor transportation, and inadequate communication systems, which can hinder access to care and coordination between healthcare providers.

3. Limited access to education and training: Healthcare providers in developing countries may have limited access to education and training on best practices for oncology care. This can lead to a lack of knowledge and skills, which can contribute to errors and poor outcomes.

4. Cultural barriers: Cultural barriers, such as stigma and lack of awareness about cancer, can make it difficult to provide effective oncology care in some developing countries. This can lead to delays in diagnosis and treatment, which can contribute to poor outcomes.

Recommendations:

1. Increase resources: Developing countries should increase resources for oncology care, including funding, equipment, and trained personnel. This can help to improve access to care and reduce the risk of errors and poor outcomes.

2. Improve infrastructure: Developing countries should invest in improving infrastructure to support effective oncology care. This includes improving facilities, transportation, and communication systems to facilitate access to care and coordination between healthcare providers.

3. Increase education and training: Healthcare providers in developing countries should have access to education and training on best practices for oncology care. This can help to improve knowledge and skills, reduce the risk of errors, and improve patient outcomes.

4. Address cultural barriers: Developing countries should address cultural barriers to effective oncology care, such as stigma and lack of awareness about cancer. This can involve educating communities about cancer prevention and treatment and addressing misconceptions and myths about the disease.

5. Despite the progress in research about patient care and safety in developing countries, there is little research about patient safety related to oncology in the majority of developing countries, therefore, conducting research is very important and highly recommended (Alshahrani et al., 2019a,b; Al-Qahtani et al., 2015; Alshahrani et al., 2020a,b; Al-Worafi, 2014; Al-Worafi, 2015; Al-Worafi, 2016; Al-Worafi et al., 2017; Al-Worafi, 2018a–d; Al-Worafi et al., 2018a–b; Al-Worafi et al., 2019; Al-Worafi, 2020a–z; Al-Worafi et al., 2020a–b; Al-Worafi et al., 2021a,b; Al-Worafi, 2022a,b; Al-Worafi, 2023; Baig et al., 2020; Elkalmi et al., 2020; Elsayed & Al-Worafi, 2020; Hasan et al., 2019; Hassan et al., 2014; Izhar et al., 2017; Lee et al., 2017; Mahmoud et al., 2020; Manan et al., 2014; Manan et al., 2016; Ming et al., 2016; Ming et al., 2020; Othman et al., 2020; Saeed et al., 2014).

In conclusion, oncology errors and related problems are a significant challenge in developing countries, where healthcare resources may be limited and oncology care may be less accessible. Addressing these challenges requires a multi-faceted approach that includes increasing resources, improving infrastructure, increasing education and training, and addressing cultural barriers. By taking these steps, developing countries can improve access to effective oncology care and reduce the risk of errors and poor outcomes.

27.7 CONCLUSION

This chapter has discussed the oncology safety issues, prevention, challenges, and recommendations for achieving the best practice in developing countries. Oncology errors and related problems are a significant challenge in developing countries, where healthcare resources may be limited and oncology care may be less accessible. Addressing these challenges requires a multi-faceted approach that includes increasing resources, improving infrastructure, increasing education and training, and addressing cultural barriers. By taking these steps, developing countries can improve access to effective oncology care and reduce the risk of errors and poor outcomes. Oncology errors and related problems can have serious consequences for patients, including delayed diagnosis, inappropriate treatment, and even death. there are many factors that can contribute to oncology errors and related problems. Healthcare providers must take steps to identify and address these issues in order to improve patient care and safety. This can involve improving communication, providing adequate training, and implementing best practices for infection control and medication management. Patients can also play a role in reducing the risk of errors by being informed and engaged in their care.

REFERENCES

Al-Qahtani, I., Almoteb, T.M., & Al-Warafi, Y. (2015). Competency of metered-dose inhaler use among Saudi community pharmacists: A Simulation method study. *RRJPPS*, 4(2), 37–31.

Alshahrani, S.M., Alakhali, K.M., & Al-Worafi, Y.M., (2019a). Medication errors in a health care facility in southern Saudi Arabia. *Tropical Journal of Pharmaceutical Research*, 18(5), pp. 1119–1122.

Alshahrani, S.M., Alavudeen, S.S., Alakhali, K.M., Al-Worafi, Y.M., Bahamdan, A.K., & Vigneshwaran, E., (2019b). Self-Medication Among King Khalid University Students, Saudi Arabia. *Risk Management and Healthcare Policy*, 12, pp. 243–249.

Alshahrani, S.M., Alakhali, K.M., Al-Worafi, Y.M., & Alshahrani, N.Z. (2020b). Awareness and use of over the counter analgesic medication: a survey in the Aseer region population, Saudi Arabia. *Int J Advan Appl Sci*, 7(3), 130–134.

Alshahrani, S.M., Alzahran, M., Alakhali, K., Vigneshwaran, E., Iqbal, M.J., Khan, N.A., ... & Alavudeen, S.S. (2020b). Association Between Diabetes Consequences and Quality of Life Among Patients With Diabetes Mellitus in the Aseer Province of Saudi Arabia. *Open Access Macedonian Journal of Medical Sciences*, 8(E), 325–330.

Al-Worafi, Y.M. (2014). Prescription writing errors at a tertiary care hospital in Yemen: prevalence, types, causes and recommendations. *Am J Pharm Health Res*, 2, 134–140.

Al-Worafi, Y.M.A. (2015). Appropriateness of metered-dose inhaler use in the Yemeni community pharmacies. *Journal of Taibah University Medical Sciences*, 10(3), 353–358.

Al-Worafi, Y.M.A. (2016). Pharmacy practice in Yemen. In *Pharmacy Practice in Developing Countries* (pp. 267–287). Academic Press.

Al-Worafi, Y.M., Kassab, Y.W., Alseragi, W.M., Almutairi, M.S., Ahmed, A., Ming, L.C., Alkhoshaiban, A.S., & Hadi, M.A., (2017). Pharmacovigilance and adverse drg reaction reporting: a perspective of community pharmacists and pharmacy technicians in Sana'a, Yemen. *Therapeutics and clinical risk management*, 13, p. 1175.

Al-Worafi, Y.M., (2018a). Knowledge, Attitude and Practice of Yemeni Physicians Toward Pharmacovigilance: A Mixed Method Study. *International Journal of Pharmacy and Pharmaceutical Sciences*, 10(10), 74–77.

Al-Worafi, Y. (2018b). Knowledge, attitude and practice of Yemeni physicians toward pharmacovigilance: A mixed method study. *Int. J. Pharm. Pharm. Sci*, 10, 74–77.

Al-Worafi, Y.M. (2018c). Dispensing errors observed by community pharmacy dispensers in IBB–YEMEN. *Asian J. Pharm. Clin. Res*, 11(11).

Al-Worafi, Y.M. (2018d). Evauation of inhaler technique among patients with asthma and COPD in Yemen. *Journal of Taibah University medical sciences*, 13(5), 488–490.

Al-Worafi, Y.M., Patel, R.P., Zaidi, S.T.R., Alseragi, W.M., Almutairi, M.S., Alkhoshaiban, A.S., & Ming, L.C. (2018a). Completeness and legibility of handwritten prescriptions in Sana'a, Yemen. *Medical Principles and Practice*, 27, 290–292.

Al-Worafi, Y.M., Alseragi, W.M., Seng, L.K., Kassab, Y.W., Yeoh, S.F., Chiau, L., … & Husain, K. (2018b). Dispensing errors in community pharmacies: a prospective study in Sana'a, Yemen. *Arch Pharm Pract*, 9(4), 1–3.

Al-Worafi, Y.M., Alseragi, W.M., & Mahmoud, M.A. (2019). Competency of metered-dose inhaler use among community pharmacy dispensers in Ibb, Yemen: A simulation method study. *Latin American Journal of Pharmacy*, 38(3), 489–494.

Al-Worafi, Y.M. (Ed.). (2020a). *Drug Safety in Developing Countries: Achievements and Challenges.*

Al-Worafi, Y.M. (2020b). Medication errors. In *Drug Safety in Developing Countries* (pp. 105–117). Academic Press.

Al-Worafi, Y.M. (2020c). Adverse drug reactions. In *Drug Safety in Developing Countries* (pp. 39–57). Academic Press.

Al-Worafi, Y.M. (2020d). Medications registration and marketing: safety-related issues. In *Drug Safety in Developing Countries* (pp. 21–28). Academic Press.

Al-Worafi, Y.M. (2020e). Pharmacovigilance. In *Drug Safety in Developing Countries* (pp. 29–38). Academic Press.

Al-Worafi, Y.M. (2020f). Drug-related problems. In *Drug safety in developing countries* (pp. 59–71). Academic Press.

Al-Worafi, Y.M. (2020g). Medications safety-related terminology. In *Drug safety in developing countries* (pp. 7–19). Academic Press.

Al-Worafi, Y.M. (2020h). Self-medication. In *Drug Safety in Developing Countries* (pp. 73–86). Academic Press.

Al-Worafi, Y.M. (2020j). Antibiotics safety issues. In *Drug Safety in Developing Countries* (pp. 87–103). Academic Press.

Al-Worafi, Y.M. (2020k). Medications safety research issues. In *Drug Safety in Developing Countries* (pp. 213–227). Academic Press.

Al-Worafi, Y.M. (2020l). Counterfeit and substandard medications. In *Drug safety in developing countries* (pp. 119–126). Academic Press.

Al-Worafi, Y.M. (2020m). Medication abuse and misuse. In *Drug safety in developing countries* (pp. 127–135). Academic Press.

Al-Worafi, Y.M. (2020n). Storage and disposal of medications. In *Drug Safety in Developing Countries* (pp. 137–142). Academic Press.

Al-Worafi, Y.M. (2020o). Safety of medications in special population. In *Drug safety in developing countries* (pp. 143–162). Academic Press.

Al-Worafi, Y.M. (2020p). Herbal medicines safety issues. In *Drug Safety in developing countries* (pp. 163–178). Academic Press.

Al-Worafi, Y.M. (2020q). Medications safety pharmacoeconomics-related issues. In *Drug Safety in Developing Countries* (pp. 187–195). Academic Press.

Al-Worafi, Y.M. (2020r). Evidence-based medications safety practice. In *Drug Safety in Developing Countries* (pp. 197–201). Academic Press.

Al-Worafi, Y.M. (2020s). Quality indicators for medications safety. In *Drug safety in developing countries* (pp. 229–242). Academic Press.

Al-Worafi, Y.M. (2020t). Drug safety in Yemen. In *Drug Safety in Developing Countries* (pp. 391–405). Academic Press.

Al-Worafi, Y.M. (2020u). Drug safety in Saudi Arabia. In *Drug Safety in Developing Countries* (pp. 407–417). Academic Press.

Al-Worafi, Y.M. (2020v). Drug safety in United Arab Emirates. In *Drug Safety in Developing Countries* (pp. 419–428). Academic Press.

Al-Worafi, Y.M. (2020w). Drug safety in Indonesia. In *Drug Safety in Developing Countries* (pp. 279–285). Academic Press.

Al-Worafi, Y.M. (2020x). Drug safety in Palestine. In *Drug Safety in Developing Countries* (pp. 471–480). Academic Press.

Al-Worafi, Y.M. (2020y). Drug safety: comparison between developing countries. In *Drug Safety in Developing Countries* (pp. 603–611). Academic Press.

Al-Worafi, Y.M. (2020z). Drug safety in developing versus developed countries. In *Drug Safety in Developing Countries* (pp. 613–615). Academic Press.

Al-Worafi, Y.M., Alseragi, W.M., Ming, L.C., & Alakhali, K.M. (2020a). Drug safety in China. In *Drug Safety in Developing Countries* (pp. 381–388). Academic Press.

Al-Worafi, Y.M., Alseragi, W.M., Alakhali, K.M., Ming, L.C., Othman, G., Halboup, A.M., ... & Elkalmi, R.M. (2020b). Knowledge, beliefs and factors affecting the use of generic medicines among patients in Ibb, Yemen: a mixed-method study. *Journal of Pharmacy Practice and Community Medicine*, 6(4).

Al-Worafi, Y.M., Elkalmi, R.M., Ming, L.C., Othman, G., Halboup, A.M., Battah, M.M., ... & Mani, V. (2021a). Dispensing errors in hospital pharmacies: A prospective study in Yemen.

Al-Worafi, Y.M., Hasan, S., Hassan, N.M., & Gaili, A.A. (2021b). Knowledge, Attitude and Experience of Pharmacist in the UAE towards Pharmacovigilance. *Research Journal of Pharmacy and Technology*, 14(1), 265–269.

Al-Worafi, Y. (2022a). *A Guide to Online Pharmacy Education: Teaching Strategies and Assessment Methods*. CRC Press.

Al-Worafi, Y.M. (2022b). Patient care errors and related problems (part I): development and validation of the model. 0000-0002-5752-2913

Al-Worafi, Y.M. (Ed.). (2023). *Clinical Case Studies on medication Safety.* Academic Press.

Baig, M.R., Al-Worafi, Y.M., Alseragi, W.M., Ming, L.C., & Siddique, A. (2020). Drug safety in India. In *Drug Safety in Developing Countries* (pp. 327–334). Academic Press.

Elkalmi, R.M., Al-Worafi, Y.M., Alseragi, W.M., Ming, L.C., & Siddique, A. (2020). Drug safety in Malaysia. In *Drug Safety in Developing Countries* (pp. 245–253). Academic Press.

Elsayed, T., & Al-Worafi, Y.M. (2020). Drug safety in Egypt. In *Drug Safety in Developing Countries* (pp. 511–523). Academic Press.

Hasan, S., Al-Omar, M.J., AlZubaidy, H., & Al-Worafi, Y.M. (2019). Use of medications in Arab Countries. *Handbook of Healthcare in the Arab World.* Cham: Springer, 42.

Hassan, Y., Abd Aziz, N., Kassab, Y.W., Elgasim, I., Shaharuddin, S., Al-Worafi, Y.M.A., ... & Ming, L.C. (2014). How to help patients to control their blood pressure? Blood pressure control and its predictor. *Archives of Pharmacy Practice,* 5(4).

Izahar, S., Lean, Q.Y., Hameed, M.A., Murugiah, M.K., Patel, R.P., Al-Worafi, Y.M., ... & Ming, L.C. (2017). Content analysis of mobile health applications on diabetes mellitus. *Frontiers in Endocrinology,* 8, 318.

Kristensen, S., & Bartels, P. (2010). Use of patient safety culture instruments and recommendations. *Aarhus, Denmark, European Society for Quality in HealthCare-Office for Quality Indicators,* 113.

Lee, K.S., Yee, S.M., Zaidi, S.T.R., Patel, R.P., Yang, Q., Al-Worafi, Y.M., & Ming, L.C., 2017. Combating sale of counterfeit and falsified medicines online: a losing battle. *Frontiers in pharmacology,* 8, p. 268.

Mahmoud, M.A., Wajid, S., Naqvi, A.A., Samreen, S., Althagfan, S.S., & Al-Worafi, Y. (2020). Self-medication with antibiotics: A cross-sectional community-based study. *Latin american journal of pharmacy,* 39(2), 348–353.

Manan, M.M., Rusli, R.A., Ang, W.C., Al-Worafi, Y.M., & Ming, L.C. (2014). Assessing the pharmaceutical care issues of antiepileptic drug therapy in hospitalised epileptic patients. *Journal of Pharmacy Practice and Research,* 44(3), 83–88.

Manan, M.M., Ibrahim, N.A., Aziz, N.A., Zulkifly, H.H., Al-Worafi, Y.M.A., & Long, C.M. (2016). Empirical use of antibiotic therapy in the prevention of early onset sepsis in neonates: a pilot study. *Archives of Medical Science,* 12(3), 603–613.

Ming, L.C., Hameed, M.A., Lee, D.D., Apidi, N.A., Lai, P.S.M., Hadi, M.A., Al-Worafi, Y.M.A., & Khan, T.M., (2016). Use of medical mobile applications among hospital pharmacists in Malaysia. *Therapeutic innovation & regulatory science,* 50(4), pp. 419–426.

Ming, L.C., Untong, N., Aliudin, N.A., Osili, N., Kifli, N., Tan, C.S., ... & Goh, H.P. (2020). Mobile health apps on COVID-19 launched in the early days of the pandemic: content analysis and review. *JMIR mHealth and uHealth,* 8(9), e19796.

Othman, G., Ali, F., Ibrahim, M.I.M., Al-Worafi, Y.M., Ansari, M., & Halboup, A.M. (2020). Assessment of Anti-Diabetic Medications Adherence among Diabetic Patients in Sana'a City, Yemen: A Cross Sectional Study. *Journal of Pharmaceutical Research International,* 32(21), 114–122.

Reynard, J., Reynolds, J., & Stevenson, P. (2009). *Practical patient safety*. OUP Oxford.

Saeed, M.S., Alkhoshaiban, A.S., Al-Worafi, Y.M.A., & Long, C.M., (2014). Perception of self-medication among university students in Saudi Arabia. *Archives of Pharmacy Practice*, 5(4), p. 149.

Salas, E., & Frush, K. (2012). *Improving patient safety through teamwork and team training*. Oxford University Press.

Vincent, C. (2011). *Patient safety*. John Wiley & Sons.

28 Patient Safety in Pharmacies

28.1 BACKGROUND

Pharmacies play a critical role in patient care and patient safety. They are responsible for dispensing medications prescribed by healthcare providers, ensuring that patients receive the right medication, in the right dose, and at the right time. Pharmacists and pharmacy technicians work together to ensure that medications are properly prepared, labeled, and stored. Patient safety is a top priority in pharmacies. Pharmacists and pharmacy technicians are trained to identify and prevent medication errors, including incorrect dosages, drug interactions, and allergies. They use computer systems and other technologies to check for potential problems and to ensure that medications are properly tracked and documented. In addition to dispensing medications, pharmacies also provide a range of other services to support patient care and safety. They may offer medication therapy management services, which involve reviewing a patient's medications, identifying potential problems, and working with the patient's healthcare team to develop a medication plan that is safe and effective. They may also provide immunizations, health screenings, and other preventive care services. Pharmacies also play a role in promoting patient education and empowerment. They can provide information about medications, potential side effects, and proper usage. They can also help patients manage chronic conditions, such as diabetes or high blood pressure, by providing resources and support. Overall, pharmacies are an essential part of the healthcare system, and they play a critical role in promoting patient care and safety. Through their expertise, technologies, and patient-centered services, they help ensure that patients receive the medications and support they need to stay healthy and manage their conditions effectively. Pharmacists have traditionally been responsible for dispensing medications and providing medication-related advice to patients. However, in recent years, there has been a growing recognition of the value that pharmacists can bring to the healthcare team, and as a result, their roles and responsibilities have expanded. Here are some of the new roles and responsibilities of pharmacists:

1. Medication Therapy Management: Pharmacists are now involved in medication therapy management (MTM), which involves reviewing a patient's medications, identifying potential problems, and working with the patient's healthcare team to develop a medication plan that is safe and effective.

2. Prescriptive Authority: In some states, pharmacists have been granted prescriptive authority, which allows them to prescribe medications for certain conditions, such as smoking cessation or travel-related illnesses.

3. Chronic Disease Management: Pharmacists play an important role in the management of chronic diseases such as diabetes, asthma, and hypertension. They work with patients to develop treatment plans, monitor their symptoms, and provide ongoing support and education.

4. Immunizations: Many pharmacists are now authorized to administer vaccines, including flu shots and other immunizations, which can help increase vaccination rates and improve public health.

5. Point-of-Care Testing: Some pharmacists are now able to perform point-of-care testing for various conditions, such as diabetes, cholesterol, and strep throat. This allows patients to receive testing and results quickly and conveniently.

6. Health Promotion: Pharmacists are increasingly involved in health promotion and disease prevention activities. They may provide health education and counseling to patients, as well as participate in community outreach programs.

7. Pharmaceutical care is a patient-centered approach to medication management that involves the pharmacist working closely with the patient and other members of the healthcare team to ensure that the patient receives safe, effective, and appropriate medication therapy. By providing pharmaceutical care, pharmacists can help to improve patient outcomes, reduce the risk of medication errors and adverse drug events, and ensure that patients receive the best possible care. It is important for pharmacists to remain vigilant and proactive in identifying and addressing potential safety risks for patients, and to continuously work toward improving patient care and safety through pharmaceutical care.

DOI: 10.1201/9781003230465-30

Overall, the expanded roles and responsibilities of pharmacists reflect a growing recognition of their expertise and value as healthcare professionals. By working collaboratively with other members of the healthcare team, pharmacists can help ensure that patients receive the highest quality care and achieve the best possible health outcomes. (Cipolle et al., 2004; Kristensen & Bartels, 2010; Reynard et al., 2009; Salas & Frush, 2012; Vincent, 2011).

28.2 PHARMACIES ERRORS AND RELATED PROBLEMS

Despite the best efforts of pharmacists and pharmacy technicians to prevent errors, medication errors can and do occur in pharmacies. These errors can result in serious harm to patients, including hospitalization, disability, or even death. Some of the common types of pharmacy errors include:

1. Dispensing Errors: Dispensing errors occur when a patient receives the wrong medication or the wrong dosage. This can happen when a medication is mislabeled, the wrong medication is dispensed, or the wrong dosage is prescribed.

2. Prescription Errors: Prescription errors can occur when a healthcare provider makes a mistake in prescribing a medication, such as writing the wrong dosage or the wrong medication. These errors can be compounded if the pharmacist or pharmacy technician also makes an error during the dispensing process.

3. Communication Errors: Communication errors can occur when there is a breakdown in communication between the healthcare provider and the pharmacy. This can happen when the healthcare provider fails to communicate important information about the patient's medication history, allergies, or other relevant information.

4. Documentation Errors: Documentation errors can occur when important information is not accurately recorded in the patient's medical record or the pharmacy's record-keeping system. This can result in confusion or errors when medications are dispensed or when healthcare providers review the patient's medication history.

To prevent these types of errors, pharmacies have implemented a range of strategies, such as computerized order entry systems, barcoding systems, and other technologies to improve accuracy and prevent errors. Additionally, pharmacists and pharmacy technicians receive extensive training on medication safety and error prevention.

However, errors can still occur, and it is important for healthcare providers and patients to be aware of the potential risks and to take steps to prevent errors. This may include double-checking medications before taking them, keeping a current list of medications and allergies, and communicating openly and effectively with healthcare providers and pharmacists.

28.3 CAUSES OF PHARMACIES ERRORS AND RELATED PROBLEMS

There are many factors that can contribute to pharmacy errors and related problems. Some of the common causes include:

1. Human Error: Human error is a common cause of pharmacy errors. Pharmacists and pharmacy technicians may make mistakes during the dispensing process, such as misreading a prescription or selecting the wrong medication from the shelf.

2. Communication Breakdowns: Communication breakdowns between healthcare providers and the pharmacy can also contribute to errors. If important information about a patient's medication history or allergies is not communicated clearly, it can lead to dispensing errors or other problems.

3. Systemic Problems: Systemic problems within the healthcare system can also contribute to pharmacy errors. This can include issues with electronic health record systems, problems with medication labeling, or staffing shortages that lead to overworked pharmacists and pharmacy technicians.

4. Patient Factors: Patients can also contribute to pharmacy errors if they fail to disclose important information about their medication history or allergies, or if they fail to follow medication instructions.

5. Look-alike or Sound-alike Medications: Look-alike or sound-alike medications can also contribute to pharmacy errors. If medications have similar names or packaging, it can lead to confusion during the dispensing process.

6. High-Volume Dispensing: High-volume dispensing can also contribute to errors. If pharmacists and pharmacy technicians are under pressure to fill a large number of prescriptions quickly, it can increase the risk of errors.

It is important to note that many pharmacy errors are preventable, and there are steps that pharmacies can take to reduce the risk of errors. This includes implementing systems and processes to prevent errors, such as barcoding and computerized order entry systems, as well as providing training to pharmacists and pharmacy technicians on medication safety and error prevention. Patients can also play a role in preventing errors by communicating openly with their healthcare providers and pharmacists, and by following medication instructions carefully.

28.4 PREVENTION OF PHARMACIES ERRORS AND RELATED PROBLEMS

Preventing pharmacy errors and related problems is crucial to ensure patient safety and optimizing health outcomes. Here are some strategies that can be used to prevent pharmacy errors:

1. Computerized Order Entry Systems: Computerized order entry systems can help reduce errors by automating the prescription ordering process. This system can flag potential errors, such as drug interactions or incorrect dosages.

2. Barcoding: Barcoding technology can help ensure that the correct medication is dispensed to the patient by verifying the medication and dosage against the patient's electronic record.

3. Double-checking: Implementing a system of double-checking can help prevent errors. This involves having a second healthcare professional to check the medication and dosage before it is dispensed to the patient.

4. Education and Training: Education and training for pharmacists and pharmacy technicians can help prevent errors by increasing their knowledge and skills related to medication safety and error prevention.

5. Patient Education: Educating patients on their medications can help prevent errors by ensuring that they understand the purpose, dosage, and potential side effects of their medications.

6. Labeling: Proper labeling of medications is crucial to prevent errors. Labels should be clear and easy to read and should include important information such as the patient's name, the medication name, dosage, and instructions for use.

7. Staffing and Workload: Adequate staffing and workload management are essential to prevent errors. Overworked pharmacists and pharmacy technicians are more likely to make mistakes, so ensuring that staffing levels are appropriate can help reduce the risk of errors.

8. Quality Assurance Programs: Quality assurance programs can help prevent errors by identifying areas of weakness in the dispensing process and implementing corrective actions.

In summary, preventing pharmacy errors requires a multifaceted approach that involves technology, education and training, patient education, labeling, staffing and workload management, and quality assurance programs. By implementing these strategies, pharmacies can help ensure patient safety and improve health outcomes.

28.5 PHARMACIES SAFETY CULTURE

Pharmacy safety culture refers to the values, attitudes, and behaviors that promote a safe and error-free environment in the pharmacy. A positive safety culture is essential for preventing errors and improving patient outcomes. Here are some key components of a strong safety culture in the pharmacy:

1. Leadership: Pharmacy leaders must set the tone for a positive safety culture by prioritizing patient safety and encouraging open communication about errors and near misses.

2. Communication: Effective communication is crucial for promoting a strong safety culture. Pharmacies should encourage open communication among staff members and provide opportunities for feedback and input from all team members.

3. Continuous Improvement: A culture of continuous improvement is essential for identifying and addressing potential safety issues. Pharmacies should have processes in place for regularly reviewing and updating policies and procedures related to medication safety.

4. Training and Education: Pharmacies should provide regular training and education for staff members on topics related to medication safety, error prevention, and quality improvement.

5. Accountability: A strong safety culture requires accountability at all levels of the organization. Staff members should be held accountable for their actions and decisions related to medication safety, and systems should be in place to identify and address potential errors or unsafe practices.

6. Patient-Centered Care: A patient-centered approach to care is essential for promoting medication safety. Pharmacists should prioritize patient safety and work closely with other healthcare providers to ensure that patients receive the most appropriate medications and dosages.

In summary, a strong safety culture is essential for promoting medication safety and error prevention in the pharmacy. By prioritizing leadership, communication, continuous improvement, training and education, accountability, and patient-centered care, pharmacies can help ensure that patients receive the highest quality care possible.

28.6 PHARMACIES ERRORS AND RELATED PROBLEMS IN DEVELOPING COUNTRIES: Challenges and Recommendations

Pharmacies errors and related problems are major issues in developing countries, where healthcare systems face various challenges such as inadequate funding, shortage of trained personnel, and poor regulatory frameworks. Some of the challenges and recommendations related to pharmacies errors in developing countries are:

1. Lack of Adequate Training and Education: Many pharmacy workers in developing countries do not have adequate training and education to handle complex prescriptions, manage drug interactions, and provide proper counseling to patients. To address this issue, there is a need for more rigorous training programs for pharmacy workers, including ongoing education and professional development.

2. Poor Quality Control: The lack of quality control measures in developing countries can lead to medication errors, including the dispensing of expired or substandard medications. To improve quality control measures, regulatory bodies should implement stricter regulations to ensure that pharmacies comply with standard quality control procedures.

3. Inadequate Access to Information: Lack of access to up-to-date information on drug interactions, side effects, and dosing guidelines can contribute to medication errors. To address this challenge, pharmacies should have access to online databases that provide accurate and up-to-date drug information.

4. Limited Use of Technology: In many developing countries, pharmacies still rely on manual systems for record-keeping and dispensing medications. The use of technology, such as electronic prescribing and medication dispensing systems, can improve accuracy and reduce errors.

5. Cultural Beliefs and Practices: In some cultures, traditional medicines are still used alongside modern medicines, which can lead to drug interactions and adverse effects. To address this challenge, there is a need for more education and awareness campaigns to promote the proper use of modern medicines.

6. Inadequate Regulatory Frameworks: Many developing countries have inadequate regulatory frameworks to monitor and regulate the operations of pharmacies. To address this challenge, regulatory bodies should be strengthened to ensure that pharmacies comply with standards and regulations.

7. Despite the progress in research about patient care and safety in many developing countries, there is little research about patient safety related to pharmacies in other countries, therefore, conducting research is very important and highly recommended (Alshahrani et al., 2019a,b; Al-Qahtani et al., 2015; Alshahrani et al., 2020a,b; Al-Worafi, 2014; Al-Worafi, 2015; Al-Worafi, 2016; Al-Worafi et al., 2017; Al-Worafi, 2018a-d; Al-Worafi et al., 2018a-b; Al-Worafi et al., 2019; Al-Worafi, 2020a-z; Al-Worafi et al., 2020a-b; Al-Worafi et al., 2021a,b; Al-Worafi, 2022a,b; Al-Worafi, 2023; Baig et al., 2020; Elkalmi et al., 2020; Elsayed & Al-Worafi, 2020; Hasan et al., 2019; Hassan et al., 2014; Izahar et al., 2017; Lee et al., 2017; Mahmoud et al., 2020; Manan et al., 2014; Manan et al., 2016; Ming et al., 2016; Ming et al., 2020; Othman et al., 2020; Saeed et al., 2014).

8. Workforce Issues: Developing countries often face challenges in recruiting and retaining qualified pharmacy professionals, due to factors such as low wages, inadequate training opportunities, and limited career advancement prospects. This can lead to shortages of pharmacy personnel and increased workload for those who remain, which can contribute to medication errors.

9. Immigration of Pharmacists: In some developing countries, skilled pharmacy professionals may migrate to other countries for better job opportunities and higher wages. This can exacerbate the shortage of pharmacy personnel in the country of origin and contribute to increased medication errors.

10. Limited Access to Healthcare: Many people in developing countries do not have adequate access to healthcare services, including pharmacies. This can lead to self-medication and the use of unregulated and potentially harmful medications, which can contribute to medication errors.

11. Lack of Patient Education: Patients in developing countries often have limited knowledge about their medications, including dosage, administration, and potential side effects. This can contribute to medication errors, as patients may not be aware of the proper way to take their medications or may not report adverse reactions.

12. Medication Counterfeiting: In some developing countries, medication counterfeiting is a significant problem, which can lead to medication errors and adverse effects. To address this issue, regulatory bodies should implement stricter regulations to prevent the distribution of counterfeit medications.

13. Workforce Issues: Developing countries often face challenges in recruiting and retaining qualified pharmacy professionals, due to factors such as low wages, inadequate training opportunities, and limited career advancement prospects. This can lead to shortages of pharmacy personnel and increased workload for those who remain, which can contribute to medication errors.

14. Immigration of Pharmacists: In some developing countries, skilled pharmacy professionals may migrate to other countries for better job opportunities and higher wages. This can exacerbate the shortage of pharmacy personnel in the country of origin and contribute to increased medication errors.

15. Limited Access to Healthcare: Many people in developing countries do not have adequate access to healthcare services, including pharmacies. This can lead to self-medication and the use of unregulated and potentially harmful medications, which can contribute to medication errors.

16. Lack of Patient Education: Patients in developing countries often have limited knowledge about their medications, including dosage, administration, and potential side effects. This can contribute to medication errors, as patients may not be aware of the proper way to take their medications or may not report adverse reactions.

17. Medication Counterfeiting: In some developing countries, medication counterfeiting is a significant problem, which can lead to medication errors and adverse effects. To address this issue, regulatory bodies should implement stricter regulations to prevent the distribution of counterfeit medications.

18. Limited Access to Diagnostic Tools: In some developing countries, there may be limited access to diagnostic tools and laboratory tests, which can lead to medication errors. This is because pharmacy personnel may not have access to important information about a patient's medical condition, which can impact the selection and dosage of medications.

19. Limited Access to Electronic Health Records (EHRs): In many developing countries, there is limited adoption of EHRs, which can lead to medication errors. This is because pharmacy personnel may not have access to important information about a patient's medication history, allergies, and medical conditions.

20. Inadequate Monitoring of Adverse Drug Reactions (ADRs): In some developing countries, there may be inadequate systems for monitoring and reporting ADRs, which can lead to underreporting and a lack of accountability. This can contribute to medication errors, as pharmacy personnel may not be aware of the potential adverse effects of certain medications.

21. Limited Access to Clinical Decision Support (CDS) Tools: In many developing countries, there is limited adoption of CDS tools, which can help pharmacy personnel make informed decisions about medication selection and dosage. This can contribute to medication errors, as pharmacy personnel may not have access to the latest evidence-based guidelines and recommendations.

22. Lack of Coordination with Other Healthcare Providers: In some developing countries, there may be limited coordination between pharmacy personnel and other healthcare providers, such as physicians and nurses. This can lead to medication errors, as pharmacy personnel may not have access to important information about a patient's medical condition and medication history.

In conclusion, pharmacies' errors and related problems are a major challenge in developing countries. To address this challenge, there is a need for concerted efforts by regulatory bodies, healthcare professionals, and governments to implement effective strategies and interventions that promote quality control, access to information, use of technology, cultural awareness, and regulatory compliance.

28.7 CONCLUSION

This chapter aims to discuss the pharmacies' safety issues, prevention, challenges, and recommendations for the best practice in developing countries. Pharmacies play a critical role in patient care and patient safety. Despite the best efforts of pharmacists and pharmacy technicians to prevent errors, medication errors can and do occur in pharmacies. These errors can result in serious harm to patients, including hospitalization, disability, or even death. To prevent these types of errors, pharmacies have implemented a range of strategies, such as computerized order entry systems, barcoding systems, and other technologies to improve accuracy and prevent errors. Additionally, pharmacists and pharmacy technicians receive extensive training on medication safety and error prevention. Pharmacies' errors and related problems are a major challenge in developing countries. To address this challenge, there is a need for concerted efforts by regulatory bodies, healthcare professionals, and governments to implement effective strategies and interventions that promote quality control, access to information, use of technology, cultural awareness, and regulatory compliance.

REFERENCES

Al-Qahtani, I., Almoteb, T.M., & Al-Warafi, Y. (2015). Competency of metered-dose inhaler use among Saudi community pharmacists: A Simulation method study. *RRJPPS*, 4(2), 37–31.

Alshahrani, S.M., Alakhali, K.M., & Al-Worafi, Y.M., (2019a). Medication errors in a health care facility in southern Saudi Arabia. *Tropical Journal of Pharmaceutical Research*, 18(5), pp. 1119–1122.

Alshahrani, S.M., Alavudeen, S.S., Alakhali, K.M., Al-Worafi, Y.M., Bahamdan, A.K., Vigneshwaran, E., (2019b). Self-Medication Among King Khalid University Students, Saudi Arabia. *Risk Management and Healthcare Policy*, 12, pp. 243–249.

Alshahrani, S.M., Alakhali, K.M., Al-Worafi, Y.M., & Alshahrani, N.Z. (2020b). Awareness and use of over the counter analgesic medication: a survey in the Aseer region population, Saudi Arabia. *Int J Advan Appl Sci*, 7(3), 130–134.

Alshahrani, S.M., Alzahran, M., Alakhali, K., Vigneshwaran, E., Iqbal, M.J., Khan, N.A., … & Alavudeen, S.S. (2020b). Association Between Diabetes Consequences and Quality of Life Among Patients With Diabetes Mellitus in the Aseer Province of Saudi Arabia. *Open Access Macedonian Journal of Medical Sciences*, 8(E), 325–330.

Al-Worafi, Y.M. (2014). Prescription writing errors at a tertiary care hospital in Yemen: prevalence, types, causes and recommendations. *Am J Pharm Health Res*, 2, 134–140.

Al-Worafi, Y.M.A. (2015). Appropriateness of metered-dose inhaler use in the Yemeni community pharmacies. *Journal of Taibah University Medical Sciences*, 10(3), 353–358.

Al-Worafi, Y.M.A., (2016). Pharmacy practice in Yemen. In *Pharmacy Practice in Developing Countries* (pp. 267–287). Academic Press.

Al-Worafi, Y.M., Kassab, Y.W., Alseragi, W.M., Almutairi, M.S., Ahmed, A., Ming, L.C., Alkhoshaiban, A.S., & Hadi, M.A., (2017). Pharmacovigilance and adverse drg reaction reporting: a perspective of community pharmacists and pharmacy technicians in Sana'a, Yemen. *Therapeutics and clinical risk management*, 13, p. 1175.

Al-Worafi, Y.M., (2018a). Knowledge, Attitude and Practice of Yemeni Physicians Toward Pharmacovigilance: A Mixed Method Study. *International Journal of Pharmacy and Pharmaceutical Sciences*, 10(10), 74–77.

Al-Worafi, Y. (2018b). Knowledge, attitude and practice of Yemeni physicians toward pharmacovigilance: A mixed method study. *Int. J. Pharm. Pharm. Sci*, 10, 74–77.

Al-Worafi, Y.M. (2018c). Dispensing errors observed by community pharmacy dispensers in IBB–YEMEN. *Asian J. Pharm. Clin. Res*, 11(11).

Al-Worafi, Y.M. (2018d). Evauation of inhaler technique among patients with asthma and COPD in Yemen. *Journal of Taibah University medical sciences*, 13(5), 488–490.

Al-Worafi, Y.M., Patel, R.P., Zaidi, S.T.R., Alseragi, W.M., Almutairi, M.S., Alkhoshaiban, A.S., & Ming, L.C. (2018a). Completeness and legibility of handwritten prescriptions in Sana'a, Yemen. *Medical Principles and Practice*, 27, 290–292.

Al-Worafi, Y.M., Alseragi, W.M., Seng, L.K., Kassab, Y.W., Yeoh, S.F., Chiau, L., … & Husain, K. (2018b). Dispensing errors in community pharmacies: a prospective study in Sana'a, Yemen. *Arch Pharm Pract*, 9(4), 1–3.

Al-Worafi, Y.M., Alseragi, W.M., & Mahmoud, M.A. (2019). Competency of metered-dose inhaler use among community pharmacy dispensers in Ibb, Yemen: A simulation method study. *Latin American Journal of Pharmacy*, 38(3), 489–494.

Al-Worafi, Y.M. (Ed.). (2020a). *Drug Safety in Developing Countries: Achievements and Challenges.*

Al-Worafi, Y.M. (2020b). Medication errors. In *Drug Safety in Developing Countries* (pp. 105–117). Academic Press.

Al-Worafi, Y.M. (2020c). Adverse drug reactions. In *Drug Safety in Developing Countries* (pp. 39–57). Academic Press.

Al-Worafi, Y.M. (2020d). Medications registration and marketing: safety-related issues. In *Drug Safety in Developing Countries* (pp. 21–28). Academic Press.

Al-Worafi, Y.M. (2020e). Pharmacovigilance. In *Drug Safety in Developing Countries* (pp. 29–38). Academic Press.

Al-Worafi, Y.M. (2020f). Drug-related problems. In *Drug safety in developing countries* (pp. 59–71). Academic Press.

Al-Worafi, Y.M. (2020g). Medications safety-related terminology. In *Drug safety in developing countries* (pp. 7–19). Academic Press.

Al-Worafi, Y.M. (2020h). Self-medication. In *Drug Safety in Developing Countries* (pp. 73–86). Academic Press.

Al-Worafi, Y.M. (2020j). Antibiotics safety issues. In *Drug Safety in Developing Countries* (pp. 87–103). Academic Press.

Al-Worafi, Y.M. (2020k). Medications safety research issues. In *Drug Safety in Developing Countries* (pp. 213–227). Academic Press.

Al-Worafi, Y.M. (2020l). Counterfeit and substandard medications. In *Drug safety in developing countries* (pp. 119–126). Academic Press.

Al-Worafi, Y.M. (2020m). Medication abuse and misuse. In *Drug safety in developing countries* (pp. 127–135). Academic Press.

Al-Worafi, Y.M. (2020n). Storage and disposal of medications. In *Drug Safety in Developing Countries* (pp. 137–142). Academic Press.

Al-Worafi, Y.M. (2020o). Safety of medications in special population. In *Drug safety in developing countries* (pp. 143–162). Academic Press.

Al-Worafi, Y.M. (2020p). Herbal medicines safety issues. In *Drug Safety in developing countries* (pp. 163–178). Academic Press.

Al-Worafi, Y.M. (2020q). Medications safety pharmacoeconomics-related issues. In *Drug Safety in Developing Countries* (pp. 187–195). Academic Press.

Al-Worafi, Y.M. (2020r). Evidence-based medications safety practice. In *Drug Safety in Developing Countries* (pp. 197–201). Academic Press.

Al-Worafi, Y.M. (2020s). Quality indicators for medications safety. In *Drug safety in developing countries* (pp. 229–242). Academic Press.

Al-Worafi, Y.M. (2020t). Drug safety in Yemen. In *Drug Safety in Developing Countries* (pp. 391–405). Academic Press.

Al-Worafi, Y.M. (2020u). Drug safety in Saudi Arabia. In *Drug Safety in Developing Countries* (pp. 407–417). Academic Press.

Al-Worafi, Y.M. (2020v). Drug safety in United Arab Emirates. In *Drug Safety in Developing Countries* (pp. 419–428). Academic Press.

Al-Worafi, Y.M. (2020w). Drug safety in Indonesia. In *Drug Safety in Developing Countries* (pp. 279–285). Academic Press.

Al-Worafi, Y.M. (2020x). Drug safety in Palestine. In *Drug Safety in Developing Countries* (pp. 471–480). Academic Press.

Al-Worafi, Y.M. (2020y). Drug safety: comparison between developing countries. In *Drug Safety in Developing Countries* (pp. 603–611). Academic Press.

Al-Worafi, Y.M. (2020z). Drug safety in developing versus developed countries. In *Drug Safety in Developing Countries* (pp. 613–615). Academic Press.

Al-Worafi, Y.M., Alseragi, W.M., Ming, L.C., & Alakhali, K.M. (2020a). Drug safety in China. In *Drug Safety in Developing Countries* (pp. 381–388). Academic Press.

Al-Worafi, Y.M., Alseragi, W.M., Alakhali, K.M., Ming, L.C., Othman, G., Halboup, A.M., … & Elkalmi, R.M. (2020b). Knowledge, beliefs and factors affecting the use of generic medicines among patients in Ibb, Yemen: a mixed-method study. *Journal of Pharmacy Practice and Community Medicine*, 6(4).

Al-Worafi, Y.M., Elkalmi, R.M., Ming, L.C., Othman, G., Halboup, A.M., Battah, M.M., … & Mani, V. (2021a). Dispensing errors in hospital pharmacies: A prospective study in Yemen.

Al-Worafi, Y.M., Hasan, S., Hassan, N.M., & Gaili, A.A. (2021b). Knowledge, Attitude and Experience of Pharmacist in the UAE towards Pharmacovigilance. *Research Journal of Pharmacy and Technology*, 14(1), 265–269.

Al-Worafi, Y. (2022a). *A Guide to Online Pharmacy Education: Teaching Strategies and Assessment Methods*. CRC Press.

Al-Worafi, Y.M. (2022b). Patient care errors and related problems (part I): development and validation of the model. 0000-0002-5752-2913

Al-Worafi, Y.M. (Ed.). (2023). *Clinical Case Studies on medication Safety*. Academic Press.

Baig, M.R., Al-Worafi, Y.M., Alseragi, W.M., Ming, L.C., & Siddique, A. (2020). Drug safety in India. In *Drug Safety in Developing Countries* (pp. 327–334). Academic Press.

Cipolle, R.J., Strand, L., & Morley, P.C. (2004). *Pharmaceutical Care Practice: The Clinician's Guide: The Clinician's Guide*. McGraw-Hill Medical.

Elkalmi, R.M., Al-Worafi, Y.M., Alseragi, W.M., Ming, L.C., & Siddique, A. (2020). Drug safety in Malaysia. In *Drug Safety in Developing Countries* (pp. 245–253). Academic Press.

Elsayed, T., & Al-Worafi, Y.M. (2020). Drug safety in Egypt. In *Drug Safety in Developing Countries* (pp. 511–523). Academic Press.

Hasan, S., Al-Omar, M.J., AlZubaidy, H., & Al-Worafi, Y.M. (2019). Use of medications in Arab Countries. *Handbook of Healthcare in the Arab World*. Cham: Springer, 42.

Hassan, Y., Abd Aziz, N., Kassab, Y.W., Elgasim, I., Shaharuddin, S., Al-Worafi, Y.M.A., … & Ming, L.C. (2014). How to help patients to control their blood pressure? Blood pressure control and its predictor. *Archives of Pharmacy Practice*, 5(4).

Izahar, S., Lean, Q.Y., Hameed, M.A., Murugiah, M.K., Patel, R.P., Al-Worafi, Y.M., … & Ming, L.C. (2017). Content analysis of mobile health applications on diabetes mellitus. *Frontiers in Endocrinology*, 8, 318.

Kristensen, S., & Bartels, P. (2010). Use of patient safety culture instruments and recommendations. *Aarhus, Denmark, European Society for Quality in HealthCare-Office for Quality Indicators*, 113.

Lee, K.S., Yee, S.M., Zaidi, S.T.R., Patel, R.P., Yang, Q., Al-Worafi, Y.M., & Ming, L.C., 2017. Combating sale of counterfeit and falsified medicines online: a losing battle. *Frontiers in pharmacology*, 8, p. 268.

Mahmoud, M.A., Wajid, S., Naqvi, A.A., Samreen, S., Althagfan, S.S., & Al-Worafi, Y. (2020). Self-medication with antibiotics: A cross-sectional community-based study. *Latin american journal of pharmacy*, 39(2), 348–353.

Manan, M.M., Rusli, R.A., Ang, W.C., Al-Worafi, Y.M., & Ming, L.C. (2014). Assessing the pharmaceutical care issues of antiepileptic drug therapy in hospitalised epileptic patients. *Journal of Pharmacy Practice and Research*, 44(3), 83–88.

Manan, M.M., Ibrahim, N.A., Aziz, N.A., Zulkifly, H.H., Al-Worafi, Y.M.A., & Long, C.M. (2016). Empirical use of antibiotic therapy in the prevention of early onset sepsis in neonates: a pilot study. *Archives of Medical Science*, 12(3), 603–613.

Ming, L.C., Hameed, M.A., Lee, D.D., Apidi, N.A., Lai, P.S.M., Hadi, M.A., Al-Worafi, Y.M.A., & Khan, T.M., (2016). Use of medical mobile applications among hospital pharmacists in Malaysia. *Therapeutic innovation & regulatory science*, 50(4), pp. 419–426.

Ming, L.C., Untong, N., Aliudin, N.A., Osili, N., Kifli, N., Tan, C.S., ... & Goh, H.P. (2020). Mobile health apps on COVID-19 launched in the early days of the pandemic: content analysis and review. *JMIR mHealth and uHealth*, 8(9), e19796.

Othman, G., Ali, F., Ibrahim, M.I.M., Al-Worafi, Y.M., Ansari, M., & Halboup, A.M. (2020). Assessment of Anti-Diabetic Medications Adherence among Diabetic Patients in Sana'a City, Yemen: A Cross Sectional Study. *Journal of Pharmaceutical Research International*, 32(21), 114–122.

Reynard, J., Reynolds, J., & Stevenson, P. (2009). *Practical patient safety*. OUP Oxford.

Saeed, M.S., Alkhoshaiban, A.S., Al-Worafi, Y.M.A., & Long, C.M., (2014). Perception of self-medication among university students in Saudi Arabia. *Archives of Pharmacy Practice*, 5(4), p. 149.

Salas, E., & Frush, K. (2012). *Improving patient safety through teamwork and team training*. Oxford University Press.

Vincent, C. (2011). *Patient safety*. John Wiley & Sons.

29 Patient Safety for Special Populations

Geriatrics

29.1 BACKGROUND

Geriatrics is a branch of medicine that focuses on the health and care of older adults. Geriatricians are medical doctors who specialize in the diagnosis, treatment, and prevention of diseases and disabilities that affect older adults. The goal of geriatric care is to promote healthy aging, prevent and manage age-related diseases and disabilities, and improve the quality of life for older adults. Geriatricians work closely with other healthcare professionals, such as nurses, social workers, physical therapists, and occupational therapists, to provide comprehensive care for older adults. Geriatric care may include preventive measures, such as vaccinations and screening tests, as well as treatments for chronic conditions, such as hypertension, diabetes, and arthritis. Geriatricians also provide support for caregivers and help older adults navigate the healthcare system. Geriatric care is becoming increasingly important as the population ages. According to the United Nations, the number of people aged 60 years and older is expected to reach 2.1 billion by 2050, up from 962 million in 2017. As a result, there is a growing need for trained professionals who can provide specialized care for older adults (Kristensen & Bartels, 2010; Reynard et al., 2009; Salas & Frush, 2012; Vincent, 2011).

29.2 PATIENT SAFETY FOR GERIATRICS: Errors and Related Problems

Patient care and safety for geriatrics is a critical aspect of geriatric medicine. Older adults may have unique needs and challenges related to their health and well-being, and healthcare providers must take these into account to ensure their patients receive the best possible care.

Here are some key considerations for patient care and safety for geriatrics:

1. Comprehensive Assessment: Older adults may have multiple chronic conditions, cognitive impairment, and functional limitations that require a comprehensive assessment to identify their health status, medical history, and medication list. Healthcare providers should take the time to conduct a thorough assessment and involve the patient and their family members in the process.

2. Medication Management: Older adults may take multiple medications, which can increase the risk of adverse drug reactions and interactions. Healthcare providers should review the patient's medication list regularly, adjust dosages as needed, and provide education on the proper use of medications.

3. Fall Prevention: Falls are a significant risk for older adults and can result in serious injuries and complications. Healthcare providers should assess patients' risk for falls and implement measures to reduce the risk, such as modifying the environment, providing assistive devices, and providing patient education on fall prevention.

4. Nutrition and Hydration: Older adults may have decreased appetite or difficulty swallowing, which can impact their nutritional status and hydration levels. Healthcare providers should assess patients' nutritional and hydration status and provide education and support as needed.

5. Communication: Older adults may have hearing or vision loss, cognitive impairment, or language barriers that can impact their ability to communicate effectively with healthcare providers. Healthcare providers should use clear, simple language, speak slowly, and ensure that the patient understands the information being provided.

By taking these considerations into account, healthcare providers can provide safe and effective care for older adults, improving their quality of life and helping them maintain their health and independence.

Patient safety is a critical concern for geriatric care due to the increased risk of errors and related problems in older adults. Here are some common types of errors and related problems that can occur in geriatric care:

1. Medication Errors: Older adults may take multiple medications, which can increase the risk of medication errors such as dosage errors, drug interactions, and adverse drug reactions. Healthcare providers should review the patient's medication list regularly, adjust dosages as needed, and provide education on the proper use of medications.

2. Falls: Falls are a significant risk for older adults and can result in serious injuries and complications. Healthcare providers should assess patients' risk for falls and implement measures to reduce the risk, such as modifying the environment, providing assistive devices, and providing patient education on fall prevention.

3. Pressure Ulcers: Older adults may have limited mobility or spend extended periods in bed or in a chair, which can increase the risk of pressure ulcers. Healthcare providers should assess patients' risk for pressure ulcers and implement measures to prevent them, such as turning and repositioning the patient, using pressure-reducing devices, and providing skin care.

4. Delirium: Delirium is a common problem in older adults and can result from various causes, including medication side effects, infections, and dehydration. Healthcare providers should be aware of the risk factors for delirium and implement measures to prevent it, such as addressing underlying medical conditions, optimizing medications, and providing hydration.

5. Infections: Older adults may have weakened immune systems, which can increase the risk of infections. Healthcare providers should implement measures to prevent infections, such as hand hygiene, vaccination, and appropriate use of antibiotics.

By being aware of these common errors and related problems in geriatric care, healthcare providers can take proactive measures to prevent them and ensure patient safety. Regular assessments, communication, and education are crucial in providing safe and effective care for older adults.

29.3 PATIENT SAFETY FOR GERIATRICS: Causes

There are several causes of patient safety concerns in geriatrics. These include:

1. Age-Related Changes: As people age, their body systems and organs undergo physiological changes that can increase the risk of adverse events, such as falls, delirium, and medication errors. Age-related changes can also impact medication absorption, distribution, and elimination, leading to adverse drug reactions and interactions.

2. Polypharmacy: Older adults may take multiple medications, which can increase the risk of medication errors and adverse drug reactions. Polypharmacy can also result in drug interactions and drug-drug, drug-disease interactions.

3. Cognitive Impairment: Older adults may have a cognitive impairment, which can impact their ability to understand and follow instructions, communicate effectively with healthcare providers, and manage their medications and healthcare needs.

4. Social Isolation: Older adults who live alone or have limited social support may be at higher risk of adverse events due to limited access to healthcare services, inadequate nutrition, and decreased mobility.

5. Comorbidities: Older adults often have multiple chronic conditions, which can increase the risk of adverse events such as falls, delirium, and medication errors. Managing comorbidities can also be complex and require multiple medications and treatments.

6. Healthcare System Factors: Healthcare system factors such as inadequate staffing, poor communication among healthcare providers, and inadequate training and education of healthcare providers can contribute to patient safety concerns for geriatrics.

By understanding the causes of patient safety concerns for geriatrics, healthcare providers can take proactive measures to prevent them and ensure safe and effective care for older adults. Regular assessments, communication, and education are crucial in identifying and addressing patient safety concerns in geriatric care.

29.4 PATIENT SAFETY FOR GERIATRICS: Prevention

Preventing patient safety concerns for geriatrics requires a proactive and comprehensive approach that takes into account the unique needs and challenges of older adults. Here are some strategies that can be used to prevent patient safety concerns in geriatric care:

1. Comprehensive Assessment: Conducting a comprehensive assessment of the patient's health status, medical history, and medication list can help identify potential safety concerns and allow

healthcare providers to develop a personalized care plan that addresses the patient's needs and preferences.

2. Medication Management: Healthcare providers should regularly review the patient's medication list and adjust dosages as needed to prevent adverse drug reactions and interactions. Patients and their families should also be educated on the proper use of medications and encouraged to ask questions and report any side effects or concerns.

3. Fall Prevention: Implementing measures to reduce the risk of falls, such as modifying the environment, providing assistive devices, and providing patient education on fall prevention, can help prevent falls and related injuries.

4. Pressure Ulcer Prevention: Implementing measures to prevent pressure ulcers, such as turning and repositioning the patient, using pressure-reducing devices, and providing skin care, can help prevent pressure ulcers and related complications.

5. Delirium Prevention: Addressing underlying medical conditions, optimizing medications, and providing hydration can help prevent delirium in older adults.

6. Infection Prevention: Implementing measures to prevent infections, such as hand hygiene, vaccination, and appropriate use of antibiotics, can help prevent infections and related complications.

7. Care Coordination: Ensuring effective communication and care coordination among healthcare providers, patients, and their families can help prevent adverse events and improve the quality of care for older adults.

By using a comprehensive and proactive approach to patient safety in geriatric care, healthcare providers can help prevent adverse events and improve outcomes for older adults. Regular assessments, communication, and education are crucial in identifying and addressing patient safety concerns in geriatric care.

29.5 PATIENT SAFETY FOR GERIATRIC IN DEVELOPING COUNTRIES: Challenges and Recommendations

Patient safety for geriatrics is a critical concern in developing countries, where access to healthcare services and resources may be limited, and the aging population is increasing. Here are some challenges and recommendations for improving patient safety for geriatrics in developing countries:

Challenges:

1. Limited Access to Healthcare: In developing countries, older adults may have limited access to healthcare services, which can increase the risk of adverse events and delayed diagnoses.

2. Limited Resources: Developing countries may have limited resources, including medical equipment, medications, and trained healthcare providers, which can impact the quality and safety of care for older adults.

3. Lack of Patient Education: Patients and their families may have limited knowledge about their medical conditions, medications, and the importance of self-care, which can increase the risk of adverse events.

4. Cultural Barriers: Cultural beliefs and practices may impact the safety and quality of care for older adults, including the use of traditional medicine, gender-based discrimination, and stigma related to certain medical conditions.

Recommendations:

1. Increase Access to Healthcare: Developing countries should invest in expanding access to healthcare services, including primary care, geriatric care, and home-based care services, to ensure that older adults receive timely and appropriate care.

2. Improve Resources: Developing countries should invest in improving healthcare infrastructure, including medical equipment, medications, and training for healthcare providers, to ensure the quality and safety of care for older adults.

3. Patient Education: Developing countries should invest in patient education programs that help patients and their families understand their medical conditions, medications, and the importance of self-care, to improve patient safety and outcomes.

4. Address Cultural Barriers: Developing countries should address cultural barriers that impact the safety and quality of care for older adults, including promoting culturally sensitive care and addressing gender-based discrimination and stigma related to medical conditions.

5. Strengthen Regulatory Frameworks: Developing countries should strengthen regulatory frameworks for healthcare services, including licensing, accreditation, and quality assurance programs, to ensure that healthcare providers adhere to best practices and standards of care.

6. Despite the progress in research about patient care and safety in developing countries, there is little research about patient safety related to geriatrics in the majority of developing countries, therefore, conducting research is very important and highly recommended (Alshahrani et al., 2019a,b; Al-Qahtani et al., 2015; Alshahrani et al., 2020a,b; Al-Worafi, 2014; Al-Worafi, 2015; Al-Worafi, 2016; Al-Worafi et al., 2017; Al-Worafi, 2018a-d; Al-Worafi et al., 2018a-b; Al-Worafi et al., 2019; Al-Worafi, 2020a-y; Al-Worafi et al., 2020a-b; Al-Worafi et al., 2021a,b; Al-Worafi, 2022a,b; Al-Worafi, 2023; Baig et al., 2020; Elkalmi et al., 2020; Elsayed & Al-Worafi, 2020; Hasan et al., 2019; Hassan et al., 2014; Izhar et al., 2017; Lee et al., 2017; Mahmoud et al., 2020; Manan et al., 2014; Manan et al., 2016; Ming et al., 2016; Ming et al., 2020; Othman et al., 2020; Saeed et al., 2014).

By addressing these challenges and implementing these recommendations, developing countries can improve patient safety for geriatrics and ensure that older adults receive timely, appropriate, and high-quality care. Regular assessments, communication, and education are crucial in identifying and addressing patient safety concerns in geriatric care.

29.6 CONCLUSION

This chapter has discussed the patient safety issues related to the geriatric population, prevention, challenges, and recommendations for the best practice in developing countries. Patient safety for geriatrics is a critical concern in developing countries, where access to healthcare services and resources may be limited, and the aging population is increasing. Healthcare providers can take proactive measures to prevent them and ensure patient safety. Regular assessments, communication, and education are crucial in providing safe and effective care for older adults.

REFERENCES

Al-Qahtani, I., Almoteb, T.M., & Al-Warafi, Y. (2015). Competency of metered-dose inhaler use among Saudi community pharmacists: a simulation method study. *RRJPPS*, 4(2), 27–31.

Alshahrani, S.M., Alakhali, K.M., & Al-Worafi, Y.M., (2019a). Medication errors in a health care facility in southern Saudi Arabia. *Tropical Journal of Pharmaceutical Research*, 18(5), 1119–1122.

Alshahrani, S.M., Alavudeen, S.S., Alakhali, K.M., Al-Worafi, Y.M., Bahamdan, A.K., & Vigneshwaran, E., (2019b). Self-medication among King Khalid University Students, Saudi Arabia. *Risk Management and Healthcare Policy*, 12, 243–249.

Alshahrani, S.M., Alakhali, K.M., Al-Worafi, Y.M., & Alshahrani, N.Z. (2020a). Awareness and use of over the counter analgesic medication: a survey in the Aseer region population, Saudi Arabia. *International Journal of Advances in Applied Sciences*, 7(3), 130–134.

Alshahrani, S.M., Alzahran, M., Alakhali, K., Vigneshwaran, E., Iqbal, M.J., Khan, N.A., ... & Alavudeen, S.S. (2020b). Association between diabetes consequences and quality of life among patients with diabetes mellitus in the Aseer Province of Saudi Arabia. *Open Access Macedonian Journal of Medical Sciences*, 8(E), 325–330.

Al-Worafi, Y.M. (2014). Prescription writing errors at a tertiary care hospital in Yemen: prevalence, types, causes and recommendations. *American Journal of Pharmacy and Health Research*, 2, 134–140.

Al-Worafi, Y.M.A. (2015). Appropriateness of metered-dose inhaler use in the Yemeni community pharmacies. *Journal of Taibah University Medical Sciences*, 10(3), 353–358.

Al-Worafi, Y.M.A., (2016). Pharmacy practice in Yemen. In *Pharmacy Practice in Developing Countries* (pp. 267–287). Academic Press.

Al-Worafi, Y.M., Kassab, Y.W., Alseragi, W.M., Almutairi, M.S., Ahmed, A., Ming, L.C., Alkhoshaiban, A.S., & Hadi, M.A., (2017). Pharmacovigilance and adverse drg reaction reporting: a perspective of community pharmacists and pharmacy technicians in Sana'a, Yemen. *Therapeutics and Clinical Risk Management*, 13, 1175.

Al-Worafi, Y.M., (2018a). Knowledge, attitude and practice of Yemeni physicians toward pharmacovigilance: a mixed method study. *International Journal of Pharmacy and Pharmaceutical Sciences*, 10(10), 74–77.

Al-Worafi, Y. (2018b). Knowledge, attitude and practice of Yemeni physicians toward pharmacovigilance: a mixed method study. *International Journal of Pharmacy and Pharmaceutical Sciences*, 10, 74–77.

Al-Worafi, Y.M. (2018c). Dispensing errors observed by community pharmacy dispensers in IBB–YEMEN. *Asian Journal of Pharmaceutical and Clinical Research*, 11(11).

Al-Worafi, Y.M. (2018d). Evauation of inhaler technique among patients with asthma and COPD in Yemen. *Journal of Taibah University Medical Sciences*, 13(5), 488–490.

Al-Worafi, Y.M., Patel, R.P., Zaidi, S.T.R., Alseragi, W.M., Almutairi, M.S., Alkhoshaiban, A.S., & Ming, L.C. (2018a). Completeness and legibility of handwritten prescriptions in Sana'a, Yemen. *Medical Principles and Practice*, 27, 290–292.

Al-Worafi, Y.M., Alseragi, W.M., Seng, L.K., Kassab, Y.W., Yeoh, S.F., Chiau, L., … & Husain, K. (2018b). Dispensing errors in community pharmacies: a prospective study in Sana'a, Yemen. *Archives of Pharmacy Practice*, 9(4), 1–3.

Al-Worafi, Y.M., Alseragi, W.M., & Mahmoud, M.A. (2019). Competency of metered-dose inhaler use among community pharmacy dispensers in Ibb, Yemen: a simulation method study. *Latin American Journal of Pharmacy*, 38(3), 489–494.

Al-Worafi, Y.M. (Ed.). (2020a). *Drug Safety in Developing Countries: Achievements and Challenges.* Academic Press.

Al-Worafi, Y.M. (2020b). Medication errors. In *Drug Safety in Developing Countries* (pp. 105–117). Academic Press.

Al-Worafi, Y.M. (2020c). Adverse drug reactions. In *Drug Safety in Developing Countries* (pp. 39–57). Academic Press.

Al-Worafi, Y.M. (2020d). Medications registration and marketing: safety-related issues. In *Drug Safety in Developing Countries* (pp. 21–28). Academic Press.

Al-Worafi, Y.M. (2020e). Pharmacovigilance. In *Drug Safety in Developing Countries* (pp. 29–38). Academic Press.

Al-Worafi, Y.M. (2020f). Drug-related problems. In *Drug Safety in Developing Countries* (pp. 59–71). Academic Press.

Al-Worafi, Y.M. (2020g). Medications safety-related terminology. In *Drug Safety in Developing Countries* (pp. 7–19). Academic Press.

Al-Worafi, Y.M. (2020h). Self-medication. In *Drug Safety in Developing Countries* (pp. 73–86). Academic Press.

Al-Worafi, Y.M. (2020i). Antibiotics safety issues. In *Drug Safety in Developing Countries* (pp. 87–103). Academic Press.

Al-Worafi, Y.M. (2020j). Medications safety research issues. In *Drug Safety in Developing Countries* (pp. 213–227). Academic Press.

Al-Worafi, Y.M. (2020k). Counterfeit and substandard medications. In *Drug Safety in Developing Countries* (pp. 119–126). Academic Press.

Al-Worafi, Y.M. (2020l). Medication abuse and misuse. In *Drug Safety in Developing Countries* (pp. 127–135). Academic Press.

Al-Worafi, Y.M. (2020m). Storage and disposal of medications. In *Drug Safety in Developing Countries* (pp. 137–142). Academic Press.

Al-Worafi, Y.M. (2020n). Safety of medications in special population. In *Drug Safety in Developing Countries* (pp. 143–162). Academic Press.

Al-Worafi, Y.M. (2020o). Herbal medicines safety issues. In *Drug Safety in Developing Countries* (pp. 163–178). Academic Press.

Al-Worafi, Y.M. (2020p). Medications safety pharmacoeconomics-related issues. In *Drug Safety in Developing Countries* (pp. 187–195). Academic Press.

Al-Worafi, Y.M. (2020q). Evidence-based medications safety practice. In *Drug Safety in Developing Countries* (pp. 197–201). Academic Press.

Al-Worafi, Y.M. (2020r). Quality indicators for medications safety. In *Drug Safety in Developing Countries* (pp. 229–242). Academic Press.

Al-Worafi, Y.M. (2020s). Drug safety in Yemen. In *Drug Safety in Developing Countries* (pp. 391–405). Academic Press.

Al-Worafi, Y.M. (2020t). Drug safety in Saudi Arabia. In *Drug Safety in Developing Countries* (pp. 407–417). Academic Press.

Al-Worafi, Y.M. (2020u). Drug safety in United Arab Emirates. In *Drug Safety in Developing Countries* (pp. 419–428). Academic Press.

Al-Worafi, Y.M. (2020v). Drug safety in Indonesia. In *Drug Safety in Developing Countries* (pp. 279–285). Academic Press.

Al-Worafi, Y.M. (2020w). Drug safety in Palestine. In *Drug Safety in Developing Countries* (pp. 471–480). Academic Press.

Al-Worafi, Y.M. (2020x). Drug safety: comparison between developing countries. In *Drug Safety in Developing Countries* (pp. 603–611). Academic Press.

Al-Worafi, Y.M. (2020y). Drug safety in developing versus developed countries. In *Drug Safety in Developing Countries* (pp. 613–615). Academic Press.

Al-Worafi, Y.M., Alseragi, W.M., Ming, L.C., & Alakhali, K.M. (2020a). Drug safety in China. In *Drug Safety in Developing Countries* (pp. 381–388). Academic Press.

Al-Worafi, Y.M., Alseragi, W.M., Alakhali, K.M., Ming, L.C., Othman, G., Halboup, A.M., ... & Elkalmi, R.M. (2020b). Knowledge, beliefs and factors affecting the use of generic medicines among patients in Ibb, Yemen: a mixed-method study. *Journal of Pharmacy Practice and Community Medicine*, 6(4), 53–56.

Al-Worafi, Y.M., Elkalmi, R.M., Ming, L.C., Othman, G., Halboup, A.M., Battah, M.M., ... & Mani, V. (2021a). Dispensing errors in hospital pharmacies: A prospective study in Yemen. *AlQalam Journal of Medical and Applied Sciences*, 4(2), 13–17.

Al-Worafi, Y.M., Hasan, S., Hassan, N.M., & Gaili, A.A. (2021b). Knowledge, attitude and experience of pharmacist in the UAE towards pharmacovigilance. *Research Journal of Pharmacy and Technology*, 14(1), 265–269.

Al-Worafi, Y. (2022a). *A Guide to Online Pharmacy Education: Teaching Strategies and Assessment Methods*. CRC Press.

Al-Worafi, Y.M. (2022b). Patient care errors and related problems (part I): development and validation of the model. 0000-0002-5752-2913

Al-Worafi, Y.M. (Ed.). (2023). *Clinical Case Studies on Medication Safety*. Academic Press.

Baig, M.R., Al-Worafi, Y.M., Alseragi, W.M., Ming, L.C., & Siddique, A. (2020). Drug safety in India. In *Drug Safety in Developing Countries* (pp. 327–334). Academic Press.

Elkalmi, R.M., Al-Worafi, Y.M., Alseragi, W.M., Ming, L.C., & Siddique, A. (2020). Drug safety in Malaysia. In *Drug Safety in Developing Countries* (pp. 245–253). Academic Press.

Elsayed, T., & Al-Worafi, Y.M. (2020). Drug safety in Egypt. In *Drug Safety in Developing Countries* (pp. 511–523). Academic Press.

Hasan, S., Al-Omar, M.J., AlZubaidy, H., & Al-Worafi, Y.M. (2019). Use of medications in Arab Countries. *Handbook of Healthcare in the Arab World*. Cham: Springer, 42.

Hassan, Y., Abd Aziz, N., Kassab, Y.W., Elgasim, I., Shaharuddin, S., Al-Worafi, Y.M.A., ... & Ming, L.C. (2014). How to help patients to control their blood pressure? Blood pressure control and its predictor. *Archives of Pharmacy Practice*, 5(4), 153–161.

Izahar, S., Lean, Q.Y., Hameed, M.A., Murugiah, M.K., Patel, R.P., Al-Worafi, Y.M., ... & Ming, L.C. (2017). Content analysis of mobile health applications on diabetes mellitus. *Frontiers in Endocrinology*, 8, 318.

Kristensen, S., & Bartels, P. (2010). Use of patient safety culture instruments and recommendations. *Aarhus, Denmark, European Society for Quality in HealthCare-Office for Quality Indicators*, 113.

Lee, K.S., Yee, S.M., Zaidi, S.T.R., Patel, R.P., Yang, Q., Al-Worafi, Y.M., & Ming, L.C., 2017. Combating sale of counterfeit and falsified medicines online: a losing battle. *Frontiers in Pharmacology*, 8, 268.

Mahmoud, M.A., Wajid, S., Naqvi, A.A., Samreen, S., Althagfan, S.S., & Al-Worafi, Y. (2020). Self-medication with antibiotics: a cross-sectional community-based study. *Latin American Journal of Pharmacy*, 39(2), 348–353.

Manan, M.M., Rusli, R.A., Ang, W.C., Al-Worafi, Y.M., & Ming, L.C. (2014). Assessing the pharmaceutical care issues of antiepileptic drug therapy in hospitalised epileptic patients. *Journal of Pharmacy Practice and Research*, 44(3), 83–88.

Manan, M.M., Ibrahim, N.A., Aziz, N.A., Zulkifly, H.H., Al-Worafi, Y.M.A., & Long, C.M. (2016). Empirical use of antibiotic therapy in the prevention of early onset sepsis in neonates: a pilot study. *Archives of Medical Science*, 12(3), 603–613.

Ming, L.C., Hameed, M.A., Lee, D.D., Apidi, N.A., Lai, P.S.M., Hadi, M.A., Al-Worafi, Y.M.A., & Khan, T.M., (2016). Use of medical mobile applications among hospital pharmacists in Malaysia. *Therapeutic Innovation & Regulatory Science*, 50(4), 419–426.

Ming, L.C., Untong, N., Aliudin, N.A., Osili, N., Kifli, N., Tan, C.S., … & Goh, H.P. (2020). Mobile health apps on COVID-19 launched in the early days of the pandemic: content analysis and review. *JMIR mHealth and uHealth*, 8(9), e19796.

Othman, G., Ali, F., Ibrahim, M.I.M., Al-Worafi, Y.M., Ansari, M., & Halboup, A.M. (2020). Assessment of anti-diabetic medications adherence among diabetic patients in Sana'a City, Yemen: a cross sectional study. *Journal of Pharmaceutical Research International*, 32(21), 114–122.

Reynard, J., Reynolds, J., & Stevenson, P. (2009). *Practical Patient Safety*. OUP Oxford.

Saeed, M.S., Alkhoshaiban, A.S., Al-Worafi, Y.M.A., & Long, C.M., (2014). Perception of self-medication among university students in Saudi Arabia. *Archives of Pharmacy Practice*, 5(4), 149.

Salas, E., & Frush, K. (2012). *Improving Patient Safety through Teamwork and Team Training*. Oxford University Press.

Vincent, C. (2011). *Patient Safety*. John Wiley & Sons.

30 Patient Safety for Special Populations

Pediatrics

30.1 BACKGROUND

Pediatrics is a branch of medicine that deals with the medical care of infants, children, and adolescents up to the age of 18. The word "pediatrics" is derived from the Greek words "pais" meaning child and "iatros" meaning doctor or healer. Pediatricians are medical doctors who specialize in the diagnosis and treatment of childhood illnesses, diseases, and disorders. They provide medical care for a wide range of conditions, including infectious diseases, genetic disorders, developmental disorders, and behavioral problems. In addition to providing medical treatment, pediatricians also play an important role in preventive care, such as immunizations, regular check-ups, and developmental screenings. They work closely with parents and caregivers to promote the health and well-being of children and to identify and address any health issues that may arise. Pediatrics is a challenging and rewarding field that requires a great deal of knowledge, skill, and compassion. Pediatricians must be able to communicate effectively with children and their families and to provide care in a manner that is both compassionate and age-appropriate. Patient care and safety are of utmost importance in pediatrics. Pediatric patients are a vulnerable population, and their safety must be the top priority of healthcare providers. Here are some key principles of patient care and safety in pediatrics:

1. Family-Centered Care: Pediatric patient care should be centered around the family. This means that healthcare providers should involve parents, guardians, and other family members in the care process and decision-making. Family-centered care promotes better communication, better patient outcomes, and better patient and family satisfaction.

2. Age-Appropriate Care: Pediatric patients have unique needs that vary according to their age, developmental level, and medical condition. Healthcare providers must provide care that is appropriate to the patient's age and developmental level. For example, a toddler may need a different approach to care than a teenager with the same medical condition.

3. Infection Control: Pediatric patients are more susceptible to infections than adults. Healthcare providers must follow strict infection control protocols to prevent the spread of infections within the hospital or clinic setting. This includes proper hand hygiene, use of personal protective equipment, and isolation precautions when necessary.

4. Medication Safety: Medication errors can be particularly dangerous in pediatrics. Healthcare providers must follow strict medication safety protocols, such as double-checking medications and dosages and using age-appropriate dosing guidelines.

5. Communication: Clear and effective communication between healthcare providers, patients, and families is essential for patient safety. Healthcare providers must ensure that patients and families understand the care plan, including any medications or treatments, and are able to ask questions and provide feedback.

6. Child Protection: Healthcare providers must be alert to signs of child abuse or neglect and take appropriate action to protect the child's safety. This includes reporting any suspected abuse or neglect to the appropriate authorities and providing support and resources to families in need.

In summary, patient care and safety in pediatrics require a comprehensive approach that includes family-centered care, age-appropriate care, infection control, medication safety, effective communication, and child protection. By following these principles, healthcare providers can ensure the best possible outcomes for pediatric patients (Kristensen & Bartels, 2010; Reynard et al., 2009; Salas & Frush, 2012; Vincent, 2011).

30.2 PATIENT SAFETY FOR PEDIATRICS: Errors and Related Problems

Patient safety is critical in pediatrics, and errors can have serious consequences for young patients. Some common errors and related problems in pediatric patient safety include:

1. Medication Errors: Medication errors are among the most common types of errors in pediatrics. They can occur during prescribing, dispensing, administering, or monitoring of medications.

Examples include incorrect dosing, wrong medication, wrong route of administration, or medication allergies.

2. Miscommunication: Miscommunication between healthcare providers, patients, and families can lead to errors in diagnosis, treatment, or medication management. For example, a healthcare provider may misunderstand a patient's symptoms, leading to an incorrect diagnosis, or a parent may misunderstand medication instructions, leading to incorrect dosing.

3. Diagnostic Errors: Diagnostic errors occur when healthcare providers fail to correctly diagnose a patient's condition. These errors can lead to delayed or incorrect treatment, which can have serious consequences for pediatric patients.

4. Infections: Pediatric patients are vulnerable to infections, and healthcare-associated infections can occur due to poor infection control practices, such as improper hand hygiene or failure to use personal protective equipment.

5. Surgical Errors: Pediatric surgical procedures are complex and require specialized skills and training. Surgical errors can include wrong-site surgery, incorrect procedure, or instrument or equipment failure.

6. Adverse Events: Adverse events can occur due to medical treatment or procedures, such as medication side effects or complications from surgery.

To address these problems and improve patient safety in pediatrics, healthcare providers must take a comprehensive approach that includes effective communication, careful medication management, infection control measures, and a focus on continuous quality improvement. This may include implementing standardized protocols and procedures, improving communication and teamwork among healthcare providers, and involving patients and families in the care process. By prioritizing patient safety, healthcare providers can help to prevent errors and ensure the best possible outcomes for pediatric patients.

30.3 PATIENT SAFETY FOR PEDIATRICS: Causes

Patient safety is a critical aspect of pediatric care, and it is important to understand the causes of patient safety incidents in order to prevent them from occurring. Some common causes of patient safety incidents in pediatrics include:

1. Communication: Poor communication between healthcare providers, patients, and families can lead to misunderstandings and errors. Communication breakdowns can occur at any point in the care process, from diagnosis to treatment and discharge.

2. Human Error: Healthcare providers are only human, and errors can occur due to a variety of factors, including fatigue, stress, distraction, and lack of knowledge or training. Examples include medication errors, diagnostic errors, and errors in surgery or other procedures.

3. Systemic Issues: Systemic issues can contribute to patient safety incidents in pediatrics. These can include problems with staffing, resources, equipment, and organizational culture. For example, inadequate staffing levels can lead to fatigue and errors, while outdated equipment can malfunction or be used improperly.

4. Patient and Family Factors: Patient and family factors can also play a role in patient safety incidents. For example, parents may fail to understand medication instructions or may be unable to administer medications properly. Patients may also be unable to communicate their symptoms effectively or may be non-compliant with treatment recommendations.

5. Environmental Factors: Environmental factors, such as noise, lighting, and distractions, can contribute to patient safety incidents. For example, a noisy hospital environment may make it difficult for healthcare providers to communicate effectively or for patients to get the rest they need.

To address these causes of patient safety incidents in pediatrics, healthcare providers must take a comprehensive approach that includes effective communication, robust training and education, appropriate staffing and resource allocation, and a focus on continuous quality improvement. By working to address these issues, healthcare providers can help to prevent patient safety incidents and ensure the best possible outcomes for pediatric patients.

30.4 PATIENT SAFETY FOR PEDIATRICS: Prevention

Preventing patient safety incidents is a critical aspect of pediatric care, and there are many strategies that healthcare providers can use to improve patient safety in pediatrics. Some effective strategies include:

1. Effective Communication: Effective communication is essential to preventing patient safety incidents in pediatrics. Healthcare providers should ensure that they communicate clearly with patients and families about their care and treatment, and should also communicate effectively with other healthcare providers to ensure that everyone is on the same page.

2. Medication Safety: Medication errors are a leading cause of patient safety incidents in pediatrics. Healthcare providers can take steps to prevent medication errors, such as using computerized order entry systems, using barcode scanning to ensure that the correct medication and dose are given, and involving parents in the medication administration process.

3. Infection Control: Pediatric patients are particularly vulnerable to infections, and healthcare providers can take steps to prevent healthcare-associated infections. This includes using proper hand hygiene, using personal protective equipment when appropriate, and ensuring that equipment is properly cleaned and disinfected.

4. Diagnostic Accuracy: Diagnostic errors can have serious consequences for pediatric patients. Healthcare providers can work to prevent diagnostic errors by taking a comprehensive approach to diagnosis, including obtaining a thorough medical history, conducting a physical exam, and ordering appropriate tests and imaging.

5. Family-Centered Care: Involving families in the care process can help to prevent patient safety incidents in pediatrics. Healthcare providers can work to involve parents and families in the care process, including encouraging questions and participation in decision-making.

6. Quality Improvement: Healthcare providers can use quality improvement methods to identify and address patient safety incidents in pediatrics. This includes collecting and analyzing data on patient safety incidents, implementing changes to prevent future incidents, and monitoring the effectiveness of those changes over time.

By implementing these and other strategies, healthcare providers can help to prevent patient safety incidents in pediatrics and ensure the best possible outcomes for young patients.

30.5 PATIENT SAFETY FOR PEDIATRICS IN DEVELOPING COUNTRIES

Patient safety is a critical issue in all healthcare settings, but it can be particularly challenging in developing countries where healthcare resources are often limited. However, there are still strategies that can be used to improve patient safety in pediatrics in these settings.

1. Basic Infrastructure and Equipment: In many developing countries, there may be a lack of basic infrastructure and equipment needed to provide safe patient care. Improving access to basic equipment, such as clean water, electricity, and appropriate medical equipment, can improve patient safety.

2. Staff Training and Education: Many healthcare providers in developing countries may lack the necessary training and education to provide safe patient care. Providing training and education on patient safety practices can help to reduce errors and improve patient outcomes.

3. Medication Safety: Medication errors are a common cause of patient safety incidents in pediatrics, and improving medication safety can be particularly challenging in developing countries where medication supply chains may be unreliable. Strategies such as using standard treatment guidelines and training healthcare providers on safe medication administration can help to improve medication safety.

4. Infection Control: Infection control is essential to prevent the spread of disease and reduce healthcare-associated infections. Improving infection control practices, such as hand hygiene and proper use of personal protective equipment, can help to improve patient safety in developing countries.

5. Family Engagement: Engaging families in the care process can help to improve patient safety in developing countries. Encouraging families to ask questions and be involved in decision-making can help to prevent errors and improve communication between healthcare providers and patients/families.

6. Strengthening Health Systems: Finally, strengthening health systems overall is critical to improving patient safety in developing countries. This includes improving access to healthcare services, strengthening healthcare infrastructure and governance, and investing in healthcare workforce development.

7. Malnutrition: Malnutrition is a major problem in many developing countries, and it can affect the health and well-being of pediatric patients. Malnourished children may be more vulnerable to infections and may not respond as well to medical treatments, which can increase the risk of patient safety incidents.

8. Lack of Access to Healthcare Services: Many children in developing countries may not have access to healthcare services, which can delay the diagnosis and treatment of medical conditions. Improving access to healthcare services can help to prevent patient safety incidents and improve outcomes for pediatric patients.

9. Limited Resources: Healthcare resources may be limited in developing countries, which can make it difficult to provide safe and effective care. Strategies such as prioritizing resources and developing cost-effective interventions can help to improve patient safety despite limited resources.

10. Language and Cultural Barriers: Language and cultural barriers can make it difficult for healthcare providers to communicate effectively with patients and families. This can increase the risk of patient safety incidents, as patients may not fully understand their care or may not feel comfortable asking questions. Healthcare providers can work to overcome these barriers by providing language interpretation services and cultural competence training.

11. Lack of Regulatory Oversight: In some developing countries, there may be limited regulatory oversight of healthcare providers and facilities. This can increase the risk of patient safety incidents, as there may be no mechanism in place to ensure that healthcare providers are providing safe and effective care. Strengthening regulatory oversight can help to improve patient safety in these settings.

12. Lack of Health Information Systems: Many developing countries have inadequate health information systems, making it difficult to track patient data, identify trends, and develop evidence-based practices. This can lead to a lack of coordinated care and increase the risk of errors.

13. Limited Availability of Vaccines: Vaccines are essential to prevent and control infectious diseases, but in some developing countries, there may be limited availability of vaccines or limited access to vaccination programs. This can increase the risk of infectious disease outbreaks, which can affect patient safety.

14. High Patient Load: Healthcare providers in developing countries may face high patient loads, which can lead to burnout, fatigue, and errors. Strategies such as improving staffing levels and workload management can help to reduce the risk of patient safety incidents.

15. Limited Access to Diagnostic Services: In many developing countries, there may be limited access to diagnostic services such as laboratory tests, imaging studies, and other diagnostic tools. This can delay the diagnosis and treatment of medical conditions, increasing the risk of patient safety incidents.

16. Lack of Standardized Protocols: In some developing countries, there may be a lack of standardized protocols and guidelines for patient care. This can lead to inconsistent care and increase the risk of errors. Developing and implementing standardized protocols and guidelines can help to improve patient safety.

17. Limited Access to Medications: Access to medications, including essential medicines, can be limited in developing countries due to a variety of factors such as cost, availability, and distribution systems. This can lead to incomplete or ineffective treatment of medical conditions, which can compromise patient safety.

18. Traditional and Complementary Medicine Practices: Traditional and complementary medicine practices are commonly used in developing countries, but they may not always be safe or effective. Lack of regulation and standardization of these practices can lead to unsafe practices, incorrect dosing, and interactions with conventional medicines, compromising patient safety.

19. Poverty and Social Determinants of Health: Poverty and social determinants of health, such as poor living conditions, lack of access to clean water and sanitation, and inadequate nutrition, can impact the health and well-being of pediatric patients in developing countries. Addressing these underlying factors can help to improve patient safety by preventing and managing illnesses and improving overall health outcomes.

20. Lack of Pediatric-Specific Training: Healthcare providers in developing countries may lack specialized training in pediatrics, which can lead to inadequate care and increase the risk of patient safety incidents. Providing training and continuing education programs that focus on pediatric-specific issues can help to improve patient safety.

21. Inadequate Infrastructure: Inadequate infrastructure, including poor transportation systems and limited access to electricity, can make it difficult to provide safe and effective care to pediatric patients in developing countries. Improving infrastructure can help to reduce the risk of patient safety incidents by improving access to healthcare services and providing essential resources and equipment.

22. Despite the progress in research about patient care and safety in developing countries, there is little research about patient safety related to the geriatrics in the majority of developing countries, therefore, conducting research is very important and highly recommended (Alshahrani et al., 2019a,b; Al-Qahtani et al., 2015; Alshahrani et al., 2020a,b; Al-Worafi, 2014; Al-Worafi, 2015; Al-Worafi, 2016; Al-Worafi et al., 2017; Al-Worafi, 2018a-d; Al-Worafi et al., 2018a-b; Al-Worafi et al., 2019; Al-Worafi, 2020a-y; Al-Worafi et al., 2020a-b; Al-Worafi et al., 2021a,b; Al-Worafi, 2022a,b; Al-Worafi, 2023; Baig et al., 2020; Elkalmi et al., 2020; Elsayed & Al-Worafi, 2020; Hasan et al., 2019; Hassan et al., 2014; Izahar et al., 2017; Lee et al., 2017; Mahmoud et al., 2020; Manan et al., 2014; Manan et al., 2016; Ming et al., 2016; Ming et al., 2020; Othman et al., 2020; Saeed et al., 2014).

Addressing these and other issues can help to improve patient safety in pediatrics in developing countries. It requires a coordinated effort involving healthcare providers, policymakers, and the community to identify and address the root causes of patient safety incidents and develop strategies to prevent them.

30.6 CONCLUSION

This chapter has discussed the patient safety issues related to the pediatric population, prevention, challenges, and recommendations for achieving the best practice in developing countries. Patient safety in pediatrics is a critical issue in healthcare, particularly in developing countries where resources and infrastructure may be limited. There are many factors that can impact patient safety, including medication errors, inadequate staffing, lack of diagnostic services, and social determinants of health. Preventing patient safety incidents requires a multifaceted approach that involves improving infrastructure, strengthening health systems, providing education and training, and promoting patient and family engagement in the care process. By addressing these issues, healthcare providers, policymakers, and the community can work together to ensure that pediatric patients receive safe and effective care, regardless of where they live.

REFERENCES

Al-Qahtani, I., Almoteb, T.M., & Al-Warafi, Y. (2015). Competency of metered-dose inhaler use among Saudi community pharmacists: a Simulation method study. *RRJPPS*, 4(2), 37–31.

Alshahrani, S.M., Alakhali, K.M., & Al-Worafi, Y.M., (2019a). Medication errors in a health care facility in southern Saudi Arabia. *Tropical Journal of Pharmaceutical Research*, 18(5), 1119–1122.

Alshahrani, S.M., Alavudeen, S.S., Alakhali, K.M., Al-Worafi, Y.M., Bahamdan, A.K., & Vigneshwaran, E., (2019b). Self-medication among King Khalid University Students, Saudi Arabia. *Risk Management and Healthcare Policy*, 12, 243–249.

Alshahrani, S.M., Alakhali, K.M., Al-Worafi, Y.M., & Alshahrani, N.Z. (2020a). Awareness and use of over the counter analgesic medication: a survey in the Aseer region population, Saudi Arabia. *International Journal of Advances in Applied Sciences*, 7(3), 130–134.

Alshahrani, S.M., Alzahran, M., Alakhali, K., Vigneshwaran, E., Iqbal, M.J., Khan, N.A., ... & Alavudeen, S.S. (2020b). Association between diabetes consequences and quality of life among patients with diabetes mellitus in the Aseer Province of Saudi Arabia. *Open Access Macedonian Journal of Medical Sciences*, 8(E), 325–330.

Al-Worafi, Y.M. (2014). Prescription writing errors at a tertiary care hospital in Yemen: prevalence, types, causes and recommendations. *American Journal of Pharmacy and Health Research*, 2, 134–140.

Al-Worafi, Y.M.A. (2015). Appropriateness of metered-dose inhaler use in the Yemeni community pharmacies. *Journal of Taibah University Medical Sciences*, 10(3), 353–358.

Al-Worafi, Y.M.A., (2016). Pharmacy practice in Yemen. In *Pharmacy Practice in Developing Countries* (pp. 267–287). Academic Press.

Al-Worafi, Y.M., Kassab, Y.W., Alseragi, W.M., Almutairi, M.S., Ahmed, A., Ming, L.C., Alkhoshaiban, A.S., & Hadi, M.A., (2017). Pharmacovigilance and adverse drg reaction reporting: a perspective of community pharmacists and pharmacy technicians in Sana'a, Yemen. *Therapeutics and Clinical Risk Management*, 13, 1175.

Al-Worafi, Y.M., (2018a). Knowledge, attitude and practice of Yemeni physicians toward pharmacovigilance: a mixed method study. *International Journal of Pharmacy and Pharmaceutical Sciences*, 10(10), 74–77.

Al-Worafi, Y. (2018b). Knowledge, attitude and practice of Yemeni physicians toward pharmacovigilance: a mixed method study. *nternational Journal of Pharmacy and Pharmaceutical Sciences*, 10, 74–77.

Al-Worafi, Y.M. (2018c). Dispensing errors observed by community pharmacy dispensers in IBB–YEMEN. *Asian Journal of Pharmaceutical and Clinical Research*, 11(11), 478–481.

Al-Worafi, Y.M. (2018d). Evauation of inhaler technique among patients with asthma and COPD in Yemen. *Journal of Taibah University Medical Sciences*, 13(5), 488–490.

Al-Worafi, Y.M., Patel, R.P., Zaidi, S.T.R., Alseragi, W.M., Almutairi, M.S., Alkhoshaiban, A.S., & Ming, L.C. (2018a). Completeness and legibility of handwritten prescriptions in Sana'a, Yemen. *Medical Principles and Practice*, 27, 290–292.

Al-Worafi, Y.M., Alseragi, W.M., Seng, L.K., Kassab, Y.W., Yeoh, S.F., Chiau, L., ... & Husain, K. (2018b). Dispensing errors in community pharmacies: a prospective study in Sana'a, Yemen. *Archives of Pharmacy Practice*, 9(4), 1–3.

Al-Worafi, Y.M., Alseragi, W.M., & Mahmoud, M.A. (2019). Competency of metered-dose inhaler use among community pharmacy dispensers in Ibb, Yemen: a simulation method study. *Latin American Journal of Pharmacy*, 38(3), 489–494.

Al-Worafi, Y.M. (Ed.). (2020a). *Drug Safety in Developing Countries: Achievements and Challenges*.

Al-Worafi, Y.M. (2020b). Medication errors. In *Drug Safety in Developing Countries* (pp. 105–117). Academic Press.

Al-Worafi, Y.M. (2020c). Adverse drug reactions. In *Drug Safety in Developing Countries* (pp. 39–57). Academic Press.

Al-Worafi, Y.M. (2020d). Medications registration and marketing: safety-related issues. In *Drug Safety in Developing Countries* (pp. 21–28). Academic Press.

Al-Worafi, Y.M. (2020e). Pharmacovigilance. In *Drug Safety in Developing Countries* (pp. 29–38). Academic Press.

Al-Worafi, Y.M. (2020f). Drug-related problems. In *Drug Safety in Developing Countries* (pp. 59–71). Academic Press.

Al-Worafi, Y.M. (2020g). Medications safety-related terminology. In *Drug Safety in Developing Countries* (pp. 7–19). Academic Press.

Al-Worafi, Y.M. (2020h). Self-medication. In *Drug Safety in Developing Countries* (pp. 73–86). Academic Press.

Al-Worafi, Y.M. (2020i). Antibiotics safety issues. In *Drug Safety in Developing Countries* (pp. 87–103). Academic Press.

Al-Worafi, Y.M. (2020j). Medications safety research issues. In *Drug Safety in Developing Countries* (pp. 213–227). Academic Press.

Al-Worafi, Y.M. (2020k). Counterfeit and substandard medications. In *Drug Safety in Developing Countries* (pp. 119–126). Academic Press.

Al-Worafi, Y.M. (2020l). Medication abuse and misuse. In *Drug Safety in Developing Countries* (pp. 127–135). Academic Press.

Al-Worafi, Y.M. (2020m). Storage and disposal of medications. In *Drug Safety in Developing Countries* (pp. 137–142). Academic Press.

Al-Worafi, Y.M. (2020n). Safety of medications in special population. In *Drug safety in Developing Countries* (pp. 143–162). Academic Press.

Al-Worafi, Y.M. (2020o). Herbal medicines safety issues. In *Drug Safety in Developing Countries* (pp. 163–178). Academic Press.

Al-Worafi, Y.M. (2020p). Medications safety pharmacoeconomics-related issues. In *Drug Safety in Developing Countries* (pp. 187–195). Academic Press.

Al-Worafi, Y.M. (2020q). Evidence-based medications safety practice. In *Drug Safety in Developing Countries* (pp. 197–201). Academic Press.

Al-Worafi, Y.M. (2020r). Quality indicators for medications safety. In *Drug Safety in Developing Countries* (pp. 229–242). Academic Press.

Al-Worafi, Y.M. (2020s). Drug safety in Yemen. In *Drug Safety in Developing Countries* (pp. 391–405). Academic Press.

Al-Worafi, Y.M. (2020t). Drug safety in Saudi Arabia. In *Drug Safety in Developing Countries* (pp. 407–417). Academic Press.

Al-Worafi, Y.M. (2020u). Drug safety in United Arab Emirates. In *Drug Safety in Developing Countries* (pp. 419–428). Academic Press.

Al-Worafi, Y.M. (2020v). Drug safety in Indonesia. In *Drug Safety in Developing Countries* (pp. 279–285). Academic Press.

Al-Worafi, Y.M. (2020w). Drug safety in Palestine. In *Drug Safety in Developing Countries* (pp. 471–480). Academic Press.

Al-Worafi, Y.M. (2020x). Drug safety: comparison between developing countries. In *Drug Safety in Developing Countries* (pp. 603–611). Academic Press.

Al-Worafi, Y.M. (2020y). Drug safety in developing versus developed countries. In *Drug Safety in Developing Countries* (pp. 613–615). Academic Press.

Al-Worafi, Y.M., Alseragi, W.M., Ming, L.C., & Alakhali, K.M. (2020a). Drug safety in China. In *Drug Safety in Developing Countries* (pp. 381–388). Academic Press.

Al-Worafi, Y.M., Alseragi, W.M., Alakhali, K.M., Ming, L.C., Othman, G., Halboup, A.M., ... & Elkalmi, R.M. (2020b). Knowledge, beliefs and factors affecting the use of generic medicines among patients in Ibb, Yemen: a mixed-method study. *Journal of Pharmacy Practice and Community Medicine*, 6(4), 53–56.

Al-Worafi, Y.M., Elkalmi, R.M., Ming, L.C., Othman, G., Halboup, A.M., Battah, M.M., ... & Mani, V. (2021a). Dispensing errors in hospital pharmacies: A prospective study in Yemen. *AlQalam Journal of Medical and Applied Sciences*, 4, 13–17.

Al-Worafi, Y.M., Hasan, S., Hassan, N.M., & Gaili, A.A. (2021b). Knowledge, attitude and experience of pharmacist in the UAE towards pharmacovigilance. *Research Journal of Pharmacy and Technology*, 14(1), 265–269.

Al-Worafi, Y. (2022a). *A Guide to Online Pharmacy Education: Teaching Strategies and Assessment Methods*. CRC Press.

Al-Worafi, Y.M. (2022b). Patient care errors and related problems (part I): development and validation of the model. (Preprint).

Al-Worafi, Y.M. (Ed.). (2023). *Clinical Case Studies on medication Safety*. Academic Press.

Baig, M.R., Al-Worafi, Y.M., Alseragi, W.M., Ming, L.C., & Siddique, A. (2020). Drug safety in India. In *Drug Safety in Developing Countries* (pp. 327–334). Academic Press.

Elkalmi, R.M., Al-Worafi, Y.M., Alseragi, W.M., Ming, L.C., & Siddique, A. (2020). Drug safety in Malaysia. In *Drug Safety in Developing Countries* (pp. 245–253). Academic Press.

Elsayed, T., & Al-Worafi, Y.M. (2020). Drug safety in Egypt. In *Drug Safety in Developing Countries* (pp. 511–523). Academic Press.

Hasan, S., Al-Omar, M.J., AlZubaidy, H., & Al-Worafi, Y.M. (2019). Use of medications in Arab Countries. *Handbook of Healthcare in the Arab World*. Cham: Springer, 42.

Hassan, Y., Abd Aziz, N., Kassab, Y.W., Elgasim, I., Shaharuddin, S., Al-Worafi, Y.M.A., ... & Ming, L.C. (2014). How to help patients to control their blood pressure? Blood pressure control and its predictor. *Archives of Pharmacy Practice*, 5(4), 153–161.

Izahar, S., Lean, Q.Y., Hameed, M.A., Murugiah, M.K., Patel, R.P., Al-Worafi, Y.M., ... & Ming, L.C. (2017). Content analysis of mobile health applications on diabetes mellitus. *Frontiers in Endocrinology*, 8, 318.

Kristensen, S., & Bartels, P. (2010). Use of patient safety culture instruments and recommendations. *Aarhus, Denmark, European Society for Quality in HealthCare-Office for Quality Indicators*, 113, 1–35.

Lee, K.S., Yee, S.M., Zaidi, S.T.R., Patel, R.P., Yang, Q., Al-Worafi, Y.M., & Ming, L.C., 2017. Combating sale of counterfeit and falsified medicines online: a losing battle. *Frontiers in Pharmacology*, 8, 268.

Mahmoud, M.A., Wajid, S., Naqvi, A.A., Samreen, S., Althagfan, S.S., & Al-Worafi, Y. (2020). Self-medication with antibiotics: a cross-sectional community-based study. *Latin American Journal of Pharmacy*, 39(2), 348–353.

Manan, M.M., Rusli, R.A., Ang, W.C., Al-Worafi, Y.M., & Ming, L.C. (2014). Assessing the pharmaceutical care issues of antiepileptic drug therapy in hospitalised epileptic patients. *Journal of Pharmacy Practice and Research*, 44(3), 83–88.

Manan, M.M., Ibrahim, N.A., Aziz, N.A., Zulkifly, H.H., Al-Worafi, Y.M.A., & Long, C.M. (2016). Empirical use of antibiotic therapy in the prevention of early onset sepsis in neonates: a pilot study. *Archives of Medical Science*, 12(3), 603–613.

Ming, L.C., Hameed, M.A., Lee, D.D., Apidi, N.A., Lai, P.S.M., Hadi, M.A., Al-Worafi, Y.M.A., & Khan, T.M., (2016). Use of medical mobile applications among hospital pharmacists in Malaysia. *Therapeutic Innovation & Regulatory Science*, 50(4), 419–426.

Ming, L.C., Untong, N., Aliudin, N.A., Osili, N., Kifli, N., Tan, C.S., … & Goh, H.P. (2020). Mobile health apps on COVID-19 launched in the early days of the pandemic: content analysis and review. *JMIR mHealth and uHealth*, 8(9), e19796.

Othman, G., Ali, F., Ibrahim, M.I.M., Al-Worafi, Y.M., Ansari, M., & Halboup, A.M. (2020). Assessment of anti-diabetic medications adherence among diabetic patients in Sana'a City, Yemen: a cross sectional study. *Journal of Pharmaceutical Research International*, 32(21), 114–122.

Reynard, J., Reynolds, J., & Stevenson, P. (2009). *Practical Patient Safety*. OUP Oxford.

Saeed, M.S., Alkhoshaiban, A.S., Al-Worafi, Y.M.A., & Long, C.M., (2014). Perception of self-medication among university students in Saudi Arabia. *Archives of Pharmacy Practice*, 5(4), 149.

Salas, E., & Frush, K. (2012). *Improving Patient Safety through Teamwork and Team Training*. Oxford University Press.

Vincent, C. (2011). *Patient Safety*. John Wiley & Sons.

31 Patient Safety for Special Populations

Pregnancy

31.1 BACKGROUND

Pregnancy is the state of carrying a developing embryo or fetus within the female reproductive system. It is a natural process that typically lasts around 40 weeks or 9 months, during which a fertilized egg implants itself in the lining of the uterus and begins to grow and develop into a baby. Pregnancy is divided into three trimesters, with each trimester consisting of approximately three months. During pregnancy, the body undergoes a wide range of physical and hormonal changes to support the growth and development of the fetus. These changes include an increase in blood volume, changes in hormone levels, and weight gain. Pregnancy can be a wonderful and exciting experience, but it can also be challenging both physically and emotionally. It is important for pregnant women to receive proper medical care and support throughout their pregnancy to ensure the health and well-being of both mother and baby. Patient care and safety are essential during pregnancy to ensure a healthy pregnancy and safe delivery. Here are some important aspects of patient care and safety during pregnancy:

1. Prenatal care: Regular prenatal care is crucial for monitoring the health of both the mother and the fetus. This involves regular check-ups with a healthcare provider, including physical exams, blood tests, and ultrasounds.

2. Nutrition: A healthy and balanced diet is important for the growth and development of the fetus. A healthcare provider can provide guidance on proper nutrition during pregnancy.

3. Exercise: Regular exercise can help maintain a healthy weight, improve mood, and reduce the risk of gestational diabetes and hypertension. However, it is important to consult with a healthcare provider before starting any exercise routine.

4. Avoiding harmful substances: Smoking, alcohol, and drugs can all be harmful to the developing fetus. It is important to avoid these substances during pregnancy.

5. Complication management: Some women may develop complications during pregnancy, such as gestational diabetes, preeclampsia, or placenta previa. These conditions require careful monitoring and management by a healthcare provider.

6. Delivery planning: Planning for delivery includes discussing options with a healthcare provider, preparing a birth plan, and understanding the signs of labor and when to go to the hospital.

Overall, patient care and safety during pregnancy involve regular prenatal care, proper nutrition and exercise, avoiding harmful substances, managing complications, and planning for delivery. It is important for pregnant women to work closely with their healthcare provider to ensure a healthy pregnancy and safe delivery (Kristensen & Bartels, 2010; Reynard et al., 2009; Salas & Frush, 2012; Vincent, 2011).

31.2 PATIENT SAFETY FOR PREGNANCY: Errors and Related Problems

Patient safety is a critical aspect of pregnancy care as it can significantly impact the health and well-being of both the mother and the developing fetus. Unfortunately, errors and related problems can occur during pregnancy and childbirth, leading to adverse outcomes. Here are some common errors and problems related to patient safety during pregnancy:

1. Medication errors: Medication errors during pregnancy can result in harm to the developing fetus. It is important for healthcare providers to carefully consider the safety and potential risks of any medication prescribed to a pregnant woman.

2. Misdiagnosis or delayed diagnosis: Failure to diagnose or a delay in the diagnosis of conditions such as gestational diabetes or preeclampsia can lead to complications during pregnancy and delivery.

3. Communication errors: Poor communication among healthcare providers or between healthcare providers and patients can result in errors or misunderstandings, leading to adverse outcomes.

DOI: 10.1201/9781003230465-33

4. Infection control: Infections during pregnancy can have serious consequences for the developing fetus. Proper infection control measures, including hand hygiene and proper sterilization of equipment, are essential for patient safety.

5. Obstetric emergencies: Obstetric emergencies such as fetal distress, cord prolapse, or placental abruption can occur suddenly and require prompt intervention to prevent adverse outcomes.

6. Surgical errors: In some cases, a cesarean section or other surgical procedure may be necessary. Errors during surgery can result in harm to the mother or the developing fetus.

To minimize these errors and problems related to patient safety during pregnancy, healthcare providers should prioritize communication and collaboration, follow evidence-based guidelines for prenatal care and delivery, and implement rigorous infection control measures. In addition, patients should be encouraged to be active participants in their care, communicate openly with their healthcare providers, and ask questions to ensure that they receive the highest quality care possible.

31.3 PATIENT SAFETY FOR PREGNANCY: Causes

There are several causes of patient safety issues during pregnancy, which can lead to adverse outcomes for both the mother and the developing fetus. Here are some common causes of patient safety issues during pregnancy:

1. Lack of standardization: Prenatal care and delivery involve many different healthcare providers, procedures, and interventions. In the absence of standardization, variations in practice can result in errors and adverse outcomes.

2. Communication breakdowns: Communication among healthcare providers or between healthcare providers and patients can be a significant barrier to patient safety. Poor communication can lead to misunderstandings, errors, and delays in treatment.

3. Systemic issues: Many patient safety issues during pregnancy are the result of broader systemic issues within the healthcare system, such as inadequate staffing, lack of resources, or poor training and education.

4. Human factors: Human factors such as fatigue, stress, and cognitive overload can impact the ability of healthcare providers to provide safe and effective care.

5. Patient factors: Patient factors such as medical history, lifestyle choices, and socioeconomic status can impact pregnancy outcomes and patient safety.

6. Inadequate risk assessment: Failure to accurately assess risk during pregnancy can result in inappropriate interventions, missed opportunities for prevention or early intervention, and adverse outcomes.

To address these causes of patient safety issues during pregnancy, healthcare providers can implement strategies such as standardization of care, improved communication and teamwork, enhanced training and education, and increased use of technology to support clinical decision-making. In addition, patients can be encouraged to take an active role in their care, communicate openly with their healthcare providers, and participate in shared decision-making.

31.4 PATIENT SAFETY FOR PREGNANCY: Prevention

Prevention is key to ensuring patient safety during pregnancy. Here are some strategies for preventing patient safety issues during pregnancy:

1. Standardization of care: Standardizing prenatal care and delivery protocols can help reduce variations in practice and prevent errors. Evidence-based guidelines can be developed and implemented to ensure consistent, high-quality care.

2. Improved communication and teamwork: Effective communication and collaboration among healthcare providers and patients can help prevent errors and improve patient safety. Healthcare providers can work together to create a culture of safety and encourage open communication with patients.

3. Risk assessment: Accurate and comprehensive risk assessment is essential for identifying patients who may be at increased risk for complications during pregnancy. Risk assessment tools can help healthcare providers identify high-risk patients and implement appropriate interventions.

4. Patient education: Patient education is an important component of preventing patient safety issues during pregnancy. Patients should be provided with information about their pregnancy, the risks associated with certain conditions, and steps they can take to promote a healthy pregnancy.

5. Use of technology: Technology can be used to support clinical decision-making and improve patient safety during pregnancy. Electronic health records can provide healthcare providers with real-time access to patient information, while decision support systems can help identify potential safety issues and provide guidance on appropriate interventions.

6. Quality improvement initiatives: Quality improvement initiatives can help identify areas for improvement in prenatal care and delivery and implement strategies to enhance patient safety. Healthcare providers can participate in quality improvement projects to identify and address patient safety issues.

Overall, prevention of patient safety issues during pregnancy requires a multi-faceted approach that involves standardization of care, improved communication and teamwork, accurate risk assessment, patient education, use of technology, and quality improvement initiatives. Healthcare providers and patients should work together to promote a culture of safety and ensure the best possible outcomes for both the mother and the developing fetus.

31.5 PATIENT SAFETY FOR PREGNANCY IN DEVELOPING COUNTRIES: Challenges and Recommendations

Patient safety during pregnancy is a critical issue in developing countries, where maternal and infant mortality rates are often higher than in developed countries. Here are some challenges and recommendations for improving patient safety during pregnancy in developing countries:

Challenges:

1. Lack of resources: Developing countries often have limited resources to provide adequate prenatal care and emergency obstetric services.

2. Limited access to healthcare: Many women in developing countries do not have access to healthcare facilities or skilled healthcare providers.

3. Poor infrastructure: Inadequate transportation and poor roads can hinder access to healthcare facilities, particularly in rural areas.

4. Cultural and social barriers: Cultural and social factors can prevent women from seeking prenatal care or emergency obstetric services.

Recommendations:

1. Improving access to healthcare: Governments and international organizations can work to improve access to healthcare facilities and skilled healthcare providers in developing countries. This can be achieved through increasing funding for healthcare, expanding healthcare facilities, and training more healthcare providers.

2. Investing in infrastructure: Infrastructure improvements, such as road construction and transportation systems, can help ensure that women have access to healthcare facilities when they need them.

3. Addressing cultural and social barriers: Efforts to address cultural and social barriers to healthcare access can include community education and outreach programs, as well as addressing gender inequality and poverty.

4. Standardizing prenatal care and delivery protocols: Standardization of care can help reduce variations in practice and improve patient safety during pregnancy. Evidence-based guidelines can be developed and implemented to ensure consistent, high-quality care.

5. Providing education and training: Education and training programs can be developed for healthcare providers and patients to improve knowledge and skills related to patient safety during pregnancy. This can include training in risk assessment, infection control, and emergency obstetric care.

6. Utilizing technology: Technology, such as telemedicine, can be used to support clinical decision-making and improve patient safety during pregnancy in developing countries. Telemedicine can provide healthcare providers with access to expert advice and support, even in remote or underserved areas.

7. Lack of adequate nutrition: Poor maternal nutrition can increase the risk of complications during pregnancy and childbirth, such as preterm birth and low birth weight. This can be addressed through education and access to nutritious food.

8. Limited access to prenatal screening and diagnostic tests: Women in developing countries may not have access to screening and diagnostic tests, such as ultrasound and blood tests, which can help identify potential complications during pregnancy. Improving access to these tests can help ensure that women receive appropriate care and treatment.

9. Inadequate management of chronic diseases: Women with chronic diseases, such as diabetes or hypertension, require specialized care during pregnancy. In developing countries, women with chronic diseases may not receive adequate care, increasing the risk of complications.

10. Lack of emergency obstetric care: In some areas of developing countries, emergency obstetric care is not readily available, leading to delays in treatment and increased risk of maternal and infant mortality.

11. Traditional birth practices: In some cultures, traditional birth practices may be preferred over modern medical care. While these practices can be safe and effective, they may not provide adequate care in cases of complications during pregnancy or childbirth.

12. Limited access to family planning: Limited access to family planning services can result in unintended pregnancies and increased risk of maternal and infant morbidity and mortality.

13. Lack of trained healthcare professionals: Many developing countries experience a shortage of trained healthcare professionals, particularly in rural areas. This can result in inadequate prenatal care and emergency obstetric services, increasing the risk of complications and mortality.

14. High rates of adolescent pregnancy: In many developing countries, adolescent pregnancy rates are higher than in developed countries. Adolescent mothers may face unique risks, such as an increased risk of preterm birth and complications during delivery.

15. Limited access to safe water and sanitation: Poor water quality and inadequate sanitation can lead to infectious diseases that can be particularly dangerous during pregnancy. Improving access to safe water and sanitation can reduce the risk of infections and improve patient safety.

16. Lack of regulation and oversight: In some developing countries, there may be a lack of regulation and oversight of healthcare providers and facilities. This can result in substandard care and an increased risk of complications during pregnancy.

17. Inadequate postpartum care: Postpartum care is critical for ensuring the health and well-being of both the mother and the infant. In developing countries, women may not receive adequate postpartum care, which can lead to complications such as postpartum hemorrhage and infections.

18. Limited access to medications: Women in developing countries may not have access to essential medications, such as antibiotics or oxytocin, which can be critical for preventing and treating complications during pregnancy and delivery.

19. Cultural and social factors: In some cultures, pregnancy and childbirth are viewed as a natural process, and medical interventions are avoided. Additionally, cultural beliefs and practices can impact women's access to healthcare and their decision-making during pregnancy and childbirth.

20. Limited access to transportation: Women in remote or rural areas may have limited access to transportation, making it difficult to reach healthcare facilities for prenatal care, delivery, or emergency obstetric services.

21. Gender inequality: In many developing countries, gender inequality can affect women's access to healthcare and decision-making during pregnancy and childbirth. Women may face barriers such as discrimination, lack of autonomy, and limited educational opportunities.

22. Lack of health education and literacy: Low health literacy and lack of health education can affect women's ability to understand and access healthcare services during pregnancy. This can result in inadequate prenatal care, delayed treatment, and increased risk of complications.

23. Economic factors: Poverty and lack of resources can impact women's access to healthcare, medications, and nutrition during pregnancy. Women may not have access to basic needs such as adequate food and clean water, which can increase the risk of complications during pregnancy and delivery.

24. Political instability and conflict: Political instability and conflict can disrupt healthcare systems and access to healthcare services, which can impact patient safety during pregnancy and childbirth.

25. Despite the progress in research about patient care and safety in developing countries, there is little research about patient safety related to the geriatrics in the majority of developing countries, therefore, conducting research is very important and highly recommended (Alshahrani et al., 2019a,b; Al-Qahtani et al., 2015; Alshahrani et al., 2020a,b; Al-Worafi, 2014; Al-Worafi, 2015; Al-Worafi, 2016; Al-Worafi et al., 2017; Al-Worafi, 2018a-d; Al-Worafi et al., 2018a-b; Al-Worafi et al., 2019; Al-Worafi, 2020a-y; Al-Worafi et al., 2020a-b; Al-Worafi et al., 2021a,b; Al-Worafi, 2022a,b; Al-Worafi, 2023; Baig et al., 2020; Elkalmi et al., 2020; Elsayed & Al-Worafi, 2020; Hasan et al., 2019; Hassan et al., 2014; Izahar et al., 2017; Lee et al., 2017; Mahmoud et al., 2020; Manan et al., 2014; Manan et al., 2016; Ming et al., 2016; Ming et al., 2020; Othman et al., 2020; Saeed et al., 2014).

Addressing these challenges will require a multi-faceted approach that involves improving healthcare infrastructure, promoting education and awareness, addressing cultural and social barriers, and addressing economic and political factors. By addressing these issues, it is possible to improve patient safety during pregnancy and childbirth in developing countries and reduce maternal and infant mortality rates.

31.6 CONCLUSION

This chapter has discussed the patient safety issues related to pregnancy, prevention, challenges, and recommendations for the best practice in developing countries. Ensuring patient safety during pregnancy is essential to reducing maternal and infant mortality rates. However, in many developing countries, there are numerous challenges that can impact patient safety, including limited access to healthcare, inadequate resources, and cultural and social barriers. These challenges can result in inadequate prenatal care, delayed treatment, and increased risk of complications during pregnancy and childbirth. To address these challenges, a comprehensive approach is needed that involves improving healthcare infrastructure, promoting education and awareness, addressing cultural and social barriers, and addressing economic and political factors. By working together to improve patient safety during pregnancy, it is possible to reduce maternal and infant mortality rates and improve the health and well-being of women and children in developing countries.

REFERENCES

Al-Qahtani, I., Almoteb, T.M., & Al-Warafi, Y. (2015). Competency of metered-dose inhaler use among Saudi community pharmacists: a Simulation method study. *RRJPPS*, 4(2), 37–31.

Alshahrani, S.M., Alakhali, K.M., & Al-Worafi, Y.M., (2019a). Medication errors in a health care facility in southern Saudi Arabia. *Tropical Journal of Pharmaceutical Research*, 18(5), 1119–1122.

Alshahrani, S.M., Alavudeen, S.S., Alakhali, K.M., Al-Worafi, Y.M., Bahamdan, A.K., & Vigneshwaran, E., (2019b). Self-medication among King Khalid University Students, Saudi Arabia. *Risk Management and Healthcare Policy*, 12, 243–249.

Alshahrani, S.M., Alakhali, K.M., Al-Worafi, Y.M., & Alshahrani, N.Z. (2020a). Awareness and use of over the counter analgesic medication: a survey in the Aseer region population, Saudi Arabia. *International Journal of Advances in Applied Sciences*, 7(3), 130–134.

Alshahrani, S.M., Alzahran, M., Alakhali, K., Vigneshwaran, E., Iqbal, M.J., Khan, N.A., … & Alavudeen, S.S. (2020b). Association between diabetes consequences and quality of life among patients with diabetes mellitus in the Aseer Province of Saudi Arabia. *Open Access Macedonian Journal of Medical Sciences*, 8(E), 325–330.

Al-Worafi, Y.M. (2014). Prescription writing errors at a tertiary care hospital in Yemen: prevalence, types, causes and recommendations. *American Journal of Pharmacy and Health Research*, 2, 134–140.

Al-Worafi, Y.M.A. (2015). Appropriateness of metered-dose inhaler use in the Yemeni community pharmacies. *Journal of Taibah University Medical Sciences*, 10(3), 353–358.

Al-Worafi, Y.M.A., (2016). Pharmacy practice in Yemen. In *Pharmacy Practice in Developing Countries* (pp. 267–287). Academic Press.

Al-Worafi, Y.M., Kassab, Y.W., Alseragi, W.M., Almutairi, M.S., Ahmed, A., Ming, L.C., Alkhoshaiban, A.S., & Hadi, M.A., (2017). Pharmacovigilance and adverse drg reaction reporting: a perspective of community pharmacists and pharmacy technicians in Sana'a, Yemen. *Therapeutics and Clinical Risk Management*, 13, 1175.

Al-Worafi, Y.M., (2018a). Knowledge, attitude and practice of Yemeni physicians toward pharmacovigilance: a mixed method study. *International Journal of Pharmacy and Pharmaceutical Sciences*, 10(10), 74–77.

Al-Worafi, Y. (2018b). Knowledge, attitude and practice of Yemeni physicians toward pharmacovigilance: a mixed method study. *International Journal of Pharmacy and Pharmaceutical Sciences*, 10, 74–77.

Al-Worafi, Y.M. (2018c). Dispensing errors observed by community pharmacy dispensers in IBB–YEMEN. *Asian Journal of Pharmaceutical and Clinical Research*, 11(11), 478–481.

Al-Worafi, Y.M. (2018d). Evauation of inhaler technique among patients with asthma and COPD in Yemen. *Journal of Taibah University Medical Sciences*, 13(5), 488–490.

Al-Worafi, Y.M., Patel, R.P., Zaidi, S.T.R., Alseragi, W.M., Almutairi, M.S., Alkhoshaiban, A.S., & Ming, L.C. (2018a). Completeness and legibility of handwritten prescriptions in Sana'a, Yemen. *Medical Principles and Practice*, 27, 290–292.

Al-Worafi, Y.M., Alseragi, W.M., Seng, L.K., Kassab, Y.W., Yeoh, S.F., Chiau, L., … & Husain, K. (2018b). Dispensing errors in community pharmacies: a prospective study in Sana'a, Yemen. *Archives of Pharmacy Practice*, 9(4), 1–3.

Al-Worafi, Y.M., Alseragi, W.M., & Mahmoud, M.A. (2019). Competency of metered-dose inhaler use among community pharmacy dispensers in Ibb, Yemen: A simulation method study. *Latin American Journal of Pharmacy*, 38(3), 489–494.

Al-Worafi, Y.M. (Ed.). (2020a). *Drug Safety in Developing Countries: Achievements and Challenges*.

Al-Worafi, Y.M. (2020b). Medication errors. In *Drug Safety in Developing Countries* (pp. 105–117). Academic Press.

Al-Worafi, Y.M. (2020c). Adverse drug reactions. In *Drug Safety in Developing Countries* (pp. 39–57). Academic Press.

Al-Worafi, Y.M. (2020d). Medications registration and marketing: safety-related issues. In *Drug Safety in Developing Countries* (pp. 21–28). Academic Press.

Al-Worafi, Y.M. (2020e). Pharmacovigilance. In *Drug Safety in Developing Countries* (pp. 29–38). Academic Press.

Al-Worafi, Y.M. (2020f). Drug-related problems. In *Drug Safety in Developing Countries* (pp. 59–71). Academic Press.

Al-Worafi, Y.M. (2020g). Medications safety-related terminology. In *Drug Safety in Developing Countries* (pp. 7–19). Academic Press.

Al-Worafi, Y.M. (2020h). Self-medication. In *Drug Safety in Developing Countries* (pp. 73–86). Academic Press.

Al-Worafi, Y.M. (2020i). Antibiotics safety issues. In *Drug Safety in Developing Countries* (pp. 87–103). Academic Press.

Al-Worafi, Y.M. (2020j). Medications safety research issues. In *Drug Safety in Developing Countries* (pp. 213–227). Academic Press.

Al-Worafi, Y.M. (2020k). Counterfeit and substandard medications. In *Drug Safety in Developing Countries* (pp. 119–126). Academic Press.

Al-Worafi, Y.M. (2020l). Medication abuse and misuse. In *Drug Safety in Developing Countries* (pp. 127–135). Academic Press.

Al-Worafi, Y.M. (2020m). Storage and disposal of medications. In *Drug Safety in Developing Countries* (pp. 137–142). Academic Press.

Al-Worafi, Y.M. (2020n). Safety of medications in special population. In *Drug Safety in Developing Countries* (pp. 143–162). Academic Press.

Al-Worafi, Y.M. (2020o). Herbal medicines safety issues. In *Drug Safety in Developing Countries* (pp. 163–178). Academic Press.

Al-Worafi, Y.M. (2020p). Medications safety pharmacoeconomics-related issues. In *Drug Safety in Developing Countries* (pp. 187–195). Academic Press.

Al-Worafi, Y.M. (2020q). Evidence-based medications safety practice. In *Drug Safety in Developing Countries* (pp. 197–201). Academic Press.

Al-Worafi, Y.M. (2020r). Quality indicators for medications safety. In *Drug Safety in Developing Countries* (pp. 229–242). Academic Press.

Al-Worafi, Y.M. (2020s). Drug safety in Yemen. In *Drug Safety in Developing Countries* (pp. 391–405). Academic Press.

Al-Worafi, Y.M. (2020t). Drug safety in Saudi Arabia. In *Drug Safety in Developing Countries* (pp. 407–417). Academic Press.

Al-Worafi, Y.M. (2020u). Drug safety in United Arab Emirates. In *Drug Safety in Developing Countries* (pp. 419–428). Academic Press.

Al-Worafi, Y.M. (2020v). Drug safety in Indonesia. In *Drug Safety in Developing Countries* (pp. 279–285). Academic Press.

Al-Worafi, Y.M. (2020w). Drug safety in Palestine. In *Drug Safety in Developing Countries* (pp. 471–480). Academic Press.

Al-Worafi, Y.M. (2020x). Drug safety: comparison between developing countries. In *Drug Safety in Developing Countries* (pp. 603–611). Academic Press.

Al-Worafi, Y.M. (2020y). Drug safety in developing versus developed countries. In *Drug Safety in Developing Countries* (pp. 613–615). Academic Press.

Al-Worafi, Y.M., Alseragi, W.M., Ming, L.C., & Alakhali, K.M. (2020a). Drug safety in China. In *Drug Safety in Developing Countries* (pp. 381–388). Academic Press.

Al-Worafi, Y.M., Alseragi, W.M., Alakhali, K.M., Ming, L.C., Othman, G., Halboup, A.M., ... & Elkalmi, R.M. (2020b). Knowledge, beliefs and factors affecting the use of generic medicines among patients in Ibb, Yemen: a mixed-method study. *Journal of Pharmacy Practice and Community Medicine*, 6(4), 53–56.

Al-Worafi, Y.M., Elkalmi, R.M., Ming, L.C., Othman, G., Halboup, A.M., Battah, M.M., ... & Mani, V. (2021a). Dispensing errors in hospital pharmacies: A prospective study in Yemen. *AlQalam Journal of Medical and Applied Sciences*, 4, 13–17.

Al-Worafi, Y.M., Hasan, S., Hassan, N.M., & Gaili, A.A. (2021b). Knowledge, attitude and experience of pharmacist in the UAE towards pharmacovigilance. *Research Journal of Pharmacy and Technology*, 14(1), 265–269.

Al-Worafi, Y. (2022a). *A Guide to Online Pharmacy Education: Teaching Strategies and Assessment Methods*. CRC Press.

Al-Worafi, Y.M. (2022b). Patient care errors and related problems (part I): development and validation of the model. (Preprint). 0000-0002-5752-2913

Al-Worafi, Y.M. (Ed.). (2023). *Clinical Case Studies on Medication Safety*. Academic Press.

Baig, M.R., Al-Worafi, Y.M., Alseragi, W.M., Ming, L.C., & Siddique, A. (2020). Drug safety in India. In *Drug Safety in Developing Countries* (pp. 327–334). Academic Press.

Elkalmi, R.M., Al-Worafi, Y.M., Alseragi, W.M., Ming, L.C., & Siddique, A. (2020). Drug safety in Malaysia. In *Drug Safety in Developing Countries* (pp. 245–253). Academic Press.

Elsayed, T., & Al-Worafi, Y.M. (2020). Drug safety in Egypt. In *Drug Safety in Developing Countries* (pp. 511–523). Academic Press.

Hasan, S., Al-Omar, M.J., AlZubaidy, H., & Al-Worafi, Y.M. (2019). Use of medications in Arab Countries. *Handbook of Healthcare in the Arab World*. Cham: Springer, 42.

Hassan, Y., Abd Aziz, N., Kassab, Y.W., Elgasim, I., Shaharuddin, S., Al-Worafi, Y.M.A., ... & Ming, L.C. (2014). How to help patients to control their blood pressure? Blood pressure control and its predictor. *Archives of Pharmacy Practice*, 5(4), 153–161.

Izahar, S., Lean, Q.Y., Hameed, M.A., Murugiah, M.K., Patel, R.P., Al-Worafi, Y.M., ... & Ming, L.C. (2017). Content analysis of mobile health applications on diabetes mellitus. *Frontiers in Endocrinology*, 8, 318.

Kristensen, S., & Bartels, P. (2010). Use of patient safety culture instruments and recommendations. *Aarhus, Denmark, European Society for Quality in HealthCare-Office for Quality Indicators*, 113.

Lee, K.S., Yee, S.M., Zaidi, S.T.R., Patel, R.P., Yang, Q., Al-Worafi, Y.M., & Ming, L.C., 2017. Combating sale of counterfeit and falsified medicines online: a losing battle. *Frontiers in Pharmacology*, 8, 268.

Mahmoud, M.A., Wajid, S., Naqvi, A.A., Samreen, S., Althagfan, S.S., & Al-Worafi, Y. (2020). Self-medication with antibiotics: a cross-sectional community-based study. *Latin American Journal of Pharmacy*, 39(2), 348–353.

Manan, M.M., Rusli, R.A., Ang, W.C., Al-Worafi, Y.M., & Ming, L.C. (2014). Assessing the pharmaceutical care issues of antiepileptic drug therapy in hospitalised epileptic patients. *Journal of Pharmacy Practice and Research*, 44(3), 83–88.

Manan, M.M., Ibrahim, N.A., Aziz, N.A., Zulkifly, H.H., Al-Worafi, Y.M.A., & Long, C.M. (2016). Empirical use of antibiotic therapy in the prevention of early onset sepsis in neonates: a pilot study. *Archives of Medical Science*, 12(3), 603–613.

Ming, L.C., Hameed, M.A., Lee, D.D., Apidi, N.A., Lai, P.S.M., Hadi, M.A., Al-Worafi, Y.M.A., & Khan, T.M., (2016). Use of medical mobile applications among hospital pharmacists in Malaysia. *Therapeutic Innovation & Regulatory Science*, 50(4), 419–426.

Ming, L.C., Untong, N., Aliudin, N.A., Osili, N., Kifli, N., Tan, C.S., ... & Goh, H.P. (2020). Mobile health apps on COVID-19 launched in the early days of the pandemic: content analysis and review. *JMIR mHealth and uHealth*, 8(9), e19796.

Othman, G., Ali, F., Ibrahim, M.I.M., Al-Worafi, Y.M., Ansari, M., & Halboup, A.M. (2020). Assessment of anti-diabetic medications adherence among diabetic patients in Sana'a City, Yemen: a cross sectional study. *Journal of Pharmaceutical Research International*, 32(21), 114–122.

Reynard, J., Reynolds, J., & Stevenson, P. (2009). *Practical Patient Safety*. OUP Oxford.

Saeed, M.S., Alkhoshaiban, A.S., Al-Worafi, Y.M.A., & Long, C.M., (2014). Perception of self-medication among university students in Saudi Arabia. *Archives of Pharmacy Practice*, 5(4), 149.

Salas, E., & Frush, K. (2012). *Improving Patient Safety through Teamwork and Team Training*. Oxford University Press.

Vincent, C. (2011). *Patient Safety*. John Wiley & Sons.

32 Patient Safety for Special Populations

Lactation

32.1 BACKGROUND

Lactation is the process of producing and secreting milk from the mammary glands of a female mammal, typically a mother after giving birth. It is an important physiological process that provides essential nutrients and immunological protection to newborn offspring. The hormone prolactin, which is secreted by the pituitary gland, stimulates lactation. Prolactin levels increase during pregnancy and remain elevated after childbirth, promoting milk production. The hormone oxytocin also plays a role in lactation by causing the milk ducts to contract and release milk. Lactation is not limited to humans, as many other mammals including cows, goats, and sheep also produce milk to feed their young. In addition to being a source of nutrition, lactation is also important for bonding and providing comfort to the infant. Patient care and safety during breastfeeding (lactation) are important to ensure the health and well-being of both the mother and the infant. Here are some important considerations:

1. Positioning and latching: Proper positioning and latching of the infant during breastfeeding can help prevent nipple soreness and ensure adequate milk transfer. A lactation consultant or healthcare provider can provide guidance on the correct positioning and latch.

2. Breast hygiene: It is important to maintain good breast hygiene during lactation. This includes washing the breasts with warm water and soap and drying them thoroughly after each feeding. Avoid using harsh soaps or lotions on the breasts, as they can cause irritation.

3. Nutrition: A breastfeeding mother should consume a well-balanced diet and drink plenty of fluids to ensure adequate milk production and maintain her own health. It is also important to avoid certain foods and substances that can be harmful to the infant, such as alcohol, caffeine, and tobacco.

4. Medications: Some medications can pass into breast milk and affect the infant. A healthcare provider should be consulted before taking any medications during lactation to ensure that they are safe for both the mother and the infant.

5. Breastfeeding and COVID-19: Breastfeeding is generally safe during the COVID-19 pandemic. However, precautions should be taken to minimize the risk of transmission. These include wearing a mask, washing hands frequently, and avoiding close contact with others who are sick.

6. Support: Breastfeeding can be challenging, and new mothers may need support and encouragement to continue breastfeeding. Family members, friends, and healthcare providers can provide emotional support and practical assistance to help ensure successful breastfeeding.

Overall, providing patient care and safety during lactation involves taking a holistic approach that considers the physical, emotional, and social well-being of both the mother and the infant (Kristensen & Bartels, 2010; Reynard et al., 2009; Salas & Frush, 2012; Vincent, 2011).

32.2 PATIENT SAFETY FOR LACTATION: Errors and Related Problems

Patient safety is a crucial aspect of healthcare delivery, and it is particularly important in lactation care. Lactation errors can have serious consequences for both the mother and the infant. Here are some of the most common lactation errors and related problems that can occur:

1. Incorrect positioning and latch: If a mother and infant are not positioned properly during breastfeeding, it can lead to problems such as sore nipples, ineffective milk transfer, and low milk supply. It is important for lactation providers to educate and assist mothers on proper positioning and latch techniques.

2. Engorgement and plugged ducts: Engorgement occurs when breasts become overly full with milk, leading to discomfort and difficulty with milk flow. Plugged ducts are a blockage in the milk duct that can cause pain, inflammation, and infection. These conditions can be prevented or managed through proper breastfeeding techniques, frequent nursing or pumping, and massage.

DOI: 10.1201/9781003230465-34

3. Mastitis: Mastitis is an infection of the breast tissue that can cause pain, fever, and flu-like symptoms. It can be caused by bacteria entering the breast through a cracked nipple or other opening. Early recognition and treatment of mastitis is essential to prevent serious complications.

4. Medication errors: Medications that are used during lactation can have potential side effects on the mother and infant. Lactation providers should be aware of any potential side effects and advise mothers on safe medication use during breastfeeding.

5. Inadequate support: Lack of support and resources can be a major barrier to successful breastfeeding. Lactation providers should be knowledgeable about community resources and provide mothers with appropriate referrals.

Overall, lactation errors and related problems can have significant impacts on the health and well-being of both mothers and infants. Proper education and support from lactation providers can help prevent and manage these issues, ultimately improving patient safety and outcomes.

32.3 PATIENT SAFETY FOR LACTATION: Causes

There are various causes of patient safety issues in lactation care. Here are some of the most common causes:

1. Lack of knowledge and training: Healthcare providers may not have adequate knowledge and training in lactation care, leading to errors in assessment, diagnosis, and treatment.

2. Inadequate communication: Poor communication between healthcare providers and patients can lead to misunderstandings, incorrect advice, and inadequate support for lactation care.

3. Cultural barriers: Cultural beliefs and practices may impact the mother's ability or willingness to breastfeed, leading to issues with lactation.

4. Breastfeeding challenges: Breastfeeding can be challenging, and mothers may face issues such as low milk supply, nipple pain, and difficulty with positioning and latch. These challenges can impact patient safety if not addressed appropriately.

5. Medication errors: Medications used during lactation can have potential side effects on the mother and infant if not used appropriately. Healthcare providers need to have an understanding of the safety of medications used during lactation.

6. Inadequate support: Mothers may not have adequate support from healthcare providers, family, or community resources to successfully breastfeed, leading to issues with lactation care.

7. Environmental factors: Environmental factors such as lack of privacy, time constraints, and unsupportive workplace policies may impact the mother's ability to breastfeed successfully.

Overall, addressing these causes through proper education and support for healthcare providers and mothers can help improve patient safety in lactation care.

32.4 PATIENT SAFETY FOR LACTATION: Prevention

Preventing patient safety issues in lactation care involves addressing the underlying causes and implementing measures to promote safe and effective breastfeeding practices. Here are some prevention strategies:

1. Education and training: Healthcare providers should receive appropriate education and training in lactation care to ensure they have the knowledge and skills to assess, diagnose, and treat lactation issues safely and effectively.

2. Communication: Providers should communicate effectively with patients to ensure that mothers have the information they need to make informed decisions about breastfeeding and receive appropriate support.

3. Cultural sensitivity: Providers should be sensitive to cultural beliefs and practices that may impact breastfeeding, and work with mothers to find culturally appropriate solutions to any lactation challenges.

4. Supportive breastfeeding practices: Providers should promote breastfeeding-friendly practices such as early and frequent skin-to-skin contact, baby-led feeding, and rooming-in to encourage successful breastfeeding.

5. Safe medication use: Providers should be knowledgeable about the safety of medications used during lactation and ensure that mothers receive appropriate advice and support in using these medications safely.

6. Adequate support: Providers should ensure that mothers have access to adequate support from healthcare providers, family, and community resources to successfully breastfeed.

7. Environmental factors: Providers should work to create a breastfeeding-friendly environment that promotes privacy, provides adequate time and support, and accommodates mothers' needs.

Overall, preventing patient safety issues in lactation care involves a multifaceted approach that addresses the underlying causes of lactation issues and promotes safe and effective breastfeeding practices

32.5 PATIENT SAFETY FOR LACTATION IN DEVELOPING COUNTRIES: Challenges and Recommendations

Patient safety for lactation in developing countries faces unique challenges due to a range of factors, including poverty, limited access to healthcare, and inadequate support for breastfeeding. Here are some challenges and recommendations for improving patient safety for lactation in developing countries:

Challenges:

1. Limited access to healthcare: Many women in developing countries do not have access to adequate healthcare services, including lactation care. This can lead to inadequate support for breastfeeding and a higher risk of lactation issues.

2. Poverty: Poverty can impact a woman's ability to access healthcare services, adequate nutrition, and safe drinking water, all of which can impact breastfeeding outcomes.

3. Lack of education and awareness: Many women in developing countries may not be aware of the benefits of breastfeeding or may lack the knowledge and skills to breastfeed effectively.

4. Cultural beliefs and practices: Cultural beliefs and practices can impact breastfeeding practices, and some traditional practices may actually be harmful to lactation.

5. Inadequate infrastructure and resources: Developing countries may lack the infrastructure and resources needed to support breastfeeding, including appropriate lactation equipment, clean water, and safe and private spaces for breastfeeding.

Recommendations:

1. Increase access to healthcare: Governments and non-governmental organizations should work to increase access to healthcare services, including lactation care, in developing countries.

2. Address poverty: Efforts to address poverty, including increasing access to education and job opportunities, can help improve breastfeeding outcomes in developing countries.

3. Promote education and awareness: Health education programs should be implemented to promote the benefits of breastfeeding and provide mothers with the knowledge and skills to breastfeed effectively.

4. Work with cultural beliefs and practices: Healthcare providers should work with cultural beliefs and practices to find culturally appropriate solutions to lactation challenges.

5. Provide adequate infrastructure and resources: Governments and organizations should work to provide adequate infrastructure and resources to support breastfeeding, including lactation equipment, clean water, and safe and private spaces for breastfeeding.

6. Support community-based breastfeeding programs: Community-based programs, such as mother-to-mother support groups, can provide valuable support and resources for breastfeeding mothers in developing countries.

7. Lack of trained healthcare providers: Many healthcare providers in developing countries may not have adequate training in lactation care, leading to a higher risk of errors and unsafe practices.

8. Limited availability of breastfeeding resources: Developing countries may lack access to breastfeeding resources, such as lactation consultants, breast pumps, and breastfeeding-friendly workplaces, which can impact breastfeeding outcomes.

9. Inadequate nutrition: Mothers in developing countries may not have access to adequate nutrition, which can impact milk production and breastfeeding outcomes.

10. Lack of legal protections: Some developing countries may lack legal protections for breast-feeding, such as workplace accommodations for lactating mothers, which can impact mothers' ability to breastfeed safely and effectively.

11. Limited access to infant formula: In some developing countries, infant formula may not be readily available or affordable, leading to a higher reliance on breastfeeding and a greater need for support.

12. Infant feeding practices: In some developing countries, there may be cultural practices or traditions that impact infant feeding, which can impact breastfeeding outcomes and patient safety.

13. Health disparities: Women in marginalized communities in developing countries may face additional challenges related to patient safety for lactation, such as discrimination, lack of access to healthcare services, and inadequate support for breastfeeding.

14. Lack of breastfeeding-friendly policies: In some developing countries, there may be a lack of policies and regulations to support breastfeeding, such as regulations for breastfeeding breaks in the workplace or laws protecting mothers' rights to breastfeed in public.

15. Limited access to clean water: Access to clean water is essential for safe breastfeeding practices, but in some developing countries, clean water may not be readily available, which can increase the risk of infection and other health problems.

16. Limited access to maternal healthcare: In addition to lactation care, women in developing countries may lack access to maternal healthcare services, such as prenatal and postnatal care, which can impact breastfeeding outcomes.

17. Lack of breastfeeding education for fathers and families: In some cultures, fathers and families may play a significant role in supporting breastfeeding, but they may not have access to adequate education and support to do so effectively.

18. Lack of support for mothers with preexisting medical conditions: Women with preexisting medical conditions, such as HIV or diabetes, may face additional challenges related to breastfeeding, but may not have access to the necessary support and resources to do so safely.

19. Inadequate monitoring and evaluation: In some developing countries, there may be a lack of monitoring and evaluation of breastfeeding practices and outcomes, which can make it difficult to identify and address patient safety issues related to lactation care.

20. Lack of support for working mothers: In some developing countries, working mothers may face challenges related to breastfeeding, such as lack of time or privacy to breastfeed or express milk during work hours.

21. Limited access to breastfeeding education for healthcare providers: Healthcare providers in developing countries may lack access to ongoing education and training in lactation care, which can impact the quality of care provided to lactating mothers.

22. Lack of support for mothers of multiples: Mothers of multiples, such as twins or triplets, may face additional challenges related to breastfeeding, such as inadequate milk production or difficulty managing multiple infants, but may not have access to the necessary support and resources.

23. Cultural taboos around breastfeeding: In some cultures, there may be taboos or stigmas surrounding breastfeeding, which can make it difficult for mothers to breastfeed safely and effectively.

24. Limited access to peer support: Peer support, such as through mother-to-mother support groups, can be a valuable resource for lactating mothers, but in some developing countries, such support may not be readily available.

25. Limited access to breastfeeding-friendly healthcare facilities: Healthcare facilities, such as hospitals and clinics, may not be equipped to support safe and effective breastfeeding practices, which can impact patient safety for lactation.

26. Despite the progress in research about the patient care and safety in developing countries, there is little research about the patient safety related to the lactation in majority of developing countries, therefore, conduct research is very important and highly recommended (Alshahrani et al., 2019a,b; Al-Qahtani et al., 2015; Alshahrani et al., 2020a,b; Al-Worafi, 2014; Al-Worafi, 2015; Al-Worafi, 2016; Al-Worafi et al., 2017; Al-Worafi, 2018a-d; Al-Worafi et al., 2018a-b; Al-Worafi et al., 2019; Al-Worafi, 2020a-y; Al-Worafi et al., 2020a-b; Al-Worafi et al., 2021a,b; Al-Worafi, 2022a,b; Al-Worafi, 2023; Baig et al., 2020; Elkalmi et al., 2020; Elsayed & Al-Worafi, 2020; Hasan et al., 2019; Hassan et al., 2014; Izahar et al., 2017; Lee et al., 2017; Mahmoud et al., 2020; Manan et al., 2014; Manan et al., 2016; Ming et al., 2016; Ming et al., 2020; Othman et al., 2020; Saeed et al., 2014).

Addressing these additional issues requires a comprehensive approach that promotes policies and practices that support safe and effective breastfeeding for all mothers, regardless of their cultural background or individual circumstances. It also requires a focus on providing adequate education and support for healthcare providers, as well as increasing access to peer support and breastfeeding-friendly resources and facilities.

32.6 CONCLUSION

This chapter has discussed the patient safety issues related to the lactation, prevention, challenges and recommendations for the best practice in developing countries. Patient safety for lactation is a critical issue, particularly in developing countries, where mothers may face a range of challenges related to breastfeeding. These challenges include inadequate access to lactation support, limited access to clean water and healthcare services, lack of legal protections, and cultural taboos around breastfeeding. To address these challenges, a comprehensive approach is needed, including policies and regulations that support safe and effective breastfeeding practices, education and support for healthcare providers, and increased access to breastfeeding-friendly resources and facilities. Additionally, addressing underlying social, economic, and cultural factors is crucial to promoting patient safety for lactation and ensuring that all mothers have the support and resources they need to breastfeed safely and effectively.

REFERENCES

Al-Qahtani, I., Almoteb, T.M., & Al-Warafi, Y. (2015). Competency of metered-dose inhaler use among Saudi community pharmacists: A Simulation method study. *RRJPPS*, 4(2), 37–31.

Alshahrani, S.M., Alakhali, K.M., & Al-Worafi, Y.M., (2019a). Medication errors in a health care facility in southern Saudi Arabia. *Tropical Journal of Pharmaceutical Research*, 18(5), 1119–1122.

Alshahrani, S.M., Alavudeen, S.S., Alakhali, K.M., Al-Worafi, Y.M., Bahamdan, A.K., & Vigneshwaran, E., (2019b). Self-medication among King Khalid University Students, Saudi Arabia. *Risk Management and Healthcare Policy*, 12, 243–249.

Alshahrani, S.M., Alakhali, K.M., Al-Worafi, Y.M., & Alshahrani, N.Z. (2020a). Awareness and use of over the counter analgesic medication: a survey in the Aseer region population, Saudi Arabia. *International Journal of Advances in Applied Sciences*, 7(3), 130–134.

Alshahrani, S.M., Alzahran, M., Alakhali, K., Vigneshwaran, E., Iqbal, M.J., Khan, N.A., … & Alavudeen, S.S. (2020b). Association between diabetes consequences and quality of life among patients with diabetes mellitus in the Aseer Province of Saudi Arabia. *Open Access Macedonian Journal of Medical Sciences*, 8(E), 325–330.

Al-Worafi, Y.M. (2014). Prescription writing errors at a tertiary care hospital in Yemen: prevalence, types, causes and recommendations. *American Journal of Pharmacy and Health Research*, 2, 134–140.

Al-Worafi, Y.M.A. (2015). Appropriateness of metered-dose inhaler use in the Yemeni community pharmacies. *Journal of Taibah University Medical Sciences*, 10(3), 353–358.

Al-Worafi, Y.M.A., (2016). Pharmacy practice in Yemen. In *Pharmacy Practice in Developing Countries* (pp. 267–287). Academic Press.

Al-Worafi, Y.M., Kassab, Y.W., Alseragi, W.M., Almutairi, M.S., Ahmed, A., Ming, L.C., Alkhoshaiban, A.S., & Hadi, M.A., (2017). Pharmacovigilance and adverse drg reaction reporting: a perspective of community pharmacists and pharmacy technicians in Sana'a, Yemen. *Therapeutics and Clinical Risk Management*, 13, 1175.

Al-Worafi, Y.M., (2018a). Knowledge, attitude and practice of Yemeni physicians toward pharmacovigilance: a mixed method study. *International Journal of Pharmacy and Pharmaceutical Sciences*, 10(10), 74–77.

Al-Worafi, Y. (2018b). Knowledge, attitude and practice of Yemeni physicians toward pharmacovigilance: a mixed method study. *International Journal of Pharmacy and Pharmaceutical Sciences*, 10, 74–77.

Al-Worafi, Y.M. (2018c). Dispensing errors observed by community pharmacy dispensers in IBB–YEMEN. *Asian Journal of Pharmaceutical and Clinical Research*, 11(11).

Al-Worafi, Y.M. (2018d). Evauation of inhaler technique among patients with asthma and COPD in Yemen. *Journal of Taibah University Medical Sciences*, 13(5), 488–490.

Al-Worafi, Y.M., Patel, R.P., Zaidi, S.T.R., Alseragi, W.M., Almutairi, M.S., Alkhoshaiban, A.S., & Ming, L.C. (2018a). Completeness and legibility of handwritten prescriptions in Sana'a, Yemen. *Medical Principles and Practice*, 27, 290–292.

Al-Worafi, Y.M., Alseragi, W.M., Seng, L.K., Kassab, Y.W., Yeoh, S.F., Chiau, L., … & Husain, K. (2018b). Dispensing errors in community pharmacies: a prospective study in Sana'a, Yemen. *Archives of Pharmacy Practice*, 9(4), 1–3.

Al-Worafi, Y.M., Alseragi, W.M., & Mahmoud, M.A. (2019). Competency of metered-dose inhaler use among community pharmacy dispensers in Ibb, Yemen: a simulation method study. *Latin American Journal of Pharmacy*, 38(3), 489–494.

Al-Worafi, Y.M. (Ed.). (2020a). *Drug Safety in Developing Countries: Achievements and Challenges.*

Al-Worafi, Y.M. (2020b). Medication errors. In *Drug Safety in Developing Countries* (pp. 105–117). Academic Press.

Al-Worafi, Y.M. (2020c). Adverse drug reactions. In *Drug Safety in Developing Countries* (pp. 39–57). Academic Press.

Al-Worafi, Y.M. (2020d). Medications registration and marketing: safety-related issues. In *Drug Safety in Developing Countries* (pp. 21–28). Academic Press.

Al-Worafi, Y.M. (2020e). Pharmacovigilance. In *Drug Safety in Developing Countries* (pp. 29–38). Academic Press.

Al-Worafi, Y.M. (2020f). Drug-related problems. In *Drug Safety in Developing Countries* (pp. 59–71). Academic Press.

Al-Worafi, Y.M. (2020g). Medications safety-related terminology. In *Drug Safety in Developing Countries* (pp. 7–19). Academic Press.

Al-Worafi, Y.M. (2020h). Self-medication. In *Drug Safety in Developing Countries* (pp. 73–86). Academic Press.

Al-Worafi, Y.M. (2020i). Antibiotics safety issues. In *Drug Safety in Developing Countries* (pp. 87–103). Academic Press.

Al-Worafi, Y.M. (2020j). Medications safety research issues. In *Drug Safety in Developing Countries* (pp. 213–227). Academic Press.

Al-Worafi, Y.M. (2020k). Counterfeit and substandard medications. In *Drug Safety in Developing Countries* (pp. 119–126). Academic Press.

Al-Worafi, Y.M. (2020l). Medication abuse and misuse. In *Drug Safety in Developing Countries* (pp. 127–135). Academic Press.

Al-Worafi, Y.M. (2020m). Storage and disposal of medications. In *Drug Safety in Developing Countries* (pp. 137–142). Academic Press.

Al-Worafi, Y.M. (2020n). Safety of medications in special population. In *Drug Safety in Developing Countries* (pp. 143–162). Academic Press.

Al-Worafi, Y.M. (2020o). Herbal medicines safety issues. In *Drug Safety in Developing Countries* (pp. 163–178). Academic Press.

Al-Worafi, Y.M. (2020p). Medications safety pharmacoeconomics-related issues. In *Drug Safety in Developing Countries* (pp. 187–195). Academic Press.

Al-Worafi, Y.M. (2020q). Evidence-based medications safety practice. In *Drug Safety in Developing Countries* (pp. 197–201). Academic Press.

Al-Worafi, Y.M. (2020r). Quality indicators for medications safety. In *Drug Safety in Developing Countries* (pp. 229–242). Academic Press.

Al-Worafi, Y.M. (2020s). Drug safety in Yemen. In *Drug Safety in Developing Countries* (pp. 391–405). Academic Press.

Al-Worafi, Y.M. (2020t). Drug safety in Saudi Arabia. In *Drug Safety in Developing Countries* (pp. 407–417). Academic Press.

Al-Worafi, Y.M. (2020u). Drug safety in United Arab Emirates. In *Drug Safety in Developing Countries* (pp. 419–428). Academic Press.

Al-Worafi, Y.M. (2020v). Drug safety in Indonesia. In *Drug Safety in Developing Countries* (pp. 279–285). Academic Press.

Al-Worafi, Y.M. (2020w). Drug safety in Palestine. In *Drug Safety in Developing Countries* (pp. 471–480). Academic Press.

Al-Worafi, Y.M. (2020x). Drug safety: comparison between developing countries. In *Drug Safety in Developing Countries* (pp. 603–611). Academic Press.

Al-Worafi, Y.M. (2020y). Drug safety in developing versus developed countries. In *Drug Safety in Developing Countries* (pp. 613–615). Academic Press.

Al-Worafi, Y.M., Alseragi, W.M., Ming, L.C., & Alakhali, K.M. (2020a). Drug safety in China. In *Drug Safety in Developing Countries* (pp. 381–388). Academic Press.

Al-Worafi, Y.M., Alseragi, W.M., Alakhali, K.M., Ming, L.C., Othman, G., Halboup, A.M., ... & Elkalmi, R.M. (2020b). Knowledge, beliefs and factors affecting the use of generic medicines among patients in Ibb, Yemen: a mixed-method study. *Journal of Pharmacy Practice and Community Medicine*, 6(4), 53–56.

Al-Worafi, Y.M., Elkalmi, R.M., Ming, L.C., Othman, G., Halboup, A.M., Battah, M.M., ... & Mani, V. (2021a). Dispensing errors in hospital pharmacies: A prospective study in Yemen. *AlQalam Journal of Medical and Applied Sciences*, 4, 13–17.

Al-Worafi, Y.M., Hasan, S., Hassan, N.M., & Gaili, A.A. (2021b). Knowledge, attitude and experience of pharmacist in the UAE towards pharmacovigilance. *Research Journal of Pharmacy and Technology*, 14(1), 265–269.

Al-Worafi, Y. (2022a). *A Guide to Online Pharmacy Education: Teaching Strategies and Assessment Methods*. CRC Press.

Al-Worafi, Y.M. (2022b). Patient care errors and related problems (part I): development and validation of the model. (Preprint). 0000-0002-5752-2913

Al-Worafi, Y.M. (Ed.). (2023). *Clinical Case Studies on Medication Safety*. Academic Press.

Baig, M.R., Al-Worafi, Y.M., Alseragi, W.M., Ming, L.C., & Siddique, A. (2020). Drug safety in India. In *Drug Safety in Developing Countries* (pp. 327–334). Academic Press.

Elkalmi, R.M., Al-Worafi, Y.M., Alseragi, W.M., Ming, L.C., & Siddique, A. (2020). Drug safety in Malaysia. In *Drug Safety in Developing Countries* (pp. 245–253). Academic Press.

Elsayed, T., & Al-Worafi, Y.M. (2020). Drug safety in Egypt. In *Drug Safety in Developing Countries* (pp. 511–523). Academic Press.

Hasan, S., Al-Omar, M.J., AlZubaidy, H., & Al-Worafi, Y.M. (2019). Use of medications in Arab countries. *Handbook of Healthcare in the Arab World*. Cham: Springer, 42.

Hassan, Y., Abd Aziz, N., Kassab, Y.W., Elgasim, I., Shaharuddin, S., Al-Worafi, Y.M.A., ... & Ming, L.C. (2014). How to help patients to control their blood pressure? Blood pressure control and its predictor. *Archives of Pharmacy Practice*, 5(4), 153–161.

Izahar, S., Lean, Q.Y., Hameed, M.A., Murugiah, M.K., Patel, R.P., Al-Worafi, Y.M., ... & Ming, L.C. (2017). Content analysis of mobile health applications on diabetes mellitus. *Frontiers in Endocrinology*, 8, 318.

Kristensen, S., & Bartels, P. (2010). Use of patient safety culture instruments and recommendations. *Aarhus, Denmark, European Society for Quality in HealthCare-Office for Quality Indicators*, 113.

Lee, K.S., Yee, S.M., Zaidi, S.T.R., Patel, R.P., Yang, Q., Al-Worafi, Y.M., & Ming, L.C., 2017. Combating sale of counterfeit and falsified medicines online: a losing battle. *Frontiers in Pharmacology*, 8, 268.

Mahmoud, M.A., Wajid, S., Naqvi, A.A., Samreen, S., Althagfan, S.S., & Al-Worafi, Y. (2020). Self-medication with antibiotics: a cross-sectional community-based study. *Latin American Journal of Pharmacy*, 39(2), 348–353.

Manan, M.M., Rusli, R.A., Ang, W.C., Al-Worafi, Y.M., & Ming, L.C. (2014). Assessing the pharmaceutical care issues of antiepileptic drug therapy in hospitalised epileptic patients. *Journal of Pharmacy Practice and Research*, 44(3), 83–88.

Manan, M.M., Ibrahim, N.A., Aziz, N.A., Zulkifly, H.H., Al-Worafi, Y.M.A., & Long, C.M. (2016). Empirical use of antibiotic therapy in the prevention of early onset sepsis in neonates: a pilot study. *Archives of Medical Science*, 12(3), 603–613.

Ming, L.C., Hameed, M.A., Lee, D.D., Apidi, N.A., Lai, P.S.M., Hadi, M.A., Al-Worafi, Y.M.A., & Khan, T.M., (2016). Use of medical mobile applications among hospital pharmacists in Malaysia. *Therapeutic Innovation & Regulatory Science*, 50(4), 419–426.

Ming, L.C., Untong, N., Aliudin, N.A., Osili, N., Kifli, N., Tan, C.S., ... & Goh, H.P. (2020). Mobile health apps on COVID-19 launched in the early days of the pandemic: content analysis and review. *JMIR mHealth and uHealth*, 8(9), e19796.

Othman, G., Ali, F., Ibrahim, M.I.M., Al-Worafi, Y.M., Ansari, M., & Halboup, A.M. (2020). Assessment of anti-diabetic medications adherence among diabetic patients in Sana'a City, Yemen: a cross sectional study. *Journal of Pharmaceutical Research International*, 32(21), 114–122.

Reynard, J., Reynolds, J., & Stevenson, P. (2009). *Practical Patient Safety*. OUP Oxford.

Saeed, M.S., Alkhoshaiban, A.S., Al-Worafi, Y.M.A., & Long, C.M., (2014). Perception of self-medication among university students in Saudi Arabia. *Archives of Pharmacy Practice*, 5(4), 149.

Salas, E., & Frush, K. (2012). *Improving Patient Safety through Teamwork and Team Training*. Oxford University Press.

Vincent, C. (2011). *Patient Safety*. John Wiley & Sons.

33 Patient Safety for Special Populations

Adolescents

33.1 BACKGROUND

Adolescents are young people who are in the stage of development between childhood and adulthood, typically between the ages of 10 and 19 years old. This period is characterized by significant physical, cognitive, emotional, and social changes, as well as a search for personal identity and a desire for independence. During adolescence, individuals may experience rapid physical growth and changes, including the development of secondary sexual characteristics. This stage is also marked by changes in cognitive abilities, such as an increased ability for abstract reasoning and the development of more complex thinking skills. Emotionally, adolescents may experience a wide range of feelings and mood swings as they navigate the challenges of adolescence. Socially, they may seek out new peer groups and relationships as they strive for independence and autonomy from their parents or caregivers.

Adolescence is a critical period of development, and the experiences that adolescents have during this time can have a lasting impact on their adult lives. As such, it is important for parents, caregivers, and educators to provide support and guidance to adolescents as they navigate the challenges of this stage of life. Patient care and safety are important considerations for adolescents, as this age group is particularly vulnerable to a variety of physical, emotional, and social challenges. Here are some key factors to consider when providing care to adolescents:

1. Communication: Effective communication is crucial when caring for adolescents. It is important to establish a rapport with the patient and to listen to their concerns and needs. Adolescents may be reluctant to share information with healthcare providers, so it is essential to create a safe and non-judgmental environment to encourage open communication.

2. Confidentiality: Adolescents value their privacy and confidentiality, and it is important to respect their rights in this regard. Healthcare providers should explain the limits of confidentiality, such as when there is a risk of harm to the patient or others, but otherwise, they should keep patient information confidential.

3. Developmental considerations: Adolescents are still developing physically, cognitively, and emotionally. Healthcare providers should take into account the unique needs of this age group, such as the need for age-appropriate explanations of medical conditions and treatments.

4. Mental health: Adolescents may be at risk for a variety of mental health conditions, such as depression, anxiety, and eating disorders. It is important to screen for these conditions and to provide appropriate support and treatment.

5. Social and environmental factors: Adolescents may be at risk for a variety of social and environmental factors that can impact their health, such as substance abuse, peer pressure, and poverty. Healthcare providers should be aware of these risk factors and provide appropriate interventions and referrals as needed.

6. Safety: Adolescents may engage in risky behaviors that can put their health and safety at risk, such as substance abuse, unprotected sex, and reckless driving. Healthcare providers should provide education and counseling on these topics and promote healthy and safe behaviors.

Overall, providing care to adolescents requires a holistic approach that takes into account their physical, emotional, and social needs. Effective communication, confidentiality, developmental considerations, mental health, social and environmental factors, and safety are all important factors to consider when providing care to adolescents (Kristensen & Bartels, 2010; Reynard et al., 2009; Salas & Frush, 2012; Vincent, 2011).

33.2 PATIENT SAFETY FOR ADOLESCENTS: Errors and Related Problems

Patient safety is an important consideration for adolescents, as they may be at risk for a variety of errors and related problems when receiving healthcare. Here are some common errors and related problems that can occur:

DOI: 10.1201/9781003230465-35

1. Medication errors: Adolescents may have difficulty following medication schedules or understanding the dosages and potential side effects of their medications. Healthcare providers should provide clear instructions and follow-up monitoring to prevent medication errors.

2. Miscommunication: Adolescents may have difficulty communicating their needs and concerns to healthcare providers, or healthcare providers may not communicate effectively with them. Miscommunication can lead to errors in diagnosis and treatment, as well as delays in care.

3. Lack of follow-up: Adolescents may not follow up with healthcare providers after receiving initial care, which can lead to missed diagnoses, untreated conditions, and complications.

4. Inadequate screening: Adolescents may not receive adequate screening for mental health conditions, substance abuse, and other risk factors, which can lead to missed diagnoses and delayed treatment.

5. Infection control: Adolescents may be at risk for infections related to healthcare settings, such as healthcare-associated infections, due to their immune systems being still developing, poor hygiene, and close contact with peers.

6. Lack of awareness of patient rights: Adolescents may not be aware of their rights as patients, including the right to informed consent, confidentiality, and access to their medical records. Healthcare providers should inform them of their rights and ensure that they are respected.

Overall, it is important for healthcare providers to be aware of the unique needs and risks of adolescents when providing care. Clear communication, follow-up monitoring, adequate screening, infection control, and awareness of patient rights are all important considerations for promoting patient safety in this population.

33.3 PATIENT SAFETY FOR ADOLESCENTS: Causes

There are several causes that can compromise patient safety for adolescents. Some of the most common causes include:

1. Communication breakdown: Adolescents may not communicate effectively about their symptoms, health concerns, or medication history, which can lead to misdiagnosis or inappropriate treatment.

2. Lack of education: Adolescents may not have enough knowledge about their health conditions, treatment options, or how to manage their health on a day-to-day basis. This can lead to poor adherence to treatment plans, missed appointments, or medication errors.

3. Risk-taking behavior: Adolescents are known for engaging in risky behaviors, such as using drugs or alcohol, not wearing seatbelts, or having unprotected sex. These behaviors can lead to injuries, illnesses, or chronic health conditions.

4. Mental health issues: Adolescents may struggle with mental health issues, such as depression, anxiety, or substance abuse, which can affect their ability to manage their health and make informed decisions about their care.

5. Social determinants of health: Adolescents from disadvantaged backgrounds may face a range of social determinants of health, such as poverty, lack of access to healthcare, or inadequate housing. These factors can impact their overall health and safety.

6. Systemic issues: The healthcare system may not be designed to meet the unique needs of adolescents, which can lead to gaps in care, miscommunication, or inadequate support.

Addressing these causes requires a multifaceted approach that involves improving communication, increasing education, addressing risk-taking behavior, providing mental health support, addressing social determinants of health, and improving the healthcare system to better meet the needs of adolescents.

33.4 PATIENT SAFETY FOR ADOLESCENTS: Prevention

Preventing patient safety issues for adolescents requires a multi-pronged approach that addresses the unique needs and challenges of this age group. Some key prevention strategies include:

1. Education: Providing adolescents with accurate and age-appropriate information about their health conditions, treatment options, and how to manage their health on a day-to-day basis can improve their understanding and engagement in their care.

2. Communication: Encouraging open and honest communication between adolescents, their families, and healthcare providers can help identify potential safety issues and ensure that the right care is provided at the right time.

3. Risk assessment: Conducting routine risk assessments, such as screenings for mental health issues, substance abuse, or risky behaviors, can help identify potential safety issues before they become a problem.

4. Support for mental health: Providing access to mental health resources, such as counseling or therapy, can help adolescents manage mental health issues that can impact their overall health and safety.

5. Patient-centered care: Adopting a patient-centered approach to care that focuses on the needs and preferences of adolescents can improve engagement and satisfaction with care, which can improve safety outcomes.

6. Addressing social determinants of health: Identifying and addressing social determinants of health, such as poverty or lack of access to healthcare, can improve overall health outcomes for adolescents and reduce the risk of safety issues.

7. Improving the healthcare system: Implementing policies and practices that are designed to meet the unique needs of adolescents, such as providing more youth-friendly environments, can improve safety outcomes and increase engagement in care.

By implementing these prevention strategies, healthcare providers can help ensure that adolescents receive safe, effective, and patient-centered care that meets their unique needs and challenges.

33.5 PATIENT SAFETY FOR ADOLESCENTS IN DEVELOPING COUNTRIES: Challenges and Recommendations

Adolescents in developing countries face numerous challenges when it comes to their safety, and patient safety is no exception. Below are some of the challenges and recommendations to address patient safety for adolescents in developing countries.

Challenges:

1. Limited access to healthcare services: Adolescents in developing countries may not have access to quality healthcare services due to limited resources, infrastructure, and healthcare professionals. This can lead to delayed or inadequate treatment, misdiagnosis, or inappropriate treatment.

2. Lack of awareness: Adolescents and their families may lack awareness about health issues and safety measures, leading to noncompliance with treatment and unsafe practices.

3. Stigma and discrimination: Adolescents may face stigma and discrimination when seeking healthcare services, particularly for sensitive issues such as sexual and reproductive health.

4. Poor medication management: There may be inadequate regulation of medication, leading to counterfeit or substandard medication, medication errors, and adverse drug reactions.

Recommendations:

1. Increase access to healthcare services: Governments, donors, and healthcare organizations should invest in building healthcare infrastructure, training healthcare professionals, and implementing policies that prioritize adolescent health.

2. Improve health education: Health education programs should be implemented to improve awareness about health issues and safety measures, as well as encourage active participation in their own health care.

3. Address stigma and discrimination: Healthcare providers should be trained to provide non-judgmental care and respect adolescents' autonomy and confidentiality. Advocacy efforts should be made to reduce stigma and discrimination against adolescents.

4. Strengthen medication management: Governments and healthcare organizations should implement regulations to ensure the quality and safety of medication. Healthcare providers should also be trained to prevent medication errors and manage adverse drug reactions.

5. Encourage youth participation: Adolescents should be involved in the development of healthcare policies and programs that affect their health. They should be encouraged to participate in healthcare decision-making and advocacy efforts to improve their own safety and well-being.

6. Lack of privacy: In many healthcare settings, privacy may be limited, and adolescents may not feel comfortable discussing sensitive issues with healthcare providers.

7. Limited mental health services: Adolescents in developing countries may not have access to mental health services, and may not receive adequate treatment for mental health issues such as depression, anxiety, and substance abuse.

8. Lack of health insurance: Many adolescents in developing countries do not have health insurance, and may face financial barriers to accessing healthcare services.

9. Cultural and social barriers: Cultural and social norms may prevent adolescents, particularly girls, from seeking healthcare services, and may lead to delayed treatment or avoidance of treatment altogether.

10. Malnutrition: Adolescents in developing countries may be at risk of malnutrition due to poverty, lack of access to nutritious food, and inadequate healthcare services.

11. Infectious diseases: Adolescents in developing countries may be at risk of infectious diseases such as malaria, tuberculosis, and HIV/AIDS, which can be exacerbated by poor living conditions, inadequate sanitation, and limited access to healthcare.

12. Violence: Adolescents may be at risk of physical, sexual, and emotional violence, including gender-based violence, which can lead to physical and mental health consequences.

13. Substance abuse: Adolescents may engage in substance abuse due to peer pressure, stress, or lack of education about the risks and consequences of drug use.

14. Limited access to clean water: Adolescents may face challenges in accessing clean and safe drinking water, which can lead to water-borne diseases such as diarrhea, cholera, and typhoid fever.

15. Road traffic accidents: Adolescents may be at risk of road traffic accidents due to inadequate infrastructure, lack of road safety measures, and risky behaviors such as speeding and drunk driving.

16. Occupational hazards: Adolescents may be engaged in hazardous work, such as mining or farming, which can lead to injuries, disabilities, and long-term health consequences.

17. Natural disasters and emergencies: Adolescents may be at risk during natural disasters and emergencies, such as earthquakes, floods, and conflict, which can lead to injuries, displacement, and mental health consequences.

18. Despite the progress in research about the patient care and safety in developing countries, there is little research about the patient safety related to the adolescents in majority of developing countries, therefore, conduct research is very important and highly recommended (Alshahrani et al., 2019a,b; Al-Qahtani et al., 2015; Alshahrani et al., 2020a,b; Al-Worafi, 2014; Al-Worafi, 2015; Al-Worafi, 2016; Al-Worafi et al., 2017; Al-Worafi, 2018a-d; Al-Worafi et al., 2018a-b; Al-Worafi et al., 2019; Al-Worafi, 2020a-y; Al-Worafi et al., 2020a-b; Al-Worafi et al., 2021a,b; Al-Worafi, 2022a,b; Al-Worafi, 2023; Baig et al., 2020; Elkalmi et al., 2020; Elsayed & Al-Worafi, 2020; Hasan et al., 2019; Hassan et al., 2014; Izahar et al., 2017; Lee et al., 2017; Mahmoud et al., 2020; Manan et al., 2014; Manan et al., 2016; Ming et al., 2016; Ming et al., 2020; Othman et al., 2020; Saeed et al., 2014).

33.6 CONCLUSION

This chapter has discussed the patient safety issues related to the adolescents population, prevention, challenges and recommendations for the best practice in developing countries.

REFERENCES

Al-Qahtani, I., Almoteb, T.M., & Al-Warafi, Y. (2015). Competency of metered-dose inhaler use among Saudi community pharmacists: A Simulation method study. *RRJPPS*, 4(2), 37–31.

Alshahrani, S.M., Alakhali, K.M., & Al-Worafi, Y.M., (2019a). Medication errors in a health care facility in southern Saudi Arabia. *Tropical Journal of Pharmaceutical Research*, 18(5), 1119–1122.

Alshahrani, S.M., Alavudeen, S.S., Alakhali, K.M., Al-Worafi, Y.M., Bahamdan, A.K., & Vigneshwaran, E., (2019b). Self-medication among King Khalid University Students, Saudi Arabia. *Risk Management and Healthcare Policy*, 12, 243–249.

Alshahrani, S.M., Alakhali, K.M., Al-Worafi, Y.M., & Alshahrani, N.Z. (2020a). Awareness and use of over the counter analgesic medication: a survey in the Aseer region population, Saudi Arabia. *International Journal of Advances in Applied Sciences*, 7(3), 130–134.

Alshahrani, S.M., Alzahran, M., Alakhali, K., Vigneshwaran, E., Iqbal, M.J., Khan, N.A., ... & Alavudeen, S.S. (2020b). Association between diabetes consequences and quality of life among patients with diabetes mellitus in the Aseer Province of Saudi Arabia. *Open Access Macedonian Journal of Medical Sciences*, 8(E), 325–330.

Al-Worafi, Y.M. (2014). Prescription writing errors at a tertiary care hospital in Yemen: prevalence, types, causes and recommendations. *American Journal of Pharmacy and Health Research*, 2, 134–140.

Al-Worafi, Y.M.A. (2015). Appropriateness of metered-dose inhaler use in the Yemeni community pharmacies. *Journal of Taibah University Medical Sciences*, 10(3), 353–358.

Al-Worafi, Y.M.A., (2016). Pharmacy practice in Yemen. In *Pharmacy Practice in Developing Countries* (pp. 267–287). Academic Press.

Al-Worafi, Y.M., Kassab, Y.W., Alseragi, W.M., Almutairi, M.S., Ahmed, A., Ming, L.C., Alkhoshaiban, A.S., & Hadi, M.A., (2017). Pharmacovigilance and adverse drg reaction reporting: a perspective of community pharmacists and pharmacy technicians in Sana'a, Yemen. *Therapeutics and Clinical Risk Management*, 13, 1175.

Al-Worafi, Y.M., (2018a). Knowledge, attitude and practice of Yemeni physicians toward pharmacovigilance: a mixed method study. *International Journal of Pharmacy and Pharmaceutical Sciences*, 10(10), 74–77.

Al-Worafi, Y. (2018b). Knowledge, attitude and practice of Yemeni physicians toward pharmacovigilance: a mixed method study. *International Journal of Pharmacy and Pharmaceutical Sciences*, 10, 74–77.

Al-Worafi, Y.M. (2018c). Dispensing errors observed by community pharmacy dispensers in IBB–YEMEN. *Asian Journal of Pharmaceutical and Clinical Research*, 11(11).

Al-Worafi, Y.M. (2018d). Evauation of inhaler technique among patients with asthma and COPD in Yemen. *Journal of Taibah University medical sciences*, 13(5), 488–490.

Al-Worafi, Y.M., Patel, R.P., Zaidi, S.T.R., Alseragi, W.M., Almutairi, M.S., Alkhoshaiban, A.S., & Ming, L.C. (2018a). Completeness and legibility of handwritten prescriptions in Sana'a, Yemen. *Medical Principles and Practice*, 27, 290–292.

Al-Worafi, Y.M., Alseragi, W.M., Seng, L.K., Kassab, Y.W., Yeoh, S.F., Chiau, L., ... & Husain, K. (2018b). Dispensing errors in community pharmacies: a prospective study in Sana'a, Yemen. *Archives of Pharmacy Practice*, 9(4), 1–3.

Al-Worafi, Y.M., Alseragi, W.M., & Mahmoud, M.A. (2019). Competency of metered-dose inhaler use among community pharmacy dispensers in Ibb, Yemen: A simulation method study. *Latin American Journal of Pharmacy*, 38(3), 489–494.

Al-Worafi, Y.M. (Ed.). (2020a). *Drug Safety in Developing Countries: Achievements and Challenges.*

Al-Worafi, Y.M. (2020b). Medication errors. In *Drug Safety in Developing Countries* (pp. 105–117). Academic Press.

Al-Worafi, Y.M. (2020c). Adverse drug reactions. In *Drug Safety in Developing Countries* (pp. 39–57). Academic Press.

Al-Worafi, Y.M. (2020d). Medications registration and marketing: safety-related issues. In *Drug Safety in Developing Countries* (pp. 21–28). Academic Press.

Al-Worafi, Y.M. (2020e). Pharmacovigilance. In *Drug Safety in Developing Countries* (pp. 29–38). Academic Press.

Al-Worafi, Y.M. (2020f). Drug-related problems. In *Drug Safety in Developing Countries* (pp. 59–71). Academic Press.

Al-Worafi, Y.M. (2020g). Medications safety-related terminology. In *Drug Safety in Developing Countries* (pp. 7–19). Academic Press.

Al-Worafi, Y.M. (2020h). Self-medication. In *Drug Safety in Developing Countries* (pp. 73–86). Academic Press.

Al-Worafi, Y.M. (2020i). Antibiotics safety issues. In *Drug Safety in Developing Countries* (pp. 87–103). Academic Press.

Al-Worafi, Y.M. (2020j). Medications safety research issues. In *Drug Safety in Developing Countries* (pp. 213–227). Academic Press.

Al-Worafi, Y.M. (2020k). Counterfeit and substandard medications. In *Drug Safety in Developing Countries* (pp. 119–126). Academic Press.

Al-Worafi, Y.M. (2020l). Medication abuse and misuse. In *Drug Safety in Developing Countries* (pp. 127–135). Academic Press.

Al-Worafi, Y.M. (2020m). Storage and disposal of medications. In *Drug Safety in Developing Countries* (pp. 137–142). Academic Press.

Al-Worafi, Y.M. (2020n). Safety of medications in special population. In *Drug Safety in Developing Countries* (pp. 143–162). Academic Press.

Al-Worafi, Y.M. (2020o). Herbal medicines safety issues. In *Drug Safety in Developing Countries* (pp. 163–178). Academic Press.

Al-Worafi, Y.M. (2020p). Medications safety pharmacoeconomics-related issues. In *Drug Safety in Developing Countries* (pp. 187–195). Academic Press.

Al-Worafi, Y.M. (2020q). Evidence-based medications safety practice. In *Drug Safety in Developing Countries* (pp. 197–201). Academic Press.

Al-Worafi, Y.M. (2020r). Quality indicators for medications safety. In *Drug Safety in Developing Countries* (pp. 229–242). Academic Press.

Al-Worafi, Y.M. (2020s). Drug safety in Yemen. In *Drug Safety in Developing Countries* (pp. 391–405). Academic Press.

Al-Worafi, Y.M. (2020t). Drug safety in Saudi Arabia. In *Drug Safety in Developing Countries* (pp. 407–417). Academic Press.

Al-Worafi, Y.M. (2020u). Drug safety in United Arab Emirates. In *Drug Safety in Developing Countries* (pp. 419–428). Academic Press.

Al-Worafi, Y.M. (2020v). Drug safety in Indonesia. In *Drug Safety in Developing Countries* (pp. 279–285). Academic Press.

Al-Worafi, Y.M. (2020w). Drug safety in Palestine. In *Drug Safety in Developing Countries* (pp. 471–480). Academic Press.

Al-Worafi, Y.M. (2020x). Drug safety: comparison between developing countries. In *Drug Safety in Developing Countries* (pp. 603–611). Academic Press.

Al-Worafi, Y.M. (2020y). Drug safety in developing versus developed countries. In *Drug Safety in Developing Countries* (pp. 613–615). Academic Press.

Al-Worafi, Y.M., Alseragi, W.M., Ming, L.C., & Alakhali, K.M. (2020a). Drug safety in China. In *Drug Safety in Developing Countries* (pp. 381–388). Academic Press.

Al-Worafi, Y.M., Alseragi, W.M., Alakhali, K.M., Ming, L.C., Othman, G., Halboup, A.M., … & Elkalmi, R.M. (2020b). Knowledge, beliefs and factors affecting the use of generic medicines among patients in Ibb, Yemen: a mixed-method study. *Journal of Pharmacy Practice and Community Medicine*, 6(4).

Al-Worafi, Y.M., Elkalmi, R.M., Ming, L.C., Othman, G., Halboup, A.M., Battah, M.M., … & Mani, V. (2021a). Dispensing errors in hospital pharmacies: A prospective study in Yemen.

Al-Worafi, Y.M., Hasan, S., Hassan, N.M., & Gaili, A.A. (2021b). Knowledge, Attitude and Experience of Pharmacist in the UAE towards Pharmacovigilance. *Research Journal of Pharmacy and Technology*, 14(1), 265–269.

Al-Worafi, Y. (2022a). *A Guide to Online Pharmacy Education: Teaching Strategies and Assessment Methods*. CRC Press.

Al-Worafi, Y.M. (2022b). Patient care errors and related problems (part I): development and validation of the model. 0000-0002-5752-2913

Al-Worafi, Y.M. (Ed.). (2023). *Clinical Case Studies on Medication Safety*. Academic Press.

Baig, M.R., Al-Worafi, Y.M., Alseragi, W.M., Ming, L.C., & Siddique, A. (2020). Drug safety in India. In *Drug Safety in Developing Countries* (pp. 327–334). Academic Press.

Elkalmi, R.M., Al-Worafi, Y.M., Alseragi, W.M., Ming, L.C., & Siddique, A. (2020). Drug safety in Malaysia. In *Drug Safety in Developing Countries* (pp. 245–253). Academic Press.

Elsayed, T., & Al-Worafi, Y.M. (2020). Drug safety in Egypt. In *Drug Safety in Developing Countries* (pp. 511–523). Academic Press.

Hasan, S., Al-Omar, M.J., AlZubaidy, H., & Al-Worafi, Y.M. (2019). Use of medications in Arab Countries. *Handbook of Healthcare in the Arab World*. Cham: Springer, 42.

Hassan, Y., Abd Aziz, N., Kassab, Y.W., Elgasim, I., Shaharuddin, S., Al-Worafi, Y.M.A., ... & Ming, L.C. (2014). How to help patients to control their blood pressure? Blood pressure control and its predictor. *Archives of Pharmacy Practice*, 5(4).

Izahar, S., Lean, Q.Y., Hameed, M.A., Murugiah, M.K., Patel, R.P., Al-Worafi, Y.M., ... & Ming, L.C. (2017). Content analysis of mobile health applications on diabetes mellitus. *Frontiers in Endocrinology*, 8, 318.

Kristensen, S., & Bartels, P. (2010). Use of patient safety culture instruments and recommendations. *Aarhus, Denmark, European Society for Quality in HealthCare-Office for Quality Indicators*, 113.

Lee, K.S., Yee, S.M., Zaidi, S.T.R., Patel, R.P., Yang, Q., Al-Worafi, Y.M., & Ming, L.C., 2017. Combating sale of counterfeit and falsified medicines online: a losing battle. *Frontiers in Pharmacology*, 8, p. 268.

Mahmoud, M.A., Wajid, S., Naqvi, A.A., Samreen, S., Althagfan, S.S., & Al-Worafi, Y. (2020). Self-medication with antibiotics: a cross-sectional community-based study. *Latin American Journal of Pharmacy*, 39(2), 348–353.

Manan, M.M., Rusli, R.A., Ang, W.C., Al-Worafi, Y.M., & Ming, L.C. (2014). Assessing the pharmaceutical care issues of antiepileptic drug therapy in hospitalised epileptic patients. *Journal of Pharmacy Practice and Research*, 44(3), 83–88.

Manan, M.M., Ibrahim, N.A., Aziz, N.A., Zulkifly, H.H., Al-Worafi, Y.M.A., & Long, C.M. (2016). Empirical use of antibiotic therapy in the prevention of early onset sepsis in neonates: a pilot study. *Archives of Medical Science*, 12(3), 603–613.

Ming, L.C., Hameed, M.A., Lee, D.D., Apidi, N.A., Lai, P.S.M., Hadi, M.A., Al-Worafi, Y.M.A., & Khan, T.M., (2016). Use of medical mobile applications among hospital pharmacists in Malaysia. *Therapeutic Innovation & Regulatory Science*, 50(4), 419–426.

Ming, L.C., Untong, N., Aliudin, N.A., Osili, N., Kifli, N., Tan, C.S., ... & Goh, H.P. (2020). Mobile health apps on COVID-19 launched in the early days of the pandemic: content analysis and review. *JMIR mHealth and uHealth*, 8(9), e19796.

Othman, G., Ali, F., Ibrahim, M.I.M., Al-Worafi, Y.M., Ansari, M., & Halboup, A.M. (2020). Assessment of anti-diabetic medications adherence among diabetic patients in Sana'a City, Yemen: a cross sectional study. *Journal of Pharmaceutical Research International*, 32(21), 114–122.

Reynard, J., Reynolds, J., & Stevenson, P. (2009). *Practical Patient Safety*. OUP Oxford.

Saeed, M.S., Alkhoshaiban, A.S., Al-Worafi, Y.M.A., & Long, C.M., (2014). Perception of self-medication among university students in Saudi Arabia. *Archives of Pharmacy Practice*, 5(4), p. 149.

Salas, E., & Frush, K. (2012). *Improving Patient Safety through Teamwork and Team Training*. Oxford University Press.

Vincent, C. (2011). *Patient Safety*. John Wiley & Sons.

34 Patient Safety during Pandemics

34.1 BACKGROUND

A pandemic is an epidemic of an infectious disease that spreads across a large region, such as multiple continents or even worldwide. Pandemics can have devastating consequences on public health, economies, and social structures. Some well-known pandemics throughout history include the Black Death (bubonic plague) in the 14th century, the Spanish flu in 1918–1919, and more recently, the COVID-19 pandemic that began in 2019. Pandemics can be caused by various infectious agents, such as bacteria, viruses, and fungi. They can spread through different modes of transmission, including respiratory droplets, direct contact with bodily fluids, or contact with contaminated objects. Examples of health pandemics are:

1. COVID-19 pandemic (ongoing)

2. HIV/AIDS pandemic (1981-present)

3. Spanish flu pandemic (1918–1920)

4. Black Death (1346–1353)

5. Cholera pandemic (1817–1824)

6. Polio pandemic (1916–1955)

7. SARS pandemic (2002–2004)

8. MERS pandemic (2012–2015)

9. Ebola pandemic (2014–2016)

10. H1N1 swine flu pandemic (2009–2010)

During a pandemic, patient care and safety become even more critical as healthcare systems face increased demand and challenges in providing care to those affected by the infectious disease. Below are some measures that can be taken to ensure patient care and safety during a pandemic:

1. Proper use of personal protective equipment (PPE): Healthcare workers should use PPE correctly to protect themselves and patients from infection. This includes wearing gloves, masks, gowns, and eye protection, as appropriate.

2. Screening patients: Patients should be screened for symptoms of the infectious disease before entering healthcare facilities to prevent transmission to other patients and healthcare workers.

3. Isolation and cohorting: Patients who test positive for the infectious disease should be isolated from other patients to prevent transmission. Cohorting is the practice of grouping patients with the same infection in the same area to prevent the spread of the disease.

4. Strict infection control measures: Healthcare facilities should implement strict infection control measures, such as frequent cleaning and disinfection, to prevent the spread of the infectious disease.

5. Communication: Healthcare providers should communicate clearly with patients and their families about the infectious disease, its transmission, and the steps being taken to ensure their safety.

6. Telemedicine: Telemedicine can be used to provide care to patients remotely, reducing the risk of transmission to both patients and healthcare workers.

7. Staff training: Healthcare workers should receive proper training on infection control measures, the proper use of PPE, and other safety measures to ensure they can provide safe care during the pandemic.

Patient care and safety during COVID-19 pandemic are of utmost importance to prevent the spread of the virus. Here are some important measures that healthcare providers can take to ensure patient safety during COVID-19 pandemic:

1. Screening: All patients should be screened for COVID-19 symptoms and risk factors before entering the healthcare facility.

DOI: 10.1201/9781003230465-36

2. Personal protective equipment (PPE): Healthcare providers should wear appropriate PPE such as gloves, face shields, gowns, and masks when treating patients with COVID-19.

3. Hand hygiene: Frequent hand hygiene, using soap and water or alcohol-based hand sanitizers, is critical to prevent the spread of COVID-19.

4. Social distancing: Patients should be encouraged to maintain social distancing in waiting rooms, and providers should minimize the number of people in exam rooms.

5. Cleaning and disinfecting: Healthcare facilities should implement enhanced cleaning and disinfecting protocols, paying special attention to high-touch surfaces and equipment.

6. Telehealth: Providers should consider using telehealth services to provide care to patients who do not require in-person visits.

7. Education: Healthcare providers should educate patients on COVID-19 prevention measures, such as hand hygiene, mask wearing, and social distancing (Kristensen & Bartels, 2010; Reynard et al., 2009; Salas & Frush, 2012; Vincent, 2011).

34.2 PATIENT SAFETY DURING PANDEMICS: Errors and Related Problems

Patient safety during pandemics can be affected by several factors, including increased workload, fatigue, stress, and communication barriers. These can lead to errors and related problems that can compromise patient safety. Here are some examples:

1. Misdiagnosis: The symptoms of some pandemics, such as COVID-19, can be similar to other diseases, making it difficult to diagnose correctly. This can lead to incorrect treatment and delayed care, which can affect patient outcomes.

2. Medication errors: The increased workload and stress during pandemics can lead to medication errors, such as administering the wrong medication or dose, which can cause harm to patients.

3. Infection control: Poor infection control practices can lead to the spread of infectious diseases, both within healthcare facilities and in the community.

4. Communication errors: Communication errors between healthcare providers, patients, and families can lead to misunderstandings and errors in care. For example, patients may not understand the instructions for self-isolation or may not report important symptoms to their healthcare providers.

5. Resource allocation: Inadequate resources, such as personal protective equipment (PPE) or ventilators, can compromise patient safety during pandemics. Healthcare providers may be forced to ration resources, which can result in difficult decisions and suboptimal care.

6. Staff burnout: The increased workload and stress during pandemics can lead to staff burnout, which can affect the quality of care provided to patients.

To prevent these errors and related problems, healthcare providers should be trained on pandemic preparedness and infection control measures, and appropriate resources should be allocated to ensure patient safety. Clear communication channels and processes should be established to ensure that patients receive appropriate care and follow-up.

34.3 PATIENT SAFETY DURING PANDEMICS: Causes

Patient safety during pandemics can be compromised due to various causes. Some of the causes are:

1. Increased workload: Healthcare providers often experience increased workload during pandemics, as they have to attend to a larger number of patients, including those with the infectious disease, and provide care in high-stress situations. This can lead to errors and lapses in patient safety.

2. Inadequate resources: Pandemics can lead to shortages of essential resources, such as personal protective equipment (PPE), ventilators, and medications, which can compromise patient safety.

3. Lack of training and education: Healthcare providers may not have adequate training or education on pandemic preparedness, infection control measures, and appropriate use of PPE, which can lead to errors and breaches in patient safety.

4. Communication barriers: Communication barriers between healthcare providers, patients, and families can lead to misunderstandings and errors in care, which can compromise patient safety. This is especially true when there are language or cultural differences.

5. Infection control breaches: Inadequate infection control practices, such as hand hygiene, disinfection, and isolation, can lead to the spread of infectious diseases within healthcare facilities and in the community.

6. Patient behaviors: During pandemics, patients may not disclose their symptoms or exposure to the disease, or they may refuse to follow recommended infection control measures, which can compromise patient safety.

7. Staff shortages: Pandemics can lead to staff shortages due to illness or quarantine, which can lead to increased workload and compromised patient safety.

It is important to address these causes of compromised patient safety during pandemics to prevent errors and ensure appropriate care for patients. This can be achieved through appropriate training and education, allocation of adequate resources, communication and collaboration between healthcare providers and patients, and implementation of infection control measures.

34.4 PATIENT SAFETY DURING PANDEMICS: Prevention

Patient safety during pandemics can be improved through prevention strategies. Here are some ways to prevent errors and ensure patient safety during pandemics:

1. Adequate training and education: Healthcare providers should receive adequate training and education on pandemic preparedness, infection control measures, appropriate use of personal protective equipment (PPE), and patient safety.

2. Communication and collaboration: Effective communication and collaboration between healthcare providers, patients, and families can help prevent errors and ensure appropriate care. Patients should be educated on pandemic prevention measures and encouraged to report symptoms or exposure.

3. Infection control measures: Strict infection control measures should be implemented to prevent the spread of infectious diseases. This includes hand hygiene, use of PPE, disinfection, and isolation.

4. Resource allocation: Adequate resources, such as PPE, ventilators, and medications, should be allocated to ensure patient safety. This can be achieved through stockpiling and distribution planning.

5. Staffing: Appropriate staffing levels should be maintained to prevent staff burnout and ensure adequate patient care.

6. Technology: Technology can be used to improve patient safety during pandemics. For example, telehealth can be used to provide remote care and reduce exposure to infectious diseases.

7. Data collection and analysis: Data collection and analysis can help identify potential patient safety issues and inform prevention strategies during pandemics.

By implementing these prevention strategies, healthcare providers can ensure patient safety during pandemics and minimize the risks of errors and complications.

34.5 PATIENT SAFETY DURING PANDEMICS IN DEVELOPING COUNTRIES:
Challenges and Recommendations

Patient safety during pandemics in developing countries faces unique challenges due to limited resources, inadequate healthcare infrastructure, and poverty. Here are some challenges and recommendations to improve patient safety during pandemics in developing countries:
   Challenges:

1. Inadequate resources: Developing countries often have limited resources to respond to pandemics, such as PPE, ventilators, and medications. This can compromise patient safety and increase the risk of transmission of infectious diseases.

2. Inadequate healthcare infrastructure: Healthcare infrastructure in developing countries may not be equipped to handle a large influx of patients during pandemics. This can lead to overcrowding and compromised patient safety.

3. Limited healthcare workforce: Developing countries often have a shortage of healthcare workers, which can affect patient safety during pandemics.

4. Poverty: Poverty can prevent patients from seeking care or following recommended infection control measures, which can compromise patient safety and increase the risk of transmission of infectious diseases.

Recommendations:

1. Increase resources: Developed countries and international organizations should provide adequate resources, such as PPE, ventilators, and medications, to developing countries to ensure patient safety during pandemics.

2. Strengthen healthcare infrastructure: Investment in healthcare infrastructure is needed to prepare for pandemics in developing countries. This includes building or upgrading hospitals and clinics, increasing the number of hospital beds, and equipping facilities with necessary medical equipment.

3. Expand healthcare workforce: Developing countries should invest in training and educating healthcare workers to increase the number of available staff during pandemics. This includes the deployment of retired healthcare workers and recruitment of volunteers.

4. Address poverty: Efforts to address poverty can help ensure patient safety during pandemics in developing countries. This includes providing financial support to vulnerable populations, such as those who have lost their jobs due to lockdowns or those who are unable to work due to illness.

5. Implement community-based interventions: Community-based interventions can help prevent the spread of infectious diseases and improve patient safety during pandemics in developing countries. This includes educating the public on infection control measures, providing access to PPE and hand hygiene products, and facilitating contact tracing and testing.

6. Limited access to healthcare: Access to healthcare may be limited in developing countries, particularly in rural or remote areas. This can prevent patients from seeking care for pandemic-related illnesses or injuries.

7. Language and cultural barriers: Language and cultural barriers can make it difficult for healthcare providers to communicate with patients during pandemics, which can affect patient safety.

8. Misinformation: Misinformation and rumors can spread quickly during pandemics, leading to confusion and distrust in healthcare providers and recommendations. This can compromise patient safety and increase the spread of infectious diseases.

9. Political instability: Political instability in developing countries can disrupt healthcare systems and compromise patient safety during pandemics. This includes issues such as a lack of government funding, corruption, and violence.

10. Lack of technology infrastructure: Developing countries may not have the technology infrastructure necessary to implement telemedicine or other remote healthcare solutions, which can make it difficult to provide care during pandemics.

11. Lack of coordination: In some developing countries, there may be a lack of coordination and communication between healthcare providers and public health officials during pandemics. This can lead to confusion and delay in response, affecting patient safety.

12. Limited transportation: Limited transportation infrastructure in some developing countries can make it difficult for patients to access healthcare facilities during pandemics. This can lead to delayed or missed care, compromising patient safety.

13. Cultural practices: Cultural practices, such as large gatherings or communal living, can increase the risk of transmission of infectious diseases during pandemics. However, changing these practices may be difficult due to cultural norms and beliefs.

14. Limited access to clean water and sanitation: Access to clean water and sanitation can be limited in developing countries, which can increase the risk of transmission of infectious diseases during pandemics. Lack of access to sanitation can also make it difficult to implement infection control measures.

15. Pre-existing health conditions: Pre-existing health conditions, such as malnutrition or chronic illnesses, can increase the risk of severe illness or death from pandemic-related illnesses. Developing countries may have higher rates of pre-existing health conditions due to limited access to healthcare.

16. Lack of data and surveillance: Developing countries may not have the infrastructure to collect and analyze data on pandemic-related illnesses and deaths, making it difficult to track the spread of disease and respond effectively.

17. Limited availability of vaccines: Developing countries may have limited access to vaccines during pandemics due to a lack of resources or global vaccine distribution inequities. This can affect patient safety and increase the spread of infectious diseases.

18. Limited availability of personal protective equipment (PPE): Developing countries may have limited access to PPE, which can put healthcare providers and patients at risk of infection during pandemics.

19. Health workforce shortages: Developing countries may have shortages of healthcare workers, which can make it difficult to provide care during pandemics. This can also lead to burnout and increased risk of errors or omissions.

20. Limited public health messaging: Developing countries may have limited resources to disseminate public health messaging during pandemics, which can affect patient behavior and compliance with public health guidelines.

21. Inadequate mental health support: Pandemics can have significant mental health impacts, including anxiety, depression, and trauma. Developing countries may have limited resources to provide mental health support during pandemics, which can affect patient safety and well-being.

22. Despite the progress in research about the patient care and safety in developing countries, there is little research about the patient safety related to the pandemics in majority of developing countries, therefore, conduct research is very important and highly recommended (Alshahrani et al., 2019a,b; Al-Qahtani et al., 2015; Alshahrani et al., 2020a,b; Al-Worafi, 2014; Al-Worafi, 2015; Al-Worafi, 2016; Al-Worafi et al., 2017; Al-Worafi, 2018a-d; Al-Worafi et al., 2018a-b; Al-Worafi et al., 2019; Al-Worafi, 2020a-z; Al-Worafi et al., 2020a-b; Al-Worafi et al., 2021a,b; Al-Worafi, 2022a,b; Al-Worafi, 2023; Baig et al., 2020; Elkalmi et al., 2020; Elsayed & Al-Worafi, 2020; Hasan et al., 2019; Hassan et al., 2014; Izahar et al., 2017; Lee et al., 2017; Mahmoud et al., 2020; Manan et al., 2014; Manan et al., 2016; Ming et al., 2016; Ming et al., 2020; Othman et al., 2020; Saeed et al., 2014).

34.6 CONCLUSION

This chapter has discussed the patient safety issues related to the pandemics, prevention, challenges and recommendations for the best practice in developing countries. Patient safety is a critical concern during pandemics in developing countries, and there are a variety of challenges that can affect patient safety. These challenges include limited access to healthcare, language and cultural barriers, misinformation, political instability, lack of technology infrastructure, lack of coordination, limited transportation, cultural practices, limited access to clean water and sanitation, pre-existing health conditions, lack of data and surveillance, limited availability of vaccines, limited availability of PPE, health workforce shortages, limited public health messaging, and inadequate mental health support. To address these challenges, it is important for developing countries to prioritize pandemic preparedness and invest in healthcare infrastructure, education, and resources. Collaboration with international organizations and developed countries can also help provide support and resources during pandemics in developing countries. By working together to address these challenges, we can improve patient safety and minimize the impact of pandemics in developing countries.

REFERENCES

Al-Qahtani, I., Almoteb, T.M., & Al-Warafi, Y. (2015). Competency of metered-dose inhaler use among Saudi community pharmacists: A Simulation method study. *RRJPPS*, 4(2), 37–31.

Alshahrani, S.M., Alakhali, K.M., & Al-Worafi, Y.M., (2019a). Medication errors in a health care facility in southern Saudi Arabia. *Tropical Journal of Pharmaceutical Research*, 18(5), pp. 1119–1122.

Alshahrani, S.M., Alavudeen, S.S., Alakhali, K.M., Al-Worafi, Y.M., Bahamdan, A.K., & Vigneshwaran, E., (2019b). Self-Medication Among King Khalid University Students, Saudi Arabia. *Risk Management and Healthcare Policy*, 12, pp. 243–249.

Alshahrani, S.M., Alakhali, K.M., Al-Worafi, Y.M., & Alshahrani, N.Z. (2020b). Awareness and use of over the counter analgesic medication: a survey in the Aseer region population, Saudi Arabia. *Int J Advan Appl Sci*, 7(3), 130–134.

Alshahrani, S.M., Alzahran, M., Alakhali, K., Vigneshwaran, E., Iqbal, M.J., Khan, N.A., … & Alavudeen, S.S. (2020b). Association Between Diabetes Consequences and Quality of Life Among Patients With Diabetes Mellitus in the Aseer Province of Saudi Arabia. *Open Access Macedonian Journal of Medical Sciences*, 8(E), 325–330.

Al-Worafi, Y.M. (2014). Prescription writing errors at a tertiary care hospital in Yemen: prevalence, types, causes and recommendations. *Am J Pharm Health Res*, 2, 134–140.

Al-Worafi, Y.M.A. (2015). Appropriateness of metered-dose inhaler use in the Yemeni community pharmacies. *Journal of Taibah University Medical Sciences*, 10(3), 353–358.

Al-Worafi, Y.M.A., (2016). Pharmacy practice in Yemen. In *Pharmacy Practice in Developing Countries* (pp. 267–287). Academic Press.

Al-Worafi, Y.M., Kassab, Y.W., Alseragi, W.M., Almutairi, M.S., Ahmed, A., Ming, L.C., Alkhoshaiban, A.S., & Hadi, M.A., (2017). Pharmacovigilance and adverse drg reaction reporting: a perspective of community pharmacists and pharmacy technicians in Sana'a, Yemen. *Therapeutics and clinical risk management*, 13, p. 1175.

Al-Worafi, Y.M., (2018a). Knowledge, Attitude and Practice of Yemeni Physicians Toward Pharmacovigilance: A Mixed Method Study. *International Journal of Pharmacy and Pharmaceutical Sciences*, 10(10), 74–77.

Al-Worafi, Y. (2018b). Knowledge, attitude and practice of Yemeni physicians toward pharmacovigilance: A mixed method study. *Int. J. Pharm. Pharm. Sci*, 10, 74–77.

Al-Worafi, Y.M. (2018c). Dispensing errors observed by community pharmacy dispensers in IBB–YEMEN. *Asian J. Pharm. Clin. Res*, 11(11).

Al-Worafi, Y.M. (2018d). Evauation of inhaler technique among patients with asthma and COPD in Yemen. *Journal of Taibah University medical sciences*, 13(5), 488–490.

Al-Worafi, Y.M., Patel, R.P., Zaidi, S.T.R., Alseragi, W.M., Almutairi, M.S., Alkhoshaiban, A.S., & Ming, L.C. (2018a). Completeness and legibility of handwritten prescriptions in Sana'a, Yemen. *Medical Principles and Practice*, 27, 290–292.

Al-Worafi, Y.M., Alseragi, W.M., Seng, L.K., Kassab, Y.W., Yeoh, S.F., Chiau, L., … & Husain, K. (2018b). Dispensing errors in community pharmacies: a prospective study in Sana'a, Yemen. *Arch Pharm Pract*, 9(4), 1–3.

Al-Worafi, Y.M., Alseragi, W.M., & Mahmoud, M.A. (2019). Competency of metered-dose inhaler use among community pharmacy dispensers in Ibb, Yemen: A simulation method study. *Latin American Journal of Pharmacy*, 38(3), 489–494.

Al-Worafi, Y.M. (Ed.). (2020a). *Drug Safety in Developing Countries: Achievements and Challenges.*

Al-Worafi, Y.M. (2020b). Medication errors. In *Drug Safety in Developing Countries* (pp. 105–117). Academic Press.

Al-Worafi, Y.M. (2020c). Adverse drug reactions. In *Drug Safety in Developing Countries* (pp. 39–57). Academic Press.

Al-Worafi, Y.M. (2020d). Medications registration and marketing: safety-related issues. In *Drug Safety in Developing Countries* (pp. 21–28). Academic Press.

Al-Worafi, Y.M. (2020e). Pharmacovigilance. In *Drug Safety in Developing Countries* (pp. 29–38). Academic Press.

Al-Worafi, Y.M. (2020f). Drug-related problems. In *Drug safety in developing countries* (pp. 59–71). Academic Press.

Al-Worafi, Y.M. (2020g). Medications safety-related terminology. In *Drug safety in developing countries* (pp. 7–19). Academic Press.

Al-Worafi, Y.M. (2020h). Self-medication. In *Drug Safety in Developing Countries* (pp. 73–86). Academic Press.

Al-Worafi, Y.M. (2020j). Antibiotics safety issues. In *Drug Safety in Developing Countries* (pp. 87–103). Academic Press.

Al-Worafi, Y.M. (2020k). Medications safety research issues. In *Drug Safety in Developing Countries* (pp. 213–227). Academic Press.

Al-Worafi, Y.M. (2020l). Counterfeit and substandard medications. In *Drug safety in developing countries* (pp. 119–126). Academic Press.

Al-Worafi, Y.M. (2020m). Medication abuse and misuse. In *Drug safety in developing countries* (pp. 127–135). Academic Press.

Al-Worafi, Y.M. (2020n). Storage and disposal of medications. In *Drug Safety in Developing Countries* (pp. 137–142). Academic Press.

Al-Worafi, Y.M. (2020o). Safety of medications in special population. In *Drug safety in developing countries* (pp. 143–162). Academic Press.

Al-Worafi, Y.M. (2020p). Herbal medicines safety issues. In *Drug Safety in developing countries* (pp. 163–178). Academic Press.

Al-Worafi, Y.M. (2020q). Medications safety pharmacoeconomics-related issues. In *Drug Safety in Developing Countries* (pp. 187–195). Academic Press.

Al-Worafi, Y.M. (2020r). Evidence-based medications safety practice. In *Drug Safety in Developing Countries* (pp. 197–201). Academic Press.

Al-Worafi, Y.M. (2020s). Quality indicators for medications safety. In *Drug safety in developing countries* (pp. 229–242). Academic Press.

Al-Worafi, Y.M. (2020t). Drug safety in Yemen. In *Drug Safety in Developing Countries* (pp. 391–405). Academic Press.

Al-Worafi, Y.M. (2020u). Drug safety in Saudi Arabia. In *Drug Safety in Developing Countries* (pp. 407–417). Academic Press.

Al-Worafi, Y.M. (2020v). Drug safety in United Arab Emirates. In *Drug Safety in Developing Countries* (pp. 419–428). Academic Press.

Al-Worafi, Y.M. (2020w). Drug safety in Indonesia. In *Drug Safety in Developing Countries* (pp. 279–285). Academic Press.

Al-Worafi, Y.M. (2020x). Drug safety in Palestine. In *Drug Safety in Developing Countries* (pp. 471–480). Academic Press.

Al-Worafi, Y.M. (2020y). Drug safety: comparison between developing countries. In *Drug Safety in Developing Countries* (pp. 603–611). Academic Press.

Al-Worafi, Y.M. (2020z). Drug safety in developing versus developed countries. In *Drug Safety in Developing Countries* (pp. 613–615). Academic Press.

Al-Worafi, Y.M., Alseragi, W.M., Ming, L.C., & Alakhali, K.M. (2020a). Drug safety in China. In *Drug Safety in Developing Countries* (pp. 381–388). Academic Press.

Al-Worafi, Y.M., Alseragi, W.M., Alakhali, K.M., Ming, L.C., Othman, G., Halboup, A.M., … & Elkalmi, R.M. (2020b). Knowledge, beliefs and factors affecting the use of generic medicines among patients in Ibb, Yemen: a mixed-method study. *Journal of Pharmacy Practice and Community Medicine*, 6(4).

Al-Worafi, Y.M., Elkalmi, R.M., Ming, L.C., Othman, G., Halboup, A.M., Battah, M.M., … & Mani, V. (2021a). Dispensing errors in hospital pharmacies: A prospective study in Yemen.

Al-Worafi, Y.M., Hasan, S., Hassan, N.M., & Gaili, A.A. (2021b). Knowledge, Attitude and Experience of Pharmacist in the UAE towards Pharmacovigilance. *Research Journal of Pharmacy and Technology*, 14(1), 265–269.

Al-Worafi, Y. (2022a). *A Guide to Online Pharmacy Education: Teaching Strategies and Assessment Methods*. CRC Press.

Al-Worafi, Y.M. (2022b). Patient care errors and related problems (part I): development and validation of the model. 0000-0002-5752-2913

Al-Worafi, Y.M. (Ed.). (2023). *Clinical Case Studies on medication Safety*. Academic Press.

Baig, M.R., Al-Worafi, Y.M., Alseragi, W.M., Ming, L.C., & Siddique, A. (2020). Drug safety in India. In *Drug Safety in Developing Countries* (pp. 327–334). Academic Press.

Elkalmi, R.M., Al-Worafi, Y.M., Alseragi, W.M., Ming, L.C., & Siddique, A. (2020). Drug safety in Malaysia. In *Drug Safety in Developing Countries* (pp. 245–253). Academic Press.

Elsayed, T., & Al-Worafi, Y.M. (2020). Drug safety in Egypt. In *Drug Safety in Developing Countries* (pp. 511–523). Academic Press.

Hasan, S., Al-Omar, M.J., AlZubaidy, H., & Al-Worafi, Y.M. (2019). Use of medications in Arab Countries. *Handbook of Healthcare in the Arab World*. Cham: Springer, 42.

Hassan, Y., Abd Aziz, N., Kassab, Y.W., Elgasim, I., Shaharuddin, S., Al-Worafi, Y.M.A., ... & Ming, L.C. (2014). How to help patients to control their blood pressure? Blood pressure control and its predictor. *Archives of Pharmacy Practice*, 5(4).

Izahar, S., Lean, Q.Y., Hameed, M.A., Murugiah, M.K., Patel, R.P., Al-Worafi, Y.M., ... & Ming, L.C. (2017). Content analysis of mobile health applications on diabetes mellitus. *Frontiers in Endocrinology*, 8, 318.

Kristensen, S., & Bartels, P. (2010). Use of patient safety culture instruments and recommendations. *Aarhus, Denmark, European Society for Quality in HealthCare-Office for Quality Indicators*, 113.

Lee, K.S., Yee, S.M., Zaidi, S.T.R., Patel, R.P., Yang, Q., Al-Worafi, Y.M., & Ming, L.C., 2017. Combating sale of counterfeit and falsified medicines online: a losing battle. *Frontiers in pharmacology*, 8, p. 268.

Mahmoud, M.A., Wajid, S., Naqvi, A.A., Samreen, S., Althagfan, S.S., & Al-Worafi, Y. (2020). Self-medication with antibiotics: A cross-sectional community-based study. *Latin american journal of pharmacy*, 39(2), 348–353.

Manan, M.M., Rusli, R.A., Ang, W.C., Al-Worafi, Y.M., & Ming, L.C. (2014). Assessing the pharmaceutical care issues of antiepileptic drug therapy in hospitalised epileptic patients. *Journal of Pharmacy Practice and Research*, 44(3), 83–88.

Manan, M.M., Ibrahim, N.A., Aziz, N.A., Zulkifly, H.H., Al-Worafi, Y.M.A., & Long, C.M. (2016). Empirical use of antibiotic therapy in the prevention of early onset sepsis in neonates: a pilot study. *Archives of Medical Science*, 12(3), 603–613.

Ming, L.C., Hameed, M.A., Lee, D.D., Apidi, N.A., Lai, P.S.M., Hadi, M.A., Al-Worafi, Y.M.A., & Khan, T.M., (2016). Use of medical mobile applications among hospital pharmacists in Malaysia. *Therapeutic innovation & regulatory science*, 50(4), pp. 419–426.

Ming, L.C., Untong, N., Aliudin, N.A., Osili, N., Kifli, N., Tan, C.S., ... & Goh, H.P. (2020). Mobile health apps on COVID-19 launched in the early days of the pandemic: content analysis and review. *JMIR mHealth and uHealth*, 8(9), e19796.

Othman, G., Ali, F., Ibrahim, M.I.M., Al-Worafi, Y.M., Ansari, M., & Halboup, A.M. (2020). Assessment of Anti-Diabetic Medications Adherence among Diabetic Patients in Sana'a City, Yemen: A Cross Sectional Study. *Journal of Pharmaceutical Research International*, 32(21), 114–122.

Reynard, J., Reynolds, J., & Stevenson, P. (2009). *Practical patient safety*. OUP Oxford.

Saeed, M.S., Alkhoshaiban, A.S., Al-Worafi, Y.M.A., & Long, C.M., (2014). Perception of self-medication among university students in Saudi Arabia. *Archives of Pharmacy Practice*, 5(4), p. 149.

Salas, E., & Frush, K. (2012). *Improving patient safety through teamwork and team training*. Oxford University Press.

Vincent, C. (2011). *Patient safety*. John Wiley & Sons.

35 Patient Safety Training

35.1 BACKGROUND

Patient safety training is an important aspect of healthcare education for healthcare professionals. It is the process of educating healthcare professionals about how to provide safe care to patients and prevent adverse events. Patient safety training covers a range of topics including infection prevention, medication safety, communication, teamwork, and error reporting. It emphasizes the importance of identifying and mitigating risks to patient safety and creating a culture of safety within healthcare organizations. Some key elements of patient safety training may include:

1. Understanding the importance of patient safety and the impact of errors on patients and healthcare organizations.

2. Learning about the systems and processes that support patient safety, such as incident reporting, root cause analysis, and quality improvement.

3. Developing skills in communication and teamwork to improve patient outcomes and reduce the risk of errors.

4. Understanding the principles of infection prevention and control to reduce the risk of healthcare-associated infections.

5. Learning about medication safety, including how to properly prescribe, dispense, and administer medications.

6. Understanding the role of technology in patient safety, including electronic health records, medication management systems, and clinical decision support.

Patient safety training can take many forms, including classroom education, simulation exercises, online learning modules, and hands-on training in clinical settings. It is important for healthcare organizations to provide ongoing patient safety training to ensure that healthcare professionals have the knowledge and skills necessary to provide safe, high-quality care to their patients (Al-Worafi, 2022a,b; Kristensen & Bartels, 2010; Reynard et al., 2009; Salas & Frush, 2012; Vincent, 2011).

35.2 PATIENT SAFETY TRAINING FOR THE MEDICAL STUDENTS

Patient safety is a critical aspect of healthcare, and it is essential that medical students receive appropriate training to ensure that they are equipped with the skills and knowledge needed to provide safe and effective care to their patients. Here are some key elements that should be included in patient safety training for medical students:

1. Understanding the principles of patient safety: Medical students should be introduced to the basic principles of patient safety, including the concepts of error, harm, and risk, and the importance of reporting incidents and near-misses.

2. Teamwork and communication: Effective communication and teamwork are crucial for ensuring patient safety. Medical students should be taught how to communicate effectively with their colleagues and patients, and how to work collaboratively as part of a healthcare team.

3. Human factors: Medical errors often arise from human factors, such as fatigue, stress, and distraction. Medical students should be taught how to recognize and manage these factors to minimize the risk of error.

4. Clinical decision-making: Medical students should be trained in clinical decision-making, including how to identify and manage uncertainty, how to use evidence-based medicine, and how to make informed decisions in the face of complexity.

5. Medication safety: Medication errors are a leading cause of harm to patients. Medical students should be taught how to prescribe and administer medications safely, including how to calculate doses and avoid adverse drug reactions.

6. Patient-centered care: Medical students should be trained to provide patient-centered care, including how to involve patients in their own care, how to respect their autonomy and preferences, and how to communicate effectively with patients and their families.

7. Quality improvement: Medical students should be taught how to identify and analyze quality problems in healthcare, how to implement improvement strategies, and how to measure the impact of these strategies on patient safety.

By including these elements in patient safety training for medical students, we can help ensure that future healthcare providers are equipped with the skills and knowledge needed to provide safe and effective care to their patients

35.3 PATIENT SAFETY TRAINING FOR THE HEALTH CARE PROFESSIONALS

Patient safety is a crucial aspect of healthcare, and it is essential that healthcare professionals receive appropriate training to ensure that they are equipped with the skills and knowledge needed to provide safe and effective care to their patients. Here are some key elements that should be included in patient safety training for healthcare professionals:

1. Understanding the principles of patient safety: Healthcare professionals should be introduced to the basic principles of patient safety, including the concepts of error, harm, and risk, and the importance of reporting incidents and near-misses.

2. Teamwork and communication: Effective communication and teamwork are crucial for ensuring patient safety. Healthcare professionals should be taught how to communicate effectively with their colleagues and patients, and how to work collaboratively as part of a healthcare team.

3. Human factors: Medical errors often arise from human factors, such as fatigue, stress, and distraction. Healthcare professionals should be taught how to recognize and manage these factors to minimize the risk of error.

4. Clinical decision-making: Healthcare professionals should be trained in clinical decision-making, including how to identify and manage uncertainty, how to use evidence-based medicine, and how to make informed decisions in the face of complexity.

5. Medication safety: Medication errors are a leading cause of harm to patients. Healthcare professionals should be taught how to prescribe and administer medications safely, including how to calculate doses and avoid adverse drug reactions.

6. Infection control: Healthcare professionals should be trained in infection control measures to prevent the spread of infections in healthcare settings.

7. Patient-centered care: Healthcare professionals should be trained to provide patient-centered care, including how to involve patients in their own care, how to respect their autonomy and preferences, and how to communicate effectively with patients and their families.

8. Quality improvement: Healthcare professionals should be taught how to identify and analyze quality problems in healthcare, how to implement improvement strategies, and how to measure the impact of these strategies on patient safety.

By including these elements in patient safety training for healthcare professionals, we can help ensure that healthcare providers are equipped with the skills and knowledge needed to provide safe and effective care to their patients. Ongoing training and education are also essential to keep healthcare professionals up to date with the latest advancements and best practices in patient safety.

35.4 RATIONALITY OF THE PATIENT SAFETY TRAINING

Patient safety training is rational for several reasons:

1. It reduces the risk of harm to patients: Patient safety training equips healthcare professionals with the skills and knowledge needed to identify and manage risks, reduce errors, and prevent harm to patients.

2. It improves the quality of care: Patient safety training emphasizes the importance of patient-centered care, teamwork, and communication, which can lead to better outcomes and improved patient satisfaction.

3. It reduces healthcare costs: Medical errors and adverse events can be costly, both in terms of patient outcomes and financial costs. Patient safety training can help reduce these costs by preventing errors and adverse events.

4. It is a legal and ethical responsibility: Healthcare professionals have a legal and ethical responsibility to provide safe and effective care to their patients. Patient safety training helps ensure that healthcare professionals are meeting these responsibilities.

5. It improves the reputation of healthcare organizations: Healthcare organizations that prioritize patient safety and invest in patient safety training are more likely to be viewed positively by patients, regulators, and the public.

In summary, patient safety training is a rational investment for healthcare organizations because it can reduce the risk of harm to patients, improve the quality of care, reduce healthcare costs, meet legal and ethical responsibilities, and improve the reputation of healthcare organizations.

35.5 IMPORTANCE OF THE PATIENT SAFETY TRAINING

Patient safety training is crucial for several reasons:

1. It reduces the risk of harm to patients: Patient safety training equips healthcare professionals with the knowledge and skills to identify and manage risks, reduce errors, and prevent harm to patients.

2. It improves the quality of care: Patient safety training emphasizes the importance of patient-centered care, teamwork, and communication, which can lead to better outcomes and improved patient satisfaction.

3. It promotes a culture of safety: Patient safety training helps create a culture of safety within healthcare organizations, where healthcare professionals prioritize patient safety and are encouraged to report incidents and near-misses.

4. It increases awareness of patient safety issues: Patient safety training raises awareness of patient safety issues among healthcare professionals, patients, and the public, which can help promote better understanding and more effective action to improve patient safety.

5. It is a legal and ethical responsibility: Healthcare professionals have a legal and ethical responsibility to provide safe and effective care to their patients. Patient safety training helps ensure that healthcare professionals are meeting these responsibilities.

6. It improves healthcare outcomes: Patient safety training can lead to improved healthcare outcomes, including reduced morbidity and mortality rates, fewer medical errors, and improved patient satisfaction.

In summary, patient safety training is essential because it reduces the risk of harm to patients, improves the quality of care, promotes a culture of safety, increases awareness of patient safety issues, meets legal and ethical responsibilities, and improves healthcare outcomes.

35.6 FACILITATORS FOR THE PATIENT SAFETY TRAINING

There are several facilitators that can help make patient safety training more effective:

1. Leadership support: Strong support from leadership can help ensure that patient safety training is given a high priority within the organization, and that resources are allocated appropriately.

2. Tailored content: Patient safety training should be tailored to the needs of specific healthcare professionals, taking into account their roles, responsibilities, and levels of experience.

3. Interactive learning: Interactive learning activities, such as role-playing exercises, case studies, and simulations, can help engage healthcare professionals and promote active learning.

4. Continuous education: Patient safety training should be ongoing, with regular updates and refresher courses to keep healthcare professionals up to date with the latest developments and best practices in patient safety.

5. Feedback and evaluation: Regular feedback and evaluation can help healthcare professionals to identify areas for improvement and adjust their practice accordingly.

6. Multi-disciplinary approach: Patient safety training should involve healthcare professionals from different disciplines and specialties, to promote teamwork and collaboration.

7. Recognition and reward: Healthcare professionals who demonstrate a commitment to patient safety should be recognized and rewarded, to encourage and motivate others to prioritize patient safety.

In summary, effective patient safety training requires leadership support, tailored content, interactive learning, continuous education, feedback and evaluation, a multi-disciplinary approach, and recognition and reward for excellence. By incorporating these facilitators, healthcare organizations can help ensure that patient safety training is effective and impactful.

35.7 BARRIERS FOR THE PATIENT SAFETY TRAINING

There are several barriers that can hinder the effectiveness of patient safety training:

1. Lack of resources: Patient safety training can require significant resources, including funding, time, and personnel. Limited resources can make it challenging to provide adequate training to all healthcare professionals who need it.

2. Resistance to change: Resistance to change can be a significant barrier to patient safety training. Healthcare professionals may be reluctant to adopt new practices or change their existing workflows, especially if they are not convinced of the benefits.

3. Lack of engagement: Healthcare professionals who are not engaged in patient safety training may not see its value or be motivated to participate fully. This can result in poor attendance, low participation, and limited uptake of new knowledge and skills.

4. Lack of alignment with organizational priorities: If patient safety training is not aligned with the broader priorities of the organization, it may not receive the necessary support and resources to be effective.

5. Lack of standardized training: Inconsistencies in patient safety training can lead to confusion and inconsistencies in practice, which can compromise patient safety.

6. Time constraints: Healthcare professionals often have demanding schedules and limited time available for training. Patient safety training may be perceived as an additional burden that competes with other priorities.

In summary, barriers to patient safety training can include limited resources, resistance to change, lack of engagement, lack of alignment with organizational priorities, lack of standardized training, and time constraints. Healthcare organizations need to identify and address these barriers to ensure that patient safety training is effective and impactful.

35.8 ONLINE PATIENT SAFETY TRAINING

Online patient safety training is an increasingly popular option for healthcare professionals who need to complete training in a convenient and flexible way. Here are some advantages and disadvantages of online patient safety training:

Advantages:

1. Convenience: Online patient safety training can be completed at any time, from any location with an internet connection, making it a convenient option for busy healthcare professionals.

2. Flexibility: Online patient safety training allows healthcare professionals to complete the training at their own pace, allowing them to balance their training with their other responsibilities.

3. Cost-effective: Online patient safety training can be more cost-effective than traditional in-person training, as it eliminates the need for travel and accommodation expenses.

4. Interactive learning: Many online patient safety training programs use interactive learning tools such as videos, quizzes, and simulations to engage healthcare professionals and reinforce learning.

5. Access to up-to-date information: Online patient safety training programs can be updated regularly to reflect the latest research and best practices in patient safety.

Disadvantages:

1. Limited interaction: Online patient safety training may lack the face-to-face interaction and collaboration opportunities that are available in traditional in-person training programs.

2. Technical issues: Technical issues such as slow internet connections or hardware problems can interrupt the learning process and cause frustration for healthcare professionals.

3. Limited hands-on experience: Some patient safety skills require hands-on practice, which may not be possible in an online training environment.

4. Limited networking opportunities: Online patient safety training may not provide opportunities for healthcare professionals to network and build relationships with colleagues from different disciplines.

In summary, online patient safety training offers several advantages, including convenience, flexibility, cost-effectiveness, interactive learning, and access to up-to-date information. However, it also has some limitations, including limited interaction, technical issues, limited hands-on experience, and limited networking opportunities. Healthcare organizations need to consider these factors when deciding whether online patient safety training is the right option for their needs.

35.9 PATIENT SAFETY TRAINING IN DEVELOPING COUNTRIES: Challenges and Recommendations

Patient safety training in developing countries faces several challenges, including limited resources, lack of infrastructure, cultural barriers, and a shortage of trained healthcare professionals. However, there are several recommendations that can help to address these challenges and promote effective patient safety training:

1. Collaborate with international organizations: Developing countries can collaborate with international organizations to access resources and expertise in patient safety training. These organizations can provide guidance and support in developing and implementing training programs.

2. Develop context-specific training: Patient safety training programs should be tailored to the specific needs and cultural context of the local healthcare system. Training should be designed to address the unique challenges faced by healthcare professionals in developing countries.

3. Emphasize teamwork and communication: Patient safety training should emphasize the importance of teamwork and effective communication among healthcare professionals. This is especially important in developing countries where healthcare professionals often work in challenging conditions and with limited resources.

4. Leverage technology: Technology can be used to overcome some of the challenges of delivering patient safety training in developing countries. For example, online training programs can be used to reach healthcare professionals in remote or hard-to-reach areas.

5. Focus on primary care: Primary care providers are often the first point of contact for patients in developing countries. Therefore, patient safety training should focus on building the capacity of primary care providers to identify and address patient safety issues.

6. Foster a culture of safety: Patient safety training should be integrated into the broader culture of safety within healthcare organizations. This can be achieved by promoting open communication, learning from errors, and encouraging healthcare professionals to report incidents and near misses.

7. Evaluate and monitor progress: Regular evaluation and monitoring of patient safety training programs can help to identify areas for improvement and ensure that the training is having a positive impact on patient safety.

8. Limited funding: Healthcare systems in developing countries often have limited funding for training programs. This can make it difficult to develop and implement effective patient safety training programs.

9. Language barriers: Healthcare professionals in developing countries may not have sufficient proficiency in the language used for training materials. This can make it difficult for them to understand and apply the concepts covered in the training.

10. Limited access to technology: Many healthcare professionals in developing countries have limited access to technology such as computers, smartphones, and high-speed internet. This can make it difficult to access online training materials and resources.

11. Limited availability of trainers: There may be a shortage of trained trainers who can deliver patient safety training programs. This can make it difficult to scale up training programs to reach a large number of healthcare professionals.

12. Resistance to change: Healthcare professionals in developing countries may be resistant to change and may not see patient safety training as a priority. This can make it difficult to encourage participation and engagement in training programs.

13. High staff turnover: Healthcare systems in developing countries may experience high rates of staff turnover, which can make it difficult to maintain consistent patient safety practices and training programs.

14. Limited infrastructure: Healthcare systems in developing countries may have limited infrastructure, including inadequate facilities and equipment. This can make it difficult for healthcare professionals to provide safe and effective care, even with training.

15. Limited access to quality healthcare: Patients in developing countries may have limited access to quality healthcare, which can increase the risk of adverse events. This can make it challenging for healthcare professionals to identify and address patient safety issues.

16. Cultural beliefs and practices: Cultural beliefs and practices can affect patient safety in developing countries. For example, patients may be reluctant to question healthcare professionals or may seek traditional remedies instead of seeking medical care. Healthcare professionals may also have different beliefs and practices that can affect patient safety.

17. Lack of regulatory oversight: Healthcare systems in developing countries may have limited regulatory oversight, which can make it difficult to enforce patient safety standards. This can result in inconsistent quality of care across different healthcare facilities.

18. Limited data on patient safety: There may be limited data on patient safety in developing countries, which can make it difficult to identify and address patient safety issues. This can also make it challenging to measure the impact of patient safety training programs.

19. Political instability: Political instability can affect patient safety training programs in developing countries. This can result in disruptions to healthcare services and a lack of continuity in training programs.

20. Limited public awareness: There may be limited public awareness of patient safety issues in developing countries. This can make it difficult to promote patient safety training programs and encourage patients to be more involved in their own care.

21. Limited resources for monitoring and evaluation: Developing countries may lack the resources and expertise to effectively monitor and evaluate patient safety training programs. This can make it difficult to assess the effectiveness of these programs and make data-driven improvements.

22. Lack of standardization: There may be a lack of standardization in patient safety training programs in developing countries. This can make it difficult for healthcare professionals to transfer knowledge and skills between different healthcare facilities.

23. Limited collaboration between healthcare professionals: Healthcare professionals in developing countries may work in isolation, which can limit opportunities for collaboration and learning. This can make it difficult to share best practices and promote a culture of continuous learning and improvement.

24. Lack of incentives: There may be a lack of incentives for healthcare professionals to participate in patient safety training programs. This can make it challenging to encourage participation and engagement in these programs.

25. Limited access to continuing education: Healthcare professionals in developing countries may have limited access to continuing education opportunities. This can make it difficult to keep up-to-date with the latest patient safety practices and guidelines.

26. Poor working conditions: Healthcare professionals in developing countries may face poor working conditions, including long hours, low pay, and a lack of resources. This can lead to burnout and a lack of motivation to participate in training programs.

27. Limited patient engagement: Patients in developing countries may not be fully engaged in their own care, which can increase the risk of adverse events. This can make it challenging for healthcare professionals to implement patient safety practices and encourage patient participation in safety initiatives.

28. Limited access to essential medicines and equipment: Developing countries may have limited access to essential medicines and equipment, which can increase the risk of adverse events. This can make it challenging for healthcare professionals to provide safe and effective care.

29. Poor communication and information sharing: Healthcare professionals in developing countries may struggle with poor communication and information sharing practices. This can increase the risk of errors and adverse events, and make it challenging to implement patient safety practices.

30. Limited awareness of patient safety: Patient safety may not be a priority for healthcare professionals and policymakers in developing countries. This can make it challenging to promote patient safety training programs and implement patient safety practices.

31. Limited research and evidence base: Developing countries may have limited research and evidence on patient safety practices and interventions. This can make it challenging to identify effective strategies for improving patient safety and implementing evidence-based practices.

32. Limited leadership and governance: Healthcare systems in developing countries may have limited leadership and governance structures in place to promote patient safety. This can make it challenging to implement patient safety training programs and enforce patient safety standards.

33. Despite the progress in research about the patient care and safety in developing countries, there is little research about the patient safety training in developing countries, therefore, conduct research is very important and highly recommended (Alshahrani et al., 2019a,b; Al-Qahtani et al., 2015; Alshahrani et al., 2020a,b; Al-Worafi, 2014; Al-Worafi, 2015; Al-Worafi, 2016; Al-Worafi et al., 2017; Al-Worafi, 2018a-d; Al-Worafi et al., 2018a-b; Al-Worafi et al., 2019; Al-Worafi, 2020a-z; Al-Worafi et al., 2020a-b; Al-Worafi et al., 2021a,b; Al-Worafi, 2022a,b; Al-Worafi, 2023; Baig et al., 2020; Elkalmi et al., 2020; Elsayed & Al-Worafi, 2020; Hasan et al., 2019; Hassan et al., 2014; Izahar et al., 2017; Lee et al., 2017; Mahmoud et al., 2020; Manan et al., 2014; Manan et al., 2016; Ming et al., 2016; Ming et al., 2020; Othman et al., 2020; Saeed et al., 2014).

35.10 CONCLUSION

This chapter has discussed the patient safety training issues in developing countries. Patient safety training is crucial for healthcare professionals to ensure safe and effective care for patients. However, developing countries face unique challenges in implementing patient safety training programs due to factors such as limited resources, inadequate infrastructure, and a lack of standardization. To address these challenges, there needs to be a concerted effort to promote patient safety and implement effective patient safety training programs in developing countries. This will require collaboration between healthcare professionals, policymakers, and other stakeholders to invest in research and evidence, promote patient engagement, improve communication and information sharing practices, and strengthen leadership and governance structures. By addressing these challenges, we can help to ensure that patients in developing countries receive the safe and effective care they deserve.

REFERENCES

Al-Qahtani, I., Almoteb, T.M., & Al-Warafi, Y. (2015). Competency of metered-dose inhaler use among Saudi community pharmacists: A Simulation method study. *RRJPPS*, 4(2), 37–31.

Alshahrani, S.M., Alakhali, K.M., & Al-Worafi, Y.M., (2019a). Medication errors in a health care facility in southern Saudi Arabia. *Tropical Journal of Pharmaceutical Research*, 18(5), pp. 1119–1122.

Alshahrani, S.M., Alavudeen, S.S., Alakhali, K.M., Al-Worafi, Y.M., Bahamdan, A.K., & Vigneshwaran, E., (2019b). Self-Medication Among King Khalid University Students, Saudi Arabia. *Risk Management and Healthcare Policy*, 12, pp. 243–249.

Alshahrani, S.M., Alakhali, K.M., Al-Worafi, Y.M., & Alshahrani, N.Z. (2020b). Awareness and use of over the counter analgesic medication: a survey in the Aseer region population, Saudi Arabia. *Int J Advan Appl Sci*, 7(3), 130–134.

Alshahrani, S.M., Alzahran, M., Alakhali, K., Vigneshwaran, E., Iqbal, M.J., Khan, N.A., ... & Alavudeen, S.S. (2020b). Association Between Diabetes Consequences and Quality of Life Among Patients With Diabetes Mellitus in the Aseer Province of Saudi Arabia. *Open Access Macedonian Journal of Medical Sciences*, 8(E), 325–330.

Al-Worafi, Y.M. (2014). Prescription writing errors at a tertiary care hospital in Yemen: prevalence, types, causes and recommendations. *Am J Pharm Health Res*, 2, 134–140.

Al-Worafi, Y.M.A. (2015). Appropriateness of metered-dose inhaler use in the Yemeni community pharmacies. *Journal of Taibah University Medical Sciences*, 10(3), 353–358.

Al-Worafi, Y.M.A., (2016). Pharmacy practice in Yemen. In *Pharmacy Practice in Developing Countries* (pp. 267–287). Academic Press.

Al-Worafi, Y.M., Kassab, Y.W., Alseragi, W.M., Almutairi, M.S., Ahmed, A., Ming, L.C., Alkhoshaiban, A.S., & Hadi, M.A., (2017). Pharmacovigilance and adverse drg reaction reporting: a perspective of community pharmacists and pharmacy technicians in Sana'a, Yemen. *Therapeutics and clinical risk management*, 13, p. 1175.

Al-Worafi, Y.M., (2018a). Knowledge, Attitude and Practice of Yemeni Physicians Toward Pharmacovigilance: A Mixed Method Study. *International Journal of Pharmacy and Pharmaceutical Sciences*, 10(10), 74–77.

Al-Worafi, Y. (2018b). Knowledge, attitude and practice of Yemeni physicians toward pharmacovigilance: A mixed method study. *Int. J. Pharm. Pharm. Sci*, 10, 74–77.

Al-Worafi, Y.M. (2018c). Dispensing errors observed by community pharmacy dispensers in IBB–YEMEN. *Asian J. Pharm. Clin. Res*, 11(11).

Al-Worafi, Y.M. (2018d). Evauation of inhaler technique among patients with asthma and COPD in Yemen. *Journal of Taibah University medical sciences*, 13(5), 488–490.

Al-Worafi, Y.M., Patel, R.P., Zaidi, S.T.R., Alseragi, W.M., Almutairi, M.S., Alkhoshaiban, A.S., & Ming, L.C. (2018a). Completeness and legibility of handwritten prescriptions in Sana'a, Yemen. *Medical Principles and Practice*, 27, 290–292.

Al-Worafi, Y.M., Alseragi, W.M., Seng, L.K., Kassab, Y.W., Yeoh, S.F., Chiau, L., ... & Husain, K. (2018b). Dispensing errors in community pharmacies: a prospective study in Sana'a, Yemen. *Arch Pharm Pract*, 9(4), 1–3.

Al-Worafi, Y.M., Alseragi, W.M., & Mahmoud, M.A. (2019). Competency of metered-dose inhaler use among community pharmacy dispensers in Ibb, Yemen: A simulation method study. *Latin American Journal of Pharmacy*, 38(3), 489–494.

Al-Worafi, Y.M. (Ed.). (2020a). *Drug Safety in Developing Countries: Achievements and Challenges*.

Al-Worafi, Y.M. (2020b). Medication errors. In *Drug Safety in Developing Countries* (pp. 105–117). Academic Press.

Al-Worafi, Y.M. (2020c). Adverse drug reactions. In *Drug Safety in Developing Countries* (pp. 39–57). Academic Press.

Al-Worafi, Y.M. (2020d). Medications registration and marketing: safety-related issues. In *Drug Safety in Developing Countries* (pp. 21–28). Academic Press.

Al-Worafi, Y.M. (2020e). Pharmacovigilance. In *Drug Safety in Developing Countries* (pp. 29–38). Academic Press.

Al-Worafi, Y.M. (2020f). Drug-related problems. In *Drug safety in developing countries* (pp. 59–71). Academic Press.

Al-Worafi, Y.M. (2020g). Medications safety-related terminology. In *Drug safety in developing countries* (pp. 7–19). Academic Press.

Al-Worafi, Y.M. (2020h). Self-medication. In *Drug Safety in Developing Countries* (pp. 73–86). Academic Press.

Al-Worafi, Y.M. (2020j). Antibiotics safety issues. In *Drug Safety in Developing Countries* (pp. 87–103). Academic Press.

Al-Worafi, Y.M. (2020k). Medications safety research issues. In *Drug Safety in Developing Countries* (pp. 213–227). Academic Press.

Al-Worafi, Y.M. (2020l). Counterfeit and substandard medications. In *Drug safety in developing countries* (pp. 119–126). Academic Press.

Al-Worafi, Y.M. (2020m). Medication abuse and misuse. In *Drug safety in developing countries* (pp. 127–135). Academic Press.

Al-Worafi, Y.M. (2020n). Storage and disposal of medications. In *Drug Safety in Developing Countries* (pp. 137–142). Academic Press.

Al-Worafi, Y.M. (2020o). Safety of medications in special population. In *Drug safety in developing countries* (pp. 143–162). Academic Press.

Al-Worafi, Y.M. (2020p). Herbal medicines safety issues. In *Drug Safety in developing countries* (pp. 163–178). Academic Press.

Al-Worafi, Y.M. (2020q). Medications safety pharmacoeconomics-related issues. In *Drug Safety in Developing Countries* (pp. 187–195). Academic Press.

Al-Worafi, Y.M. (2020r). Evidence-based medications safety practice. In *Drug Safety in Developing Countries* (pp. 197–201). Academic Press.

Al-Worafi, Y.M. (2020s). Quality indicators for medications safety. In *Drug safety in developing countries* (pp. 229–242). Academic Press.

Al-Worafi, Y.M. (2020t). Drug safety in Yemen. In *Drug Safety in Developing Countries* (pp. 391–405). Academic Press.

Al-Worafi, Y.M. (2020u). Drug safety in Saudi Arabia. In *Drug Safety in Developing Countries* (pp. 407–417). Academic Press.

Al-Worafi, Y.M. (2020v). Drug safety in United Arab Emirates. In *Drug Safety in Developing Countries* (pp. 419–428). Academic Press.

Al-Worafi, Y.M. (2020w). Drug safety in Indonesia. In *Drug Safety in Developing Countries* (pp. 279–285). Academic Press.

Al-Worafi, Y.M. (2020x). Drug safety in Palestine. In *Drug Safety in Developing Countries* (pp. 471–480). Academic Press.

Al-Worafi, Y.M. (2020y). Drug safety: comparison between developing countries. In *Drug Safety in Developing Countries* (pp. 603–611). Academic Press.

Al-Worafi, Y.M. (2020z). Drug safety in developing versus developed countries. In *Drug Safety in Developing Countries* (pp. 613–615). Academic Press.

Al-Worafi, Y.M., Alseragi, W.M., Ming, L.C., & Alakhali, K.M. (2020a). Drug safety in China. In *Drug Safety in Developing Countries* (pp. 381–388). Academic Press.

Al-Worafi, Y.M., Alseragi, W.M., Alakhali, K.M., Ming, L.C., Othman, G., Halboup, A.M., … & Elkalmi, R.M. (2020b). Knowledge, beliefs and factors affecting the use of generic medicines among patients in Ibb, Yemen: a mixed-method study. *Journal of Pharmacy Practice and Community Medicine*, 6(4).

Al-Worafi, Y.M., Elkalmi, R.M., Ming, L.C., Othman, G., Halboup, A.M., Battah, M.M., … & Mani, V. (2021a). Dispensing errors in hospital pharmacies: A prospective study in Yemen.

Al-Worafi, Y.M., Hasan, S., Hassan, N.M., & Gaili, A.A. (2021b). Knowledge, Attitude and Experience of Pharmacist in the UAE towards Pharmacovigilance. *Research Journal of Pharmacy and Technology*, 14(1), 265–269.

Al-Worafi, Y. (2022a). *A Guide to Online Pharmacy Education: Teaching Strategies and Assessment Methods*. CRC Press.

Al-Worafi, Y.M. (2022b). Patient care errors and related problems (part I): development and validation of the model. 0000-0002-5752-2913

Al-Worafi, Y.M. (Ed.). (2023). *Clinical Case Studies on medication Safety*. Academic Press.

Baig, M.R., Al-Worafi, Y.M., Alseragi, W.M., Ming, L.C., & Siddique, A. (2020). Drug safety in India. In *Drug Safety in Developing Countries* (pp. 327–334). Academic Press.

Elkalmi, R.M., Al-Worafi, Y.M., Alseragi, W.M., Ming, L.C., & Siddique, A. (2020). Drug safety in Malaysia. In *Drug Safety in Developing Countries* (pp. 245–253). Academic Press.

Elsayed, T., & Al-Worafi, Y.M. (2020). Drug safety in Egypt. In *Drug Safety in Developing Countries* (pp. 511–523). Academic Press.

Hasan, S., Al-Omar, M.J., AlZubaidy, H., & Al-Worafi, Y.M. (2019). Use of medications in Arab Countries. *Handbook of Healthcare in the Arab World*. Cham: Springer, 42.

Hassan, Y., Abd Aziz, N., Kassab, Y.W., Elgasim, I., Shaharuddin, S., Al-Worafi, Y.M.A., … & Ming, L.C. (2014). How to help patients to control their blood pressure? Blood pressure control and its predictor. *Archives of Pharmacy Practice*, 5(4).

Izahar, S., Lean, Q.Y., Hameed, M.A., Murugiah, M.K., Patel, R.P., Al-Worafi, Y.M., … & Ming, L.C. (2017). Content analysis of mobile health applications on diabetes mellitus. *Frontiers in Endocrinology*, 8, 318.

Kristensen, S., & Bartels, P. (2010). Use of patient safety culture instruments and recommendations. *Aarhus, Denmark, European Society for Quality in HealthCare-Office for Quality Indicators*, 113.

Lee, K.S., Yee, S.M., Zaidi, S.T.R., Patel, R.P., Yang, Q., Al-Worafi, Y.M., & Ming, L.C., 2017. Combating sale of counterfeit and falsified medicines online: a losing battle. *Frontiers in pharmacology*, 8, p. 268.

Mahmoud, M.A., Wajid, S., Naqvi, A.A., Samreen, S., Althagfan, S.S., & Al-Worafi, Y. (2020). Self-medication with antibiotics: A cross-sectional community-based study. *Latin american journal of pharmacy*, 39(2), 348–353.

Manan, M.M., Rusli, R.A., Ang, W.C., Al-Worafi, Y.M., & Ming, L.C. (2014). Assessing the pharmaceutical care issues of antiepileptic drug therapy in hospitalised epileptic patients. *Journal of Pharmacy Practice and Research*, 44(3), 83–88.

Manan, M.M., Ibrahim, N.A., Aziz, N.A., Zulkifly, H.H., Al-Worafi, Y.M.A., & Long, C.M. (2016). Empirical use of antibiotic therapy in the prevention of early onset sepsis in neonates: a pilot study. *Archives of Medical Science*, 12(3), 603–613.

Ming, L.C., Hameed, M.A., Lee, D.D., Apidi, N.A., Lai, P.S.M., Hadi, M.A., Al-Worafi, Y.M.A., & Khan, T.M., (2016). Use of medical mobile applications among hospital pharmacists in Malaysia. *Therapeutic innovation & regulatory science*, 50(4), pp. 419–426.

Ming, L.C., Untong, N., Aliudin, N.A., Osili, N., Kifli, N., Tan, C.S., … & Goh, H.P. (2020). Mobile health apps on COVID-19 launched in the early days of the pandemic: content analysis and review. *JMIR mHealth and uHealth*, 8(9), e19796.

Othman, G., Ali, F., Ibrahim, M.I.M., Al-Worafi, Y.M., Ansari, M., & Halboup, A.M. (2020). Assessment of Anti-Diabetic Medications Adherence among Diabetic Patients in Sana'a City, Yemen: A Cross Sectional Study. *Journal of Pharmaceutical Research International*, 32(21), 114–122.

Reynard, J., Reynolds, J., & Stevenson, P. (2009). *Practical patient safety*. OUP Oxford.

Saeed, M.S., Alkhoshaiban, A.S., Al-Worafi, Y.M.A., & Long, C.M., (2014). Perception of self-medication among university students in Saudi Arabia. *Archives of Pharmacy Practice*, 5(4), p. 149.

Salas, E., & Frush, K. (2012). *Improving patient safety through teamwork and team training*. Oxford University Press.

Vincent, C. (2011). *Patient safety*. John Wiley & Sons.

36 Patient Safety

Antimicrobial-Resistance and Interventions

36.1 BACKGROUND

Antimicrobial therapy is an important aspect of patient care and safety, particularly in the treatment and prevention of infectious diseases. Antimicrobials include antibiotics, antivirals, antifungals, and antiparasitic agents, which are used to kill or inhibit the growth of microorganisms that cause infection. However, the overuse and misuse of antimicrobial agents can lead to the emergence of antibiotic-resistant bacteria, which pose a significant threat to patient safety. Therefore, it is crucial for healthcare professionals to use antimicrobial agents judiciously and in accordance with established guidelines. To ensure patient safety and prevent the spread of antibiotic-resistant bacteria, healthcare professionals should:

1. Use antimicrobial agents only when they are necessary and appropriate for the treatment of a specific infection.

2. Choose the most appropriate antimicrobial agent based on the susceptibility of the micro-organism, the site of infection, and the patient's medical history.

3. Use the correct dose and duration of treatment, as recommended by established guidelines.

4. Monitor patients for adverse effects and adjust treatment accordingly.

5. Implement infection prevention and control measures to minimize the risk of transmission of resistant organisms.

6. Educate patients and their families about the appropriate use of antimicrobial agents and the importance of completing the full course of treatment.

Antimicrobial resistance (AMR) is a global health challenge that occurs when microorganisms (such as bacteria, viruses, fungi, and parasites) develop resistance to antimicrobial drugs, making infections harder to treat and potentially life-threatening. AMR can occur naturally or due to human activities such as overuse and misuse of antibiotics, poor infection prevention and control practices, and inadequate sanitation and hygiene.

Interventions to address AMR can be broadly categorized into three main areas:

1. Prevention: Preventing the spread of infections is the most effective way to reduce the need for antimicrobial use. Prevention measures include vaccination, good hygiene practices (such as handwashing and safe food preparation), and infection prevention and control measures in healthcare settings.

2. Rational use of antimicrobials: Appropriate use of antimicrobials can help reduce the development of resistance. This includes prescribing antibiotics only when they are needed, using the right antibiotic for the type of infection, and completing the full course of treatment as prescribed.

3. Research and innovation: Developing new antimicrobial drugs, vaccines, and diagnostics is essential for addressing AMR. This requires investment in research and development, as well as regulatory frameworks that incentivize the development of new treatments.

Overall, a comprehensive approach is needed to address AMR, which involves coordinated action across different sectors such as health, agriculture, and environment (Kristensen & Bartels, 2010; Murray et al., 2022; Reynard et al., 2009; Salas & Frush, 2012; Vincent, 2011).

36.2 PATIENT SAFETY: Antimicrobial-Resistance

Antimicrobial resistance (AMR) is the ability of microorganisms, such as bacteria, viruses, fungi, and parasites, to resist the effects of antimicrobial drugs, such as antibiotics, antivirals, antifungals, and antiparasitics. This resistance can occur naturally or as a result of the misuse or overuse of antimicrobial agents.

AMR is a global public health threat that can lead to prolonged illness, increased healthcare costs, and even death. The emergence of resistant microorganisms has made some previously treatable infections more difficult or impossible to treat, leading to an increased risk of complications and

DOI: 10.1201/9781003230465-38

mortality. The misuse of antimicrobial agents, such as the overuse of antibiotics, is a major factor contributing to the emergence of AMR. Overuse of antimicrobials can lead to the development of resistant strains of bacteria, as those bacteria that are able to survive exposure to the drugs are able to reproduce and pass on their resistant traits to their offspring. To combat AMR, it is important to use antimicrobial agents judiciously, follow established guidelines for their use, and implement infection prevention and control measures. This includes promoting the appropriate use of antibiotics and other antimicrobial agents, investing in research to develop new drugs, and supporting global efforts to combat AMR. Effective management of AMR requires a coordinated and collaborative approach between healthcare professionals, policymakers, researchers, and the public. By working together, we can help to preserve the effectiveness of antimicrobial agents and protect the health of patients and communities around the world.

36.3 ANTIMICROBIAL-RESISTANCE IN DEVELOPING COUNTRIES

Antimicrobial resistance (AMR) is a global problem, but it poses a particularly significant threat to developing countries. Developing countries often lack the resources and infrastructure necessary to effectively manage and prevent AMR. In these countries, factors such as poor sanitation, limited access to clean water, and inadequate healthcare systems can contribute to the spread of infectious diseases and the overuse and misuse of antimicrobial agents. These conditions can also contribute to the emergence and spread of resistant microorganisms. In addition, the availability of antimicrobial agents over the counter without a prescription is common in some developing countries, which can lead to their overuse and misuse, further contributing to the development of AMR. The consequences of AMR in developing countries can be particularly severe, as these countries often have higher rates of infectious diseases and limited access to effective treatments. This can result in prolonged illness, increased healthcare costs, and higher mortality rates.

To address AMR in developing countries, it is important to improve access to effective healthcare and to promote the appropriate use of antimicrobial agents. This includes investing in healthcare infrastructure and systems, improving sanitation and hygiene, promoting public awareness and education, and strengthening regulatory frameworks to promote the responsible use of antimicrobial agents. Collaboration between developed and developing countries is also important to address the global threat of AMR. Developed countries can provide resources, expertise, and support to help developing countries improve their healthcare systems and implement effective strategies to prevent and manage AMR.

36.4 CAUSES OF ANTIMICROBIAL-RESISTANCE

Antimicrobial resistance (AMR) is a complex problem that can arise from a variety of factors. Some of the main causes of AMR include:

1. Overuse and misuse of antimicrobial agents: Overuse and misuse of antibiotics, antivirals, antifungals, and antiparasitic agents can contribute to the development of resistant microorganisms. When these drugs are used excessively or inappropriately, they can create an environment in which resistant organisms can thrive.

2. Inadequate infection prevention and control measures: Poor sanitation and hygiene practices can contribute to the spread of infectious diseases and the emergence and spread of resistant microorganisms.

3. Lack of access to effective healthcare: In many parts of the world, access to effective healthcare is limited, which can lead to the overuse and misuse of antimicrobial agents and the spread of resistant microorganisms.

4. Inadequate surveillance and monitoring of AMR: The lack of comprehensive surveillance and monitoring systems can make it difficult to track the emergence and spread of resistant microorganisms, making it harder to take effective action to prevent and control AMR.

5. Limited research and development of new antimicrobial agents: There is a need for continued research and development of new antimicrobial agents to ensure that effective treatments are available to combat resistant microorganisms.

6. Environmental factors: Environmental contamination with antimicrobial agents and resistant microorganisms can contribute to the development and spread of AMR.

To address AMR, it is important to implement a multifaceted approach that addresses these and other factors. This includes promoting the appropriate use of antimicrobial agents, improving infection prevention and control measures, investing in research and development of new antimicrobial agents, and strengthening surveillance and monitoring systems to track the emergence and spread of resistant microorganisms

36.5 PREVENTION

Prevention is key to addressing the growing problem of antimicrobial resistance (AMR). There are several strategies that can be employed to prevent the development and spread of AMR, including:

1. Promoting appropriate use of antimicrobial agents: This includes prescribing and using antibiotics, antivirals, antifungals, and antiparasitic agents only when they are needed and in the right dose and duration.

2. Improving infection prevention and control measures: This includes promoting good hand hygiene, ensuring clean water and sanitation, and implementing appropriate infection control practices in healthcare settings.

3. Strengthening surveillance and monitoring systems: This includes developing comprehensive surveillance systems to monitor the emergence and spread of resistant microorganisms and tracking patterns of antimicrobial use.

4. Investing in research and development of new antimicrobial agents: This includes supporting the development of new drugs, vaccines, and other technologies to combat resistant microorganisms.

5. Educating healthcare professionals, patients, and the public: This includes promoting awareness about the appropriate use of antimicrobial agents and the risks of AMR, and encouraging patients to take antibiotics and other antimicrobial agents only when they are needed.

6. Improving healthcare systems and access to healthcare: This includes strengthening healthcare infrastructure, improving access to effective healthcare, and addressing socioeconomic factors that can contribute to the spread of infectious diseases.

Overall, addressing AMR requires a comprehensive and coordinated approach that involves healthcare professionals, policymakers, researchers, and the public. By working together to prevent the development and spread of AMR, we can help to ensure that effective antimicrobial agents remain available to combat infectious diseases and protect public health.

36.6 INTERVENTIONS

There are several interventions that can be implemented to address antimicrobial resistance (AMR), including:

1. Antibiotic stewardship programs: These programs aim to optimize the use of antibiotics by promoting appropriate prescribing and reducing overuse and misuse. This can involve interventions such as prescribing guidelines, education and training for healthcare professionals, and regular monitoring of antibiotic use.

2. Infection prevention and control measures: These measures aim to reduce the transmission of infectious diseases and limit the development and spread of resistant microorganisms. This can involve interventions such as promoting hand hygiene, ensuring clean water and sanitation, and implementing appropriate infection control practices in healthcare settings.

3. Vaccination programs: Vaccines can help to prevent the spread of infectious diseases and reduce the need for antimicrobial agents. This can help to limit the development and spread of resistant microorganisms.

4. Development of new antimicrobial agents: There is a need for continued research and development of new antimicrobial agents to ensure that effective treatments are available to combat resistant microorganisms.

5. Education and public awareness campaigns: These campaigns can help to promote awareness about the appropriate use of antimicrobial agents and the risks of AMR. This can involve

interventions such as public education campaigns, healthcare professional training, and social marketing campaigns.

6. International collaboration and cooperation: Addressing AMR requires a coordinated global response that involves collaboration and cooperation between countries and regions. This can involve interventions such as sharing surveillance and monitoring data, promoting research and development of new antimicrobial agents, and supporting capacity building in developing countries.

Overall, addressing AMR requires a multifaceted and coordinated approach that involves a range of interventions across multiple sectors. By implementing these interventions, we can help to reduce the development and spread of resistant microorganisms and ensure that effective antimicrobial agents remain available to combat infectious diseases and protect public health.

36.7 ANTIMICROBIAL SAFETY ISSUES IN DEVELOPING COUNTRIES: Challenges and Recommendations

Antimicrobial resistance (AMR) is a global challenge, but developing countries face unique challenges in addressing this issue. Some of the main challenges and recommendations for improving antimicrobial safety in developing countries are:
    Challenges:

1. Limited access to effective healthcare: In many developing countries, access to healthcare is limited, which can lead to the overuse and misuse of antimicrobial agents and the spread of resistant microorganisms.

2. Poor sanitation and hygiene practices: Poor sanitation and hygiene practices can contribute to the spread of infectious diseases and the emergence and spread of resistant microorganisms.

3. Limited resources for surveillance and monitoring of AMR: Many developing countries lack the resources and infrastructure needed to monitor the emergence and spread of resistant microorganisms.

4. Limited research and development of new antimicrobial agents: There is a need for continued research and development of new antimicrobial agents, but many developing countries lack the resources and expertise needed to support this work.

Recommendations:

1. Improving access to effective healthcare: This includes strengthening healthcare infrastructure, improving access to effective treatments, and addressing socioeconomic factors that can contribute to the spread of infectious diseases.

2. Promoting infection prevention and control measures: This includes promoting good hand hygiene, ensuring clean water and sanitation, and implementing appropriate infection control practices in healthcare settings.

3. Strengthening surveillance and monitoring systems: This includes developing comprehensive surveillance systems to monitor the emergence and spread of resistant microorganisms and tracking patterns of antimicrobial use.

4. Investing in research and development of new antimicrobial agents: This includes supporting the development of new drugs, vaccines, and other technologies to combat resistant microorganisms.

5. Improving education and awareness: This includes promoting awareness about the appropriate use of antimicrobial agents and the risks of AMR, and encouraging patients to take antibiotics and other antimicrobial agents only when they are needed.

6. International collaboration and cooperation: Addressing AMR requires a coordinated global response that involves collaboration and cooperation between countries and regions. This can involve interventions such as sharing surveillance and monitoring data, promoting research and development of new antimicrobial agents, and supporting capacity building in developing countries.

7. Limited availability of diagnostic tools: Many developing countries lack access to diagnostic tools that can help healthcare professionals accurately diagnose and treat infections. Without these tools, healthcare professionals may resort to prescribing broad-spectrum antimicrobial agents, which can contribute to the development of resistance.

8. High burden of infectious diseases: Many developing countries have a high burden of infectious diseases, which can contribute to the overuse and misuse of antimicrobial agents and the development and spread of resistant microorganisms.

9. Lack of regulation and enforcement: Some developing countries may have weak or nonexistent regulations and enforcement mechanisms for the appropriate use of antimicrobial agents. This can lead to the sale and use of counterfeit or substandard drugs, as well as inappropriate prescribing practices.

10. Agricultural use of antimicrobial agents: In many developing countries, antimicrobial agents are widely used in agriculture to promote growth and prevent disease in livestock. This can contribute to the development and spread of resistant microorganisms in both animals and humans.

11. Limited access to clean water and sanitation: Poor sanitation and lack of access to clean water can contribute to the spread of infectious diseases and the development and spread of resistant microorganisms.

12. Limited funding and resources: Many developing countries lack the funding and resources needed to address AMR effectively. This can include limited funding for research and development of new antimicrobial agents, limited resources for surveillance and monitoring, and limited resources for promoting appropriate use of antimicrobial agents.

13. Limited availability of alternative treatments: In many developing countries, antimicrobial agents may be the only available treatment option for infectious diseases. This can contribute to the overuse and misuse of these agents, as well as the development and spread of resistance.

14. Inadequate infection prevention and control practices: Inadequate infection prevention and control practices in healthcare facilities can contribute to the spread of resistant microorganisms. This can include inadequate hand hygiene, inadequate sterilization of medical equipment, and inadequate isolation of patients with resistant infections.

15. Lack of public awareness: In some developing countries, there may be limited public awareness about the risks of AMR and the appropriate use of antimicrobial agents. This can contribute to inappropriate use of these agents and the development and spread of resistance.

16. Limited access to healthcare in rural areas: In many developing countries, access to healthcare is limited in rural areas. This can lead to delays in diagnosis and treatment of infectious diseases, as well as the use of inappropriate or ineffective treatments.

17. Limited availability of vaccines: Vaccines can help to prevent infectious diseases and reduce the need for antimicrobial agents. However, in many developing countries, access to vaccines may be limited due to cost or lack of infrastructure.

18. Climate change and environmental factors: Climate change and other environmental factors can contribute to the spread of infectious diseases and the development and spread of resistant microorganisms. For example, changes in temperature and rainfall patterns can affect the distribution and prevalence of vector-borne diseases.

19. Strengthen regulatory frameworks: Developing countries should strengthen their regulatory frameworks for antimicrobials by implementing and enforcing laws and regulations that promote the rational use of antimicrobials. This includes regulations for the prescription, dispensing, and sale of antimicrobials, as well as regulations for the quality control of antimicrobials.

20. Improve antimicrobial stewardship: Developing countries should implement antimicrobial stewardship programs in healthcare settings to promote the appropriate use of antimicrobials. This includes educating healthcare providers and patients on the appropriate use of antimicrobials, developing guidelines for the use of antimicrobials, and monitoring antimicrobial use and resistance patterns.

21. Increase access to diagnostics: Developing countries should increase access to diagnostic tests to enable rapid and accurate diagnosis of infectious diseases. This will help to reduce unnecessary use of antimicrobials and improve patient outcomes.

22. Promote infection prevention and control: Developing countries should promote infection prevention and control measures in healthcare settings to prevent the spread of infectious diseases. This includes measures such as hand hygiene, environmental cleaning, and the use of personal protective equipment.

23. Develop surveillance systems: Developing countries should develop surveillance systems for antimicrobial use and resistance to monitor the effectiveness of antimicrobial safety interventions and identify emerging patterns of resistance.

24. Increase public awareness: Developing countries should increase public awareness of the dangers of antimicrobial resistance and the importance of using antimicrobials appropriately. This includes education campaigns aimed at healthcare providers, patients, and the general public.

25. Despite the progress in research about the patient care and safety in developing countries, there is little research about the patient safety related to the antimicrobial-resistance and interventions in majority of developing countries, therefore, conduct research is very important and highly recommended (Alshahrani et al., 2019a,b; Al-Qahtani et al., 2015; Alshahrani et al., 2020a,b; Al-Worafi, 2014; Al-Worafi, 2015; Al-Worafi, 2016; Al-Worafi et al., 2017; Al-Worafi, 2018a-d; Al-Worafi et al., 2018a-b; Al-Worafi et al., 2019; Al-Worafi, 2020a-z; Al-Worafi et al., 2020a-b; Al-Worafi et al., 2021a,b; Al-Worafi, 2022a,b; Al-Worafi, 2023; Baig et al., 2020; Elkalmi et al., 2020; Elsayed & Al-Worafi, 2020; Hasan et al., 2019; Hassan et al., 2014; Izahar et al., 2017; Lee et al., 2017; Mahmoud et al., 2020; Manan et al., 2014; Manan et al., 2016; Ming et al., 2016; Ming et al., 2020; Othman et al., 2020; Saeed et al., 2014).

36.8 CONCLUSION

This chapter has discussed the patient safety issues related to the antimicrobial-resistance and interventions, challenges and recommendations for the best practice in developing countries. Addressing AMR in developing countries requires a comprehensive and coordinated approach that involves healthcare professionals, policymakers, researchers, and the public. By working together to implement these recommendations, we can help to prevent the development and spread of resistant microorganisms and ensure that effective antimicrobial agents remain available to combat infectious diseases and protect public health. Antimicrobial safety interventions are essential in developing countries to prevent the emergence and spread of antimicrobial resistance and ensure the safe and effective use of antimicrobials. These interventions include strengthening regulatory frameworks, implementing antimicrobial stewardship programs, increasing access to diagnostics, promoting infection prevention and control, developing surveillance systems, and increasing public awareness. A multifaceted approach that encompasses regulatory, clinical, and public health interventions is crucial for addressing the complex challenge of antimicrobial resistance in developing countries. By taking action to promote antimicrobial safety, developing countries can help to preserve the effectiveness of antimicrobials and improve the health outcomes of their populations.

REFERENCES

Al-Qahtani, I., Almoteb, T.M., & Al-Warafi, Y. (2015). Competency of metered-dose inhaler use among Saudi community pharmacists: A Simulation method study. *RRJPPS*, 4(2), 37–31.

Alshahrani, S.M., Alakhali, K.M., & Al-Worafi, Y.M., (2019a). Medication errors in a health care facility in southern Saudi Arabia. *Tropical Journal of Pharmaceutical Research*, 18(5), pp. 1119–1122.

Alshahrani, S.M., Alavudeen, S.S., Alakhali, K.M., Al-Worafi, Y.M., Bahamdan, A.K., & Vigneshwaran, E., (2019b). Self-Medication Among King Khalid University Students, Saudi Arabia. *Risk Management and Healthcare Policy*, 12, pp. 243–249.

Alshahrani, S.M., Alakhali, K.M., Al-Worafi, Y.M., & Alshahrani, N.Z. (2020b). Awareness and use of over the counter analgesic medication: a survey in the Aseer region population, Saudi Arabia. *Int J Advan Appl Sci*, 7(3), 130–134.

Alshahrani, S.M., Alzahran, M., Alakhali, K., Vigneshwaran, E., Iqbal, M.J., Khan, N.A., ... & Alavudeen, S.S. (2020b). Association Between Diabetes Consequences and Quality of Life Among Patients With Diabetes Mellitus in the Aseer Province of Saudi Arabia. *Open Access Macedonian Journal of Medical Sciences*, 8(E), 325–330.

Al-Worafi, Y.M. (2014). Prescription writing errors at a tertiary care hospital in Yemen: prevalence, types, causes and recommendations. *Am J Pharm Health Res*, 2, 134–140.

Al-Worafi, Y.M.A. (2015). Appropriateness of metered-dose inhaler use in the Yemeni community pharmacies. *Journal of Taibah University Medical Sciences*, 10(3), 353–358.

Al-Worafi, Y.M.A., (2016). Pharmacy practice in Yemen. In *Pharmacy Practice in Developing Countries* (pp. 267–287). Academic Press.

Al-Worafi, Y.M., Kassab, Y.W., Alseragi, W.M., Almutairi, M.S., Ahmed, A., Ming, L.C., Alkhoshaiban, A.S., & Hadi, M.A., (2017). Pharmacovigilance and adverse drg reaction reporting: a perspective of community pharmacists and pharmacy technicians in Sana'a, Yemen. *Therapeutics and clinical risk management*, 13, p. 1175.

Al-Worafi, Y.M., (2018a). Knowledge, Attitude and Practice of Yemeni Physicians Toward Pharmacovigilance: A Mixed Method Study. *International Journal of Pharmacy and Pharmaceutical Sciences*, 10(10), 74–77.

Al-Worafi, Y. (2018b). Knowledge, attitude and practice of Yemeni physicians toward pharmacovigilance: A mixed method study. *Int. J. Pharm. Pharm. Sci*, 10, 74–77.

Al-Worafi, Y.M. (2018c). Dispensing errors observed by community pharmacy dispensers in IBB–YEMEN. *Asian J. Pharm. Clin. Res*, 11(11).

Al-Worafi, Y.M. (2018d). Evauation of inhaler technique among patients with asthma and COPD in Yemen. *Journal of Taibah University medical sciences*, 13(5), 488–490.

Al-Worafi, Y.M., Patel, R.P., Zaidi, S.T.R., Alseragi, W.M., Almutairi, M.S., Alkhoshaiban, A.S., & Ming, L.C. (2018a). Completeness and legibility of handwritten prescriptions in Sana'a, Yemen. *Medical Principles and Practice*, 27, 290–292.

Al-Worafi, Y.M., Alseragi, W.M., Seng, L.K., Kassab, Y.W., Yeoh, S.F., Chiau, L., ... & Husain, K. (2018b). Dispensing errors in community pharmacies: a prospective study in Sana'a, Yemen. *Arch Pharm Pract*, 9(4), 1–3.

Al-Worafi, Y.M., Alseragi, W.M., & Mahmoud, M.A. (2019). Competency of metered-dose inhaler use among community pharmacy dispensers in Ibb, Yemen: A simulation method study. *Latin American Journal of Pharmacy*, 38(3), 489–494.

Al-Worafi, Y.M. (Ed.). (2020a). *Drug Safety in Developing Countries: Achievements and Challenges.*

Al-Worafi, Y.M. (2020b). Medication errors. In *Drug Safety in Developing Countries* (pp. 105–117). Academic Press.

Al-Worafi, Y.M. (2020c). Adverse drug reactions. In *Drug Safety in Developing Countries* (pp. 39–57). Academic Press.

Al-Worafi, Y.M. (2020d). Medications registration and marketing: safety-related issues. In *Drug Safety in Developing Countries* (pp. 21–28). Academic Press.

Al-Worafi, Y.M. (2020e). Pharmacovigilance. In *Drug Safety in Developing Countries* (pp. 29–38). Academic Press.

Al-Worafi, Y.M. (2020f). Drug-related problems. In *Drug safety in developing countries* (pp. 59–71). Academic Press.

Al-Worafi, Y.M. (2020g). Medications safety-related terminology. In *Drug safety in developing countries* (pp. 7–19). Academic Press.

Al-Worafi, Y.M. (2020h). Self-medication. In *Drug Safety in Developing Countries* (pp. 73–86). Academic Press.

Al-Worafi, Y.M. (2020j). Antibiotics safety issues. In *Drug Safety in Developing Countries* (pp. 87–103). Academic Press.

Al-Worafi, Y.M. (2020k). Medications safety research issues. In *Drug Safety in Developing Countries* (pp. 213–227). Academic Press.

Al-Worafi, Y.M. (2020l). Counterfeit and substandard medications. In *Drug safety in developing countries* (pp. 119–126). Academic Press.

Al-Worafi, Y.M. (2020m). Medication abuse and misuse. In *Drug safety in developing countries* (pp. 127–135). Academic Press.

Al-Worafi, Y.M. (2020n). Storage and disposal of medications. In *Drug Safety in Developing Countries* (pp. 137–142). Academic Press.

Al-Worafi, Y.M. (2020o). Safety of medications in special population. In *Drug safety in developing countries* (pp. 143–162). Academic Press.

Al-Worafi, Y.M. (2020p). Herbal medicines safety issues. In *Drug Safety in developing countries* (pp. 163–178). Academic Press.

Al-Worafi, Y.M. (2020q). Medications safety pharmacoeconomics-related issues. In *Drug Safety in Developing Countries* (pp. 187–195). Academic Press.

Al-Worafi, Y.M. (2020r). Evidence-based medications safety practice. In *Drug Safety in Developing Countries* (pp. 197–201). Academic Press.

Al-Worafi, Y.M. (2020s). Quality indicators for medications safety. In *Drug safety in developing countries* (pp. 229–242). Academic Press.

Al-Worafi, Y.M. (2020t). Drug safety in Yemen. In *Drug Safety in Developing Countries* (pp. 391–405). Academic Press.

Al-Worafi, Y.M. (2020u). Drug safety in Saudi Arabia. In *Drug Safety in Developing Countries* (pp. 407–417). Academic Press.

Al-Worafi, Y.M. (2020v). Drug safety in United Arab Emirates. In *Drug Safety in Developing Countries* (pp. 419–428). Academic Press.

Al-Worafi, Y.M. (2020w). Drug safety in Indonesia. In *Drug Safety in Developing Countries* (pp. 279–285). Academic Press.

Al-Worafi, Y.M. (2020x). Drug safety in Palestine. In *Drug Safety in Developing Countries* (pp. 471–480). Academic Press.

Al-Worafi, Y.M. (2020y). Drug safety: comparison between developing countries. In *Drug Safety in Developing Countries* (pp. 603–611). Academic Press.

Al-Worafi, Y.M. (2020z). Drug safety in developing versus developed countries. In *Drug Safety in Developing Countries* (pp. 613–615). Academic Press.

Al-Worafi, Y.M., Alseragi, W.M., Ming, L.C., & Alakhali, K.M. (2020a). Drug safety in China. In *Drug Safety in Developing Countries* (pp. 381–388). Academic Press.

Al-Worafi, Y.M., Alseragi, W.M., Alakhali, K.M., Ming, L.C., Othman, G., Halboup, A.M., ... & Elkalmi, R.M. (2020b). Knowledge, beliefs and factors affecting the use of generic medicines among patients in Ibb, Yemen: a mixed-method study. *Journal of Pharmacy Practice and Community Medicine*, 6(4).

Al-Worafi, Y.M., Elkalmi, R.M., Ming, L.C., Othman, G., Halboup, A.M., Battah, M.M., ... & Mani, V. (2021a). Dispensing errors in hospital pharmacies: A prospective study in Yemen.

Al-Worafi, Y.M., Hasan, S., Hassan, N.M., & Gaili, A.A. (2021b). Knowledge, Attitude and Experience of Pharmacist in the UAE towards Pharmacovigilance. *Research Journal of Pharmacy and Technology*, 14(1), 265–269.

Al-Worafi, Y. (2022a). *A Guide to Online Pharmacy Education: Teaching Strategies and Assessment Methods*. CRC Press.

Al-Worafi, Y.M. (2022b). Patient care errors and related problems (part I): development and validation of the model. 0000-0002-5752-2913

Al-Worafi, Y.M. (Ed.). (2023). *Clinical Case Studies on medication Safety*. Academic Press.

Baig, M.R., Al-Worafi, Y.M., Alseragi, W.M., Ming, L.C., & Siddique, A. (2020). Drug safety in India. In *Drug Safety in Developing Countries* (pp. 327–334). Academic Press.

Elkalmi, R.M., Al-Worafi, Y.M., Alseragi, W.M., Ming, L.C., & Siddique, A. (2020). Drug safety in Malaysia. In *Drug Safety in Developing Countries* (pp. 245–253). Academic Press.

Elsayed, T., & Al-Worafi, Y.M. (2020). Drug safety in Egypt. In *Drug Safety in Developing Countries* (pp. 511–523). Academic Press.

Hasan, S., Al-Omar, M.J., AlZubaidy, H., & Al-Worafi, Y.M. (2019). Use of medications in Arab Countries. *Handbook of Healthcare in the Arab World*. Cham: Springer, 42.

Hassan, Y., Abd Aziz, N., Kassab, Y.W., Elgasim, I., Shaharuddin, S., Al-Worafi, Y.M.A., ... & Ming, L.C. (2014). How to help patients to control their blood pressure? Blood pressure control and its predictor. *Archives of Pharmacy Practice*, 5(4).

Izahar, S., Lean, Q.Y., Hameed, M.A., Murugiah, M.K., Patel, R.P., Al-Worafi, Y.M., ... & Ming, L.C. (2017). Content analysis of mobile health applications on diabetes mellitus. *Frontiers in Endocrinology*, 8, 318.

Kristensen, S., & Bartels, P. (2010). Use of patient safety culture instruments and recommendations. *Aarhus, Denmark, European Society for Quality in HealthCare-Office for Quality Indicators*, 113.

Lee, K.S., Yee, S.M., Zaidi, S.T.R., Patel, R.P., Yang, Q., Al-Worafi, Y.M., & Ming, L.C., 2017. Combating sale of counterfeit and falsified medicines online: a losing battle. *Frontiers in pharmacology*, 8, p. 268.

Mahmoud, M.A., Wajid, S., Naqvi, A.A., Samreen, S., Althagfan, S.S., & Al-Worafi, Y. (2020). Self-medication with antibiotics: A cross-sectional community-based study. *Latin american journal of pharmacy*, 39(2), 348–353.

Manan, M.M., Rusli, R.A., Ang, W.C., Al-Worafi, Y.M., & Ming, L.C. (2014). Assessing the pharmaceutical care issues of antiepileptic drug therapy in hospitalised epileptic patients. *Journal of Pharmacy Practice and Research*, 44(3), 83–88.

Manan, M.M., Ibrahim, N.A., Aziz, N.A., Zulkifly, H.H., Al-Worafi, Y.M.A., & Long, C.M. (2016). Empirical use of antibiotic therapy in the prevention of early onset sepsis in neonates: a pilot study. *Archives of Medical Science*, 12(3), 603–613.

Ming, L.C., Hameed, M.A., Lee, D.D., Apidi, N.A., Lai, P.S.M., Hadi, M.A., Al-Worafi, Y.M.A., & Khan, T.M., (2016). Use of medical mobile applications among hospital pharmacists in Malaysia. *Therapeutic innovation & regulatory science*, 50(4), pp. 419–426.

Ming, L.C., Untong, N., Aliudin, N.A., Osili, N., Kifli, N., Tan, C.S., ... & Goh, H.P. (2020). Mobile health apps on COVID-19 launched in the early days of the pandemic: content analysis and review. *JMIR mHealth and uHealth*, 8(9), e19796.

Murray, C.J., Ikuta, K.S., Sharara, F., Swetschinski, L., Aguilar, G.R., Gray, A., ... & Naghavi, M. (2022). Global burden of bacterial antimicrobial resistance in 2019: a systematic analysis. *The Lancet*, 399(10325), 629–655.

Othman, G., Ali, F., Ibrahim, M.I.M., Al-Worafi, Y.M., Ansari, M., & Halboup, A.M. (2020). Assessment of Anti-Diabetic Medications Adherence among Diabetic Patients in Sana'a City, Yemen: A Cross Sectional Study. *Journal of Pharmaceutical Research International*, 32(21), 114–122.

Reynard, J., Reynolds, J., & Stevenson, P. (2009). *Practical patient safety*. OUP Oxford.

Saeed, M.S., Alkhoshaiban, A.S., Al-Worafi, Y.M.A., & Long, C.M., (2014). Perception of self-medication among university students in Saudi Arabia. *Archives of Pharmacy Practice*, 5(4), p. 149.

Salas, E., & Frush, K. (2012). *Improving patient safety through teamwork and team training*. Oxford University Press.

Vincent, C. (2011). *Patient safety*. John Wiley & Sons.

37 Patient Safety

Dermatology, Beauty and Cosmetic Medicine

37.1 BACKGROUND

Dermatology is the branch of medicine that deals with the study and treatment of the skin, hair, and nails. Dermatologists are medical doctors who specialize in diagnosing and treating skin conditions, such as acne, eczema, psoriasis, and skin cancer. Beauty and cosmetic medicine, on the other hand, focus on enhancing a person's appearance. This can include non-surgical treatments, such as skin rejuvenation, laser hair removal, and Botox injections, as well as surgical procedures like breast augmentation, liposuction, and facelifts. While there is some overlap between dermatology and cosmetic medicine, they are distinct fields with different goals. Dermatology focuses on treating medical conditions related to the skin, hair, and nails, while cosmetic medicine focuses on improving a person's appearance through non-surgical or surgical procedures. It is important to note that while many cosmetic procedures are safe and effective, they do carry some risks, and patients should always seek out qualified professionals with appropriate training and experience. Patient care and safety are critical components of dermatology, beauty, and cosmetic medicine. Here are some key points to keep in mind:

1. Communication: Clear and effective communication between the patient and the provider is essential to ensure that the patient's needs and expectations are met. It is important to discuss any potential risks and complications associated with the procedure or treatment before proceeding.

2. Qualifications: Only qualified and licensed professionals should perform cosmetic procedures. Ensure that the provider has the proper training and certifications to perform the treatment or procedure.

3. Sanitation and hygiene: Proper sanitation and hygiene should be maintained in the clinic or treatment room. Instruments should be sterilized or disposed of properly, and surfaces should be cleaned and disinfected.

4. Skin type and sensitivity: Skin type and sensitivity vary from patient to patient. It is important to assess the patient's skin type and sensitivity before performing any cosmetic procedure or treatment. This can help determine the appropriate products and techniques to use and reduce the risk of adverse reactions.

5. Allergies: Patients should be asked about any allergies or sensitivities they have to specific products or ingredients. This information can help avoid adverse reactions and minimize risks.

6. Aftercare: Patients should be given clear instructions for aftercare, including any necessary medications, skincare products, or activities to avoid. This can help prevent complications and ensure optimal results.

7. Follow-up: It is important to schedule follow-up appointments to monitor the patient's progress and address any concerns or complications that may arise.

Overall, patient care and safety should be the top priority in dermatology, beauty, and cosmetic medicine. Providers should take the necessary steps to ensure that their patients are informed, comfortable, and receive the best possible care (Kristensen & Bartels, 2010; Reynard et al., 2009; Salas & Frush, 2012; Vincent, 2011).

37.2 PATIENT SAFETY: Dermatology

Patient safety is a critical aspect of dermatology, and healthcare professionals should take all necessary steps to ensure that patients are safe and receive optimal care. Here are some key points to consider regarding patient safety in dermatology:

1. Proper diagnosis: A proper diagnosis is essential to ensure that the patient receives appropriate treatment. The healthcare professional should take a comprehensive medical history and perform a thorough physical examination to ensure that the correct diagnosis is made.

2. Informed consent: Informed consent is essential for any treatment or procedure. The healthcare professional should provide the patient with detailed information about the treatment, including potential risks and complications, to help the patient make an informed decision.

DOI: 10.1201/9781003230465-39

3. Sterilization and hygiene: The healthcare professional should ensure that all instruments and equipment used during procedures are sterilized or disposed of properly. Proper hygiene measures should be taken to minimize the risk of infection.

4. Proper medication management: The healthcare professional should carefully review the patient's medical history and medication list to ensure that any prescribed medications do not interact with other medications the patient is taking.

5. Proper use of technology: Technology, such as lasers, can be effective in treating certain skin conditions. However, healthcare professionals should ensure that the technology is used properly and that the patient is protected from any potential harm.

6. Monitoring for adverse reactions: Healthcare professionals should monitor patients closely for any adverse reactions to treatments or medications. If an adverse reaction occurs, the healthcare professional should take immediate action to address the situation.

7. Follow-up care: Follow-up care is essential to ensure that the patient is recovering properly and to address any issues that may arise. Healthcare professionals should provide clear instructions for aftercare and schedule follow-up appointments as necessary.

Overall, healthcare professionals in dermatology should take all necessary steps to ensure patient safety, including proper diagnosis, informed consent, sterilization and hygiene, proper medication management, proper use of technology, monitoring for adverse reactions, and follow-up care.

37.3 PATIENT SAFETY: Beauty and Cosmetic Medicine

Patient safety is essential in beauty and cosmetic medicine. The following are some important considerations for ensuring patient safety in beauty:

1. Proper qualifications: Only qualified and licensed professionals should perform cosmetic procedures. It is essential to verify that the provider has the appropriate training and certifications to perform the treatment or procedure.

2. Informed consent: Informed consent is necessary for any treatment or procedure. The provider should provide the patient with detailed information about the treatment, including potential risks and complications, to help the patient make an informed decision.

3. Sanitation and hygiene: Proper sanitation and hygiene should be maintained in the clinic or treatment room. Instruments should be sterilized or disposed of properly, and surfaces should be cleaned and disinfected.

4. Skin type and sensitivity: Skin type and sensitivity vary from patient to patient. It is necessary to assess the patient's skin type and sensitivity before performing any cosmetic procedure or treatment. This can help determine the appropriate products and techniques to use and reduce the risk of adverse reactions.

5. Allergies: Patients should be asked about any allergies or sensitivities they have to specific products or ingredients. This information can help avoid adverse reactions and minimize risks.

6. Proper use of technology: Technology, such as lasers, can be effective in treating certain beauty concerns. However, the provider should ensure that the technology is used properly, and the patient is protected from any potential harm.

7. Follow-up care: Follow-up care is essential to ensure that the patient is recovering properly and to address any issues that may arise. Providers should provide clear instructions for aftercare and schedule follow-up appointments as necessary.

8. Proper qualifications: Only qualified and licensed professionals should perform cosmetic procedures. It is essential to verify that the provider has the appropriate training and certifications to perform the treatment or procedure.

9. Informed consent: Informed consent is necessary for any treatment or procedure. The provider should provide the patient with detailed information about the treatment, including potential risks and complications, to help the patient make an informed decision.

10. Sanitation and hygiene: Proper sanitation and hygiene should be maintained in the clinic or treatment room. Instruments should be sterilized or disposed of properly, and surfaces should be cleaned and disinfected.

11. Proper diagnosis: A proper diagnosis is essential to ensure that the patient receives appropriate treatment. The healthcare professional should take a comprehensive medical history and perform a thorough physical examination to ensure that the correct diagnosis is made.

12. Allergies: Patients should be asked about any allergies or sensitivities they have to specific products or ingredients. This information can help avoid adverse reactions and minimize risks.

13. Proper medication management: The healthcare professional should carefully review the patient's medical history and medication list to ensure that any prescribed medications do not interact with other medications the patient is taking.

14. Monitoring for adverse reactions: Healthcare professionals should monitor patients closely for any adverse reactions to treatments or medications. If an adverse reaction occurs, the healthcare professional should take immediate action to address the situation.

15. Follow-up care: Follow-up care is essential to ensure that the patient is recovering properly and to address any issues that may arise. Healthcare professionals should provide clear instructions for aftercare and schedule follow-up appointments as necessary.

In summary, patient safety is critical in cosmetic medicine. Providers should take necessary steps to ensure that patients are informed, comfortable, and receive the best possible care. This includes proper qualifications, informed consent, sanitation and hygiene, proper diagnosis, allergy screening, proper medication management, proper use of technology, monitoring for adverse reactions, and follow-up care.

37.4 PATIENT SAFETY: Dermatology, Beauty and Cosmetic Medicine: Errors and Related Problems

Patient safety is an essential aspect of dermatology, beauty, and cosmetic medicine. However, errors and related problems can occur, which can result in adverse outcomes for the patient. The following are some common errors and related problems that can occur:

1. Adverse reactions: Adverse reactions to cosmetic products, medications, or treatments can occur, resulting in skin irritation, infections, or other complications.

2. Misdiagnosis: Misdiagnosis can occur in dermatology, leading to incorrect treatment or delayed treatment. This can result in the worsening of the patient's condition or even permanent scarring.

3. Infection: Infection can occur during cosmetic procedures or treatments, particularly if proper sanitation and hygiene practices are not followed.

4. Over-treatment: Over-treatment can occur in cosmetic medicine when the healthcare professional applies too much of a product or treatment. This can lead to complications such as scarring, hyperpigmentation, and skin damage.

5. Under-treatment: Under-treatment can occur when the healthcare professional fails to provide enough of a product or treatment. This can result in the failure to achieve the desired results, leading to patient dissatisfaction.

6. Unqualified providers: Unqualified providers can perform cosmetic procedures or treatments, which can lead to serious complications or adverse outcomes.

7. Inadequate informed consent: Inadequate informed consent can occur when the healthcare professional fails to provide the patient with enough information about the treatment, including potential risks and complications.

8. Use of unapproved products: The use of unapproved products or medications can result in adverse reactions or complications.

9. Lack of follow-up care: Lack of follow-up care can result in delayed treatment or complications that could have been prevented or addressed earlier.

In summary, errors and related problems can occur in dermatology, beauty, and cosmetic medicine, leading to adverse outcomes for the patient. It is essential to take necessary precautions and follow best practices to ensure patient safety, including proper diagnosis, qualified providers, informed consent, sanitation and hygiene, appropriate use of products and medications, and follow-up care.

37.5 DERMATOLOGY, BEAUTY AND COSMETIC MEDICINE ERRORS AND RELATED PROBLEMS: Causes

There are various causes of dermatology, beauty, and cosmetic medicine errors and related problems. Some of the common causes are:

1. Lack of proper training and experience: One of the main causes of errors in dermatology, beauty, and cosmetic medicine is a lack of proper training and experience. Practitioners who are not adequately trained or who lack experience may make mistakes during procedures, leading to unwanted outcomes.

2. Poor communication: Poor communication between the practitioner and the patient can also lead to errors. Patients may not fully understand the risks and benefits of a particular procedure, or they may fail to disclose important medical information, which can result in adverse reactions.

3. Improper use of equipment: The improper use of equipment during procedures can lead to injuries or other complications. If equipment is not properly maintained, cleaned, or sterilized, it can also cause infections and other problems.

4. Inadequate preparation: Inadequate preparation for a procedure can also lead to errors. Practitioners who do not properly assess the patient's skin or who fail to adequately prepare the patient for a procedure may cause unwanted outcomes.

5. Unethical behavior: Unethical behavior, such as performing procedures that are not medically necessary or charging patients excessive fees, can also lead to problems in dermatology, beauty, and cosmetic medicine.

6. Lack of regulation: The lack of regulation in the beauty and cosmetic medicine industry can also contribute to errors and problems. Without proper oversight, practitioners may not be held to a high standard of care, leading to increased risk for patients.

7. Cultural and societal pressures: Cultural and societal pressures can also contribute to errors and problems in dermatology, beauty, and cosmetic medicine. Patients may feel pressured to undergo procedures to conform to certain beauty standards or societal expectations, even if they are not suitable candidates for the procedure.

37.6 DERMATOLOGY, BEAUTY AND COSMETIC MEDICINE ERRORS AND RELATED PROBLEMS: Prevention

There are several ways to prevent dermatology, beauty, and cosmetic medicine errors and related problems:

1. Adequate training and experience: Practitioners should have adequate training and experience before performing procedures. They should also engage in ongoing education to stay up-to-date with the latest techniques and best practices.

2. Effective communication: Practitioners should communicate effectively with patients, providing them with clear information about the risks and benefits of a procedure, and ensuring that patients understand the procedure and what to expect.

3. Proper use of equipment: Practitioners should ensure that all equipment is properly maintained, cleaned, and sterilized. They should also use equipment properly during procedures to minimize the risk of injury or complications.

4. Thorough preparation: Practitioners should thoroughly prepare for procedures, including assessing the patient's skin and medical history, and ensuring that the patient is a suitable candidate for the procedure.

5. Ethical behavior: Practitioners should always act ethically, performing only medically necessary procedures and charging fair fees. They should also prioritize patient safety and satisfaction.

6. Regulation and oversight: The beauty and cosmetic medicine industry should be subject to regulation and oversight to ensure that practitioners are held to a high standard of care.

7. Patient empowerment: Patients should be empowered to make informed decisions about their care. This includes having access to information about procedures, the risks and benefits of each procedure, and the qualifications of practitioners performing the procedures.

By following these practices, dermatology, beauty, and cosmetic medicine errors and related problems can be minimized, leading to better outcomes for patients.

37.7 PATIENT SAFETY: Dermatology, Beauty and Cosmetic Medicine in Developing Countries

Dermatology, beauty, and cosmetic medicine in developing countries face unique challenges in ensuring patient safety. Some of the challenges include:

1. Limited resources: Developing countries may lack the resources necessary to provide adequate training and oversight for practitioners in the beauty and cosmetic medicine industry.

2. Lack of regulation: Many developing countries may lack regulations and oversight for the beauty and cosmetic medicine industry, leaving patients vulnerable to unscrupulous practitioners and unsafe procedures.

3. Cultural and societal pressures: Patients in developing countries may face cultural and societal pressures to conform to certain beauty standards or undergo certain procedures, even if they are not suitable candidates or do not fully understand the risks involved.

4. Limited access to information: Patients in developing countries may have limited access to information about procedures, risks, and qualifications of practitioners.

To improve patient safety in dermatology, beauty, and cosmetic medicine in developing countries, several recommendations can be made:

1. Increase awareness: The importance of patient safety in dermatology, beauty, and cosmetic medicine should be highlighted through public education campaigns.

2. Establish regulations: Governments and professional organizations should establish regulations and oversight for the beauty and cosmetic medicine industry to ensure that practitioners are held to a high standard of care.

3. Improve training and education: Practitioners should receive adequate training and education to ensure they are capable of providing safe and effective treatments.

4. Promote ethical behavior: Practitioners should be encouraged to act ethically and prioritize patient safety and satisfaction.

5. Empower patients: Patients should be empowered with access to information about procedures, risks, and qualifications of practitioners, and encouraged to make informed decisions about their care.

6. Foster collaboration: Collaboration between government, professional organizations, and practitioners can help to promote patient safety and improve access to care.

7. Lack of standardized protocols: The lack of standardized protocols for procedures and treatments may increase the risk of errors and complications.

8. Limited access to quality products: Some developing countries may have limited access to quality products, such as injectables or skincare products, which may increase the risk of adverse reactions.

9. Limited access to medical care: Patients in remote or rural areas may have limited access to medical care and may rely on untrained or unqualified practitioners for beauty and cosmetic treatments.

10. Lack of continuity of care: Patients may receive treatments from multiple practitioners, which can make it difficult to track their medical history and ensure proper follow-up care.

11. Language and cultural barriers: Patients and practitioners may face language and cultural barriers that can hinder communication and increase the risk of misunderstandings.

12. Limited funding for research: Limited funding for research and development in the beauty and cosmetic medicine industry may result in a lack of evidence-based practices and treatments.

13. Counterfeit products: In some developing countries, counterfeit beauty and cosmetic products may be prevalent. These products may be ineffective or even dangerous, and patients may not be able to easily differentiate between genuine and counterfeit products.

14. Lack of medical insurance: Many patients in developing countries may not have access to medical insurance, which can make it difficult for them to seek medical care for any complications or adverse reactions that may arise from beauty and cosmetic treatments.

15. Stigma around seeking medical care: In some cultures, there may be a stigma around seeking medical care for beauty or cosmetic concerns, which can discourage patients from seeking appropriate care and advice.

16. Limited resources for adverse event reporting: Developing countries may have limited resources for reporting and tracking adverse events related to beauty and cosmetic treatments, which can make it difficult to identify and address safety issues.

17. Unregulated providers: In some developing countries, there may be unregulated or unlicensed providers offering beauty and cosmetic treatments. These providers may lack the necessary training or experience to perform treatments safely and effectively.

18. Limited access to follow-up care: Patients in developing countries may have limited access to follow-up care or aftercare instructions, which can increase the risk of complications or adverse reactions.

19. Lack of access to technology: In some developing countries, there may be a lack of access to technology such as lasers or advanced imaging equipment, which can limit the availability of certain treatments and increase the risk of adverse events.

20. Lack of transparency: Patients may not always be provided with transparent information about the qualifications, experience, and safety record of practitioners, which can make it difficult for them to make informed decisions about their care.

21. Cultural practices and traditions: Cultural practices and traditions may impact patient safety in dermatology, beauty, and cosmetic medicine. For example, certain herbal remedies or traditional practices may not be safe or effective, and patients may be reluctant to disclose their use of these remedies to healthcare providers.

22. Limited research: Limited research and data on the safety and efficacy of beauty and cosmetic treatments in certain populations can make it difficult to develop evidence-based practices and guidelines.

23. Lack of collaboration: Collaboration between healthcare providers, regulators, and industry stakeholders may be limited, which can impede efforts to improve patient safety and address emerging safety issues.

24. Limited resources for patient education: Patients in developing countries may have limited access to resources for education and information about beauty and cosmetic treatments, which can make it difficult for them to make informed decisions and reduce their risk of adverse events.

25. Despite the progress in research about the patient care and safety in developing countries, there is little research about the patient safety related to dermatology, beauty and cosmetic medicine in majority of developing countries, therefore, conduct research is very important and highly recommended (Alshahrani et al., 2019a,b; Al-Qahtani et al., 2015; Alshahrani et al., 2020a,b; Al-Worafi, 2014; Al-Worafi, 2015; Al-Worafi, 2016; Al-Worafi et al., 2017;

Al-Worafi, 2018a-d; Al-Worafi et al., 2018a-b; Al-Worafi et al., 2019; Al-Worafi, 2020a-z; Al-Worafi et al., 2020a-b; Al-Worafi et al., 2021a,b; Al-Worafi, 2022a,b; Al-Worafi, 2023; Baig et al., 2020; Elkalmi et al., 2020; Elsayed & Al-Worafi, 2020; Hasan et al., 2019; Hassan et al., 2014; Izahar et al., 2017; Lee et al., 2017; Mahmoud et al., 2020; Manan et al., 2014; Manan et al., 2016; Ming et al., 2016; Ming et al., 2020; Othman et al., 2020; Saeed et al., 2014).

37.8 CONCLUSION

This chapter has discussed the patient safety issues related to the dermatology, beauty, and cosmetic medicine, prevention, challenges and recommendations for the best practice in developing countries. Patient safety in dermatology, beauty, and cosmetic medicine in developing countries is a complex issue that requires a multi-faceted approach to address. A range of issues, such as limited access to quality products, lack of standardization and regulation, limited access to medical care, and cultural barriers, can impact patient safety in these settings. Addressing these issues may require increased investment in training and education, regulation and oversight, and public awareness campaigns. By working together, healthcare providers, policymakers, and industry stakeholders can improve patient safety and ensure that all patients have access to safe, effective, and high-quality dermatological, beauty, and cosmetic medicine treatments.

REFERENCES

Al-Qahtani, I., Almoteb, T.M., & Al-Warafi, Y. (2015). Competency of metered-dose inhaler use among Saudi community pharmacists: A Simulation method study. *RRJPPS*, 4(2), 37–31.

Alshahrani, S.M., Alakhali, K.M., & Al-Worafi, Y.M., (2019a). Medication errors in a health care facility in southern Saudi Arabia. *Tropical Journal of Pharmaceutical Research*, 18(5), pp. 1119–1122.

Alshahrani, S.M., Alavudeen, S.S., Alakhali, K.M., Al-Worafi, Y.M., Bahamdan, A.K., & Vigneshwaran, E., (2019b). Self-Medication Among King Khalid University Students, Saudi Arabia. *Risk Management and Healthcare Policy*, 12, pp. 243–249.

Alshahrani, S.M., Alakhali, K.M., Al-Worafi, Y.M., & Alshahrani, N.Z. (2020b). Awareness and use of over the counter analgesic medication: a survey in the Aseer region population, Saudi Arabia. *Int J Advan Appl Sci*, 7(3), 130–134.

Alshahrani, S.M., Alzahran, M., Alakhali, K., Vigneshwaran, E., Iqbal, M.J., Khan, N.A., ... & Alavudeen, S.S. (2020b). Association Between Diabetes Consequences and Quality of Life Among Patients With Diabetes Mellitus in the Aseer Province of Saudi Arabia. *Open Access Macedonian Journal of Medical Sciences*, 8(E), 325–330.

Al-Worafi, Y.M. (2014). Prescription writing errors at a tertiary care hospital in Yemen: prevalence, types, causes and recommendations. *Am J Pharm Health Res*, 2, 134–140.

Al-Worafi, Y.M.A. (2015). Appropriateness of metered-dose inhaler use in the Yemeni community pharmacies. *Journal of Taibah University Medical Sciences*, 10(3), 353–358.

Al-Worafi, Y.M.A., (2016). Pharmacy practice in Yemen. In *Pharmacy Practice in Developing Countries* (pp. 267–287). Academic Press.

Al-Worafi, Y.M., Kassab, Y.W., Alseragi, W.M., Almutairi, M.S., Ahmed, A., Ming, L.C., Alkhoshaiban, A.S., & Hadi, M.A., (2017). Pharmacovigilance and adverse drg reaction reporting: a perspective of community pharmacists and pharmacy technicians in Sana'a, Yemen. *Therapeutics and clinical risk management*, 13, p. 1175.

Al-Worafi, Y.M., (2018a). Knowledge, Attitude and Practice of Yemeni Physicians Toward Pharmacovigilance: A Mixed Method Study. *International Journal of Pharmacy and Pharmaceutical Sciences*, 10(10), 74–77.

Al-Worafi, Y. (2018b). Knowledge, attitude and practice of Yemeni physicians toward pharmacovigilance: A mixed method study. *Int. J. Pharm. Pharm. Sci*, 10, 74–77.

Al-Worafi, Y.M. (2018c). Dispensing errors observed by community pharmacy dispensers in IBB–YEMEN. *Asian J. Pharm. Clin. Res*, 11(11).

Al-Worafi, Y.M. (2018d). Evauation of inhaler technique among patients with asthma and COPD in Yemen. *Journal of Taibah University medical sciences*, 13(5), 488–490.

Al-Worafi, Y.M., Patel, R.P., Zaidi, S.T.R., Alseragi, W.M., Almutairi, M.S., Alkhoshaiban, A.S., & Ming, L.C. (2018a). Completeness and legibility of handwritten prescriptions in Sana'a, Yemen. *Medical Principles and Practice*, 27, 290–292.

Al-Worafi, Y.M., Alseragi, W.M., Seng, L.K., Kassab, Y.W., Yeoh, S.F., Chiau, L., ... & Husain, K. (2018b). Dispensing errors in community pharmacies: a prospective study in Sana'a, Yemen. *Arch Pharm Pract*, 9(4), 1–3.

Al-Worafi, Y.M., Alseragi, W.M., & Mahmoud, M.A. (2019). Competency of metered-dose inhaler use among community pharmacy dispensers in Ibb, Yemen: A simulation method study. *Latin American Journal of Pharmacy*, 38(3), 489–494.

Al-Worafi, Y.M. (Ed.). (2020a). *Drug Safety in Developing Countries: Achievements and Challenges*.

Al-Worafi, Y.M. (2020b). Medication errors. In *Drug Safety in Developing Countries* (pp. 105–117). Academic Press.

Al-Worafi, Y.M. (2020c). Adverse drug reactions. In *Drug Safety in Developing Countries* (pp. 39–57). Academic Press.

Al-Worafi, Y.M. (2020d). Medications registration and marketing: safety-related issues. In *Drug Safety in Developing Countries* (pp. 21–28). Academic Press.

Al-Worafi, Y.M. (2020e). Pharmacovigilance. In *Drug Safety in Developing Countries* (pp. 29–38). Academic Press.

Al-Worafi, Y.M. (2020f). Drug-related problems. In *Drug safety in developing countries* (pp. 59–71). Academic Press.

Al-Worafi, Y.M. (2020g). Medications safety-related terminology. In *Drug safety in developing countries* (pp. 7–19). Academic Press.

Al-Worafi, Y.M. (2020h). Self-medication. In *Drug Safety in Developing Countries* (pp. 73–86). Academic Press.

Al-Worafi, Y.M. (2020j). Antibiotics safety issues. In *Drug Safety in Developing Countries* (pp. 87–103). Academic Press.

Al-Worafi, Y.M. (2020k). Medications safety research issues. In *Drug Safety in Developing Countries* (pp. 213–227). Academic Press.

Al-Worafi, Y.M. (2020l). Counterfeit and substandard medications. In *Drug safety in developing countries* (pp. 119–126). Academic Press.

Al-Worafi, Y.M. (2020m). Medication abuse and misuse. In *Drug safety in developing countries* (pp. 127–135). Academic Press.

Al-Worafi, Y.M. (2020n). Storage and disposal of medications. In *Drug Safety in Developing Countries* (pp. 137–142). Academic Press.

Al-Worafi, Y.M. (2020o). Safety of medications in special population. In *Drug safety in developing countries* (pp. 143–162). Academic Press.

Al-Worafi, Y.M. (2020p). Herbal medicines safety issues. In *Drug Safety in developing countries* (pp. 163–178). Academic Press.

Al-Worafi, Y.M. (2020q). Medications safety pharmacoeconomics-related issues. In *Drug Safety in Developing Countries* (pp. 187–195). Academic Press.

Al-Worafi, Y.M. (2020r). Evidence-based medications safety practice. In *Drug Safety in Developing Countries* (pp. 197–201). Academic Press.

Al-Worafi, Y.M. (2020s). Quality indicators for medications safety. In *Drug safety in developing countries* (pp. 229–242). Academic Press.

Al-Worafi, Y.M. (2020t). Drug safety in Yemen. In *Drug Safety in Developing Countries* (pp. 391–405). Academic Press.

Al-Worafi, Y.M. (2020u). Drug safety in Saudi Arabia. In *Drug Safety in Developing Countries* (pp. 407–417). Academic Press.

Al-Worafi, Y.M. (2020v). Drug safety in United Arab Emirates. In *Drug Safety in Developing Countries* (pp. 419–428). Academic Press.

Al-Worafi, Y.M. (2020w). Drug safety in Indonesia. In *Drug Safety in Developing Countries* (pp. 279–285). Academic Press.

Al-Worafi, Y.M. (2020x). Drug safety in Palestine. In *Drug Safety in Developing Countries* (pp. 471–480). Academic Press.

Al-Worafi, Y.M. (2020y). Drug safety: comparison between developing countries. In *Drug Safety in Developing Countries* (pp. 603–611). Academic Press.

Al-Worafi, Y.M. (2020z). Drug safety in developing versus developed countries. In *Drug Safety in Developing Countries* (pp. 613–615). Academic Press.

Al-Worafi, Y.M., Alseragi, W.M., Ming, L.C., & Alakhali, K.M. (2020a). Drug safety in China. In *Drug Safety in Developing Countries* (pp. 381–388). Academic Press.

Al-Worafi, Y.M., Alseragi, W.M., Alakhali, K.M., Ming, L.C., Othman, G., Halboup, A.M., … & Elkalmi, R.M. (2020b). Knowledge, beliefs and factors affecting the use of generic medicines among patients in Ibb, Yemen: a mixed-method study. *Journal of Pharmacy Practice and Community Medicine*, 6(4).

Al-Worafi, Y.M., Elkalmi, R.M., Ming, L.C., Othman, G., Halboup, A.M., Battah, M.M., … & Mani, V. (2021a). Dispensing errors in hospital pharmacies: A prospective study in Yemen.

Al-Worafi, Y.M., Hasan, S., Hassan, N.M., & Gaili, A.A. (2021b). Knowledge, Attitude and Experience of Pharmacist in the UAE towards Pharmacovigilance. *Research Journal of Pharmacy and Technology*, 14(1), 265–269.

Al-Worafi, Y. (2022a). *A Guide to Online Pharmacy Education: Teaching Strategies and Assessment Methods*. CRC Press.

Al-Worafi, Y.M. (2022b). Patient care errors and related problems (part I): development and validation of the model. 0000-0002-5752-2913

Al-Worafi, Y.M. (Ed.). (2023). *Clinical Case Studies on medication Safety*. Academic Press.

Baig, M.R., Al-Worafi, Y.M., Alseragi, W.M., Ming, L.C., & Siddique, A. (2020). Drug safety in India. In *Drug Safety in Developing Countries* (pp. 327–334). Academic Press.

Elkalmi, R.M., Al-Worafi, Y.M., Alseragi, W.M., Ming, L.C., & Siddique, A. (2020). Drug safety in Malaysia. In *Drug Safety in Developing Countries* (pp. 245–253). Academic Press.

Elsayed, T., & Al-Worafi, Y.M. (2020). Drug safety in Egypt. In *Drug Safety in Developing Countries* (pp. 511–523). Academic Press.

Hasan, S., Al-Omar, M.J., AlZubaidy, H., & Al-Worafi, Y.M. (2019). Use of medications in Arab Countries. *Handbook of Healthcare in the Arab World*. Cham: Springer, 42.

Hassan, Y., Abd Aziz, N., Kassab, Y.W., Elgasim, I., Shaharuddin, S., Al-Worafi, Y.M.A., ... & Ming, L.C. (2014). How to help patients to control their blood pressure? Blood pressure control and its predictor. *Archives of Pharmacy Practice*, 5(4).

Izahar, S., Lean, Q.Y., Hameed, M.A., Murugiah, M.K., Patel, R.P., Al-Worafi, Y.M., ... & Ming, L.C. (2017). Content analysis of mobile health applications on diabetes mellitus. *Frontiers in Endocrinology*, 8, 318.

Kristensen, S., & Bartels, P. (2010). Use of patient safety culture instruments and recommendations. *Aarhus, Denmark, European Society for Quality in HealthCare-Office for Quality Indicators*, 113.

Lee, K.S., Yee, S.M., Zaidi, S.T.R., Patel, R.P., Yang, Q., Al-Worafi, Y.M., & Ming, L.C., 2017. Combating sale of counterfeit and falsified medicines online: a losing battle. *Frontiers in pharmacology*, 8, p. 268.

Mahmoud, M.A., Wajid, S., Naqvi, A.A., Samreen, S., Althagfan, S.S., & Al-Worafi, Y. (2020). Self-medication with antibiotics: A cross-sectional community-based study. *Latin american journal of pharmacy*, 39(2), 348–353.

Manan, M.M., Rusli, R.A., Ang, W.C., Al-Worafi, Y.M., & Ming, L.C. (2014). Assessing the pharmaceutical care issues of antiepileptic drug therapy in hospitalised epileptic patients. *Journal of Pharmacy Practice and Research*, 44(3), 83–88.

Manan, M.M., Ibrahim, N.A., Aziz, N.A., Zulkifly, H.H., Al-Worafi, Y.M.A., & Long, C.M. (2016). Empirical use of antibiotic therapy in the prevention of early onset sepsis in neonates: a pilot study. *Archives of Medical Science*, 12(3), 603–613.

Ming, L.C., Hameed, M.A., Lee, D.D., Apidi, N.A., Lai, P.S.M., Hadi, M.A., Al-Worafi, Y.M.A., & Khan, T.M., (2016). Use of medical mobile applications among hospital pharmacists in Malaysia. *Therapeutic innovation & regulatory science*, 50(4), pp. 419–426.

Ming, L.C., Untong, N., Aliudin, N.A., Osili, N., Kifli, N., Tan, C.S., ... & Goh, H.P. (2020). Mobile health apps on COVID-19 launched in the early days of the pandemic: content analysis and review. *JMIR mHealth and uHealth*, 8(9), e19796.

Othman, G., Ali, F., Ibrahim, M.I.M., Al-Worafi, Y.M., Ansari, M., & Halboup, A.M. (2020). Assessment of Anti-Diabetic Medications Adherence among Diabetic Patients in Sana'a City, Yemen: A Cross Sectional Study. *Journal of Pharmaceutical Research International*, 32(21), 114–122.

Reynard, J., Reynolds, J., & Stevenson, P. (2009). *Practical patient safety*. OUP Oxford.

Saeed, M.S., Alkhoshaiban, A.S., Al-Worafi, Y.M.A., & Long, C.M., (2014). Perception of self-medication among university students in Saudi Arabia. *Archives of Pharmacy Practice*, 5(4), p. 149.

Salas, E., & Frush, K. (2012). *Improving patient safety through teamwork and team training*. Oxford University Press.

Vincent, C. (2011). *Patient safety*. John Wiley & Sons.

38 Technology for Patient Safety

38.1 BACKGROUND

Technology has revolutionized healthcare, making it more efficient, effective, and accessible. Here are some examples of technology in healthcare:

1. Electronic Health Records (EHRs): EHRs are digital versions of a patient's medical history, including diagnoses, medications, and treatment plans. This technology allows for easier and more accurate tracking of a patient's health status.

2. Telemedicine: Telemedicine uses video conferencing technology to provide remote medical care. This technology is particularly useful for patients who live in remote areas or have limited mobility.

3. Wearable Technology: Wearable technology, such as fitness trackers and smartwatches, can be used to monitor a patient's health and track their activity levels. This information can be used to identify potential health problems and make treatment recommendations.

4. Medical Imaging: Medical imaging technologies such as X-rays, MRI, and CT scans provide detailed images of the inside of the body, helping doctors diagnose and treat a wide range of conditions.

5. Robotic Surgery: Robotic surgery uses advanced robots to perform complex surgeries with greater precision and accuracy than human surgeons.

6. Artificial Intelligence: AI is being used to analyze large amounts of medical data, helping doctors make more accurate diagnoses and treatment plans.

7. 3D Printing: 3D printing technology can be used to create customized prosthetics, implants, and other medical devices, improving patient outcomes and reducing costs.

Overall, technology is transforming healthcare and has the potential to improve patient outcomes and reduce costs.

There are many technologies that are used in healthcare to improve patient care and safety. Here are some examples:

1. Electronic Medical Records (EMRs): EMRs are digital versions of a patient's medical record that allow healthcare professionals to easily access and update patient information. This can improve patient safety by reducing the risk of medical errors caused by miscommunication or incomplete information.

2. Medication Management Systems: These systems help healthcare professionals to manage and track medications for patients, ensuring that patients receive the correct medication, dosage, and frequency. This can help to reduce medication errors and improve patient outcomes.

3. Patient Monitoring Systems: Patient monitoring systems can track vital signs such as heart rate, blood pressure, and oxygen levels, and alert healthcare professionals if there are any changes that may indicate a potential health issue. This can help to detect health problems early and prevent complications.

4. Fall Prevention Systems: Fall prevention systems use sensors and alarms to alert healthcare professionals when a patient is at risk of falling. This can reduce the risk of injury and improve patient safety.

5. Remote Patient Monitoring: Remote patient monitoring allows patients to be monitored from their homes, using wearable devices or other technologies. This can be particularly useful for patients with chronic conditions, allowing them to receive care and support while maintaining their independence.

6. Patient Identification Systems: Patient identification systems use technologies such as barcodes, RFID, or biometric identification to ensure that patients receive the correct treatment and medication. This can reduce the risk of medical errors and improve patient safety.

Overall, technology plays a crucial role in improving patient care and safety in healthcare settings. By reducing errors and improving communication and monitoring, these technologies can help to improve patient outcomes and ensure that patients receive the best possible care (Kristensen & Bartels, 2010; Reynard et al., 2009; Salas & Frush, 2012; Vincent, 2011).

38.2 APPLICATIONS OF TECHNOLOGY IN PATIENT SAFETY

Technology has played a critical role in improving patient safety in healthcare. Some applications and examples of technology in patient safety include:

1. Electronic Health Records (EHRs): EHRs are digital records of patient health information that allow healthcare providers to access and share patient information across different settings. EHRs help improve patient safety by reducing errors due to illegible handwriting, ensuring accurate and complete documentation, and providing alerts and reminders for medication interactions and allergies.

2. Barcode Medication Administration (BCMA): BCMA is a technology that uses barcodes to identify patients and medications at the bedside. By scanning the patient's wristband and the medication barcode, BCMA ensures that the right medication is given to the right patient at the right time, reducing medication errors.

3. Clinical Decision Support Systems (CDSS): CDSS are computer-based systems that provide healthcare providers with real-time clinical knowledge and patient-specific information to support decision-making. CDSS can help prevent medication errors, diagnose conditions, and manage chronic diseases.

4. Telemedicine: Telemedicine allows healthcare providers to diagnose and treat patients remotely, reducing the need for in-person visits and minimizing the risk of healthcare-associated infections. Telemedicine can also improve access to care for patients in rural or underserved areas.

5. Patient Portals: Patient portals are secure online portals that allow patients to access their health information, communicate with their healthcare providers, and manage their care. Patient portals can help patients stay informed about their health status, track medications and test results, and participate in their care.

6. Telehealth: Telehealth technology allows healthcare providers to remotely monitor patients and provide virtual consultations. Telehealth can help to reduce the risk of infections in hospitals and improve access to care for patients who are unable to travel to a healthcare facility.

7. Patient Monitoring Systems: Patient monitoring systems use sensors to track a patient's vital signs and alert healthcare providers to any changes or abnormalities. These systems can help to identify potential problems before they become serious.

8. Hand hygiene monitoring systems: Hand hygiene monitoring systems help to promote hand hygiene compliance among healthcare providers. These systems use sensors to track hand hygiene compliance and provide real-time feedback to providers. Medication Dispensing Systems: Medication dispensing systems can help to reduce errors and improve medication adherence by providing patients with the right dose of medication at the right time. These systems can also alert healthcare providers to missed doses or potential medication interactions.

9. Remote Patient Monitoring: Remote patient monitoring allows healthcare providers to monitor patients' health remotely using wearable devices and mobile apps. This technology can help to identify potential health problems before they become serious and reduce the need for hospitalizations.

10. Automated Alert Systems: Automated alert systems can help to reduce the risk of medical errors by alerting healthcare providers to potential problems or deviations from best practices. For example, an automated alert system can remind healthcare providers to administer a medication at a specific time or alert them to a potential drug interaction.

11. Surgical Navigation Systems: Surgical navigation systems use 3D imaging technology to guide surgeons during procedures, reducing the risk of errors and improving surgical outcomes. These systems can also help to minimize the amount of radiation exposure during surgeries.

12. Virtual Reality (VR) and Augmented Reality (AR) Technology: VR and AR technology can be used to simulate surgical procedures and train healthcare providers in a safe and controlled environment. This technology can help to improve surgical skills and reduce the risk of errors during procedures.

13. Patient Engagement Tools: Patient engagement tools, such as mobile apps and patient portals, can help to improve patient education and communication. These tools can help patients to better understand their health conditions and treatment options, which can lead to better health outcomes and reduced medical errors.

Wearable technologies are electronic devices that are worn on the body, typically as accessories or clothing, and that can track or monitor a wide range of health-related metrics. These devices have become increasingly popular in recent years as consumers have become more interested in tracking their health and fitness.

Fitness Trackers: Fitness trackers, such as Fitbit and Garmin, are wearable devices that track physical activity, heart rate, and sleep patterns. These devices can help people to monitor their exercise habits and improve their overall fitness.

Smartwatches: Smartwatches, such as the Apple Watch and Samsung Galaxy Watch, are wearable devices that offer a wide range of health-related features, including heart rate monitoring, ECG tracking, and fall detection. These devices can also be used to track fitness goals, monitor sleep patterns, and receive notifications about medication reminders and other health-related information.

Medical Alert Devices: Medical alert devices, such as Life Alert and Medical Guardian, are wearable devices that can be used to alert healthcare providers or emergency responders in the event of a medical emergency. These devices can be especially useful for seniors or people with chronic medical conditions.

Smart Clothing: Smart clothing, such as the Hexoskin shirt and the OMsignal bra, contains sensors that can track heart rate, respiration, and other vital signs. This technology can be used to monitor patients in hospital settings or to track the health of athletes during training and competition.

Wearable Blood Glucose Monitors: Wearable blood glucose monitors, such as the Dexcom G6 and the FreeStyle Libre, allow people with diabetes to monitor their blood sugar levels without the need for frequent finger pricks. These devices can provide continuous monitoring of blood sugar levels, which can help people with diabetes to manage their condition more effectively

Wearable technologies have significant potential for improving patient safety by enabling continuous monitoring of patients and alerting healthcare providers to potential problems. Here are some examples of wearable technologies used for patient safety:

1. Fall Detection Devices: Wearable fall detection devices, such as the Lively Mobile Plus and the Philips Lifeline, can help to reduce the risk of falls in older adults. These devices can detect falls and automatically alert caregivers or emergency responders, helping to ensure that patients receive prompt medical attention.

2. Continuous Vital Sign Monitoring Devices: Wearable devices that continuously monitor patients' vital signs, such as heart rate, blood pressure, and oxygen saturation, can provide early warning signs of potential health problems. These devices can alert healthcare providers to potential problems before they become serious, allowing for early intervention.

3. Patient Location Tracking Devices: Wearable devices that track the location of patients, such as the CarePredict Tempo, can help to prevent wandering in patients with dementia or Alzheimer's disease. These devices can alert caregivers or family members if a patient leaves a designated area, helping to prevent falls, injuries, or other medical emergencies.

4. Medication Adherence Devices: Wearable devices that remind patients to take their medication, such as the MedMinder and the Hero Pill Dispenser, can help to improve medication adherence and reduce the risk of medication errors. These devices can be programmed to dispense medication at specific times, and can also alert caregivers or healthcare providers if a patient misses a dose.

5. Postoperative Monitoring Devices: Wearable devices that monitor patients' recovery after surgery, such as the Pulse Oximeter and the EMOTIV headset, can help to ensure that patients are recovering safely and without complications. These devices can provide early warning signs of potential problems, such as infection or bleeding, and can alert healthcare providers to potential problems before they become serious.

Overall, wearable technologies have significant potential for improving patient safety by providing continuous monitoring of patients and alerting healthcare providers to potential problems. As these devices become more advanced and affordable, they are likely to become an increasingly important tool in healthcare.

38.3 ARTIFICIAL INTELLIGENCE (AI) IN PATIENT SAFETY

Artificial intelligence (AI) has the potential to revolutionize patient care and safety by improving the accuracy and efficiency of diagnosis, treatment, and monitoring. Here are some examples of how AI is being used in patient care and safety:

1. Diagnosis: AI can be used to analyze large amounts of data, such as medical images and patient records, to help healthcare providers make more accurate and timely diagnoses. For example, AI algorithms can analyze medical images to detect early signs of diseases such as cancer, or predict the likelihood of certain diseases based on patient characteristics and family history.

2. Treatment: AI can also be used to personalize treatment plans for individual patients based on their unique characteristics and medical history. For example, AI can analyze patient data to predict the likelihood of a patient responding to a particular treatment or to identify potential side effects of certain medications.

3. Monitoring: AI can be used to continuously monitor patients in real-time and detect early signs of potential health problems. For example, AI algorithms can analyze patient vital signs and alert healthcare providers if there are any changes that could indicate a medical emergency.

4. Medical Research: AI can also be used to accelerate medical research by analyzing large amounts of data and identifying potential new treatments or cures for diseases. For example, AI algorithms can analyze genomic data to identify potential targets for new drugs, or identify patients who may be eligible for clinical trials.

5. Patient Safety: AI can be used to improve patient safety by reducing the risk of medical errors and adverse events. For example, AI algorithms can help to identify patients who are at risk of developing infections or other complications while in the hospital, or identify potential medication errors before they occur.

Overall, AI has the potential to transform patient care and safety by providing healthcare providers with new tools and insights that can improve diagnosis, treatment, and monitoring. As AI technology continues to evolve and become more advanced, it is likely to become an increasingly important tool in healthcare.

38.4 ADVANTAGES OF TECHNOLOGIES IN PATIENT SAFETY

The use of technology has revolutionized patient safety in many ways, offering numerous advantages that improve patient outcomes and prevent errors. Here are some of the key advantages of technologies in patient safety:

1. Improved accuracy and efficiency: With technology, healthcare providers can enter, access and process patient data more accurately and efficiently, reducing the risk of errors in diagnosis, treatment, and medication administration.

2. Enhanced communication: Technology enables healthcare professionals to communicate more easily with one another, improving the coordination of care and reducing the risk of miscommunication or delayed responses.

3. Early detection of health issues: Technologies such as electronic health records (EHRs) and telemedicine allow healthcare providers to monitor patients remotely and identify potential health issues before they become serious.

4. Real-time tracking: Tracking systems and sensors can monitor patient movements, medication use, and other vital signs in real-time, enabling healthcare providers to respond immediately to any changes in a patient's condition.

5. Reduced medication errors: Electronic medication administration systems (eMARs) and barcode scanning can help ensure that patients receive the right medication at the right dose and at the right time, reducing the risk of medication errors.

6. Improved patient engagement: Technology can improve patient engagement by enabling patients to access their health information, communicate with their healthcare providers, and receive personalized education and support.

Overall, technology has the potential to enhance patient safety, improve quality of care, and reduce medical errors. However, it is important to note that technology is not a substitute for human expertise and judgment. Healthcare providers must still exercise good clinical judgment and follow best practices to ensure safe and effective patient care.

38.5 DISADVANTAGES OF TECHNOLOGIES IN PATIENT SAFETY

While technology has numerous advantages in patient safety, it also has some potential disadvantages. Here are some of the key disadvantages of technologies in patient safety:

1. Technical difficulties: Technology can malfunction, causing errors in patient care, and may require technical support to resolve the issue.

2. Cost: The cost of implementing and maintaining technology can be significant, which may make it difficult for some healthcare organizations to adopt new technologies.

3. Cybersecurity risks: Electronic health records and other digital systems are vulnerable to cyber-attacks, which can compromise patient data and cause harm to patients.

4. User error: Technology requires proper training and education to use correctly, and user error can lead to errors in patient care.

5. Dependence on technology: Over-reliance on technology can lead to complacency and a lack of critical thinking, which can increase the risk of errors in patient care.

6. Privacy concerns: The use of technology can raise concerns about patient privacy and data security, especially if patient data is stored in the cloud or accessed remotely.

Overall, while technology has numerous advantages in patient safety, it is important to be aware of the potential disadvantages and to take steps to mitigate them. Healthcare organizations should carefully consider the costs and risks associated with new technologies before implementing them and should provide adequate training and support to ensure that healthcare providers use technology safely and effectively.

38.6 TECHNOLOGIES IN PATIENT SAFETY: Facilitators

Technologies have a significant impact on patient safety and can facilitate the implementation of safety measures in healthcare. Here are some of the ways that technologies act as facilitators for patient safety:

1. Automation of safety processes: Technologies can automate safety processes, such as medication ordering and administration, to reduce the risk of errors.

2. Integration of safety tools: Technologies can integrate safety tools, such as checklists and protocols, into electronic health records to help healthcare providers follow safety guidelines.

3. Access to real-time data: Technologies provide healthcare providers with access to real-time patient data, such as vital signs and lab results, allowing for timely interventions and improved patient outcomes.

4. Standardization of care: Technologies can help standardize care by providing healthcare providers with evidence-based protocols and guidelines, reducing variability in care delivery.

5. Enhanced communication: Technologies facilitate communication between healthcare providers and patients, improving patient engagement and allowing for timely interventions.

6. Data analytics: Technologies can help healthcare organizations analyze patient safety data to identify areas for improvement and to monitor the effectiveness of safety interventions.

Overall, technologies can facilitate the implementation of patient safety measures and improve patient outcomes. Healthcare organizations should consider adopting technologies that align with their patient safety goals and provide adequate training and support to healthcare providers to ensure safe and effective use of these technologies.

There are several facilitators that can promote the effective use of technologies in patient safety. Here are some of the key facilitators for the use of technologies in patient safety:

1. Leadership support: Strong leadership support for the adoption of new technologies is essential for their successful implementation.

2. User engagement: Healthcare providers should be involved in the design and selection of new technologies, ensuring that they meet their needs and that they are easy to use.

3. Education and training: Adequate education and training should be provided to healthcare providers to ensure that they use new technologies safely and effectively.

4. Standardization: Standardizing the use of new technologies across healthcare settings can help ensure consistent and effective use.

5. Interoperability: Technologies should be designed to be interoperable, allowing for easy data sharing and communication between healthcare providers.

6. Data analytics: Using data analytics to monitor and evaluate the effectiveness of new technologies can help identify areas for improvement and promote continuous quality improvement.

7. Financial incentives: Providing financial incentives, such as reimbursement for the use of new technologies, can encourage healthcare organizations to adopt and use them effectively.

Overall, effective implementation of technologies in patient safety requires a collaborative approach that involves healthcare providers, patients, leadership, and other stakeholders. By addressing facilitators such as user engagement, education and training, and data analytics, healthcare organizations can promote the successful use of technologies in patient safety and improve patient outcomes.

38.7 TECHNOLOGIES IN PATIENT SAFETY: Barriers

While technologies have the potential to improve patient safety, there are several barriers that can prevent their successful implementation. Here are some of the key barriers to implementing technologies in patient safety:

1. Cost: The cost of implementing new technologies can be a significant barrier, especially for smaller healthcare organizations or those with limited budgets.

2. Resistance to change: Healthcare providers may be resistant to changing their practices, particularly if they are used to using manual systems and processes.

3. Technical challenges: The technical complexity of some technologies, such as electronic health records, can make their implementation challenging, and technical problems may arise during their use.

4. Lack of interoperability: Incompatibility between different technologies used in healthcare can prevent effective data sharing and communication between healthcare providers, hindering patient safety efforts.

5. Cybersecurity risks: Healthcare organizations may be hesitant to adopt new technologies due to concerns about cybersecurity and data breaches.

6. Training and support: Adequate training and support are necessary to ensure that healthcare providers use technologies safely and effectively, and a lack of training and support can prevent successful implementation.

Overall, the barriers to implementing technologies in patient safety are complex and multifaceted. Healthcare organizations must carefully consider these barriers when adopting new technologies and take steps to address them to ensure the successful implementation of patient safety technologies.

38.8 PATIENT SAFETY TECHNOLOGIES IN DEVELOPING COUNTRIES: Challenges and Recommendations

Patient safety technologies have the potential to improve healthcare outcomes in developing countries, but there are several challenges that must be overcome to effectively implement them.

Here are some of the key challenges and recommendations for patient safety technologies in developing countries:

Challenges:

1. Lack of infrastructure: Developing countries often lack the necessary infrastructure, such as reliable electricity and internet connectivity, to support the implementation of patient safety technologies.

2. Limited resources: Healthcare systems in developing countries may have limited financial and human resources, making it difficult to invest in patient safety technologies.

3. Cultural and language barriers: Cultural and language differences may make it difficult to effectively communicate the importance of patient safety technologies and how to use them.

4. Limited technical expertise: There may be a lack of technical expertise in developing countries to effectively implement and maintain patient safety technologies.

Recommendations:

1. Partnership and collaboration: Developing partnerships and collaborations between healthcare organizations in developing and developed countries can provide access to technical expertise, financial resources, and other forms of support.

2. Customization and localization: Patient safety technologies should be customized and localized to meet the specific needs of healthcare systems in developing countries, taking into account cultural and language differences.

3. Capacity building: Investing in the training and development of healthcare providers and technical staff can improve their technical expertise and ensure that patient safety technologies are used effectively.

4. Prioritization: Prioritizing patient safety technologies in national healthcare policies and strategies can increase the resources and support available for their implementation.

5. Sustainability: Patient safety technologies should be designed with sustainability in mind, taking into account the long-term costs and maintenance requirements to ensure their continued use.

6. Limited access to healthcare: In many developing countries, a large portion of the population lives in rural or remote areas with limited access to healthcare facilities. This can make it difficult to implement patient safety technologies that require regular monitoring and maintenance.

7. Regulatory and legal barriers: Regulatory and legal barriers can make it difficult to import or use certain types of patient safety technologies in developing countries, particularly if they are not approved by local regulatory authorities.

8. Lack of awareness: Lack of awareness about patient safety technologies among healthcare providers, patients, and policymakers can hinder their adoption and implementation.

9. Resistance to change: Healthcare providers and patients may be resistant to changing established practices and may not see the value in adopting new patient safety technologies.

10. Data privacy concerns: Data privacy concerns may be a barrier to the implementation of patient safety technologies, particularly if patients are hesitant to share their personal health information.

11. Maintenance and repair: Maintenance and repair of patient safety technologies can be a challenge in developing countries due to limited resources, lack of technical expertise, and limited access to spare parts.

12. Limited internet access: Many developing countries have limited access to high-speed internet, which can make it difficult to implement patient safety technologies that rely on connectivity.

13. Power outages: Power outages and fluctuations in electricity supply are common in some developing countries, which can make it challenging to operate and maintain patient safety technologies that require electricity.

14. Lack of coordination: Lack of coordination between healthcare providers and institutions can result in fragmentation of patient care and hinder the implementation of patient safety technologies that require data sharing and collaboration.

15. Inadequate policies and regulations: Some developing countries may lack adequate policies and regulations to support the implementation of patient safety technologies or may have policies that are not enforced effectively.

16. Limited research: Limited research on the effectiveness and implementation of patient safety technologies in developing countries can hinder their adoption and lead to uncertainty about their benefits.

17. Socioeconomic factors: Socioeconomic factors such as poverty, illiteracy, and cultural beliefs can affect the uptake and utilization of patient safety technologies.

18. Limited resources for procurement: Procuring and maintaining patient safety technologies can be costly, and healthcare systems in developing countries may have limited financial resources to invest in them.

19. Limited supply chain and logistics: The supply chain and logistics infrastructure in developing countries may be inadequate to support the timely and efficient delivery of patient safety technologies, spare parts, and consumables.

20. Limited human resources: Developing countries often face a shortage of trained healthcare professionals, which can make it difficult to implement patient safety technologies that require specialized knowledge and skills.

21. Poor infrastructure for waste management: Inadequate infrastructure for waste management can result in the improper disposal of medical equipment and supplies, which can be hazardous to both patients and the environment.

22. Political instability: Political instability, conflict, and violence can disrupt healthcare systems and hinder the implementation of patient safety technologies.

23. Limited public awareness and participation: The success of patient safety technologies relies on the participation and engagement of patients and the public. Limited public awareness and participation in developing countries can hinder the adoption and sustainability of these technologies.

24. Despite the progress in research about the patient care and safety in developing countries, there is little research about the impact of technologies in patient safety, therefore, conduct research is very important and highly recommended (Alshahrani et al., 2019a,b; Al-Qahtani et al., 2015; Alshahrani et al., 2020a,b; Al-Worafi, 2014; Al-Worafi, 2015; Al-Worafi, 2016; Al-Worafi et al., 2017; Al-Worafi, 2018a-d; Al-Worafi et al., 2018a-b; Al-Worafi et al., 2019; Al-Worafi, 2020a-z; Al-Worafi et al., 2020a-b; Al-Worafi et al., 2021a,b; Al-Worafi, 2022a,b; Al-Worafi, 2023; Baig et al., 2020; Elkalmi et al., 2020; Elsayed & Al-Worafi, 2020; Hasan et al., 2019; Hassan et al., 2014; Izahar et al., 2017; Lee et al., 2017; Mahmoud et al., 2020; Manan et al., 2014; Manan et al., 2016; Ming et al., 2016; Ming et al., 2020; Othman et al., 2020; Saeed et al., 2014).

To overcome these challenges, healthcare organizations and policymakers in developing countries should focus on building capacity, developing sustainable models for procurement and maintenance, improving the supply chain and logistics infrastructure, investing in human resources, promoting public awareness and participation, and fostering stable political environments. International partnerships and collaborations can also be valuable in addressing these challenges and supporting the implementation of patient safety technologies in developing countries.

38.9 CONCLUSION

This chapter has discussed the patient safety issues related to the technology for patient safety, its applications, advantages, disadvantages, facilitators, barriers and recommendations for the best practice in developing countries. Patient safety technologies have the potential to improve healthcare outcomes and reduce the incidence of medical errors. However, their implementation in developing countries can be challenging due to a range of barriers and challenges, including limited resources, inadequate infrastructure, regulatory barriers, and cultural and socioeconomic factors. To successfully implement patient safety technologies in developing countries, healthcare organizations and policymakers must prioritize investments in healthcare infrastructure, build capacity, improve supply chain and logistics infrastructure, promote public awareness and participation, and foster stable political environments. International partnerships and collaborations can also be valuable in addressing these challenges and supporting the adoption and sustainable use of patient safety technologies in developing countries. Despite the challenges, the potential benefits of patient safety technologies make their implementation a critical priority for improving healthcare outcomes and promoting patient safety in developing countries.

REFERENCES

Al-Qahtani, I., Almoteb, T.M., & Al-Warafi, Y. (2015). Competency of metered-dose inhaler use among Saudi community pharmacists: A Simulation method study. *RRJPPS*, 4(2), 37–31.

Alshahrani, S.M., Alakhali, K.M., & Al-Worafi, Y.M., (2019a). Medication errors in a health care facility in southern Saudi Arabia. *Tropical Journal of Pharmaceutical Research*, 18(5), pp. 1119–1122.

Alshahrani, S.M., Alavudeen, S.S., Alakhali, K.M., Al-Worafi, Y.M., Bahamdan, A.K., & Vigneshwaran, E., (2019b). Self-Medication Among King Khalid University Students, Saudi Arabia. *Risk Management and Healthcare Policy*, 12, pp. 243–249.

Alshahrani, S.M., Alakhali, K.M., Al-Worafi, Y.M., & Alshahrani, N.Z. (2020b). Awareness and use of over the counter analgesic medication: a survey in the Aseer region population, Saudi Arabia. *Int J Advan Appl Sci*, 7(3), 130–134.

Alshahrani, S.M., Alzahran, M., Alakhali, K., Vigneshwaran, E., Iqbal, M.J., Khan, N.A., ... & Alavudeen, S.S. (2020b). Association Between Diabetes Consequences and Quality of Life Among Patients With Diabetes Mellitus in the Aseer Province of Saudi Arabia. *Open Access Macedonian Journal of Medical Sciences*, 8(E), 325–330.

Al-Worafi, Y.M. (2014). Prescription writing errors at a tertiary care hospital in Yemen: prevalence, types, causes and recommendations. *Am J Pharm Health Res*, 2, 134–140.

Al-Worafi, Y.M.A. (2015). Appropriateness of metered-dose inhaler use in the Yemeni community pharmacies. *Journal of Taibah University Medical Sciences*, 10(3), 353–358.

Al-Worafi, Y.M.A., (2016). Pharmacy practice in Yemen. In *Pharmacy Practice in Developing Countries* (pp. 267–287). Academic Press.

Al-Worafi, Y.M., Kassab, Y.W., Alseragi, W.M., Almutairi, M.S., Ahmed, A., Ming, L.C., Alkhoshaiban, A.S., & Hadi, M.A., (2017). Pharmacovigilance and adverse drg reaction reporting: a perspective of community pharmacists and pharmacy technicians in Sana'a, Yemen. *Therapeutics and clinical risk management*, 13, p. 1175.

Al-Worafi, Y.M., (2018a). Knowledge, Attitude and Practice of Yemeni Physicians Toward Pharmacovigilance: A Mixed Method Study. *International Journal of Pharmacy and Pharmaceutical Sciences*, 10(10), 74–77.

Al-Worafi, Y. (2018b). Knowledge, attitude and practice of Yemeni physicians toward pharmacovigilance: A mixed method study. *Int. J. Pharm. Pharm. Sci*, 10, 74–77.

Al-Worafi, Y.M. (2018c). Dispensing errors observed by community pharmacy dispensers in IBB–YEMEN. *Asian J. Pharm. Clin. Res*, 11(11).

Al-Worafi, Y.M. (2018d). Evauation of inhaler technique among patients with asthma and COPD in Yemen. *Journal of Taibah University medical sciences*, 13(5), 488–490.

Al-Worafi, Y.M., Patel, R.P., Zaidi, S.T.R., Alseragi, W.M., Almutairi, M.S., Alkhoshaiban, A.S., & Ming, L.C. (2018a). Completeness and legibility of handwritten prescriptions in Sana'a, Yemen. *Medical Principles and Practice*, 27, 290–292.

Al-Worafi, Y.M., Alseragi, W.M., Seng, L.K., Kassab, Y.W., Yeoh, S.F., Chiau, L., … & Husain, K. (2018b). Dispensing errors in community pharmacies: a prospective study in Sana'a, Yemen. *Arch Pharm Pract*, 9(4), 1–3.

Al-Worafi, Y.M., Alseragi, W.M., & Mahmoud, M.A. (2019). Competency of metered-dose inhaler use among community pharmacy dispensers in Ibb, Yemen: A simulation method study. *Latin American Journal of Pharmacy*, 38(3), 489–494.

Al-Worafi, Y.M. (Ed.). (2020a). *Drug Safety in Developing Countries: Achievements and Challenges*.

Al-Worafi, Y.M. (2020b). Medication errors. In *Drug Safety in Developing Countries* (pp. 105–117). Academic Press.

Al-Worafi, Y.M. (2020c). Adverse drug reactions. In *Drug Safety in Developing Countries* (pp. 39–57). Academic Press.

Al-Worafi, Y.M. (2020d). Medications registration and marketing: safety-related issues. In *Drug Safety in Developing Countries* (pp. 21–28). Academic Press.

Al-Worafi, Y.M. (2020e). Pharmacovigilance. In *Drug Safety in Developing Countries* (pp. 29–38). Academic Press.

Al-Worafi, Y.M. (2020f). Drug-related problems. In *Drug safety in developing countries* (pp. 59–71). Academic Press.

Al-Worafi, Y.M. (2020g). Medications safety-related terminology. In *Drug safety in developing countries* (pp. 7–19). Academic Press.

Al-Worafi, Y.M. (2020h). Self-medication. In *Drug Safety in Developing Countries* (pp. 73–86). Academic Press.

Al-Worafi, Y.M. (2020j). Antibiotics safety issues. In *Drug Safety in Developing Countries* (pp. 87–103). Academic Press.

Al-Worafi, Y.M. (2020k). Medications safety research issues. In *Drug Safety in Developing Countries* (pp. 213–227). Academic Press.

Al-Worafi, Y.M. (2020l). Counterfeit and substandard medications. In *Drug safety in developing countries* (pp. 119–126). Academic Press.

Al-Worafi, Y.M. (2020m). Medication abuse and misuse. In *Drug safety in developing countries* (pp. 127–135). Academic Press.

Al-Worafi, Y.M. (2020n). Storage and disposal of medications. In *Drug Safety in Developing Countries* (pp. 137–142). Academic Press.

Al-Worafi, Y.M. (2020o). Safety of medications in special population. In *Drug safety in developing countries* (pp. 143–162). Academic Press.

Al-Worafi, Y.M. (2020p). Herbal medicines safety issues. In *Drug Safety in developing countries* (pp. 163–178). Academic Press.

Al-Worafi, Y.M. (2020q). Medications safety pharmacoeconomics-related issues. In *Drug Safety in Developing Countries* (pp. 187–195). Academic Press.

Al-Worafi, Y.M. (2020r). Evidence-based medications safety practice. In *Drug Safety in Developing Countries* (pp. 197–201). Academic Press.

Al-Worafi, Y.M. (2020s). Quality indicators for medications safety. In *Drug safety in developing countries* (pp. 229–242). Academic Press.

Al-Worafi, Y.M. (2020t). Drug safety in Yemen. In *Drug Safety in Developing Countries* (pp. 391–405). Academic Press.

Al-Worafi, Y.M. (2020u). Drug safety in Saudi Arabia. In *Drug Safety in Developing Countries* (pp. 407–417). Academic Press.

Al-Worafi, Y.M. (2020v). Drug safety in United Arab Emirates. In *Drug Safety in Developing Countries* (pp. 419–428). Academic Press.

Al-Worafi, Y.M. (2020w). Drug safety in Indonesia. In *Drug Safety in Developing Countries* (pp. 279–285). Academic Press.

Al-Worafi, Y.M. (2020x). Drug safety in Palestine. In *Drug Safety in Developing Countries* (pp. 471–480). Academic Press.

Al-Worafi, Y.M. (2020y). Drug safety: comparison between developing countries. In *Drug Safety in Developing Countries* (pp. 603–611). Academic Press.

Al-Worafi, Y.M. (2020z). Drug safety in developing versus developed countries. In *Drug Safety in Developing Countries* (pp. 613–615). Academic Press.

Al-Worafi, Y.M., Alseragi, W.M., Ming, L.C., & Alakhali, K.M. (2020a). Drug safety in China. In *Drug Safety in Developing Countries* (pp. 381–388). Academic Press.

Al-Worafi, Y.M., Alseragi, W.M., Alakhali, K.M., Ming, L.C., Othman, G., Halboup, A.M., … & Elkalmi, R.M. (2020b). Knowledge, beliefs and factors affecting the use of generic medicines among patients in Ibb, Yemen: a mixed-method study. *Journal of Pharmacy Practice and Community Medicine*, 6(4).

Al-Worafi, Y.M., Elkalmi, R.M., Ming, L.C., Othman, G., Halboup, A.M., Battah, M.M., … & Mani, V. (2021a). Dispensing errors in hospital pharmacies: A prospective study in Yemen.

Al-Worafi, Y.M., Hasan, S., Hassan, N.M., & Gaili, A.A. (2021b). Knowledge, Attitude and Experience of Pharmacist in the UAE towards Pharmacovigilance. *Research Journal of Pharmacy and Technology*, 14(1), 265–269.

Al-Worafi, Y. (2022a). *A Guide to Online Pharmacy Education: Teaching Strategies and Assessment Methods*. CRC Press.

Al-Worafi, Y.M. (2022b). Patient care errors and related problems (part I): development and validation of the model. 0000-0002-5752-2913

Al-Worafi, Y.M. (Ed.). (2023). *Clinical Case Studies on medication Safety*. Academic Press.

Baig, M.R., Al-Worafi, Y.M., Alseragi, W.M., Ming, L.C., & Siddique, A. (2020). Drug safety in India. In *Drug Safety in Developing Countries* (pp. 327–334). Academic Press.

Elkalmi, R.M., Al-Worafi, Y.M., Alseragi, W.M., Ming, L.C., & Siddique, A. (2020). Drug safety in Malaysia. In *Drug Safety in Developing Countries* (pp. 245–253). Academic Press.

Elsayed, T., & Al-Worafi, Y.M. (2020). Drug safety in Egypt. In *Drug Safety in Developing Countries* (pp. 511–523). Academic Press.

Hasan, S., Al-Omar, M.J., AlZubaidy, H., & Al-Worafi, Y.M. (2019). Use of medications in Arab Countries. *Handbook of Healthcare in the Arab World*. Cham: Springer, 42.

Hassan, Y., Abd Aziz, N., Kassab, Y.W., Elgasim, I., Shaharuddin, S., Al-Worafi, Y.M.A., ... & Ming, L.C. (2014). How to help patients to control their blood pressure? Blood pressure control and its predictor. *Archives of Pharmacy Practice*, 5(4).

Izahar, S., Lean, Q.Y., Hameed, M.A., Murugiah, M.K., Patel, R.P., Al-Worafi, Y.M., ... & Ming, L.C. (2017). Content analysis of mobile health applications on diabetes mellitus. *Frontiers in Endocrinology*, 8, 318.

Kristensen, S., & Bartels, P. (2010). Use of patient safety culture instruments and recommendations. *Aarhus, Denmark, European Society for Quality in HealthCare-Office for Quality Indicators*, 113.

Lee, K.S., Yee, S.M., Zaidi, S.T.R., Patel, R.P., Yang, Q., Al-Worafi, Y.M., & Ming, L.C., 2017. Combating sale of counterfeit and falsified medicines online: a losing battle. *Frontiers in pharmacology*, 8, p. 268.

Mahmoud, M.A., Wajid, S., Naqvi, A.A., Samreen, S., Althagfan, S.S., & Al-Worafi, Y. (2020). Self-medication with antibiotics: A cross-sectional community-based study. *Latin american journal of pharmacy*, 39(2), 348–353.

Manan, M.M., Rusli, R.A., Ang, W.C., Al-Worafi, Y.M., & Ming, L.C. (2014). Assessing the pharmaceutical care issues of antiepileptic drug therapy in hospitalised epileptic patients. *Journal of Pharmacy Practice and Research*, 44(3), 83–88.

Manan, M.M., Ibrahim, N.A., Aziz, N.A., Zulkifly, H.H., Al-Worafi, Y.M.A., & Long, C.M. (2016). Empirical use of antibiotic therapy in the prevention of early onset sepsis in neonates: a pilot study. *Archives of Medical Science*, 12(3), 603–613.

Ming, L.C., Hameed, M.A., Lee, D.D., Apidi, N.A., Lai, P.S.M., Hadi, M.A., Al-Worafi, Y.M.A., & Khan, T.M., (2016). Use of medical mobile applications among hospital pharmacists in Malaysia. *Therapeutic innovation & regulatory science*, 50(4), pp. 419–426.

Ming, L.C., Untong, N., Aliudin, N.A., Osili, N., Kifli, N., Tan, C.S., ... & Goh, H.P. (2020). Mobile health apps on COVID-19 launched in the early days of the pandemic: content analysis and review. *JMIR mHealth and uHealth*, 8(9), e19796.

Othman, G., Ali, F., Ibrahim, M.I.M., Al-Worafi, Y.M., Ansari, M., & Halboup, A.M. (2020). Assessment of Anti-Diabetic Medications Adherence among Diabetic Patients in Sana'a City, Yemen: A Cross Sectional Study. *Journal of Pharmaceutical Research International*, 32(21), 114–122.

Reynard, J., Reynolds, J., & Stevenson, P. (2009). *Practical patient safety*. OUP Oxford.

Saeed, M.S., Alkhoshaiban, A.S., Al-Worafi, Y.M.A., & Long, C.M., (2014). Perception of self-medication among university students in Saudi Arabia. *Archives of Pharmacy Practice*, 5(4), p. 149.

Salas, E., & Frush, K. (2012). *Improving patient safety through teamwork and team training*. Oxford University Press.

Vincent, C. (2011). *Patient safety*. John Wiley & Sons.

39 Evidence-based Patient Safety

39.1 BACKGROUND

Evidence-based medicine (EBM) is an approach to healthcare that emphasizes the use of the best available evidence from clinical research in making decisions about patient care. It involves the conscientious, explicit, and judicious use of current best evidence in making decisions about the care of individual patients. EBM aims to integrate individual clinical expertise with the best available external clinical evidence from systematic research. The practice of evidence-based medicine involves several steps, including formulating a clear and answerable clinical question, searching for the best available evidence, critically appraising the evidence for its validity and usefulness, applying the evidence to the individual patient's circumstances, and evaluating the effectiveness and efficiency of the chosen intervention. The use of EBM has become increasingly important in healthcare, as it provides a structured and rigorous approach to decision-making that can improve patient outcomes and reduce variability in clinical practice. However, it is important to note that EBM is not a one-size-fits-all approach, and clinical judgement and expertise remain crucial components of healthcare decision-making. Evidence-based patient safety is an approach to improving the safety and quality of healthcare that involves using the best available evidence from research to identify and implement strategies that can reduce the risk of harm to patients. The key principles of evidence-based patient safety include:

1. Identifying and analyzing adverse events: This involves collecting and analyzing data on adverse events, near misses, and other indicators of patient harm, in order to understand the root causes of errors and identify opportunities for improvement.

2. Developing and implementing evidence-based interventions: Based on the analysis of adverse events, evidence-based interventions can be developed and implemented to reduce the risk of harm to patients. Examples of such interventions include standardized protocols for medication administration, checklists for surgical procedures, and training programs for healthcare providers.

3. Continuous monitoring and evaluation: Regular monitoring and evaluation of patient safety initiatives is necessary to ensure that they are effective and sustainable over time. This involves ongoing data collection, analysis, and feedback, as well as continuous improvement and refinement of interventions.

4. Involving patients and families: Patient and family involvement is essential for effective patient safety initiatives. Patients and families can provide valuable insights into their experiences and perspectives, and can help identify areas where improvements can be made.

5. Communication and teamwork: Effective communication and teamwork among healthcare providers is essential for patient safety. Strategies such as standardized handoff procedures, team training, and regular feedback and debriefing can improve communication and teamwork and reduce the risk of errors.

6. Health information technology: The use of health information technology (HIT) can improve patient safety by reducing errors related to medication administration, diagnostic testing, and other aspects of care. HIT can also facilitate the collection and analysis of data related to adverse events and patient outcomes.

7. Cultural competence: Cultural competence is the ability of healthcare providers to understand and respond to the cultural and linguistic needs of patients and families.

The use of evidence-based patient safety practices has been shown to reduce the risk of adverse events and improve patient outcomes. However, it requires a commitment to continuous improvement, ongoing monitoring and evaluation, and collaboration among healthcare providers, patients, and families (Kristensen & Bartels, 2010; Reynard et al., 2009; Salas & Frush, 2012; Vincent, 2011).

39.2 RATIONALITY OF EVIDENCE-BASED PATIENT SAFETY

Evidence-based medicine (EBM) is a rational approach to medical decision-making that emphasizes the use of the best available scientific evidence to inform clinical practice. The rationality of EBM

DOI: 10.1201/9781003230465-41

stems from its commitment to following a systematic and transparent process for evaluating the validity and reliability of scientific evidence, as well as its recognition of the importance of clinical expertise and patient values in making treatment decisions. EBM starts with a clinical question that arises in the course of patient care. The question is then formulated into a structured format known as the PICO framework (Patient, Intervention, Comparison, Outcome). This allows the clinician to identify the key elements of the question and the information needed to answer it. The clinician then searches the medical literature for relevant studies, critically appraises their methodology, and synthesizes the evidence to answer the question. The rationality of EBM lies in its emphasis on the use of high-quality, unbiased scientific evidence, rather than relying on anecdote or opinion. EBM recognizes that scientific evidence is not infallible, but it provides the best available guide for clinical decision-making. EBM also recognizes the importance of clinical expertise, which is used to interpret the evidence in the context of the individual patient's situation, and patient values, which are used to guide treatment decisions that are consistent with the patient's goals and preferences. In summary, the rationality of evidence-based medicine lies in its systematic and transparent approach to evaluating scientific evidence, its recognition of the importance of clinical expertise and patient values in making treatment decisions, and its commitment to providing the best available guidance for clinical practice. Patient safety is a critical aspect of healthcare that aims to prevent harm to patients from errors, accidents, and infections. Evidence-based patient safety is a rational approach to improving patient safety that emphasizes the use of the best available scientific evidence to identify and implement interventions that have been shown to be effective in reducing harm to patients. The rationality of evidence-based patient safety lies in its commitment to following a systematic and transparent process for evaluating the validity and reliability of scientific evidence, and its use of this evidence to inform interventions that have the greatest potential to reduce harm to patients. Evidence-based patient safety starts with the identification of a patient safety problem, such as a high rate of medication errors or healthcare-associated infections. The problem is then evaluated using a structured process that involves identifying the underlying causes and the potential solutions. The best available scientific evidence is then used to identify interventions that have been shown to be effective in reducing harm in similar situations. The rationality of evidence-based patient safety lies in its emphasis on the use of high-quality, unbiased scientific evidence, rather than relying on anecdote or opinion. This approach recognizes that patient safety is a complex problem that requires a systematic and evidence-based approach to identify and address its underlying causes. It also recognizes the importance of continuous monitoring and evaluation to ensure that interventions are effective and sustainable. In summary, the rationality of evidence-based patient safety lies in its systematic and transparent approach to identifying patient safety problems, its use of the best available scientific evidence to identify effective interventions, and its commitment to continuous monitoring and evaluation to ensure that interventions are effective and sustainable. By using this approach, healthcare organizations can improve patient safety and reduce the risk of harm to patients.

39.3 IMPORTANCE OF EVIDENCE-BASED PATIENT SAFETY

Evidence-based patient safety is of critical importance in healthcare for several reasons:

1. Reducing harm to patients: Evidence-based patient safety interventions have been shown to be effective in reducing harm to patients, such as healthcare-associated infections, medication errors, and falls. By implementing these interventions, healthcare organizations can improve patient safety and reduce the risk of harm to patients.

2. Improving healthcare quality: Evidence-based patient safety interventions are also associated with improvements in healthcare quality, such as improved communication and teamwork among healthcare providers. By improving quality, healthcare organizations can enhance patient experiences and outcomes.

3. Enhancing patient trust: Patients and their families place a great deal of trust in healthcare providers to provide safe and effective care. By implementing evidence-based patient safety interventions, healthcare organizations can demonstrate their commitment to providing high-quality care and build trust with their patients.

4. Reducing healthcare costs: Healthcare-associated harm is associated with significant costs, such as increased hospital length of stay, readmissions, and litigation. Evidence-based patient safety interventions can reduce these costs by preventing harm and improving healthcare quality.

5. Meeting regulatory requirements: Healthcare organizations are increasingly subject to regulatory requirements related to patient safety, such as accreditation standards and reporting requirements. Implementing evidence-based patient safety interventions can help organizations meet these requirements and avoid penalties or sanctions.

6. Addressing healthcare disparities: Evidence-based patient safety interventions can help address healthcare disparities by ensuring that all patients receive the same high-quality, safe, and effective care, regardless of their race, ethnicity, or socioeconomic status.

7. Enhancing healthcare workforce satisfaction: Evidence-based patient safety interventions can improve the work environment for healthcare providers by reducing stress and burnout, and improving teamwork and communication. This can result in greater job satisfaction and retention among healthcare providers.

8. Encouraging a culture of safety: Evidence-based patient safety interventions can help create a culture of safety within healthcare organizations by emphasizing the importance of reporting errors, near misses, and adverse events, and by promoting open and honest communication among healthcare providers.

9. Improving public health: Evidence-based patient safety interventions can contribute to improving public health by preventing the spread of infectious diseases, reducing the overuse of antibiotics, and promoting vaccination and other preventive measures.

10. Advancing healthcare research: Evidence-based patient safety interventions can contribute to the advancement of healthcare research by generating new knowledge about the effectiveness of different interventions, and by identifying areas where further research is needed to improve patient safety.

In summary, evidence-based patient safety is important in healthcare because it can reduce harm to patients, improve healthcare quality, enhance patient trust, reduce healthcare costs, and meet regulatory requirements. By implementing evidence-based patient safety interventions, healthcare organizations can improve patient safety and provide high-quality, safe, and effective care.

39.4 FACILITATORS FOR THE EVIDENCE-BASED PATIENT SAFETY

There are several facilitators for evidence-based patient safety, including:

1. Leadership support: Strong leadership support is essential for implementing evidence-based patient safety interventions. Leaders can provide the necessary resources, establish policies and procedures, and promote a culture of safety within the organization.

2. Staff engagement: Staff engagement is critical for the success of evidence-based patient safety interventions. Staff members who are involved in the planning, implementation, and evaluation of interventions are more likely to be invested in their success and to provide feedback that can improve their effectiveness.

3. Education and training: Education and training are important for ensuring that staff members have the knowledge and skills necessary to implement evidence-based patient safety interventions effectively. This includes training on the principles of patient safety, as well as on specific interventions such as hand hygiene, medication safety, and infection control.

4. Data collection and analysis: Data collection and analysis are essential for monitoring the effectiveness of evidence-based patient safety interventions. This includes tracking the incidence of adverse events and near misses, as well as collecting data on the implementation and outcomes of interventions.

5. Collaboration and partnerships: Collaboration and partnerships can facilitate the implementation of evidence-based patient safety interventions. This includes partnerships with other healthcare organizations, professional associations, and regulatory agencies, as well as collaboration among different departments and disciplines within the organization.

6. Continuous quality improvement: Continuous quality improvement is essential for ensuring that evidence-based patient safety interventions are effective and sustainable. This includes ongoing monitoring and evaluation of interventions, as well as regular review of policies and procedures to identify areas for improvement.

In summary, facilitators for evidence-based patient safety include leadership support, staff engagement, education and training, data collection and analysis, collaboration and partnerships, and continuous quality improvement. By addressing these facilitators, healthcare organizations can successfully implement evidence-based patient safety interventions and improve patient safety.

39.5 BARRIERS FOR THE EVIDENCE-BASED PATIENT SAFETY

There are several barriers to implementing evidence-based patient safety interventions, including:

1. Lack of resources: One of the main barriers to implementing evidence-based patient safety interventions is a lack of resources, including funding, staff, and time. Implementing interventions can be costly, and healthcare organizations may not have the resources necessary to support them.

2. Resistance to change: Resistance to change can be a barrier to implementing evidence-based patient safety interventions. Healthcare providers may be resistant to changing their practices, or may not see the value in implementing new interventions.

3. Lack of awareness and knowledge: Healthcare providers may not be aware of evidence-based patient safety interventions, or may not have the necessary knowledge or skills to implement them effectively.

4. Inadequate data systems: Inadequate data systems can be a barrier to implementing evidence-based patient safety interventions. Healthcare organizations may not have the necessary data systems in place to collect and analyze data on adverse events and near misses, or to monitor the effectiveness of interventions.

5. Regulatory barriers: Regulatory barriers can be a barrier to implementing evidence-based patient safety interventions. Healthcare organizations may be subject to regulations that limit their ability to implement certain interventions or require them to implement interventions that may not be evidence-based.

6. Lack of collaboration and communication: Lack of collaboration and communication can be a barrier to implementing evidence-based patient safety interventions. Healthcare providers may work in silos and not share information or best practices with one another, which can impede the implementation of interventions.

In summary, barriers to implementing evidence-based patient safety interventions include a lack of resources, resistance to change, lack of awareness and knowledge, inadequate data systems, regulatory barriers, and lack of collaboration and communication. By addressing these barriers, healthcare organizations can successfully implement evidence-based patient safety interventions and improve patient safety.

39.6 EVIDENCE-BASED PATIENT SAFETY ERRORS AND RELATED PROBLEMS

There are several evidence-based patient safety errors and related problems that can occur in healthcare, including:

1. Medication errors: Medication errors are a common patient safety error in healthcare, and can include administering the wrong medication or dose, prescribing the wrong medication or dose, or failing to monitor patients for adverse reactions to medication.

2. Healthcare-associated infections (HAIs): HAIs are infections that patients acquire while receiving healthcare services, and are a significant patient safety issue. Examples include central line-associated bloodstream infections, catheter-associated urinary tract infections, and surgical site infections.

3. Diagnostic errors: Diagnostic errors occur when healthcare providers fail to correctly identify a patient's condition or disease, or when they incorrectly diagnose a patient with a condition or disease. These errors can result in delayed or inappropriate treatment, which can negatively impact patient outcomes.

4. Falls: Falls are a common patient safety problem, particularly among older adults. Falls can result in injuries such as fractures, head injuries, and lacerations, and can lead to prolonged hospital stays or increased healthcare costs.

5. Pressure injuries: Pressure injuries, also known as bedsores or pressure ulcers, are a common patient safety issue among patients who are immobile or have limited mobility. These injuries can be painful and can increase the risk of infection and other complications.

6. Communication errors: Communication errors can occur between healthcare providers, between healthcare providers and patients, or between healthcare providers and families. These errors can result in misunderstandings, delays in treatment, or inappropriate treatment.

In summary, evidence-based patient safety errors and related problems include medication errors, healthcare-associated infections, diagnostic errors, falls, pressure injuries, and communication errors. Addressing these errors and problems requires the implementation of evidence-based patient safety interventions that are tailored to the specific needs of patients and healthcare organizations.

39.7 EVIDENCE-BASED PATIENT SAFETY IN DEVELOPING COUNTRIES: Challenges and Recommendations

Evidence-based patient safety is an important issue in developing countries, where patients often face significant challenges in accessing quality healthcare. Some of the challenges faced by developing countries in implementing evidence-based patient safety include:

1. Limited resources: Developing countries often have limited financial and human resources to invest in patient safety initiatives, which can make it difficult to implement evidence-based practices.

2. Lack of infrastructure: Many developing countries lack the necessary infrastructure, such as reliable power and water supplies, to support patient safety initiatives.

3. Inadequate training and education: Healthcare providers in developing countries may not have access to adequate training and education on patient safety, which can make it difficult for them to implement evidence-based practices.

4. Cultural and linguistic barriers: Cultural and linguistic barriers can make it difficult to communicate patient safety information to patients and healthcare providers in developing countries.

5. Limited data and information systems: Many developing countries lack the necessary data and information systems to track patient safety incidents and monitor the effectiveness of patient safety initiatives.

To address these challenges, several recommendations can be made for developing countries:

1. Develop national patient safety strategies: Developing countries should develop national patient safety strategies that prioritize evidence-based patient safety interventions and outline clear objectives and targets.

2. Invest in training and education: Healthcare providers in developing countries should have access to ongoing training and education on patient safety, including evidence-based practices.

3. Improve infrastructure: Developing countries should invest in improving infrastructure, such as reliable power and water supplies, to support patient safety initiatives.

4. Address cultural and linguistic barriers: Patient safety information should be communicated in a culturally and linguistically appropriate manner, taking into account the local context.

5. Strengthen data and information systems: Developing countries should invest in strengthening data and information systems to track patient safety incidents and monitor the effectiveness of patient safety initiatives.

6. Misidentification of patients: Patients can be misidentified, leading to medication errors, incorrect procedures, and other patient safety issues. This can happen due to inadequate patient identification processes or incomplete medical records.

7. Inadequate hand hygiene: Healthcare workers who do not practice adequate hand hygiene can transmit infections between patients, leading to healthcare-associated infections and other patient safety issues.

8. Surgical errors: Errors during surgery can lead to patient harm, including wrong-site surgery, retained surgical instruments, and anesthesia errors.

9. Adverse drug reactions: Patients may experience adverse drug reactions to medications, which can be life-threatening. Healthcare providers must monitor patients for potential adverse reactions and adjust medications accordingly.

10. Equipment failure: Equipment failure can result in patient harm or delay in treatment. Healthcare providers should have procedures in place for the maintenance and replacement of equipment.

11. Inadequate staffing: Understaffing can lead to inadequate patient monitoring and missed changes in patient condition, leading to delayed treatment and negative patient outcomes.

12. Inadequate communication with patients: Inadequate communication with patients can lead to misunderstandings, lack of informed consent, and other patient safety issues.

13. Inadequate pain management: Inadequate pain management can lead to patient harm and decreased patient satisfaction. Healthcare providers must monitor patients for pain and adjust treatment accordingly.

14. Patient elopement: Patients may leave the healthcare facility without permission, putting themselves at risk for harm. Healthcare providers must have measures in place to prevent patient elopement.

15. Inadequate patient discharge planning: Inadequate patient discharge planning can lead to readmissions and other negative patient outcomes. Healthcare providers must have procedures in place for effective discharge planning, including education on self-care and medication management.

16. Healthcare-associated infections: Healthcare-associated infections (HAIs) can occur as a result of invasive procedures, contaminated equipment, or poor infection control practices. These infections can lead to prolonged hospital stays, increased healthcare costs, and even death.

17. Falls: Patients may fall in healthcare facilities, leading to injuries such as fractures and head trauma. Healthcare providers must assess patients for fall risk and implement preventative measures.

18. Pressure ulcers: Patients who are immobilized or have limited mobility may develop pressure ulcers, which can be painful and lead to serious infections. Healthcare providers must assess patients for pressure ulcer risk and implement preventative measures.

19. Medication errors: Medication errors can occur at any point in the medication process, including prescribing, dispensing, and administration. These errors can result in harm to the patient, including adverse drug reactions and death.

20. Diagnostic errors: Diagnostic errors can occur when healthcare providers fail to recognize or properly diagnose a patient's condition. These errors can lead to delayed treatment and negative patient outcomes.

21. Inadequate infection control: Inadequate infection control practices can lead to the spread of infections among patients and healthcare workers. This can include poor hand hygiene, inadequate sterilization of equipment, and inadequate isolation precautions.

22. Inadequate pain assessment: Healthcare providers may fail to assess a patient's pain adequately, leading to inadequate pain management and negative patient outcomes.

23. Lack of informed consent: Patients may not fully understand the risks and benefits of a procedure or treatment, leading to lack of informed consent. This can result in patient harm and legal issues.

24. Inadequate patient education: Patients may not receive adequate education on their condition, treatment, and self-care, leading to negative patient outcomes and readmissions.

25. Healthcare worker fatigue: Healthcare workers who are fatigued may be more prone to errors and may provide lower quality care, leading to negative patient outcomes.

26. Despite the progress in research about the patient care and safety in developing countries, there is little research about the evidence-based patient safety in majority of developing countries, therefore, conduct research is very important and highly recommended (Alshahrani et al., 2019a,b; Al-Qahtani et al., 2015; Alshahrani et al., 2020a,b; Al-Worafi, 2014; Al-Worafi, 2015; Al-Worafi, 2016; Al-Worafi et al., 2017; Al-Worafi, 2018a-d; Al-Worafi et al., 2018a-b; Al-Worafi et al., 2019; Al-Worafi, 2020a-z; Al-Worafi et al., 2020a-b; Al-Worafi et al., 2021a,b; Al-Worafi, 2022a,b; Al-Worafi, 2023; Baig et al., 2020; Elkalmi et al., 2020; Elsayed & Al-Worafi, 2020; Hasan et al., 2019; Hassan et al., 2014; Izahar et al., 2017; Lee et al., 2017; Mahmoud et al., 2020; Manan et al., 2014; Manan et al., 2016; Ming et al., 2016; Ming et al., 2020; Othman et al., 2020; Saeed et al., 2014).

39.8 CONCLUSION

This chapter has discussed the evidence-based patient safety, challenges and recommendations for the best practice in developing countries. Evidence-based patient safety is an important aspect of healthcare delivery. Evidence-based practices are based on scientific research and are aimed at improving patient outcomes by preventing harm, reducing errors, and improving the quality of care. Evidence-based patient safety issues can occur at any point in the healthcare process and are diverse, ranging from medication errors to inadequate hand hygiene. Effective implementation of evidence-based patient safety practices requires a commitment to continuous quality improvement, the use of data to inform decision-making, and collaboration among healthcare providers, patients, and families. By adopting evidence-based patient safety practices, healthcare providers can improve patient outcomes, reduce healthcare costs, and enhance patient satisfaction.

REFERENCES

Al-Qahtani, I., Almoteb, T.M., & Al-Warafi, Y. (2015). Competency of metered-dose inhaler use among Saudi community pharmacists: A Simulation method study. *RRJPPS*, 4(2), 37–31.

Alshahrani, S.M., Alakhali, K.M., & Al-Worafi, Y.M., (2019a). Medication errors in a health care facility in southern Saudi Arabia. *Tropical Journal of Pharmaceutical Research*, 18(5), pp. 1119–1122.

Alshahrani, S.M., Alavudeen, S.S., Alakhali, K.M., Al-Worafi, Y.M., Bahamdan, A.K., & Vigneshwaran, E., (2019b). Self-Medication Among King Khalid University Students, Saudi Arabia. *Risk Management and Healthcare Policy*, 12, pp. 243–249.

Alshahrani, S.M., Alakhali, K.M., Al-Worafi, Y.M., & Alshahrani, N.Z. (2020b). Awareness and use of over the counter analgesic medication: a survey in the Aseer region population, Saudi Arabia. *Int J Advan Appl Sci*, 7(3), 130–134.

Alshahrani, S.M., Alzahran, M., Alakhali, K., Vigneshwaran, E., Iqbal, M.J., Khan, N.A., ... & Alavudeen, S.S. (2020b). Association Between Diabetes Consequences and Quality of Life Among Patients With Diabetes Mellitus in the Aseer Province of Saudi Arabia. *Open Access Macedonian Journal of Medical Sciences*, 8(E), 325–330.

Al-Worafi, Y.M. (2014). Prescription writing errors at a tertiary care hospital in Yemen: prevalence, types, causes and recommendations. *Am J Pharm Health Res*, 2, 134–140.

Al-Worafi, Y.M.A. (2015). Appropriateness of metered-dose inhaler use in the Yemeni community pharmacies. *Journal of Taibah University Medical Sciences*, 10(3), 353–358.

Al-Worafi, Y.M.A., (2016). Pharmacy practice in Yemen. In *Pharmacy Practice in Developing Countries* (pp. 267–287). Academic Press.

Al-Worafi, Y.M., Kassab, Y.W., Alseragi, W.M., Almutairi, M.S., Ahmed, A., Ming, L.C., Alkhoshaiban, A.S., & Hadi, M.A., (2017). Pharmacovigilance and adverse drg reaction reporting: a perspective of community pharmacists and pharmacy technicians in Sana'a, Yemen. *Therapeutics and clinical risk management*, 13, p. 1175.

Al-Worafi, Y.M., (2018a). Knowledge, Attitude and Practice of Yemeni Physicians Toward Pharmacovigilance: A Mixed Method Study. *International Journal of Pharmacy and Pharmaceutical Sciences*, 10(10), 74–77.

Al-Worafi, Y. (2018b). Knowledge, attitude and practice of Yemeni physicians toward pharmacovigilance: A mixed method study. *Int. J. Pharm. Pharm. Sci*, 10, 74–77.

Al-Worafi, Y.M. (2018c). Dispensing errors observed by community pharmacy dispensers in IBB–YEMEN. *Asian J. Pharm. Clin. Res*, 11(11).

Al-Worafi, Y.M. (2018d). Evauation of inhaler technique among patients with asthma and COPD in Yemen. *Journal of Taibah University medical sciences*, 13(5), 488–490.

Al-Worafi, Y.M., Patel, R.P., Zaidi, S.T.R., Alseragi, W.M., Almutairi, M.S., Alkhoshaiban, A.S., & Ming, L.C. (2018a). Completeness and legibility of handwritten prescriptions in Sana'a, Yemen. *Medical Principles and Practice*, 27, 290–292.

Al-Worafi, Y.M., Alseragi, W.M., Seng, L.K., Kassab, Y.W., Yeoh, S.F., Chiau, L., ... & Husain, K. (2018b). Dispensing errors in community pharmacies: a prospective study in Sana'a, Yemen. *Arch Pharm Pract*, 9(4), 1–3.

Al-Worafi, Y.M., Alseragi, W.M., & Mahmoud, M.A. (2019). Competency of metered-dose inhaler use among community pharmacy dispensers in Ibb, Yemen: A simulation method study. *Latin American Journal of Pharmacy*, 38(3), 489–494.

Al-Worafi, Y.M. (Ed.). (2020a). *Drug Safety in Developing Countries: Achievements and Challenges*.

Al-Worafi, Y.M. (2020b). Medication errors. In *Drug Safety in Developing Countries* (pp. 105–117). Academic Press.

Al-Worafi, Y.M. (2020c). Adverse drug reactions. In *Drug Safety in Developing Countries* (pp. 39–57). Academic Press.

Al-Worafi, Y.M. (2020d). Medications registration and marketing: safety-related issues. In *Drug Safety in Developing Countries* (pp. 21–28). Academic Press.

Al-Worafi, Y.M. (2020e). Pharmacovigilance. In *Drug Safety in Developing Countries* (pp. 29–38). Academic Press.

Al-Worafi, Y.M. (2020f). Drug-related problems. In *Drug safety in developing countries* (pp. 59–71). Academic Press.

Al-Worafi, Y.M. (2020g). Medications safety-related terminology. In *Drug safety in developing countries* (pp. 7–19). Academic Press.

Al-Worafi, Y.M. (2020h). Self-medication. In *Drug Safety in Developing Countries* (pp. 73–86). Academic Press.

Al-Worafi, Y.M. (2020j). Antibiotics safety issues. In *Drug Safety in Developing Countries* (pp. 87–103). Academic Press.

Al-Worafi, Y.M. (2020k). Medications safety research issues. In *Drug Safety in Developing Countries* (pp. 213–227). Academic Press.

Al-Worafi, Y.M. (2020l). Counterfeit and substandard medications. In *Drug safety in developing countries* (pp. 119–126). Academic Press.

Al-Worafi, Y.M. (2020m). Medication abuse and misuse. In *Drug safety in developing countries* (pp. 127–135). Academic Press.

Al-Worafi, Y.M. (2020n). Storage and disposal of medications. In *Drug Safety in Developing Countries* (pp. 137–142). Academic Press.

Al-Worafi, Y.M. (2020o). Safety of medications in special population. In *Drug safety in developing countries* (pp. 143–162). Academic Press.

Al-Worafi, Y.M. (2020p). Herbal medicines safety issues. In *Drug Safety in developing countries* (pp. 163–178). Academic Press.

Al-Worafi, Y.M. (2020q). Medications safety pharmacoeconomics-related issues. In *Drug Safety in Developing Countries* (pp. 187–195). Academic Press.

Al-Worafi, Y.M. (2020r). Evidence-based medications safety practice. In *Drug Safety in Developing Countries* (pp. 197–201). Academic Press.

Al-Worafi, Y.M. (2020s). Quality indicators for medications safety. In *Drug safety in developing countries* (pp. 229–242). Academic Press.

Al-Worafi, Y.M. (2020t). Drug safety in Yemen. In *Drug Safety in Developing Countries* (pp. 391–405). Academic Press.

Al-Worafi, Y.M. (2020u). Drug safety in Saudi Arabia. In *Drug Safety in Developing Countries* (pp. 407–417). Academic Press.

Al-Worafi, Y.M. (2020v). Drug safety in United Arab Emirates. In *Drug Safety in Developing Countries* (pp. 419–428). Academic Press.

Al-Worafi, Y.M. (2020w). Drug safety in Indonesia. In *Drug Safety in Developing Countries* (pp. 279–285). Academic Press.

Al-Worafi, Y.M. (2020x). Drug safety in Palestine. In *Drug Safety in Developing Countries* (pp. 471–480). Academic Press.

Al-Worafi, Y.M. (2020y). Drug safety: comparison between developing countries. In *Drug Safety in Developing Countries* (pp. 603–611). Academic Press.

Al-Worafi, Y.M. (2020z). Drug safety in developing versus developed countries. In *Drug Safety in Developing Countries* (pp. 613–615). Academic Press.

Al-Worafi, Y.M., Alseragi, W.M., Ming, L.C., & Alakhali, K.M. (2020a). Drug safety in China. In *Drug Safety in Developing Countries* (pp. 381–388). Academic Press.

Al-Worafi, Y.M., Alseragi, W.M., Alakhali, K.M., Ming, L.C., Othman, G., Halboup, A.M., … & Elkalmi, R.M. (2020b). Knowledge, beliefs and factors affecting the use of generic medicines among patients in Ibb, Yemen: a mixed-method study. *Journal of Pharmacy Practice and Community Medicine*, 6(4).

Al-Worafi, Y.M., Elkalmi, R.M., Ming, L.C., Othman, G., Halboup, A.M., Battah, M.M., … & Mani, V. (2021a). Dispensing errors in hospital pharmacies: A prospective study in Yemen.

Al-Worafi, Y.M., Hasan, S., Hassan, N.M., & Gaili, A.A. (2021b). Knowledge, Attitude and Experience of Pharmacist in the UAE towards Pharmacovigilance. *Research Journal of Pharmacy and Technology*, 14(1), 265–269.

Al-Worafi, Y. (2022a). *A Guide to Online Pharmacy Education: Teaching Strategies and Assessment Methods*. CRC Press.

Al-Worafi, Y.M. (2022b). Patient care errors and related problems (part I): development and validation of the model. 0000-0002-5752-2913

Al-Worafi, Y.M. (Ed.). (2023). *Clinical Case Studies on medication Safety*. Academic Press.

Baig, M.R., Al-Worafi, Y.M., Alseragi, W.M., Ming, L.C., & Siddique, A. (2020). Drug safety in India. In *Drug Safety in Developing Countries* (pp. 327–334). Academic Press.

Elkalmi, R.M., Al-Worafi, Y.M., Alseragi, W.M., Ming, L.C., & Siddique, A. (2020). Drug safety in Malaysia. In *Drug Safety in Developing Countries* (pp. 245–253). Academic Press.

Elsayed, T., & Al-Worafi, Y.M. (2020). Drug safety in Egypt. In *Drug Safety in Developing Countries* (pp. 511–523). Academic Press.

Hasan, S., Al-Omar, M.J., AlZubaidy, H., & Al-Worafi, Y.M. (2019). Use of medications in Arab Countries. *Handbook of Healthcare in the Arab World*. Cham: Springer, 42.

Hassan, Y., Abd Aziz, N., Kassab, Y.W., Elgasim, I., Shaharuddin, S., Al-Worafi, Y.M.A., … & Ming, L.C. (2014). How to help patients to control their blood pressure? Blood pressure control and its predictor. *Archives of Pharmacy Practice*, 5(4).

Izahar, S., Lean, Q.Y., Hameed, M.A., Murugiah, M.K., Patel, R.P., Al-Worafi, Y.M., … & Ming, L.C. (2017). Content analysis of mobile health applications on diabetes mellitus. *Frontiers in Endocrinology*, 8, 318.

Kristensen, S., & Bartels, P. (2010). Use of patient safety culture instruments and recommendations. *Aarhus, Denmark, European Society for Quality in HealthCare-Office for Quality Indicators*, 113.

Lee, K.S., Yee, S.M., Zaidi, S.T.R., Patel, R.P., Yang, Q., Al-Worafi, Y.M., & Ming, L.C., 2017. Combating sale of counterfeit and falsified medicines online: a losing battle. *Frontiers in pharmacology*, 8, p. 268.

Mahmoud, M.A., Wajid, S., Naqvi, A.A., Samreen, S., Althagfan, S.S., & Al-Worafi, Y. (2020). Self-medication with antibiotics: A cross-sectional community-based study. *Latin american journal of pharmacy*, 39(2), 348–353.

Manan, M.M., Rusli, R.A., Ang, W.C., Al-Worafi, Y.M., & Ming, L.C. (2014). Assessing the pharmaceutical care issues of antiepileptic drug therapy in hospitalised epileptic patients. *Journal of Pharmacy Practice and Research*, 44(3), 83–88.

Manan, M.M., Ibrahim, N.A., Aziz, N.A., Zulkifly, H.H., Al-Worafi, Y.M.A., & Long, C.M. (2016). Empirical use of antibiotic therapy in the prevention of early onset sepsis in neonates: a pilot study. *Archives of Medical Science*, 12(3), 603–613.

Ming, L.C., Hameed, M.A., Lee, D.D., Apidi, N.A., Lai, P.S.M., Hadi, M.A., Al-Worafi, Y.M.A., & Khan, T.M., (2016). Use of medical mobile applications among hospital pharmacists in Malaysia. *Therapeutic innovation & regulatory science*, 50(4), pp. 419–426.

Ming, L.C., Untong, N., Aliudin, N.A., Osili, N., Kifli, N., Tan, C.S., … & Goh, H.P. (2020). Mobile health apps on COVID-19 launched in the early days of the pandemic: content analysis and review. *JMIR mHealth and uHealth*, 8(9), e19796.

Othman, G., Ali, F., Ibrahim, M.I.M., Al-Worafi, Y.M., Ansari, M., & Halboup, A.M. (2020).

Assessment of Anti-Diabetic Medications Adherence among Diabetic Patients in Sana'a City, Yemen: A Cross Sectional Study. *Journal of Pharmaceutical Research International*, 32(21), 114–122.

Reynard, J., Reynolds, J., & Stevenson, P. (2009). *Practical patient safety*. OUP Oxford.

Saeed, M.S., Alkhoshaiban, A.S., Al-Worafi, Y.M.A., & Long, C.M., (2014). Perception of self-medication among university students in Saudi Arabia. *Archives of Pharmacy Practice*, 5(4), p. 149.

Salas, E., & Frush, K. (2012). *Improving patient safety through teamwork and team training*. Oxford University Press.

Vincent, C. (2011). *Patient safety*. John Wiley & Sons.

SECTION 3
PATIENT SAFETY RESEARCH

40 Patient Safety Research

History and Importance

40.1 BACKGROUND

Patient safety research is a field of study that focuses on identifying and reducing the risk of harm to patients during medical care. The goal of patient safety research is to develop strategies and interventions that can prevent medical errors and improve the quality of care provided to patients. Patient safety research can cover a wide range of topics, including medication safety, surgical safety, infection control, communication and teamwork among healthcare providers, and the use of technology in healthcare. Researchers in this field use various methods to gather and analyze data, such as medical record reviews, surveys, interviews, and simulation studies. Patient safety research is essential for improving the quality and safety of healthcare for patients. By identifying and addressing the root causes of medical errors and adverse events, healthcare providers can deliver better care and reduce the risk of harm to patients. World Health Organization described the patient safety as "Patient Safety is a health care discipline that emerged with the evolving complexity in health care systems and the resulting rise of patient harm in health care facilities. It aims to prevent and reduce risks, errors and harm that occur to patients during provision of health care. A cornerstone of the discipline is a continuous improvement based on learning from errors and adverse events; Patient safety is fundamental to delivering quality essential health services" (WHO, 2019). Patient safety-related issues such as medications safety are a major concern in developing countries as well as developed countries; it is associated with treatment outcomes, increase the morbidity and mortality, an increase in the cost of illness, increase the length of hospital stay, increase the admission to the emergency department as well as visiting the healthcare facilities; decrease the quality of life among patients and public, decrease the satisfaction towards the health care services and systems, increase the health expenditure (Al-Worafi, 2020; WHO, 2019). Patient safety issues such as medical errors, medication errors, surgical errors, adverse drug reactions, drug related problems are affecting patients, patients families and health care system, therefore, the collaboration between the health care profes-sionals, health care researchers, health care educators, health care colleges & centres and policy makers are very important and the key to success in improve the patient care, improve the patient safety practice and prevent harm due to patient safety issues such as medical errors, medication errors and others (WHO, 2019; Al-Worafi, 2020).

40.2 HISTORY OF PATIENT SAFETY RESEARCH

The history of patient safety research dates back to the mid-twentieth century, with the publication of a series of reports that highlighted the prevalence of medical errors and the need for improved patient safety measures. It is reported that the term primum non nocere (first, do no harm) is attributed by some historians to Galen and was introduced to American and British medical culture by Worthington Hooker in 1847 (Hooker, 1847; Ilan & Fowler, 2005). Dr Harvey Cushing, a pioneer in surgery and neurosurgery, published detailed descriptions of harm caused to his patients secondary to his own performance at the beginning of the 20th century (Pinkus, 2001; Ilan & Fowler, 2005). However, it is believed that Drug Related Problems had a very long history since the ancient's times (Al-Worafi, 2020b) and literature reported that during the Greek period "a court physician called Glaucos, who took care of a mad man named Hephaestus. According to Arries, Glaucos prescribed him a wrong medication, and Hephaestus died" (Siculus, 1933; Somville et al., 2010). Adverse drug reactions have been reported for more than two thousand years (Al-Worafi, 2020c). History can be summarized as:

- Ancient times: The Hippocratic Oath, a pledge taken by physicians to uphold ethical standards and "do no harm", is developed in ancient Greece.

- 1860s: Florence Nightingale, a British nurse and social reformer, advocates for improved hospital hygiene and infection control practices.

- 1900s: The Flexner Report, a landmark study of medical education in the United States, prompts the closure of many substandard medical schools and the development of more rigorous standards for medical training.

DOI: 10.1201/9781003230465-43

- 1920s: The Hawthorne Studies, a series of experiments on worker productivity and behavior, lead to the discovery of the "Hawthorne effect" - the phenomenon of people changing their behavior when they know they are being observed.

- 1950s: The American Medical Association creates the Committee on the Cost of Medical Care, which publishes a report entitled "Accidents in Medical Care" that highlights the prevalence of medical errors and the need for improved patient safety measures.

- 1978: A study conducted by researchers at Harvard Medical School led by Dr. Lucian Leape finds that medical errors are much more common than previously thought, with 36% of hospital admissions resulting in adverse events.

- 1983: The Joint Commission on Accreditation of Healthcare Organizations (JCAHO) requires hospitals to implement quality assurance programs to reduce the risk of medical errors.

- 1991: The Harvard Medical Practice Study, led by Dr. Lucian Leape, estimates that there are 180,000 preventable deaths in U.S. hospitals each year.

- 1999: The Institute of Medicine (IOM) publishes the report "To Err Is Human: Building a Safer Health System," which estimates that between 44,000 and 98,000 Americans die each year as a result of medical errors.

- 2001: The IOM publishes the report "Crossing the Quality Chasm: A New Health System for the 21st Century," which calls for a major overhaul of the healthcare system to improve patient safety and quality of care.

- 2004: The World Alliance for Patient Safety is established by the World Health Organization (WHO) to promote international cooperation and collaboration in patient safety research and initiatives.

- 2006: The Joint Commission implements a new National Patient Safety Goal that requires healthcare organizations to implement medication reconciliation processes to reduce the risk of medication errors.

- 2013: The National Patient Safety Foundation becomes the Institute for Healthcare Improvement (IHI), with a renewed focus on improving patient safety through research, education, and advocacy.

- 2019: The WHO launches the third Global Patient Safety Challenge, "Medication Without Harm," with the goal of reducing medication-related harm by 50% over the next five years.

40.3 IMPORTANCE OF PATIENT SAFETY RESEARCH

Patient safety research are very important for health care professionals, students, researchers, policy makers, patients and public. Patient safety research is crucial for a number of reasons:

Improving Patient Outcomes: Research on patient care and safety can help identify best practices and interventions that can improve patient outcomes. By understanding how different factors, such as medical treatments, hospital environments, and patient demographics, can affect patient health and wellbeing, healthcare providers can make more informed decisions about how to treat patients and reduce the risk of adverse events. Reducing Medical Errors: Research on patient safety can help identify areas where medical errors are more likely to occur, such as during medication administration, surgical procedures, or patient handoffs between healthcare providers. By understanding the causes of medical errors, healthcare providers can develop strategies to prevent them, such as improving communication among providers, implementing checklists, and using technology to reduce human error. Enhancing Patient Experience: Patient care research can also help healthcare providers understand how to create a better patient experience. By identifying what patients value most in their interactions with healthcare providers, such as empathy, clear communication, and respect for their preferences and values, providers can work to create a more patient-centered approach to care. Informing Policy and Practice: Patient care and safety research can also inform healthcare policy and practice at the local, national, and international levels. By identifying trends and patterns in patient care and safety, researchers can help policymakers and healthcare leaders make informed decisions about how to allocate resources, implement interventions, and improve the overall quality of care. The following are some key reasons why patient safety research is so vital (Al-Worafi, 2020a-d; Al-Worafi 2022a-d):

1. Reducing medical errors: Research into patient safety can help to identify the root causes of medical errors and develop strategies to prevent them. This can lead to improved patient outcomes and fewer adverse events.

2. Improving healthcare processes: Patient safety research can help to identify inefficiencies and areas for improvement in healthcare processes. This can lead to the development of best practices and streamlined workflows, which can improve the quality of care and reduce the risk of errors.

3. Enhancing healthcare provider training: Patient safety research can inform the development of training programs for healthcare providers, which can improve their knowledge, skills, and attitudes towards patient safety.

4. Informing policy and practice: Research into patient safety can inform policy and practice at all levels of the healthcare system, from local hospitals to national regulatory bodies. This can lead to changes in regulations, standards, and guidelines that improve patient safety.

5. Engaging patients and families: Patient safety research can engage patients and families in the process of improving healthcare safety. This can help to promote shared decision-making, patient-centered care, and a culture of safety.

6. Identifying and reducing healthcare disparities: Patient safety research can help to identify disparities in access to care and outcomes among different patient populations. By understanding these disparities, researchers can develop strategies to reduce them and improve equity in healthcare.

7. Improving medication safety: Medication errors are a significant cause of patient harm in healthcare. Patient safety research can help to identify the root causes of medication errors and develop strategies to prevent them, such as improved medication reconciliation processes and medication management systems.

8. Enhancing communication and teamwork: Effective communication and teamwork among healthcare providers are critical to ensuring patient safety. Patient safety research can help to identify barriers to effective communication and teamwork and develop strategies to improve these skills.

9. Preventing healthcare-associated infections: Healthcare-associated infections are a significant cause of morbidity and mortality in healthcare settings. Patient safety research can help to identify strategies to prevent these infections, such as improved hand hygiene practices and infection control protocols.

10. Addressing the impact of new technologies on patient safety: New technologies such as electronic health records, telemedicine, and artificial intelligence have the potential to improve patient care but also present new risks to patient safety. Patient safety research can help to identify these risks and develop strategies to mitigate them.

11. Improving diagnostic accuracy: Diagnostic errors are a significant cause of patient harm in healthcare, and patient safety research can help to identify the root causes of diagnostic errors and develop strategies to improve diagnostic accuracy. This could involve changes to the diagnostic process or the development of new diagnostic tools.

12. Addressing provider burnout: Burnout among healthcare providers can have a negative impact on patient safety, as it can lead to errors and poor patient outcomes. Patient safety research can help to identify the causes of provider burnout and develop strategies to address it, such as improving work-life balance, providing emotional support, and promoting a culture of well-being.

13. Improving patient engagement: Patients who are actively involved in their care tend to have better outcomes and experience fewer adverse events. Patient safety research can help to

identify strategies to improve patient engagement, such as providing patients with access to their health information or involving them in the development of care plans.

14. Enhancing patient-centered care: Patient-centered care involves tailoring care to meet patients' individual needs and preferences, and it has been shown to improve patient outcomes and satisfaction. Patient safety research can help to identify strategies to promote patient-centered care, such as improving communication with patients or involving them in shared decision-making.

15. Addressing the impact of social determinants of health: Social determinants of health, such as income, education, and access to healthcare, can have a significant impact on patient outcomes and safety. Patient safety research can help to identify ways to address these social determinants of health and promote equity in healthcare.

In summary, patient safety research is critical to improving the quality and safety of patient care. By identifying the root causes of errors, improving healthcare processes, enhancing provider training, informing policy and practice, and engaging patients and families, patient safety research can make a significant impact on healthcare safety and quality.

40.4 CONCLUSION

This chapter has discussed the history and importance of patient safety research. Patient safety research is a vital area of healthcare research that can improve the quality and safety of patient care. By identifying the root causes of medical errors, improving healthcare processes, enhancing provider training, informing policy and practice, engaging patients and families, and addressing a range of other issues, patient safety research can make a significant impact on healthcare safety and quality. Through ongoing research and collaboration among healthcare providers, researchers, policymakers, and patients.

REFERENCES

Al-Worafi, Y.M. (Ed.). (2020). *Drug Safety in Developing Countries: Achievements and Challenges.* Academic Press.

Al-Worafi, Y.M. (2020b). Drug-related problems. In *Drug Safety in Developing Countries* (pp. 105–117). Academic Press.

Al-Worafi, Y.M. (2020c). Adverse drug reactions. In *Drug Safety in Developing Countries* (pp. 39–57). Academic Press.

Al-Worafi, Y.M. (2020d). Medications safety research issues. In *Drug Safety in Developing Countries* (pp. 213–227). Academic Press.

Al-Worafi, Y. (2022a). *A Guide to Online Pharmacy Education: Teaching Strategies and Assessment Methods.* CRC Press.

Al-Worafi, Y. (2022b). History and Importance. In *A Guide to Online Pharmacy Education: Teaching Strategies and Assessment Methods.* CRC Press.

Al-Worafi, Y. (2022c). Terminologies. In *A Guide to Online Pharmacy Education: Teaching Strategies and Assessment Methods.* CRC Press.

Al-Worafi, Y. (2022d). Research Methods and Methodology. In *A Guide to Online Pharmacy Education: Teaching Strategies and Assessment Methods.* CRC Press.

Hooker W. (1847). Physician and patient. New York (NY)7 Baker and physician and patient. *New York (NY)7 Baker and Scribner.*

Ilan, R., & Fowler, R. (2005). Brief history of patient safety culture and science. *Journal of critical care,* 20(1), 2–5.

Pinkus, R.L.B. (2001). Mistakes as a social construct: an historical approach. *Kennedy Institute of Ethics Journal*, 11(2), 117–133.

Siculus, D., (1933). Diodorus Siculus. *Life [edit]*, 7, p. 2.

Somville, F.J.M.P., Broos, P.L.O., & Van Hee, R. (2010). Some notes on medical liability in ancient times. *Acta Chirurgica Belgica*, 110(3), 405–409.

World Health Orgainization (WHO) (2019). Available at: https://www.who.int/news-room/fact-sheets/detail/patient-safety

41 Patient Safety Research

Literature Review

41.1 BACKGROUND

A literature review is a comprehensive summary and analysis of existing published research on a particular topic or field of study. The purpose of a literature review is to identify what has already been studied about the topic and to evaluate the strengths and weaknesses of the existing research. A literature review typically begins with a research question or problem statement, which helps to focus the review on a specific topic. The review then involves searching for and gathering relevant articles, books, and other sources of information on the topic. The literature is then analyzed and synthesized to identify key themes, trends, and patterns in the research. The review may also include a critical evaluation of the quality and relevance of the studies reviewed. A well-written literature review should provide a clear and concise summary of the existing research on the topic and highlight any gaps in the literature. It can also help to identify areas for future research and provide a foundation for the development of new research studies. Literature reviews are commonly used in academic research papers, dissertations, and theses, as well as in professional reports and policy documents (Galvan & Galvan, 2017).

41.2 RATIONALITY OF LITERATURE REVIEW

A literature review is an essential component of academic research, and its rationality lies in its ability to provide a comprehensive overview of the current state of knowledge on a particular research topic. The literature review serves as a critical evaluation of existing literature, identifying gaps, inconsistencies, and areas where further research is needed. A well-conducted literature review helps researchers to identify relevant theoretical frameworks, methodologies, and research methods that can be applied to their own research questions. It also allows researchers to establish the context of their research within the existing body of knowledge, enabling them to demonstrate the originality and significance of their work. Furthermore, a literature review helps to avoid duplication of research efforts, as researchers can identify previous studies that have already investigated similar research questions. This enables researchers to build on previous findings, rather than repeating previous research efforts, which saves time and resources. In the field of patient safety, a literature review is crucial for several reasons. Firstly, it enables researchers to identify and summarize the current state of knowledge on patient safety, including the various factors that contribute to errors and adverse events in healthcare. This knowledge can inform the development of interventions and strategies aimed at improving patient safety. Secondly, a literature review can help to identify gaps in the current knowledge base, highlighting areas where further research is needed. For example, a literature review may identify gaps in the understanding of how specific healthcare settings or patient populations are impacted by safety incidents. Thirdly, a literature review can help to identify best practices and evidence-based interventions that have been effective in improving patient safety. This information can be used to inform the development of policies and guidelines aimed at reducing the incidence of adverse events in healthcare. Finally, a literature review can help to raise awareness of patient safety issues among healthcare providers, policymakers, and the general public. By summarizing and disseminating the latest research findings, a literature review can help to promote a culture of safety in healthcare, where patient safety is prioritized and integrated into all aspects of healthcare delivery. Overall, a literature review is critical in patient safety research as it provides a comprehensive and critical evaluation of the current state of knowledge, identifies gaps and opportunities for further research, and helps to inform the development of evidence-based interventions to improve patient safety in healthcare.

41.3 IMPORTANCE OF LITERATURE REVIEW

A literature review is an essential component of academic research, and its importance cannot be overstated. Below are some of the key reasons why literature reviews are critical to research:

1. Establishes the context of the research: A literature review provides a summary and evaluation of the current state of knowledge on a particular topic, enabling researchers to position their research within the broader context of the field.

DOI: 10.1201/9781003230465-44

2. Identifies gaps and opportunities for further research: By critically evaluating existing literature, researchers can identify areas where further research is needed, as well as gaps in the current knowledge base.

3. Helps to refine research questions and hypotheses: Literature reviews can help researchers to clarify their research questions and hypotheses by identifying key concepts, theoretical frameworks, and methodologies that are relevant to their research.

4. Identifies relevant sources and evidence: Literature reviews provide an overview of the key sources and evidence related to a particular topic, enabling researchers to identify the most relevant and reliable sources of information.

5. Facilitates critical thinking and analysis: Literature reviews require critical thinking and analysis, which helps researchers to develop their own ideas and arguments based on the existing literature.

6. Supports the development of a theoretical framework: Literature reviews are essential for the development of a theoretical framework, which is the conceptual basis for research studies.

7. Demonstrates the originality and significance of the research: By summarizing and evaluating existing literature, researchers can demonstrate the originality and significance of their own research, highlighting how it contributes to the broader body of knowledge in the field.

In the field of patient safety, a literature review is critical for several reasons:

1. Identifies key factors contributing to patient safety incidents: A literature review can help identify the factors contributing to patient safety incidents, such as communication breakdowns, medication errors, and system failures. This information can be used to inform the development of interventions and strategies aimed at improving patient safety.

2. Evaluates the effectiveness of patient safety interventions: A literature review can help to evaluate the effectiveness of patient safety interventions, enabling healthcare providers to identify evidence-based interventions that have been effective in improving patient safety.

3. Identifies gaps and opportunities for further research: A literature review can help to identify gaps in the current knowledge base, highlighting areas where further research is needed. This can inform the development of research studies aimed at improving patient safety.

4. Supports the development of patient safety policies and guidelines: Literature reviews can inform the development of patient safety policies and guidelines, based on evidence-based best practices.

5. Promotes a culture of safety in healthcare: By summarizing and disseminating the latest research findings, a literature review can help to raise awareness of patient safety issues among healthcare providers, policymakers, and the general public. This can help to promote a culture of safety in healthcare, where patient safety is prioritized and integrated into all aspects of healthcare delivery.

In summary, a literature review is critical in patient safety research, as it helps to identify factors contributing to patient safety incidents, evaluate the effectiveness of interventions, identify gaps in the current knowledge base, inform the development of patient safety policies and guidelines, and promote a culture of safety in healthcare.

41.4 ADVANTAGES OF LITERATURE REVIEW

There are several advantages of conducting a literature review:

1. Establishes the current state of knowledge: A literature review provides an overview of the current state of knowledge on a particular topic, enabling researchers to position their research within the broader context of the field.

2. Identifies gaps and opportunities for further research: By critically evaluating existing literature, researchers can identify areas where further research is needed, as well as gaps in the current knowledge base.

3. Helps to refine research questions and hypotheses: Literature reviews can help researchers to clarify their research questions and hypotheses by identifying key concepts, theoretical frameworks, and methodologies that are relevant to their research.

4. Identifies relevant sources and evidence: Literature reviews provide an overview of the key sources and evidence related to a particular topic, enabling researchers to identify the most relevant and reliable sources of information.

5. Facilitates critical thinking and analysis: Literature reviews require critical thinking and analysis, which helps researchers to develop their own ideas and arguments based on the existing literature.

6. Supports the development of a theoretical framework: Literature reviews are essential for the development of a theoretical framework, which is the conceptual basis for research studies.

7. Demonstrates the originality and significance of the research: By summarizing and evaluating existing literature, researchers can demonstrate the originality and significance of their own research, highlighting how it contributes to the broader body of knowledge in the field.

8. Saves time and resources: Conducting a literature review can save time and resources by avoiding duplication of research efforts and identifying areas where further research is needed.

In summary, conducting a literature review provides numerous advantages, including establishing the current state of knowledge, identifying gaps and opportunities for further research, refining research questions and hypotheses, identifying relevant sources and evidence, facilitating critical thinking and analysis, supporting the development of a theoretical framework, demonstrating the originality and significance of the research, and saving time and resources.

41.5 DISADVANTAGES OF LITERATURE REVIEW

While literature reviews have numerous advantages, there are also some potential disadvantages to consider:

1. Limited perspective: Literature reviews are limited by the scope and quality of the literature that is available. If key studies are missed or the literature is biased, the conclusions drawn from the review may be limited or inaccurate.

2. Time-consuming: Conducting a thorough literature review can be time-consuming, as it requires significant effort to identify and evaluate relevant sources of information.

3. Subjectivity: Literature reviews can be subjective, as they rely on the interpretation of the researcher. Different researchers may draw different conclusions from the same body of literature, depending on their interpretation and analysis.

4. Publication bias: Literature reviews may be subject to publication bias, as studies that show positive or statistically significant results are more likely to be published than studies that do not. This can lead to an over-representation of positive results in the literature.

5. Outdated information: Literature reviews can quickly become outdated, as new studies and information are constantly being published. It is important to update literature reviews regularly to ensure that they reflect the most current state of knowledge on a particular topic.

6. Lack of original research: Literature reviews do not involve the collection of new data, but rather a synthesis and analysis of existing data. While this can provide valuable insights and knowledge, it is not the same as conducting original research.

In summary, while literature reviews have numerous advantages, there are also potential disadvantages to consider, including limited perspective, time-consuming nature, subjectivity, publication bias, outdated information, and lack of original research. It is important for researchers to be aware of these potential limitations and to take steps to address them when conducting literature reviews.

41.6 FACILITATORS OF LITERATURE REVIEW

Literature reviews are important components of academic research projects. They serve as a means of examining and synthesizing existing literature on a particular topic or research question. Some key facilitators of literature review include:

1. Access to relevant literature: Facilitating literature review requires access to relevant literature that is specific to the research topic. This may include academic journals, books, reports, and other resources. Researchers need to have access to online databases or physical libraries that contain relevant literature.

2. Familiarity with search strategies: Effective literature review requires familiarity with search strategies, such as Boolean operators, keywords, and phrases. Researchers should be able to formulate effective search strategies to obtain the most relevant and up-to-date literature.

3. Critical reading skills: Literature review involves critically reading and evaluating the literature. Researchers should have the ability to assess the quality of the literature, identify gaps in knowledge, and draw connections between different studies.

4. Time management skills: Literature review is a time-consuming process that requires effective time management. Researchers need to allocate enough time to search for relevant literature, read and evaluate the literature, and write the literature review.

5. Organizational skills: Literature review requires effective organization of the literature. Researchers should be able to categorize and synthesize the literature based on themes, research questions, and key findings.

6. Collaboration and feedback: Collaborating with colleagues and seeking feedback from peers and mentors can help improve the quality of the literature review. It provides an opportunity to receive constructive criticism and suggestions for improvement.

Overall, successful literature review requires a combination of access to relevant literature, effective search strategies, critical reading and evaluation skills, time management and organizational skills, and collaboration with others.

41.7 BARRIERS TO LITERATURE REVIEW

While literature reviews are important components of academic research, there are several barriers that researchers may face in conducting them effectively. Some of these barriers include:

1. Limited access to literature: One of the main barriers to literature review is limited access to relevant literature. This may be due to limited resources or access to online databases, journals, or libraries. This can make it challenging to find the most relevant and up-to-date literature.

2. Overwhelming amount of literature: Another barrier to literature review is the overwhelming amount of literature that exists on a particular topic. Sorting through large volumes of literature to find the most relevant sources can be time-consuming and challenging.

3. Lack of time: Literature review is a time-consuming process, and researchers may face time constraints due to other research and academic commitments. This can make it difficult to allocate enough time to conduct a thorough literature review.

4. Difficulty in synthesizing the literature: Literature reviews require the ability to synthesize the literature into a cohesive narrative. This can be challenging for researchers who may struggle to identify common themes or draw connections between different studies.

5. Limited expertise: Conducting a literature review may require expertise in a particular field or subject matter. Researchers who lack expertise in a particular area may find it challenging to evaluate the quality of the literature or identify relevant sources.

6. Bias in the literature: Bias in the literature can be a significant barrier to conducting a comprehensive literature review. Researchers must be aware of potential bias in the literature and take steps to address it by evaluating the quality of the sources and considering alternative perspectives.

Overall, conducting a thorough literature review requires researchers to overcome several barriers, including limited access to literature, time constraints, overwhelming amounts of literature, difficulty synthesizing the literature, limited expertise, and potential bias in the literature.

41.8 QUALITY OF LITERATURE REVIEW

The quality of a literature review is critical to the success of a research project. A high-quality literature review should be comprehensive, well-organized, and based on credible sources. Here are some factors that contribute to the quality of a literature review:

1. Comprehensive coverage: A high-quality literature review should cover all relevant research on the topic. This includes both published and unpublished sources. The review should be systematic and follow a well-defined search strategy to ensure that no relevant studies are missed.

2. Critical evaluation of sources: A high-quality literature review should critically evaluate each source included. Researchers should assess the quality of the studies and identify any biases or limitations. This helps to ensure that only credible and relevant sources are included in the review.

3. Clear organization: A high-quality literature review should be well-organized and clearly written. The review should follow a logical structure and be divided into clear sections, such as introduction, methodology, results, and discussion. This makes it easy for readers to understand the key findings and conclusions.

4. Integration of studies: A high-quality literature review should integrate the findings from different studies. The review should identify common themes and trends in the literature and synthesize the findings to provide an overall picture of the current state of research on the topic.

5. Implications for future research: A high-quality literature review should also provide insights into areas for future research. The review should identify gaps in the literature and suggest potential avenues for further investigation.

6. Credibility and reliability of sources: A high-quality literature review should be based on credible and reliable sources. Researchers should use reputable journals, books, and databases to ensure that the information presented in the review is accurate and up-to-date.

In summary, a high-quality literature review should be comprehensive, well-organized, and based on credible sources. It should integrate the findings from different studies, critically evaluate sources, and provide implications for future research.

41.9 LITERATURE REVIEW IN DEVELOPING COUNTRIES: Challenges and Recommendations

Literature reviews are an important aspect of research in developing countries, as they provide a basis for understanding the current state of knowledge and identifying gaps in research that can be addressed through new studies. However, conducting literature reviews in developing countries can pose unique challenges. Patient safety research in developing countries has made significant achievements in recent years. Many developing countries have conducted many researches about the various issues of patient safety and care research (Alshahrani et al., 2019a,b; Al-Qahtani et al., 2015; Alshahrani et al., 2020a,b; Al-Worafi, 2014; Al-Worafi, 2015; Al-Worafi, 2016; Al-Worafi et al., 2017; Al-Worafi, 2018a-d;Al-Worafi et al., 2018a-b; Al-Worafi et al., 2019; Al-Worafi, 2020a-z; Al-Worafi et al., 2020a-b; Al-Worafi et al., 2021a,b; Al-Worafi, 2022a-e; Al-Worafi, 2023; Baig et al., 2020; Elkalmi et al., 2020; Elsayed & Al-Worafi, 2020; Hasan et al., 2019; Hassan et al., 2014; Izahar et al., 2017; Lee et al., 2017; Mahmoud et al., 2020; Manan et al., 2014; Manan et al., 2016; Ming et al., 2016; Ming et al., 2020; Othman et al., 2020; Saeed et al., 2014), however, there are many challenges and recommendations for conducting literature reviews in developing countries such as:

1. Limited access to literature: One of the main challenges of conducting literature reviews in developing countries is limited access to literature. Researchers may not have access to online databases or physical libraries that contain relevant literature. To address this challenge, researchers should explore alternative sources of information, such as government reports, conference proceedings, and grey literature. They should also consider collaborating with researchers from other institutions or countries who may have access to relevant literature.

2. Poor infrastructure: Developing countries may lack the necessary infrastructure, such as reliable electricity and internet access, to conduct effective literature reviews. Researchers should consider working with local institutions that have better infrastructure, such as universities or research centers, to access necessary resources.

3. Limited funding: Researchers in developing countries may have limited funding to conduct literature reviews. To address this challenge, researchers should seek out funding opportunities from government agencies, non-governmental organizations, or international organizations that support research in developing countries.

4. Language barriers: Conducting literature reviews in developing countries may require proficiency in multiple languages. Researchers should consider collaborating with bilingual colleagues or translators to help overcome language barriers.

5. Limited local research: Developing countries may have limited local research on a particular topic, which can make it challenging to conduct a comprehensive literature review. Researchers should consider broadening their search to include studies from other countries or regions, or conducting new studies to address gaps in local research.

6. Lack of standardization: There may be a lack of standardization in research methods and reporting in developing countries. Researchers should be aware of these limitations and take steps to critically evaluate the quality of the studies included in their literature reviews.

7. Cultural differences: Cultural differences between the researcher and the study population may impact the interpretation of the literature. Researchers should consider the cultural context of the literature they review and how it may impact the applicability of the findings to their study population.

8. Limited resources for data collection: Developing countries may have limited resources for data collection, which can make it challenging to gather sufficient data to conduct a comprehensive literature review. Researchers should consider using multiple sources of data, including secondary data sources, to help overcome this challenge.

9. Lack of expertise: Researchers in developing countries may have limited expertise in conducting literature reviews, which can impact the quality of the review. Researchers should seek out training opportunities or mentorship from experienced researchers to help develop their skills in conducting literature reviews.

10. Political instability: Political instability in developing countries can impact the availability of literature and make it challenging for researchers to access information. Researchers should be aware of the political climate in the country and take steps to ensure their safety and the safety of their data.

11. Ethics and research integrity: Developing countries may have different ethical standards and regulations for conducting research, which can impact the quality of the literature review. Researchers should be aware of local regulations and guidelines for conducting research and ensure that their study is conducted ethically and with integrity.

In summary, conducting literature reviews in developing countries can pose unique challenges, including limited access to literature, poor infrastructure, limited funding, language barriers, limited local research, and a lack of standardization in research methods and reporting. To address these challenges, researchers should seek out alternative sources of information, collaborate with others, broaden their search, and critically evaluate the quality of studies included in their literature reviews.

41.10 CONCLUSION

This chapter has discussed the patient safety research issues related to the literature review, importance, facilitators, barriers, challenges and recommendations for the best practice in developing countries. Conducting literature reviews in developing countries can pose several unique challenges. These challenges may include limited access to literature, poor infrastructure, limited funding, language barriers, limited local research, a lack of standardization, cultural differences, limited resources for data collection, lack of expertise, political instability, and ethics and research integrity. To overcome these challenges, researchers should consider seeking out alternative sources of information, collaborating with others, broadening their search, critically evaluating the quality of studies included in their literature reviews, and seeking out training and mentorship opportunities. By addressing these challenges, researchers can conduct comprehensive and high-quality literature reviews that help to advance the state of knowledge in their respective fields, despite the challenges they may face in their developing countries.

REFERENCES

Al-Qahtani, I., Almoteb, T.M., & Al-Warafi, Y. (2015). Competency of metered-dose inhaler use among Saudi community pharmacists: A Simulation method study. *RRJPPS*, 4(2), 37–31.

Alshahrani, S.M., Alakhali, K.M., & Al-Worafi, Y.M., (2019a). Medication errors in a health care facility in southern Saudi Arabia. *Tropical Journal of Pharmaceutical Research*, 18(5), pp. 1119–1122.

Alshahrani, S.M., Alavudeen, S.S., Alakhali, K.M., Al-Worafi, Y.M., Bahamdan, A.K., & Vigneshwaran, E., (2019b). Self-Medication Among King Khalid University Students, Saudi Arabia. *Risk Management and Healthcare Policy*, 12, pp. 243–249.

Alshahrani, S.M., Alakhali, K.M., Al-Worafi, Y.M., & Alshahrani, N.Z. (2020a). Awareness and use of over the counter analgesic medication: a survey in the Aseer region population, Saudi Arabia. *Int J Advan Appl Sci*, 7(3), 130–134.

Alshahrani, S.M., Alzahran, M., Alakhali, K., Vigneshwaran, E., Iqbal, M.J., Khan, N.A., … & Alavudeen, S.S. (2020b). Association Between Diabetes Consequences and Quality of Life Among Patients With Diabetes Mellitus in the Aseer Province of Saudi Arabia. *Open Access Macedonian Journal of Medical Sciences*, 8(E), 325–330.

Al-Worafi, Y.M. (2014). Prescription writing errors at a tertiary care hospital in Yemen: prevalence, types, causes and recommendations. *Am J Pharm Health Res*, 2, 134–140.

Al-Worafi, Y.M.A. (2015). Appropriateness of metered-dose inhaler use in the Yemeni community pharmacies. *Journal of Taibah University Medical Sciences*, 10(3), 353–358.

Al-Worafi, Y.M.A., (2016). Pharmacy practice in Yemen. In *Pharmacy Practice in Developing Countries* (pp. 267–287). Academic Press.

Al-Worafi, Y.M., Kassab, Y.W., Alseragi, W.M., Almutairi, M.S., Ahmed, A., Ming, L.C., Alkhoshaiban, A.S., & Hadi, M.A., (2017). Pharmacovigilance and adverse drg reaction reporting: a perspective of community pharmacists and pharmacy technicians in Sana'a, Yemen. *Therapeutics and clinical risk management*, 13, p. 1175.

Al-Worafi, Y.M., (2018a). Knowledge, Attitude and Practice of Yemeni Physicians Toward Pharmacovigilance: A Mixed Method Study. *International Journal of Pharmacy and Pharmaceutical Sciences*, 10(10), 74–77.

Al-Worafi, Y. (2018b). Knowledge, attitude and practice of Yemeni physicians toward pharmacovigilance: A mixed method study. *Int. J. Pharm. Pharm. Sci*, 10, 74–77.

Al-Worafi, Y.M. (2018c). Dispensing errors observed by community pharmacy dispensers in IBB–YEMEN. *Asian J. Pharm. Clin. Res*, 11(11).

Al-Worafi, Y.M. (2018d). Evauation of inhaler technique among patients with asthma and COPD in Yemen. *Journal of Taibah University medical sciences*, 13(5), 488–490.

Al-Worafi, Y.M., Patel, R.P., Zaidi, S.T.R., Alseragi, W.M., Almutairi, M.S., Alkhoshaiban, A.S., & Ming, L.C. (2018a). Completeness and legibility of handwritten prescriptions in Sana'a, Yemen. *Medical Principles and Practice*, 27, 290–292.

Al-Worafi, Y.M., Alseragi, W.M., Seng, L.K., Kassab, Y.W., Yeoh, S.F., Chiau, L., … & Husain, K. (2018b). Dispensing errors in community pharmacies: a prospective study in Sana'a, Yemen. *Arch Pharm Pract*, 9(4), 1–3.

Al-Worafi, Y.M., Alseragi, W.M., & Mahmoud, M.A. (2019). Competency of metered-dose inhaler use among community pharmacy dispensers in Ibb, Yemen: A simulation method study. *Latin American Journal of Pharmacy*, 38(3), 489–494.

Al-Worafi, Y.M. (Ed.). (2020a). *Drug Safety in Developing Countries: Achievements and Challenges.*

Al-Worafi, Y.M. (2020b). Medication errors. In *Drug Safety in Developing Countries* (pp. 105–117). Academic Press.

Al-Worafi, Y.M. (2020c). Adverse drug reactions. In *Drug Safety in Developing Countries* (pp. 39–57). Academic Press.

Al-Worafi, Y.M. (2020d). Medications registration and marketing: safety-related issues. In *Drug Safety in Developing Countries* (pp. 21–28). Academic Press.

Al-Worafi, Y.M. (2020e). Pharmacovigilance. In *Drug Safety in Developing Countries* (pp. 29–38). Academic Press.

Al-Worafi, Y.M. (2020f). Drug-related problems. In *Drug safety in developing countries* (pp. 59–71). Academic Press.

Al-Worafi, Y.M. (2020g). Medications safety-related terminology. In *Drug safety in developing countries* (pp. 7–19). Academic Press.

Al-Worafi, Y.M. (2020h). Self-medication. In *Drug Safety in Developing Countries* (pp. 73–86). Academic Press.

Al-Worafi, Y.M. (2020j). Antibiotics safety issues. In *Drug Safety in Developing Countries* (pp. 87–103). Academic Press.

Al-Worafi, Y.M. (2020k). Medications safety research issues. In *Drug Safety in Developing Countries* (pp. 213–227). Academic Press.

Al-Worafi, Y.M. (2020l). Counterfeit and substandard medications. In *Drug safety in developing countries* (pp. 119–126). Academic Press.

Al-Worafi, Y.M. (2020m). Medication abuse and misuse. In *Drug safety in developing countries* (pp. 127–135). Academic Press.

Al-Worafi, Y.M. (2020n). Storage and disposal of medications. In *Drug Safety in Developing Countries* (pp. 137–142). Academic Press.

Al-Worafi, Y.M. (2020o). Safety of medications in special population. In *Drug safety in developing countries* (pp. 143–162). Academic Press.

Al-Worafi, Y.M. (2020p). Herbal medicines safety issues. In *Drug Safety in developing countries* (pp. 163–178). Academic Press.

Al-Worafi, Y.M. (2020q). Medications safety pharmacoeconomics-related issues. In *Drug Safety in Developing Countries* (pp. 187–195). Academic Press.

Al-Worafi, Y.M. (2020r). Evidence-based medications safety practice. In *Drug Safety in Developing Countries* (pp. 197–201). Academic Press.

Al-Worafi, Y.M. (2020s). Quality indicators for medications safety. In *Drug safety in developing countries* (pp. 229–242). Academic Press.

Al-Worafi, Y.M. (2020t). Drug safety in Yemen. In *Drug Safety in Developing Countries* (pp. 391–405). Academic Press.

Al-Worafi, Y.M. (2020u). Drug safety in Saudi Arabia. In *Drug Safety in Developing Countries* (pp. 407–417). Academic Press.

Al-Worafi, Y.M. (2020v). Drug safety in United Arab Emirates. In *Drug Safety in Developing Countries* (pp. 419–428). Academic Press.

Al-Worafi, Y.M. (2020w). Drug safety in Indonesia. In *Drug Safety in Developing Countries* (pp. 279–285). Academic Press.

Al-Worafi, Y.M. (2020x). Drug safety in Palestine. In *Drug Safety in Developing Countries* (pp. 471–480). Academic Press.

Al-Worafi, Y.M. (2020y). Drug safety: comparison between developing countries. In *Drug Safety in Developing Countries* (pp. 603–611). Academic Press.

Al-Worafi, Y.M. (2020z). Drug safety in developing versus developed countries. In *Drug Safety in Developing Countries* (pp. 613–615). Academic Press.

Al-Worafi, Y.M., Alseragi, W.M., Ming, L.C., & Alakhali, K.M. (2020a). Drug safety in China. In *Drug Safety in Developing Countries* (pp. 381–388). Academic Press.

Al-Worafi, Y.M., Alseragi, W.M., Alakhali, K.M., Ming, L.C., Othman, G., Halboup, A.M., … & Elkalmi, R.M. (2020b). Knowledge, beliefs and factors affecting the use of generic medicines among patients in Ibb, Yemen: a mixed-method study. *Journal of Pharmacy Practice and Community Medicine*, 6(4).

Al-Worafi, Y.M., Elkalmi, R.M., Ming, L.C., Othman, G., Halboup, A.M., Battah, M.M., … & Mani, V. (2021a). Dispensing errors in hospital pharmacies: A prospective study in Yemen.

Al-Worafi, Y.M., Hasan, S., Hassan, N.M., & Gaili, A.A. (2021b). Knowledge, Attitude and Experience of Pharmacist in the UAE towards Pharmacovigilance. *Research Journal of Pharmacy and Technology*, 14(1), 265–269.

Al-Worafi, Y. (2022a). *A Guide to Online Pharmacy Education: Teaching Strategies and Assessment Methods*. CRC Press.

Al-Worafi, Y. (2022b). History and Importance. In *A Guide to Online Pharmacy Education: Teaching Strategies and Assessment Methods*. CRC Press.

Al-Worafi, Y. (2022c). *Terminologies. In A Guide to Online Pharmacy Education: Teaching Strategies and Assessment Methods*. CRC Press.

Al-Worafi, Y. (2022d). Research Methods and Methodology. In *A Guide to Online Pharmacy Education: Teaching Strategies and Assessment Methods*. CRC Press.

Al-Worafi, Y.M. (2022e). Patient care errors and related problems (part I): development and validation of the model. 0000-0002-5752-2913

Al-Worafi, Y.M. (Ed.). (2023). *Clinical Case Studies on medication Safety*. Academic Press.

Baig, M.R., Al-Worafi, Y.M., Alseragi, W.M., Ming, L.C., & Siddique, A. (2020). Drug safety in India. In *Drug Safety in Developing Countries* (pp. 327–334). Academic Press.

Elkalmi, R.M., Al-Worafi, Y.M., Alseragi, W.M., Ming, L.C., & Siddique, A. (2020). Drug safety in Malaysia. In *Drug Safety in Developing Countries* (pp. 245–253). Academic Press.

Elsayed, T., & Al-Worafi, Y.M. (2020). Drug safety in Egypt. In *Drug Safety in Developing Countries* (pp. 511–523). Academic Press.

Galvan, J.L., & Galvan, M.C. (2017). *Writing literature reviews: A guide for students of the social and behavioral sciences.* Routledge.

Hasan, S., Al-Omar, M.J., AlZubaidy, H., & Al-Worafi, Y.M. (2019). Use of medications in Arab Countries. *Handbook of Healthcare in the Arab World.* Cham: Springer, 42.

Hassan, Y., Abd Aziz, N., Kassab, Y.W., Elgasim, I., Shaharuddin, S., Al-Worafi, Y.M.A., ... & Ming, L.C. (2014). How to help patients to control their blood pressure? Blood pressure control and its predictor. *Archives of Pharmacy Practice,* 5(4).

Izahar, S., Lean, Q.Y., Hameed, M.A., Murugiah, M.K., Patel, R.P., Al-Worafi, Y.M., ... & Ming, L.C. (2017). Content analysis of mobile health applications on diabetes mellitus. *Frontiers in Endocrinology,* 8, 318.

Lee, K.S., Yee, S.M., Zaidi, S.T.R., Patel, R.P., Yang, Q., Al-Worafi, Y.M., & Ming, L.C., 2017. Combating sale of counterfeit and falsified medicines online: a losing battle. *Frontiers in pharmacology,* 8, p. 268.

Mahmoud, M.A., Wajid, S., Naqvi, A.A., Samreen, S., Althagfan, S.S., & Al-Worafi, Y. (2020). Self-medication with antibiotics: A cross-sectional community-based study. *Latin american journal of pharmacy,* 39(2), 348–353.

Manan, M.M., Rusli, R.A., Ang, W.C., Al-Worafi, Y.M., & Ming, L.C. (2014). Assessing the pharmaceutical care issues of antiepileptic drug therapy in hospitalised epileptic patients. *Journal of Pharmacy Practice and Research,* 44(3), 83–88.

Manan, M.M., Ibrahim, N.A., Aziz, N.A., Zulkifly, H.H., Al-Worafi, Y.M.A., & Long, C.M. (2016). Empirical use of antibiotic therapy in the prevention of early onset sepsis in neonates: a pilot study. *Archives of Medical Science,* 12(3), 603–613.

Ming, L.C., Hameed, M.A., Lee, D.D., Apidi, N.A., Lai, P.S.M., Hadi, M.A., Al-Worafi, Y.M.A., & Khan, T.M., (2016). Use of medical mobile applications among hospital pharmacists in Malaysia. *Therapeutic innovation & regulatory science,* 50(4), pp. 419–426.

Ming, L.C., Untong, N., Aliudin, N.A., Osili, N., Kifli, N., Tan, C.S., ... & Goh, H.P. (2020). Mobile health apps on COVID-19 launched in the early days of the pandemic: content analysis and review. *JMIR mHealth and uHealth,* 8(9), e19796.

Othman, G., Ali, F., Ibrahim, M.I.M., Al-Worafi, Y.M., Ansari, M., & Halboup, A.M. (2020). Assessment of Anti-Diabetic Medications Adherence among Diabetic Patients in Sana'a City, Yemen: A Cross Sectional Study. *Journal of Pharmaceutical Research International,* 32(21), 114–122.

Saeed, M.S., Alkhoshaiban, A.S., Al-Worafi, Y.M.A., & Long, C.M., (2014). Perception of self-medication among university students in Saudi Arabia. *Archives of Pharmacy Practice,* 5(4), p. 149.

42 Patient Safety Research

Qualitative Methods

42.1 BACKGROUND

Qualitative research is a method of inquiry that aims to understand the subjective experiences, perspectives, and meanings of individuals or groups. Unlike quantitative research, which focuses on numerical data and statistical analysis, qualitative research involves collecting and analyzing non-numerical data, such as observations, interviews, and written documents. Qualitative research often uses an iterative and flexible approach to data collection and analysis, allowing researchers to adapt their methods and research questions as they gain a deeper understanding of the phenomenon under study. This approach can be particularly useful for exploring complex or sensitive topics, or for understanding the experiences and perspectives of underrepresented or marginalized groups (Taylor et al., 2015).

Some common methods used in qualitative research include:

■ Interviews: One-on-one conversations with participants to gather detailed information about their experiences and perspectives.

■ Focus groups: Group discussions with several participants to gather a range of perspectives on a particular topic.

■ Observations: Systematic observation of behavior or interactions in naturalistic settings to understand social processes and behaviors.

■ Document analysis: Review of written or visual materials (such as diaries, photographs, or social media posts) to gain insights into the experiences and perspectives of individuals or groups.

Qualitative research can be used in many fields, including psychology, sociology, anthropology, education, and healthcare. When conducted rigorously, qualitative research can provide rich and nuanced insights into complex phenomena, and can help researchers better understand the perspectives and experiences of the individuals and communities they study.

42.2 RATIONALITY OF QUALITATIVE RESEARCH

Qualitative research can be a highly rational and rigorous method of inquiry, despite some common misconceptions that it may be less objective or systematic than quantitative research. Here are some key reasons why qualitative research can be considered rational:

1. Clearly defined research questions: Just like in quantitative research, qualitative research requires a clear and well-defined research question or set of questions. This ensures that the research is focused and purposeful.

2. Systematic data collection and analysis: Qualitative researchers use systematic and rigorous methods for collecting and analyzing data, such as detailed note-taking during interviews or observations, or coding and organizing data in a systematic manner. This helps to ensure that the data is collected and analyzed in a rigorous and transparent way.

3. Transparency and reflexivity: Qualitative researchers are typically transparent about their methods and assumptions, and often engage in a process of reflexivity, which involves reflecting on their own perspectives, biases, and assumptions throughout the research process. This helps to ensure that the research is transparent and objective.

4. Validity and reliability: Qualitative research can be assessed for its validity and reliability, just like quantitative research. For example, researchers can assess the validity of their findings by checking for consistency across different sources of data, or by using member checking, which involves sharing findings with participants to ensure accuracy and completeness.

5. Contribution to knowledge: Qualitative research can contribute to the development of theory and knowledge, just like quantitative research. By providing detailed and nuanced insights into complex phenomena, qualitative research can help to expand our understanding of the world around us.

In summary, qualitative research can be a highly rational and systematic method of inquiry, as long as it is conducted rigorously and transparently.

DOI: 10.1201/9781003230465-45

Qualitative research can be a highly valuable approach in patient safety, as it can provide rich insights into the experiences, perspectives, and behaviors of patients, healthcare providers, and other stakeholders involved in healthcare delivery. This type of research can help identify root causes of errors, explore the impact of safety interventions, and generate ideas for improving safety culture and communication in healthcare organizations. One of the key strengths of qualitative research is its ability to capture the complexity and diversity of human experiences and interactions, which can be difficult to quantify using quantitative methods. For example, qualitative research can provide a detailed understanding of how patients perceive their care, how healthcare providers navigate complex clinical situations, or how safety culture is manifested in everyday practices.

Another advantage of qualitative research in patient safety is that it can help identify and explore unexpected or emergent issues that may not have been previously considered. Through open-ended interviews, focus groups, and other qualitative methods, researchers can uncover new perspectives and insights that may not have been apparent through surveys or other quantitative approaches.

Here are some ways in which qualitative research can contribute to patient safety:

1. Understanding the patient perspective: Qualitative research can provide insights into patients' experiences of care and their perceptions of safety. This can help to identify areas of care that may need improvement, and to inform the development of patient-centered approaches to care.

2. Exploring organizational culture and practices: Qualitative research can help to identify organizational and cultural factors that may contribute to patient safety incidents, such as communication breakdowns or resistance to change. This can inform efforts to improve safety culture and implement effective interventions.

3. Identifying barriers and facilitators to safe care: Qualitative research can help to identify barriers and facilitators to safe care, such as workload, staffing, or training issues. This can inform strategies for improving patient safety and reducing the risk of adverse events.

4. Co-creating solutions with patients and healthcare providers: Qualitative research can involve patients and healthcare providers in the research process, allowing them to provide input and co-create solutions for improving patient safety. This can increase the relevance and accept-ability of interventions, and improve the likelihood of successful.

42.3 IMPORTANCE OF QUALITATIVE RESEARCH

Qualitative research is important because it provides a deep understanding of complex phenomena, including human experiences, behaviors, and perspectives. It involves collecting data through methods such as interviews, observations, and focus groups, and then analyzing this data to identify themes and patterns.

Here are some of the key reasons why qualitative research is important:

1. It helps us understand human experiences: Qualitative research allows us to delve deeply into people's experiences and perspectives, which can be difficult to capture with quantitative methods. By exploring people's thoughts, feelings, and behaviors, qualitative research can help us understand why people behave in certain ways and what motivates them.

2. It provides a rich and nuanced understanding: Qualitative research allows us to collect data in natural settings, which can provide a more accurate and complete picture of the phenomenon being studied. By analyzing this data in-depth, we can identify subtle patterns and nuances that may not be apparent through quantitative research alone.

3. It helps us generate new insights and hypotheses: Qualitative research is often exploratory in nature, which means that it can generate new ideas and hypotheses for future research. By exploring a phenomenon in-depth, researchers can uncover new perspectives and ideas that may not have been previously considered.

4. It can inform policy and practice: Qualitative research can provide valuable insights into the needs and experiences of patients, consumers, and other stakeholders. This information can be used to develop policies and programs that better meet their needs and improve their outcomes.

5. It can be used to evaluate interventions: Qualitative research can be used to evaluate the effectiveness of interventions and programs. By collecting data before and after an intervention, researchers can assess the impact of the intervention on people's experiences and outcomes.

Overall, qualitative research is an important tool for understanding complex phenomena and generating new insights and hypotheses. It can inform policy and practice, and help us develop interventions and programs that better meet the needs of individuals and communities.

Qualitative research is particularly important in patient safety because it provides valuable insights into the experiences, perspectives, and behaviors of patients, healthcare providers, and other stakeholders involved in healthcare delivery. Here are some of the key reasons why qualitative research is important in patient safety:

1. It helps identify the root causes of errors: Qualitative research can help identify the underlying factors that contribute to errors in healthcare. By exploring the experiences and perspectives of those involved in healthcare delivery, researchers can uncover the complex interactions and system-level issues that contribute to safety incidents.

2. It can inform the development of safety interventions: Qualitative research can be used to develop and evaluate safety interventions that are more effective at addressing the needs and experiences of patients and healthcare providers. By involving patients and healthcare providers in the development of safety interventions, researchers can ensure that they are more relevant and acceptable.

3. It provides a deeper understanding of safety culture: Safety culture is an important aspect of patient safety, and qualitative research can provide valuable insights into how safety culture is manifested in everyday practices. By exploring the experiences and perspectives of healthcare providers and patients, researchers can identify the cultural norms and values that influence safety practices in healthcare organizations.

4. It can help improve communication and teamwork: Effective communication and teamwork are critical components of patient safety, and qualitative research can help identify the factors that contribute to communication breakdowns and ineffective teamwork. By exploring the experiences and perspectives of healthcare providers, researchers can develop strategies to improve communication and teamwork in healthcare organizations.

5. It can inform policy and practice: Qualitative research can provide valuable insights into the needs and experiences of patients and healthcare providers, which can inform the development of policies and practices that better meet their needs. By involving patients and healthcare providers in the development of policies and practices, researchers can ensure that they are more relevant and acceptable.

Overall, qualitative research is an important tool for improving patient safety. It can help identify the root causes of errors, inform the development of safety interventions, provide a deeper understanding of safety culture, improve communication and teamwork, and inform policy and practice.

42.4 ADVANTAGES OF QUALITATIVE RESEARCH

Qualitative research offers several advantages over quantitative research, as it focuses on exploring and understanding the complexity of human experiences, behaviors, and perspectives. Here are some of the key advantages of qualitative research:

1. Provides in-depth understanding: Qualitative research is designed to provide a deeper understanding of the phenomenon being studied. By collecting data through methods such as interviews, observations, and focus groups, and analyzing it in-depth, researchers can identify underlying patterns and themes that may not be apparent through quantitative research alone.

2. Captures complexity and diversity: Qualitative research is particularly useful for studying complex phenomena, such as human behavior and experiences, which are difficult to capture through quantitative research methods. Qualitative research can help capture the diversity of perspectives and experiences of different groups of people, providing a more nuanced understanding of the phenomenon being studied.

3. Flexible and adaptable: Qualitative research is flexible and adaptable, allowing researchers to change their approach as they learn more about the phenomenon being studied. This flexibility allows researchers to adjust their research methods to better capture the data they need to answer their research questions.

4. Builds rapport with participants: Qualitative research often involves building a rapport with participants, which can lead to a greater willingness to share information and experiences. This can lead to more insightful and meaningful data that would not have been captured through other research methods.

5. Generates new insights and hypotheses: Qualitative research is often exploratory in nature, which means that it can generate new insights and hypotheses for future research. By exploring a phenomenon in-depth, researchers can uncover new perspectives and ideas that may not have been previously considered.

Overall, qualitative research offers several advantages over quantitative research, including a deeper understanding of the phenomenon being studied, flexibility and adaptability, and the generation of new insights and hypotheses. These advantages make qualitative research a valuable tool for researchers across a wide range of fields.

42.5 DISADVANTAGES OF QUALITATIVE RESEARCH

Qualitative research has several disadvantages, including:

1. Subjectivity: Qualitative research is often based on the researcher's interpretation of data, making it subjective. This means that different researchers may draw different conclusions from the same data.

2. Limited generalizability: Qualitative research often involves a small sample size, making it difficult to generalize findings to a larger population. This can limit the applicability of the research.

3. Time-consuming: Qualitative research typically involves collecting data through in-depth interviews, focus groups, and observations. This can be time-consuming and expensive.

4. Difficulty with replication: Because qualitative research is often based on unique experiences and perspectives, it can be challenging to replicate the findings. This can make it difficult to test the validity of the research.

5. Limited statistical analysis: Qualitative research often does not involve statistical analysis, making it difficult to quantify and measure findings. This can make it challenging to compare results across studies.

6. Potential for bias: Qualitative research may be subject to bias if the researcher has a preconceived idea of what the research should find. This can affect the interpretation of the data and the conclusions drawn from it.

42.6 FACILITATORS OF QUALITATIVE RESEARCH

Qualitative research has several facilitators, including:

1. In-depth exploration: Qualitative research allows for a more in-depth exploration of a research question or topic. It can provide rich and detailed data that can help researchers understand complex phenomena.

2. Flexibility: Qualitative research is flexible and can be adapted to suit the needs of the research question or study. Researchers can modify their research methods and data collection techniques to ensure they are capturing the most relevant and valuable data.

3. Rich data: Qualitative research generates rich, descriptive data that can help researchers understand the context and meaning behind people's experiences and perspectives.

4. Participant voice: Qualitative research often involves direct interaction with participants, allowing them to share their perspectives and experiences in their own words. This can provide valuable insights into their beliefs, attitudes, and behaviors.

5. Validity: Qualitative research can be valid, even without statistical analysis. Researchers can use a variety of methods to ensure the accuracy and credibility of their findings, such as member checking and triangulation.

6. Holistic understanding: Qualitative research provides a holistic understanding of a phenomenon, considering the context and environment in which it occurs. This can help researchers identify important factors that may not be captured in quantitative research.

42.7 BARRIERS OF QUALITATIVE RESEARCH

Qualitative research can face several barriers, including:

1. Limited resources: Qualitative research can be time-consuming and expensive, requiring significant resources in terms of funding, personnel, and time. This can make it difficult for researchers to conduct qualitative studies, particularly in low-resource settings.

2. Bias: Qualitative research can be subject to bias, particularly if the researcher has preconceived ideas about the research topic or participants. Researchers must take steps to mitigate bias, such as using multiple data sources and triangulating data.

3. Limited generalizability: Qualitative research typically involves a small sample size, making it difficult to generalize findings to larger populations. This can limit the applicability of the research.

4. Access to participants: Qualitative research often requires direct interaction with participants, which can be challenging if participants are difficult to access, located in remote areas, or have busy schedules.

5. Ethical considerations: Qualitative research involves direct interaction with participants, which can raise ethical concerns about informed consent, confidentiality, and privacy. Researchers must take steps to ensure that participants are fully informed about the research and their rights, and that their privacy is protected.

6. Analyzing and interpreting data: Qualitative research generates rich and complex data, which can be challenging to analyze and interpret. Researchers must be skilled in qualitative data analysis techniques to ensure that their findings are accurate and credible.

42.8 QUALITY OF QUALITATIVE RESEARCH

The quality of qualitative research can be assessed using several criteria, including:

1. Credibility: This refers to the extent to which the research findings accurately reflect the experiences and perspectives of the participants. Researchers can enhance credibility by using multiple data sources, triangulating data, and ensuring that the research methods and findings are consistent with the participants' experiences.

2. Transferability: This refers to the extent to which the research findings can be applied to other settings or populations. Researchers can enhance transferability by providing a detailed description of the research context and methods, and by comparing their findings with those of other studies.

3. Dependability: This refers to the stability and consistency of the research findings over time. Researchers can enhance dependability by ensuring that the research methods and findings are well-documented and transparent, and by using a systematic and rigorous approach to data analysis.

4. Confirmability: This refers to the degree to which the research findings are supported by the data and are not influenced by the researchers' biases or assumptions. Researchers can enhance confirmability by using a systematic and transparent approach to data collection and analysis, and by documenting the research process and decision-making.

5. Ethics: This refers to the ethical considerations involved in the research, such as informed consent, confidentiality, and privacy. Researchers must ensure that their research is conducted in an ethical manner and that the rights and well-being of the participants are protected.

Overall, the quality of qualitative research depends on the rigor and transparency of the research methods, the credibility of the research findings, and the ethical considerations involved in the research.

42.9 ONLINE QUALITATIVE RESEARCH

Online qualitative research refers to research methods that use online platforms to collect data from participants. Online qualitative research methods include online focus groups, interviews, and observations.

Some advantages of online qualitative research include:

1. Convenience: Online qualitative research allows participants to participate in research from the comfort of their own home, at a time that is convenient for them.

2. Cost-effective: Online qualitative research can be cost-effective compared to in-person research methods, as it eliminates the need for travel, venue hire, and other associated costs.

3. Larger sample size: Online qualitative research can reach a larger sample size than in-person research methods, as it can include participants from different geographic locations.

4. Rich data: Online qualitative research can generate rich data, including text, audio, and video recordings, which can provide a detailed understanding of participants' experiences and perspectives.

5. Reduced social desirability bias: Online qualitative research can reduce social desirability bias, as participants may feel more comfortable sharing their opinions and experiences online, compared to face-to-face interactions.

Some disadvantages of online qualitative research include:

1. Limited control over the research environment: Researchers have limited control over the research environment, and may not be able to control external factors that could influence the research findings.

2. Technical issues: Online qualitative research is dependent on technology, and technical issues such as poor internet connection or software glitches can impact the quality of the data collected.

3. Limited non-verbal cues: Online qualitative research may limit the ability to observe non-verbal cues, which can be important in understanding participants' experiences and perspectives.

4. Limited engagement: Online qualitative research may limit participant engagement compared to in-person research methods, as participants may not feel as connected to the research process.

Overall, online qualitative research can be a useful research method, but researchers should consider the advantages and disadvantages before choosing this method.

42.10 QUALITATIVE RESEARCH IN DEVELOPING COUNTRIES: Challenges and Recommendations

Patient safety research in developing countries has made significant achievements in recent years. Many developing countries have conducted many researches about the various issues of patient safety and care research (Alshahrani et al., 2019a,b; Al-Qahtani et al., 2015; Alshahrani et al., 2020a,b; Al-Worafi, 2014; Al-Worafi, 2015; Al-Worafi, 2016; Al-Worafi et al., 2017; Al-Worafi, 2018a-d; Al-Worafi et al., 2018a-b; Al-Worafi et al., 2019; Al-Worafi, 2020a-z; Al-Worafi et al., 2020a-b; Al-Worafi et al., 2021a,b; Al-Worafi, 2022a-e; Al-Worafi, 2023; Baig et al., 2020; Elkalmi et al., 2020; Elsayed & Al-Worafi, 2020; Hasan et al., 2019; Hassan et al., 2014; Izahar et al., 2017; Lee et al., 2017; Mahmoud et al., 2020; Manan et al., 2014; Manan et al., 2016; Ming et al., 2016; Ming et al., 2020; Othman et al., 2020; Saeed et al., 2014), however, there are many however, there are many challenges and recommendations for conducting qualitative research in developing countries such as:

1. Understand the local context: Before conducting any research in a developing country, it is essential to have a good understanding of the local context. Researchers should take the time to learn about the culture, language, and customs of the community they are studying. This can help ensure that the research is culturally appropriate and respectful.

2. Establish trust and rapport with participants: Building trust and rapport with participants is crucial in qualitative research. Researchers should take the time to establish relationships with participants and show respect for their knowledge and experiences.

3. Address language barriers: Language barriers can be a significant obstacle in qualitative research. Researchers should consider hiring local translators or interpreters to help facilitate communication with participants.

4. Consider ethical concerns: Researchers should be aware of potential ethical concerns when conducting research in developing countries. This may include issues such as informed consent, confidentiality, and the potential for exploitation. Researchers should take steps to ensure that their research is conducted in an ethical manner.

5. Adapt research methods to the local context: Researchers should be willing to adapt their research methods to the local context. This may involve using different data collection techniques or modifying research questions to better align with local knowledge and experiences.

6. Work with local partners: Working with local partners can be a valuable way to gain insights into the local context and build trust with participants. Local partners can also help researchers navigate logistical challenges and provide guidance on cultural norms and customs.

7. Ensure access to resources: Researchers should be aware of potential resource limitations in developing countries and take steps to ensure that participants have access to the resources they need. This may involve providing transportation or offering compensation for participation in the study.

8. Limited infrastructure: Developing countries may have limited infrastructure, such as transportation, electricity, or internet access. This can make it challenging for researchers to collect and analyze data, as well as communicate with participants and stakeholders.

9. Political instability and conflict: Political instability and conflict can create challenges for researchers, including restricted access to certain areas or groups, safety concerns, and potential interference from government or military officials.

10. Power imbalances: Power imbalances between researchers and participants can create ethical concerns and make it difficult to establish trust and rapport. Researchers should be aware of their own positionality and take steps to minimize any power differentials.

11. Data security and privacy: Data security and privacy can be a concern in developing countries, where regulations and enforcement may be weaker. Researchers should take steps to ensure that participants' data is protected and that confidentiality is maintained.

12. Limited research capacity: Developing countries may have limited research capacity, including trained researchers and access to resources such as funding, equipment, and software. Researchers should consider collaborating with local institutions and building research capacity in the communities they work with.

13. Cultural norms and beliefs: Cultural norms and beliefs can affect how participants respond to research questions and how researchers interpret data. Researchers should be aware of cultural norms and beliefs and adapt their research methods accordingly.

14. Language dialects and accents: In some developing countries, there may be multiple dialects and accents within a single language, making it challenging for researchers to communicate with participants or for participants to communicate with each other. Researchers may need to use different data collection techniques or work with local translators to overcome these language barriers.

15. Limited access to healthcare: In some developing countries, access to healthcare may be limited, which can affect participants' health and wellbeing. Researchers should be aware of potential health risks and take steps to minimize any negative impacts on participants.

16. Gender and social inequalities: Gender and social inequalities can affect participation in research and influence the data collected. Researchers should be aware of potential biases and take steps to ensure that their research is inclusive and respectful of all participants.

17. Historical and cultural trauma: Historical and cultural trauma can affect participants' experiences and perspectives, and may make it challenging for researchers to collect data. Researchers should be aware of these traumas and work to ensure that their research does not further harm participants or perpetuate historical injustices.

18. Limited funding: Funding for research in developing countries may be limited, making it challenging for researchers to cover the costs of data collection and analysis. Researchers should be creative in seeking funding sources and finding ways to work within limited budgets.

19. Environmental factors: Environmental factors, such as natural disasters or climate change, can affect participants' experiences and make it challenging for researchers to collect data. Researchers should be aware of these factors and adapt their research methods accordingly.

20. Limited access to technology: In some developing countries, access to technology may be limited, which can affect data collection and analysis. Researchers should be aware of potential technology limitations and work to find alternative methods for data collection and analysis.

21. Language barriers within a country: In some developing countries, there may be multiple languages spoken within a single country, making it challenging for researchers to communicate with participants or for participants to communicate with each other. Researchers may need to use different data collection techniques or work with local translators to overcome these language barriers.

Overall, researchers conducting qualitative research in developing countries need to be aware of the unique challenges and contexts of their research settings and be prepared to adapt their methods and approaches accordingly. By doing so, they can ensure that their research is respectful, meaningful, and contributes to positive social change.

42.11 CONCLUSION

This chapter has discussed the patient safety research issues related to the qualitative research, importance, facilitators, barriers, challenges and recommendations for the best practice in developing countries.

In conclusion, qualitative research in developing countries presents a unique set of challenges that researchers must be aware of and prepared to address. These challenges can range from limited infrastructure and political instability to power imbalances and language barriers, and may require researchers to be flexible, adaptable, and sensitive to the cultural and historical contexts of their research settings. Despite these challenges, conducting qualitative research in developing countries can also offer rich insights into the experiences and perspectives of marginalized and underrepresented groups, and can contribute to positive social change. To ensure that their research is respectful, meaningful, and contributes to positive social change, researchers must work collaboratively with participants and stakeholders, be mindful of potential biases and power differentials, and be committed to building research capacity and promoting ethical research practices. By doing so, researchers can contribute to a more just and equitable world.

REFERENCES

Al-Qahtani, I., Almoteb, T.M., & Al-Warafi, Y. (2015). Competency of metered-dose inhaler use among Saudi community pharmacists: A Simulation method study. *RRJPPS*, 4(2), 37–31.

Alshahrani, S.M., Alakhali, K.M., & Al-Worafi, Y.M., (2019a). Medication errors in a health care facility in southern Saudi Arabia. *Tropical Journal of Pharmaceutical Research*, 18(5), pp. 1119–1122.

Alshahrani, S.M., Alavudeen, S.S., Alakhali, K.M., Al-Worafi, Y.M., Bahamdan, A.K., & Vigneshwaran, E., (2019b). Self-Medication Among King Khalid University Students, Saudi Arabia. *Risk Management and Healthcare Policy*, 12, pp. 243–249.

Alshahrani, S.M., Alakhali, K.M., Al-Worafi, Y.M., & Alshahrani, N.Z. (2020a). Awareness and use of over the counter analgesic medication: a survey in the Aseer region population, Saudi Arabia. *Int J Advan Appl Sci*, 7(3), 130–134.

Alshahrani, S.M., Alzahran, M., Alakhali, K., Vigneshwaran, E., Iqbal, M.J., Khan, N.A., ... & Alavudeen, S.S. (2020b). Association Between Diabetes Consequences and Quality of Life Among Patients With Diabetes Mellitus in the Aseer Province of Saudi Arabia. *Open Access Macedonian Journal of Medical Sciences*, 8(E), 325–330.

Al-Worafi, Y.M. (2014). Prescription writing errors at a tertiary care hospital in Yemen: prevalence, types, causes and recommendations. *Am J Pharm Health Res*, 2, 134–140.

Al-Worafi, Y.M.A. (2015). Appropriateness of metered-dose inhaler use in the Yemeni community pharmacies. *Journal of Taibah University Medical Sciences*, 10(3), 353–358.

Al-Worafi, Y.M.A., (2016). Pharmacy practice in Yemen. In *Pharmacy Practice in Developing Countries* (pp. 267–287). Academic Press.

Al-Worafi, Y.M., Kassab, Y.W., Alseragi, W.M., Almutairi, M.S., Ahmed, A., Ming, L.C., Alkhoshaiban, A.S., & Hadi, M.A., (2017). Pharmacovigilance and adverse drg reaction reporting: a perspective of community pharmacists and pharmacy technicians in Sana'a, Yemen. *Therapeutics and clinical risk management*, 13, p. 1175.

Al-Worafi, Y.M., (2018a). Knowledge, Attitude and Practice of Yemeni Physicians Toward Pharmacovigilance: A Mixed Method Study. *International Journal of Pharmacy and Pharmaceutical Sciences*, 10(10), 74–77.

Al-Worafi, Y. (2018b). Knowledge, attitude and practice of Yemeni physicians toward pharmacovigilance: A mixed method study. *Int. J. Pharm. Pharm. Sci*, 10, 74–77.

Al-Worafi, Y.M. (2018c). Dispensing errors observed by community pharmacy dispensers in IBB–YEMEN. *Asian J. Pharm. Clin. Res*, 11(11).

Al-Worafi, Y.M. (2018d). Evauation of inhaler technique among patients with asthma and COPD in Yemen. *Journal of Taibah University medical sciences*, 13(5), 488–490.

Al-Worafi, Y.M., Patel, R.P., Zaidi, S.T.R., Alseragi, W.M., Almutairi, M.S., Alkhoshaiban, A.S., & Ming, L.C. (2018a). Completeness and legibility of handwritten prescriptions in Sana'a, Yemen. *Medical Principles and Practice*, 27, 290–292.

Al-Worafi, Y.M., Alseragi, W.M., Seng, L.K., Kassab, Y.W., Yeoh, S.F., Chiau, L., … & Husain, K. (2018b). Dispensing errors in community pharmacies: a prospective study in Sana'a, Yemen. *Arch Pharm Pract*, 9(4), 1–3.

Al-Worafi, Y.M., Alseragi, W.M., & Mahmoud, M.A. (2019). Competency of metered-dose inhaler use among community pharmacy dispensers in Ibb, Yemen: A simulation method study. *Latin American Journal of Pharmacy*, 38(3), 489–494.

Al-Worafi, Y.M. (Ed.). (2020a). *Drug Safety in Developing Countries: Achievements and Challenges.*

Al-Worafi, Y.M. (2020b). Medication errors. In *Drug Safety in Developing Countries* (pp. 105–117). Academic Press.

Al-Worafi, Y.M. (2020c). Adverse drug reactions. In *Drug Safety in Developing Countries* (pp. 39–57). Academic Press.

Al-Worafi, Y.M. (2020d). Medications registration and marketing: safety-related issues. In *Drug Safety in Developing Countries* (pp. 21–28). Academic Press.

Al-Worafi, Y.M. (2020e). Pharmacovigilance. In *Drug Safety in Developing Countries* (pp. 29–38). Academic Press.

Al-Worafi, Y.M. (2020f). Drug-related problems. In *Drug safety in developing countries* (pp. 59–71). Academic Press.

Al-Worafi, Y.M. (2020g). Medications safety-related terminology. In *Drug safety in developing countries* (pp. 7–19). Academic Press.

Al-Worafi, Y.M. (2020h). Self-medication. In *Drug Safety in Developing Countries* (pp. 73–86). Academic Press.

Al-Worafi, Y.M. (2020j). Antibiotics safety issues. In *Drug Safety in Developing Countries* (pp. 87–103). Academic Press.

Al-Worafi, Y.M. (2020k). Medications safety research issues. In *Drug Safety in Developing Countries* (pp. 213–227). Academic Press.

Al-Worafi, Y.M. (2020l). Counterfeit and substandard medications. In *Drug safety in developing countries* (pp. 119–126). Academic Press.

Al-Worafi, Y.M. (2020m). Medication abuse and misuse. In *Drug safety in developing countries* (pp. 127–135). Academic Press.

Al-Worafi, Y.M. (2020n). Storage and disposal of medications. In *Drug Safety in Developing Countries* (pp. 137–142). Academic Press.

Al-Worafi, Y.M. (2020o). Safety of medications in special population. In *Drug safety in developing countries* (pp. 143–162). Academic Press.

Al-Worafi, Y.M. (2020p). Herbal medicines safety issues. In *Drug Safety in developing countries* (pp. 163–178). Academic Press.

Al-Worafi, Y.M. (2020q). Medications safety pharmacoeconomics-related issues. In *Drug Safety in Developing Countries* (pp. 187–195). Academic Press.

Al-Worafi, Y.M. (2020r). Evidence-based medications safety practice. In *Drug Safety in Developing Countries* (pp. 197–201). Academic Press.

Al-Worafi, Y.M. (2020s). Quality indicators for medications safety. In *Drug safety in developing countries* (pp. 229–242). Academic Press.

Al-Worafi, Y.M. (2020t). Drug safety in Yemen. In *Drug Safety in Developing Countries* (pp. 391–405). Academic Press.

Al-Worafi, Y.M. (2020u). Drug safety in Saudi Arabia. In *Drug Safety in Developing Countries* (pp. 407–417). Academic Press.

Al-Worafi, Y.M. (2020v). Drug safety in United Arab Emirates. In *Drug Safety in Developing Countries* (pp. 419–428). Academic Press.

Al-Worafi, Y.M. (2020w). Drug safety in Indonesia. In *Drug Safety in Developing Countries* (pp. 279–285). Academic Press.

Al-Worafi, Y.M. (2020x). Drug safety in Palestine. In *Drug Safety in Developing Countries* (pp. 471–480). Academic Press.

Al-Worafi, Y.M. (2020y). Drug safety: comparison between developing countries. In *Drug Safety in Developing Countries* (pp. 603–611). Academic Press.

Al-Worafi, Y.M. (2020z). Drug safety in developing versus developed countries. In *Drug Safety in Developing Countries* (pp. 613–615). Academic Press.

Al-Worafi, Y.M., Alseragi, W.M., Ming, L.C., & Alakhali, K.M. (2020a). Drug safety in China. In *Drug Safety in Developing Countries* (pp. 381–388). Academic Press.

Al-Worafi, Y.M., Alseragi, W.M., Alakhali, K.M., Ming, L.C., Othman, G., Halboup, A.M., ... & Elkalmi, R.M. (2020b). Knowledge, beliefs and factors affecting the use of generic medicines among patients in Ibb, Yemen: a mixed-method study. *Journal of Pharmacy Practice and Community Medicine*, 6(4).

Al-Worafi, Y.M., Elkalmi, R.M., Ming, L.C., Othman, G., Halboup, A.M., Battah, M.M., ... & Mani, V. (2021a). Dispensing errors in hospital pharmacies: A prospective study in Yemen.

Al-Worafi, Y.M., Hasan, S., Hassan, N.M., & Gaili, A.A. (2021b). Knowledge, Attitude and Experience of Pharmacist in the UAE towards Pharmacovigilance. *Research Journal of Pharmacy and Technology*, 14(1), 265–269.

Al-Worafi, Y. (2022a). *A Guide to Online Pharmacy Education: Teaching Strategies and Assessment Methods*. CRC Press.

Al-Worafi, Y. (2022b). History and Importance. In *A Guide to Online Pharmacy Education: Teaching Strategies and Assessment Methods*. CRC Press.

Al-Worafi, Y. (2022c). Terminologies. In *A Guide to Online Pharmacy Education: Teaching Strategies and Assessment Methods*. CRC Press.

Al-Worafi, Y. (2022d). Research Methods and Methodology. In *A Guide to Online Pharmacy Education: Teaching Strategies and Assessment Methods*. CRC Press.

Al-Worafi, Y.M. (2022e). Patient care errors and related problems (part I): development and validation of the model. 0000-0002-5752-2913

Al-Worafi, Y.M. (Ed.). (2023). *Clinical Case Studies on medication Safety*. Academic Press.

Baig, M.R., Al-Worafi, Y.M., Alseragi, W.M., Ming, L.C., & Siddique, A. (2020). Drug safety in India. In *Drug Safety in Developing Countries* (pp. 327–334). Academic Press.

Elkalmi, R.M., Al-Worafi, Y.M., Alseragi, W.M., Ming, L.C., & Siddique, A. (2020). Drug safety in Malaysia. In *Drug Safety in Developing Countries* (pp. 245–253). Academic Press.

Elsayed, T., & Al-Worafi, Y.M. (2020). Drug safety in Egypt. In *Drug Safety in Developing Countries* (pp. 511–523). Academic Press.

Hasan, S., Al-Omar, M.J., AlZubaidy, H., & Al-Worafi, Y.M. (2019). Use of medications in Arab Countries. *Handbook of Healthcare in the Arab World*. Cham: Springer, 42.

Hassan, Y., Abd Aziz, N., Kassab, Y.W., Elgasim, I., Shaharuddin, S., Al-Worafi, Y.M.A., ... & Ming, L.C. (2014). How to help patients to control their blood pressure? Blood pressure control and its predictor. *Archives of Pharmacy Practice*, 5(4).

Izahar, S., Lean, Q.Y., Hameed, M.A., Murugiah, M.K., Patel, R.P., Al-Worafi, Y.M., ... & Ming, L.C. (2017). Content analysis of mobile health applications on diabetes mellitus. *Frontiers in Endocrinology*, 8, 318.

Lee, K.S., Yee, S.M., Zaidi, S.T.R., Patel, R.P., Yang, Q., Al-Worafi, Y.M., & Ming, L.C., 2017. Combating sale of counterfeit and falsified medicines online: a losing battle. *Frontiers in pharmacology*, 8, p. 268.

Mahmoud, M.A., Wajid, S., Naqvi, A.A., Samreen, S., Althagfan, S.S., & Al-Worafi, Y. (2020). Self-medication with antibiotics: A cross-sectional community-based study. *Latin american journal of pharmacy*, 39(2), 348–353.

Manan, M.M., Rusli, R.A., Ang, W.C., Al-Worafi, Y.M., & Ming, L.C. (2014). Assessing the pharmaceutical care issues of antiepileptic drug therapy in hospitalised epileptic patients. *Journal of Pharmacy Practice and Research*, 44(3), 83–88.

Manan, M.M., Ibrahim, N.A., Aziz, N.A., Zulkifly, H.H., Al-Worafi, Y.M.A., & Long, C.M. (2016). Empirical use of antibiotic therapy in the prevention of early onset sepsis in neonates: a pilot study. *Archives of Medical Science*, 12(3), 603–613.

Ming, L.C., Hameed, M.A., Lee, D.D., Apidi, N.A., Lai, P.S.M., Hadi, M.A., Al-Worafi, Y.M.A., & Khan, T.M., (2016). Use of medical mobile applications among hospital pharmacists in Malaysia. *Therapeutic innovation & regulatory science*, 50(4), pp. 419–426.

Ming, L.C., Untong, N., Aliudin, N.A., Osili, N., Kifli, N., Tan, C.S., ... & Goh, H.P. (2020). Mobile health apps on COVID-19 launched in the early days of the pandemic: content analysis and review. *JMIR mHealth and uHealth*, 8(9), e19796.

Othman, G., Ali, F., Ibrahim, M.I.M., Al-Worafi, Y.M., Ansari, M., & Halboup, A.M. (2020). Assessment of Anti-Diabetic Medications Adherence among Diabetic Patients in Sana'a City, Yemen: A Cross Sectional Study. *Journal of Pharmaceutical Research International*, 32(21), 114–122.

Saeed, M.S., Alkhoshaiban, A.S., Al-Worafi, Y.M.A., & Long, C.M., (2014). Perception of self-medication among university students in Saudi Arabia. *Archives of Pharmacy Practice*, 5(4), p. 149.

Taylor, S.J., Bogdan, R., & DeVault, M. (2015). *Introduction to qualitative research methods: A guidebook and resource*. John Wiley & Sons.

43 Patient Safety Research

Quantitative Methods

43.1 BACKGROUND

Quantitative research is a research method that relies on collecting and analyzing numerical data to answer research questions or test hypotheses. This method involves the use of structured surveys, questionnaires, or experiments to collect data from a large sample of participants. Quantitative research is characterized by the use of statistical analysis to identify patterns, relationships, and correlations between variables. The aim is to identify generalizable results that can be applied to a larger population. Some of the key features of quantitative research include:

1. Objective measurement: The research focuses on numerical data that can be objectively measured and analyzed.

2. Large sample size: The research typically involves a large sample size, with statistical techniques used to ensure that the results are representative of the population.

3. Statistical analysis: The data collected is analyzed using statistical techniques to identify patterns, relationships, and correlations between variables.

4. Replicability: Quantitative research aims to produce results that can be replicated in future studies.

Quantitative research is commonly used in social sciences, such as psychology, sociology, and education, as well as in business and marketing research (Polgar & Thomas, 2011). Quantitative research can be used to investigate patient safety issues in healthcare settings. Some examples of quantitative research in patient safety include:

1. Incident reporting and analysis: Quantitative methods can be used to analyze incident reports and identify patterns and trends in patient safety incidents. This can help healthcare organizations to identify areas for improvement and develop strategies to reduce the risk of patient harm.

2. Survey research: Surveys can be used to gather data on healthcare professionals' attitudes, beliefs, and practices related to patient safety. This information can be used to identify areas where education and training may be needed to improve patient safety.

3. Observational studies: Observational studies can be used to identify factors that contribute to patient safety incidents, such as communication breakdowns, workflow issues, or equipment failures.

4. Randomized controlled trials: Randomized controlled trials can be used to evaluate the effectiveness of interventions designed to improve patient safety, such as checklists or standardized protocols.

5. Data analysis: Quantitative methods can be used to analyze large datasets, such as electronic health records, to identify patterns and trends in patient safety incidents and outcomes.

Overall, quantitative research can provide valuable insights into patient safety issues and help healthcare organizations to develop strategies to improve patient safety and reduce the risk of harm.

43.2 RATIONALITY OF QUANTITATIVE RESEARCH

Quantitative research is considered a rational and scientific approach to research because it is based on the principles of objectivity, reliability, and validity. Here are some reasons why quantitative research is considered a rational approach to research:

1. Objectivity: Quantitative research relies on objective measurements and data that can be observed and measured using standardized tools and techniques. This reduces the potential for researcher bias and ensures that the data collected is reliable.

2. Reliability: Quantitative research involves the use of statistical analysis to ensure that the results are reliable and accurate. The use of large sample sizes and standardized tools and techniques further enhances the reliability of the data.

DOI: 10.1201/9781003230465-46

3. Validity: Quantitative research aims to ensure that the data collected is valid, meaning that it measures what it is intended to measure. Validity can be established through the use of appropriate research designs, sampling methods, and data collection tools.

4. Replicability: Quantitative research is designed to produce results that are replicable, meaning that the findings can be repeated in other studies. This increases the confidence in the accuracy and generalizability of the research findings.

5. Generalizability: Quantitative research aims to produce results that are generalizable to larger populations. This is achieved through the use of representative samples and statistical techniques that allow for the extrapolation of findings to larger populations.

Overall, the use of objective, reliable, and valid data, combined with the use of statistical analysis, makes quantitative research a rational and scientific approach to research. It allows researchers to draw meaningful conclusions based on empirical evidence and to produce results that can be replicated and generalized to larger populations.

Quantitative research is a rational approach to investigating patient safety issues in healthcare settings. Here are some reasons why:

1. Objectivity: Quantitative research relies on objective measurements and data that can be observed and measured using standardized tools and techniques. This reduces the potential for researcher bias and ensures that the data collected is reliable.

2. Reliability: Quantitative research involves the use of statistical analysis to ensure that the results are reliable and accurate. The use of large sample sizes and standardized tools and techniques further enhances the reliability of the data.

3. Validity: Quantitative research aims to ensure that the data collected is valid, meaning that it measures what it is intended to measure. Validity can be established through the use of appropriate research designs, sampling methods, and data collection tools.

4. Replicability: Quantitative research is designed to produce results that are replicable, meaning that the findings can be repeated in other studies. This increases the confidence in the accuracy and generalizability of the research findings.

5. Generalizability: Quantitative research aims to produce results that are generalizable to larger populations. This is achieved through the use of representative samples and statistical techniques that allow for the extrapolation of findings to larger populations.

6. Evidence-based practice: The objective and scientific approach of quantitative research provides healthcare organizations with evidence-based data to inform patient safety policies and practices.

Overall, the use of objective, reliable, and valid data, combined with the use of statistical analysis, makes quantitative research a rational and scientific approach to investigating patient safety issues in healthcare settings. It allows researchers to draw meaningful conclusions based on empirical evidence and to produce results that can inform evidence-based practice and improve patient safety.

43.3 IMPORTANCE OF QUANTITATIVE RESEARCH

Quantitative research plays an important role in many areas of study, including social sciences, natural sciences, and healthcare. Here are some reasons why quantitative research is important:

1. Objectivity: Quantitative research relies on objective measurements and data that can be observed and measured using standardized tools and techniques. This reduces the potential for researcher bias and ensures that the data collected is reliable.

2. Reliability: Quantitative research involves the use of statistical analysis to ensure that the results are reliable and accurate. The use of large sample sizes and standardized tools and techniques further enhances the reliability of the data.

3. Validity: Quantitative research aims to ensure that the data collected is valid, meaning that it measures what it is intended to measure. Validity can be established through the use of appropriate research designs, sampling methods, and data collection tools.

4. Generalizability: Quantitative research aims to produce results that are generalizable to larger populations. This is achieved through the use of representative samples and statistical techniques that allow for the extrapolation of findings to larger populations.

5. Replicability: Quantitative research is designed to produce results that are replicable, meaning that the findings can be repeated in other studies. This increases the confidence in the accuracy and generalizability of the research findings.

6. Evidence-based practice: The objective and scientific approach of quantitative research provides evidence-based data to inform policies, practices, and decision-making in many fields, including healthcare, education, and business.

7. Testing of hypotheses: Quantitative research provides a rigorous and systematic approach to testing hypotheses and theories, allowing researchers to make evidence-based conclusions and recommendations.

Overall, the importance of quantitative research lies in its ability to provide objective, reliable, and valid data to inform evidence-based practice and decision-making in many areas of study. It plays a crucial role in advancing knowledge, testing hypotheses, and improving outcomes in many fields.

Quantitative research plays a crucial role in investigating and improving patient safety in healthcare settings. Here are some reasons why quantitative research is important in patient safety:

1. Objectivity: Quantitative research relies on objective measurements and data that can be observed and measured using standardized tools and techniques. This reduces the potential for researcher bias and ensures that the data collected is reliable.

2. Reliability: Quantitative research involves the use of statistical analysis to ensure that the results are reliable and accurate. The use of large sample sizes and standardized tools and techniques further enhances the reliability of the data.

3. Validity: Quantitative research aims to ensure that the data collected is valid, meaning that it measures what it is intended to measure. Validity can be established through the use of appropriate research designs, sampling methods, and data collection tools.

4. Generalizability: Quantitative research aims to produce results that are generalizable to larger populations. This is achieved through the use of representative samples and statistical techniques that allow for the extrapolation of findings to larger populations.

5. Evidence-based practice: The objective and scientific approach of quantitative research provides healthcare organizations with evidence-based data to inform patient safety policies and practices.

6. Identification of patient safety issues: Quantitative research can help identify patterns and trends in patient safety incidents, allowing healthcare organizations to address underlying issues and improve patient outcomes.

7. Evaluation of interventions: Quantitative research can be used to evaluate the effectiveness of interventions aimed at improving patient safety, allowing healthcare organizations to make evidence-based decisions about the most effective strategies for improving patient outcomes.

Overall, the importance of quantitative research in patient safety lies in its ability to provide objective, reliable, and valid data to inform evidence-based practice and decision-making in healthcare organizations. It plays a crucial role in identifying patient safety issues, evaluating interventions, and improving outcomes for patients.

43.4 ADVANTAGES OF QUANTITATIVE RESEARCH

Quantitative research has several advantages, including:

1. Objectivity: Quantitative research relies on objective measurements and data that can be observed and measured using standardized tools and techniques. This reduces the potential for researcher bias and ensures that the data collected is reliable.

2. Reliability: Quantitative research involves the use of statistical analysis to ensure that the results are reliable and accurate. The use of large sample sizes and standardized tools and techniques further enhances the reliability of the data.

3. Generalizability: Quantitative research aims to produce results that are generalizable to larger populations. This is achieved through the use of representative samples and statistical techniques that allow for the extrapolation of findings to larger populations.

4. Replicability: Quantitative research is designed to produce results that are replicable, meaning that the findings can be repeated in other studies. This increases the confidence in the accuracy and generalizability of the research findings.

5. Efficiency: Quantitative research can be conducted quickly and efficiently, allowing researchers to collect and analyze data on a large scale.

6. Cost-effectiveness: The use of standardized tools and techniques in quantitative research can reduce the cost of data collection and analysis, making it a cost-effective approach to research.

7. Testing of hypotheses: Quantitative research provides a rigorous and systematic approach to testing hypotheses and theories, allowing researchers to make evidence-based conclusions and recommendations.

Overall, the advantages of quantitative research lie in its ability to provide objective, reliable, and valid data efficiently and cost-effectively, and to produce results that are generalizable and replicable. This makes it a valuable approach to research in many fields, including healthcare, social sciences, and natural sciences.

43.5 DISADVANTAGES OF QUANTITATIVE RESEARCH

While quantitative research has many advantages, it also has several potential disadvantages, including:

1. Limited depth: Quantitative research typically focuses on a narrow set of variables and uses standardized measures and tools, which can limit the depth of understanding of complex phenomena.

2. Lack of context: Quantitative research often focuses on statistical analysis of data, which can lead to a lack of understanding of the social, cultural, and environmental contexts in which phenomena occur.

3. Reductionism: Quantitative research tends to reduce complex phenomena into simple categories or numerical values, which can oversimplify the complexity of real-world phenomena.

4. Difficulty in measuring subjective experiences: Quantitative research is often unable to capture subjective experiences, emotions, and perspectives, which can be important in understanding certain phenomena.

5. Potential for researcher bias: While the use of standardized tools and techniques can reduce the potential for researcher bias, it is still possible for researchers to influence the data through the design of the study, data collection, or data analysis.

6. Ethics: The use of quantitative research can raise ethical issues, such as privacy concerns, informed consent, and potential harm to participants.

7. Limited scope: Quantitative research often focuses on specific variables or outcomes, which may limit the scope of the study and its ability to address broader issues.

Overall, the disadvantages of quantitative research lie in its potential limitations in capturing the complexity of real-world phenomena and its potential for researcher bias, and ethical issues. However, these limitations can often be addressed through careful research design, data collection, and data analysis techniques.

43.6 FACILI4TATORS OF QUANTITATIVE RESEARCH

There are several factors that can facilitate the conduct of quantitative research, including:

1. Clear research question: A well-defined research question can provide a clear focus for the study, guide the research design and data collection methods, and ensure that the research is feasible and achievable.

2. Availability of data: Access to high-quality data, such as large datasets or medical records, can facilitate the conduct of quantitative research and reduce the cost and time required for data collection.

3. Suitable research design: A suitable research design, such as a randomized controlled trial or cohort study, can provide a rigorous and systematic approach to data collection and analysis, and help ensure the validity and reliability of the research findings.

4. Appropriate sampling strategy: An appropriate sampling strategy, such as random sampling or stratified sampling, can help ensure that the sample is representative of the population of interest and reduce the potential for bias in the research findings.

5. Standardized data collection tools: The use of standardized data collection tools, such as questionnaires or checklists, can improve the reliability and validity of the data and facilitate comparisons between studies.

6. Statistical software: The availability of statistical software, such as SPSS or SAS, can facilitate the analysis of large datasets and complex statistical models, and help ensure the accuracy and reliability of the research findings.

7. Expertise and resources: The availability of expertise and resources, such as research assistants, statisticians, or funding, can facilitate the conduct of quantitative research and ensure that the research is conducted to a high standard.

Overall, the facilitators of quantitative research lie in the availability of clear research questions, high-quality data, suitable research design, appropriate sampling strategy, standardized data collection tools, statistical software, expertise, and resources. These factors can help ensure that the research is rigorous, reliable, and valid, and can lead to meaningful and impactful research findings.

43.7 BARRIERS OF QUANTITATIVE RESEARCH

There are several potential barriers to conducting quantitative research, including:

1. Limited access to data: Access to high-quality data can be a significant barrier to conducting quantitative research, particularly in fields such as healthcare, where patient data is often protected by privacy regulations or institutional policies.

2. Cost and time: Conducting quantitative research can be expensive and time-consuming, particularly when large samples are required, or when the study involves multiple data collection points or follow-up periods.

3. Participant recruitment: Recruitment of participants can be challenging, particularly when the study involves vulnerable or hard-to-reach populations or when the study requires a large sample size.

4. Ethical considerations: Quantitative research can raise ethical considerations, such as issues related to informed consent, participant confidentiality, and the potential for harm to participants.

5. Lack of suitable research design: The selection of an inappropriate research design can result in biased or unreliable findings, and can limit the ability to draw meaningful conclusions from the study.

6. Limited generalizability: The findings from a quantitative study may not be generalizable to other populations or settings, which can limit the impact and relevance of the research.

7. Researcher bias: Researchers may introduce bias into the study through the design of the study, data collection, or data analysis, which can undermine the validity and reliability of the research findings.

Overall, the barriers to conducting quantitative research lie in the challenges related to data access, cost and time, participant recruitment, ethical considerations, suitable research design, limited generalizability, and potential for researcher bias. These barriers can be addressed through careful study design, selection of appropriate methods and measures, and appropriate consideration of ethical and practical issues.

43.8 QUALITY OF QUANTITATIVE RESEARCH

The quality of quantitative research can be assessed using several criteria, including:

1. Validity: Validity refers to the degree to which the research measures what it is intended to measure. For quantitative research, this includes internal validity (the extent to which the study design and analysis minimize the risk of error or bias) and external validity (the extent to which the findings can be generalized to other populations or settings).

2. Reliability: Reliability refers to the consistency and stability of the research findings over time and across different measures or raters. This includes the measurement reliability (the extent to which the measures are consistent) and the inter-rater reliability (the extent to which different raters produce consistent results).

3. Sample size and representativeness: The sample size and representativeness of the sample can impact the generalizability and power of the study. A larger sample size and a more representative sample can increase the statistical power and the external validity of the research findings.

4. Research design: The research design should be appropriate for the research question and the research objectives. A well-designed study should have a clear and well-defined research question, appropriate methods for data collection, and appropriate methods for data analysis.

5. Data analysis: The data analysis should be appropriate for the research question and the research objectives. This includes the use of appropriate statistical methods, appropriate interpretation of the statistical results, and appropriate reporting of the research findings.

6. Ethical considerations: The research should be conducted ethically, including obtaining informed consent from participants, ensuring participant confidentiality, and minimizing the risk of harm to participants.

7. Reporting: The research should be reported in a clear and transparent manner, including a clear description of the research design, methods, and results, and a discussion of the limitations and implications of the research findings.

Overall, the quality of quantitative research can be assessed based on the validity, reliability, sample size and representativeness, research design, data analysis, ethical considerations, and reporting. These criteria can be used to evaluate the quality of the research findings and their relevance and usefulness for informing clinical practice or policy decisions.

43.9 ONLINE QUANTITATIVE RESEARCH

Online quantitative research refers to the use of online platforms and tools to collect data for quantitative research studies. This can include surveys, questionnaires, experiments, and other types of quantitative research methods. Some advantages of online quantitative research include:

1. Cost-effectiveness: Online research can be more cost-effective than traditional methods of data collection, such as telephone or in-person interviews. Researchers can save on costs related to travel, printing, and mailing of surveys.

2. Convenience: Online research allows participants to complete surveys or questionnaires at their own convenience, without the need to schedule appointments or travel to a research site.

3. Reach: Online research can reach a wider audience, including participants from different geographic locations and with different backgrounds and demographics.

4. Real-time data collection: Online research allows for real-time data collection, which can be useful for tracking changes over time or for measuring responses to time-sensitive events or interventions.

5. Standardization: Online research can improve the standardization of data collection, as it allows for the use of standardized questions and response options.

However, there are also some limitations and potential drawbacks of online quantitative research, including:

1. Limited access to certain populations: Online research may not be accessible to certain populations, such as those who do not have access to the internet or those who are not comfortable using online tools.

2. Sampling bias: Online research may suffer from sampling bias, as participants who are more likely to complete online surveys may be different from those who are less likely to participate.

3. Response bias: Online research may be subject to response bias, as participants may not take the survey seriously or may be more likely to give socially desirable responses.

4. Security and privacy concerns: Online research may raise security and privacy concerns, particularly if sensitive or personal information is being collected.

5. Technical issues: Online research may be subject to technical issues, such as internet connectivity problems or compatibility issues with different devices or browsers.

Overall, online quantitative research can be a useful tool for collecting data for quantitative research studies, but it is important to consider the advantages and limitations of this approach and to design the study in a way that minimizes potential biases and limitations.

43.10 QUANTITATIVE RESEARCH IN DEVELOPING COUNTRIES: Challenges and Recommendations

Patient safety research in developing countries has made significant achievements in recent years. Many developing countries have conducted many researches about the various issues of patient safety and care research (Alshahrani et al., 2019a,b; Al-Qahtani et al., 2015; Alshahrani et al., 2020a,b; Al-Worafi, 2014; Al-Worafi, 2015; Al-Worafi, 2016; Al-Worafi et al., 2017; Al-Worafi, 2018a-d; Al-Worafi et al., 2018a-b; Al-Worafi et al., 2019; Al-Worafi, 2020a-z; Al-Worafi et al., 2020a-b; Al-Worafi et al., 2021a,b; Al-Worafi, 2022a-e; Al-Worafi, 2023; Baig et al., 2020; Elkalmi et al., 2020; Elsayed & Al-Worafi, 2020; Hasan et al., 2019; Hassan et al., 2014; Izahar et al., 2017; Lee et al., 2017; Mahmoud et al., 2020; Manan et al., 2014; Manan et al., 2016; Ming et al., 2016; Ming et al., 2020; Othman et al., 2020; Saeed et al., 2014), however, there are many however, there are many challenges and recommendations for conducting quantitative research in developing countries such as:

1. Access to data: One of the main challenges in developing countries is the limited availability and quality of data. National statistical agencies in many developing countries lack the resources to collect, maintain and analyze data at a granular level. Researchers may need to collect their own data, which can be time-consuming and costly.

2. Sample size and representativeness: Obtaining a representative sample is crucial for accurate results. In developing countries, it can be challenging to obtain a large enough sample size due to a lack of infrastructure, poor communication, or distrust of outsiders.

3. Language barriers: Language barriers can make data collection and analysis difficult, especially if the research team does not speak the local language.

4. Cultural differences: Cultural differences may impact the validity and reliability of data collection. It is essential to understand cultural norms and tailor research methods accordingly.

5. Ethical concerns: Conducting research in developing countries raises ethical concerns, such as informed consent, confidentiality, and potential exploitation.

Recommendations:

1. Collaborate with local institutions: Collaborating with local universities, research institutions, or non-governmental organizations (NGOs) can help researchers overcome language and cultural barriers, access data, and establish relationships with local communities.

2. Build trust and engage with local communities: Researchers should take the time to build trust with local communities and stakeholders, engage with them, and explain the research objectives and potential benefits.

3. Consider alternative data sources: Researchers can consider alternative data sources, such as administrative records or data from mobile phones, to supplement their research.

4. Use mixed-methods approaches: Combining quantitative and qualitative methods can provide a more comprehensive understanding of the research topic and help to triangulate findings.

5. Follow ethical guidelines: Researchers should follow ethical guidelines, such as obtaining informed consent, protecting participants' confidentiality, and avoiding any potential exploitation of vulnerable populations.

6. Carefully select your research topic and design: It is important to choose a research topic that is relevant and meaningful to the local community and to design the research in a way that is sensitive to cultural, social, and economic factors.

7. Work with local partners: Collaborate with local organizations, community leaders, and researchers who have knowledge and experience in the local context. This can help ensure that the research is culturally appropriate and addresses the needs and concerns of the local community.

8. Be aware of power dynamics: Research can create power imbalances between the researchers and the participants, especially in developing countries where poverty and inequality are prevalent. Researchers should be aware of these dynamics and take steps to minimize them, such as providing informed consent, ensuring confidentiality, and respecting the participants' autonomy.

9. Use appropriate methods: Quantitative research methods such as surveys and experiments can be effective in developing countries, but they need to be adapted to the local context. For example, surveys may need to be translated into local languages, and experiments may need to be conducted in a way that is culturally appropriate.

10. Ensure data quality: Quality control is critical in quantitative research. Researchers should take steps to ensure the validity and reliability of their data, such as pretesting survey instruments and using trained data collectors.

11. Communicate findings and engage stakeholders: It is important to communicate research findings to the local community and engage stakeholders in the research process. This can help ensure that the research has a positive impact on the community and can inform future research and policy decisions.

12. Address language barriers: Researchers should ensure that language barriers do not prevent participation in the study. This can be done by providing translations of study materials, using trained interpreters, or recruiting bilingual staff.

13. Address issues of access: Researchers should consider issues of access to technology and infrastructure when conducting quantitative research in developing countries. This may include providing participants with mobile devices or internet access, or conducting surveys and data collection in person.

14. Consider the impact of cultural norms: Cultural norms and beliefs can affect the way research is conducted and the interpretation of findings. Researchers should be aware of these norms and consider how they may impact the study design, recruitment, and data analysis.

15. Ensure diversity in the research sample: It is important to ensure diversity in the research sample to ensure that findings are representative of the population of interest. This may require targeted recruitment efforts or oversampling of underrepresented groups.

16. Address issues of power and privilege: Researchers should consider their own power and privilege in the research process, particularly in the context of developing countries where poverty and inequality are prevalent. This may require a critical reflection on the research process and the involvement of local partners in decision-making.

17. Use appropriate statistical techniques: Statistical techniques should be selected based on the research question and data type, and should be appropriate for the sample size and level of variability in the data. Researchers should consult with a statistician or data analyst to ensure appropriate statistical analysis.

18. Address issues of data storage and management: Researchers should ensure that data is stored securely and that appropriate data management protocols are in place. This may include using encrypted data storage and limiting access to data to authorized personnel only.

19. Address issues of sustainability: Researchers should consider the long-term impact of their research on the local community, and consider ways to ensure that the benefits of the research are sustained over time. This may require involving local partners in the design and implementation of the research, or developing capacity-building initiatives to build local research capacity.

43.11 CONCLUSION

This chapter has discussed the patient safety research issues related to the quantitative research, importance, facilitators, barriers, challenges and recommendations for the best practice in developing countries. conducting quantitative research in developing countries requires careful consideration of a range of ethical, cultural, and practical issues. Researchers should work in partnership with local organizations and community members to ensure that the research is culturally appropriate and addresses the needs and concerns of the local community. They should also be aware of power dynamics and take steps to minimize these imbalances. Finally, they should use appropriate methods, ensure data quality, address ethical concerns, and communicate findings to stakeholders to ensure that the research has a positive impact on the community and informs future research and policy decisions. By following these recommendations, researchers can conduct high-quality quantitative research that is ethical, culturally sensitive, and has a positive impact on the local community.

REFERENCES

Al-Qahtani, I., Almoteb, T.M., & Al-Warafi, Y. (2015). Competency of metered-dose inhaler use among Saudi community pharmacists: A Simulation method study. *RRJPPS*, 4(2), 37–31.

Alshahrani, S.M., Alakhali, K.M., & Al-Worafi, Y.M., (2019a). Medication errors in a health care facility in southern Saudi Arabia. *Tropical Journal of Pharmaceutical Research*, 18(5), pp. 1119–1122.

Alshahrani, S.M., Alavudeen, S.S., Alakhali, K.M., Al-Worafi, Y.M., Bahamdan, A.K., & Vigneshwaran, E., (2019b). Self-Medication Among King Khalid University Students, Saudi Arabia. *Risk Management and Healthcare Policy*, 12, pp. 243–249.

Alshahrani, S.M., Alakhali, K.M., Al-Worafi, Y.M., & Alshahrani, N.Z. (2020a). Awareness and use of over the counter analgesic medication: a survey in the Aseer region population, Saudi Arabia. *Int J Advan Appl Sci*, 7(3), 130–134.

Alshahrani, S.M., Alzahran, M., Alakhali, K., Vigneshwaran, E., Iqbal, M.J., Khan, N.A., … & Alavudeen, S.S. (2020b). Association Between Diabetes Consequences and Quality of Life Among Patients With Diabetes Mellitus in the Aseer Province of Saudi Arabia. *Open Access Macedonian Journal of Medical Sciences*, 8(E), 325–330.

Al-Worafi, Y.M. (2014). Prescription writing errors at a tertiary care hospital in Yemen: prevalence, types, causes and recommendations. *Am J Pharm Health Res*, 2, 134–140.

Al-Worafi, Y.M.A. (2015). Appropriateness of metered-dose inhaler use in the Yemeni community pharmacies. *Journal of Taibah University Medical Sciences*, 10(3), 353–358.

Al-Worafi, Y.M.A., (2016). Pharmacy practice in Yemen. In *Pharmacy Practice in Developing Countries* (pp. 267–287). Academic Press.

Al-Worafi, Y.M., Kassab, Y.W., Alseragi, W.M., Almutairi, M.S., Ahmed, A., Ming, L.C., Alkhoshaiban, A.S., & Hadi, M.A., (2017). Pharmacovigilance and adverse drg reaction reporting: a perspective of community pharmacists and pharmacy technicians in Sana'a, Yemen. *Therapeutics and clinical risk management*, 13, p. 1175.

Al-Worafi, Y.M., (2018a). Knowledge, Attitude and Practice of Yemeni Physicians Toward Pharmacovigilance: A Mixed Method Study. *International Journal of Pharmacy and Pharmaceutical Sciences*, 10(10), 74–77.

Al-Worafi, Y. (2018b). Knowledge, attitude and practice of Yemeni physicians toward pharmacovigilance: A mixed method study. *Int. J. Pharm. Pharm. Sci*, 10, 74–77.

Al-Worafi, Y.M. (2018c). Dispensing errors observed by community pharmacy dispensers in IBB–YEMEN. *Asian J. Pharm. Clin. Res*, 11(11).

Al-Worafi, Y.M. (2018d). Evauation of inhaler technique among patients with asthma and COPD in Yemen. *Journal of Taibah University medical sciences*, 13(5), 488–490.

Al-Worafi, Y.M., Patel, R.P., Zaidi, S.T.R., Alseragi, W.M., Almutairi, M.S., Alkhoshaiban, A.S., & Ming, L.C. (2018a). Completeness and legibility of handwritten prescriptions in Sana'a, Yemen. *Medical Principles and Practice*, 27, 290–292.

Al-Worafi, Y.M., Alseragi, W.M., Seng, L.K., Kassab, Y.W., Yeoh, S.F., Chiau, L., ... & Husain, K. (2018b). Dispensing errors in community pharmacies: a prospective study in Sana'a, Yemen. *Arch Pharm Pract*, 9(4), 1–3.

Al-Worafi, Y.M., Alseragi, W.M., & Mahmoud, M.A. (2019). Competency of metered-dose inhaler use among community pharmacy dispensers in Ibb, Yemen: A simulation method study. *Latin American Journal of Pharmacy*, 38(3), 489–494.

Al-Worafi, Y.M. (Ed.). (2020a). *Drug Safety in Developing Countries: Achievements and Challenges*.

Al-Worafi, Y.M. (2020b). Medication errors. In *Drug Safety in Developing Countries* (pp. 105–117). Academic Press.

Al-Worafi, Y.M. (2020c). Adverse drug reactions. In *Drug Safety in Developing Countries* (pp. 39–57). Academic Press.

Al-Worafi, Y.M. (2020d). Medications registration and marketing: safety-related issues. In *Drug Safety in Developing Countries* (pp. 21–28). Academic Press.

Al-Worafi, Y.M. (2020e). Pharmacovigilance. In *Drug Safety in Developing Countries* (pp. 29–38). Academic Press.

Al-Worafi, Y.M. (2020f). Drug-related problems. In *Drug safety in developing countries* (pp. 59–71). Academic Press.

Al-Worafi, Y.M. (2020g). Medications safety-related terminology. In *Drug safety in developing countries* (pp. 7–19). Academic Press.

Al-Worafi, Y.M. (2020h). Self-medication. In *Drug Safety in Developing Countries* (pp. 73–86). Academic Press.

Al-Worafi, Y.M. (2020j). Antibiotics safety issues. In *Drug Safety in Developing Countries* (pp. 87–103). Academic Press.

Al-Worafi, Y.M. (2020k). Medications safety research issues. In *Drug Safety in Developing Countries* (pp. 213–227). Academic Press.

Al-Worafi, Y.M. (2020l). Counterfeit and substandard medications. In *Drug safety in developing countries* (pp. 119–126). Academic Press.

Al-Worafi, Y.M. (2020m). Medication abuse and misuse. In *Drug safety in developing countries* (pp. 127–135). Academic Press.

Al-Worafi, Y.M. (2020n). Storage and disposal of medications. In *Drug Safety in Developing Countries* (pp. 137–142). Academic Press.

Al-Worafi, Y.M. (2020o). Safety of medications in special population. In *Drug safety in developing countries* (pp. 143–162). Academic Press.

Al-Worafi, Y.M. (2020p). Herbal medicines safety issues. In *Drug Safety in developing countries* (pp. 163–178). Academic Press.

Al-Worafi, Y.M. (2020q). Medications safety pharmacoeconomics-related issues. In *Drug Safety in Developing Countries* (pp. 187–195). Academic Press.

Al-Worafi, Y.M. (2020r). Evidence-based medications safety practice. In *Drug Safety in Developing Countries* (pp. 197–201). Academic Press.

Al-Worafi, Y.M. (2020s). Quality indicators for medications safety. In *Drug safety in developing countries* (pp. 229–242). Academic Press.

Al-Worafi, Y.M. (2020t). Drug safety in Yemen. In *Drug Safety in Developing Countries* (pp. 391–405). Academic Press.

Al-Worafi, Y.M. (2020u). Drug safety in Saudi Arabia. In *Drug Safety in Developing Countries* (pp. 407–417). Academic Press.

Al-Worafi, Y.M. (2020v). Drug safety in United Arab Emirates. In *Drug Safety in Developing Countries* (pp. 419–428). Academic Press.

Al-Worafi, Y.M. (2020w). Drug safety in Indonesia. In *Drug Safety in Developing Countries* (pp. 279–285). Academic Press.

Al-Worafi, Y.M. (2020x). Drug safety in Palestine. In *Drug Safety in Developing Countries* (pp. 471–480). Academic Press.

Al-Worafi, Y.M. (2020y). Drug safety: comparison between developing countries. In *Drug Safety in Developing Countries* (pp. 603–611). Academic Press.

Al-Worafi, Y.M. (2020z). Drug safety in developing versus developed countries. In *Drug Safety in Developing Countries* (pp. 613–615). Academic Press.

Al-Worafi, Y.M., Alseragi, W.M., Ming, L.C., & Alakhali, K.M. (2020a). Drug safety in China. In *Drug Safety in Developing Countries* (pp. 381–388). Academic Press.

Al-Worafi, Y.M., Alseragi, W.M., Alakhali, K.M., Ming, L.C., Othman, G., Halboup, A.M., … & Elkalmi, R.M. (2020b). Knowledge, beliefs and factors affecting the use of generic medicines among patients in Ibb, Yemen: a mixed-method study. *Journal of Pharmacy Practice and Community Medicine*, 6(4).

Al-Worafi, Y.M., Elkalmi, R.M., Ming, L.C., Othman, G., Halboup, A.M., Battah, M.M., … & Mani, V. (2021a). Dispensing errors in hospital pharmacies: A prospective study in Yemen.

Al-Worafi, Y.M., Hasan, S., Hassan, N.M., & Gaili, A.A. (2021b). Knowledge, Attitude and Experience of Pharmacist in the UAE towards Pharmacovigilance. *Research Journal of Pharmacy and Technology*, 14(1), 265–269.

Al-Worafi, Y. (2022a). *A Guide to Online Pharmacy Education: Teaching Strategies and Assessment Methods*. CRC Press.

Al-Worafi, Y. (2022b). History and Importance. In *A Guide to Online Pharmacy Education: Teaching Strategies and Assessment Methods*. CRC Press.

Al-Worafi, Y. (2022c). Terminologies. In *A Guide to Online Pharmacy Education: Teaching Strategies and Assessment Methods*. CRC Press.

Al-Worafi, Y. (2022d). Research Methods and Methodology. In *A Guide to Online Pharmacy Education: Teaching Strategies and Assessment Methods*. CRC Press.

Al-Worafi, Y.M. (2022e). Patient care errors and related problems (part I): development and validation of the model. 0000-0002-5752-2913

Al-Worafi, Y.M. (Ed.). (2023). *Clinical Case Studies on medication Safety*. Academic Press.

Baig, M.R., Al-Worafi, Y.M., Alseragi, W.M., Ming, L.C., & Siddique, A. (2020). Drug safety in India. In *Drug Safety in Developing Countries* (pp. 327–334). Academic Press.

Elkalmi, R.M., Al-Worafi, Y.M., Alseragi, W.M., Ming, L.C., & Siddique, A. (2020). Drug safety in Malaysia. In *Drug Safety in Developing Countries* (pp. 245–253). Academic Press.

Elsayed, T., & Al-Worafi, Y.M. (2020). Drug safety in Egypt. In *Drug Safety in Developing Countries* (pp. 511–523). Academic Press.

Hasan, S., Al-Omar, M.J., AlZubaidy, H., & Al-Worafi, Y.M. (2019). Use of medications in Arab Countries. *Handbook of Healthcare in the Arab World*. Cham: Springer, 42.

Hassan, Y., Abd Aziz, N., Kassab, Y.W., Elgasim, I., Shaharuddin, S., Al-Worafi, Y.M.A., ... & Ming, L.C. (2014). How to help patients to control their blood pressure? Blood pressure control and its predictor. *Archives of Pharmacy Practice*, 5(4).

Izahar, S., Lean, Q.Y., Hameed, M.A., Murugiah, M.K., Patel, R.P., Al-Worafi, Y.M., ... & Ming, L.C. (2017). Content analysis of mobile health applications on diabetes mellitus. *Frontiers in Endocrinology*, 8, 318.

Lee, K.S., Yee, S.M., Zaidi, S.T.R., Patel, R.P., Yang, Q., Al-Worafi, Y.M., & Ming, L.C., 2017. Combating sale of counterfeit and falsified medicines online: a losing battle. *Frontiers in pharmacology*, 8, p. 268.

Mahmoud, M.A., Wajid, S., Naqvi, A.A., Samreen, S., Althagfan, S.S., & Al-Worafi, Y. (2020). Self-medication with antibiotics: A cross-sectional community-based study. *Latin american journal of pharmacy*, 39(2), 348–353.

Manan, M.M., Rusli, R.A., Ang, W.C., Al-Worafi, Y.M., & Ming, L.C. (2014). Assessing the pharmaceutical care issues of antiepileptic drug therapy in hospitalised epileptic patients. *Journal of Pharmacy Practice and Research*, 44(3), 83–88.

Manan, M.M., Ibrahim, N.A., Aziz, N.A., Zulkifly, H.H., Al-Worafi, Y.M.A., & Long, C.M. (2016). Empirical use of antibiotic therapy in the prevention of early onset sepsis in neonates: a pilot study. *Archives of Medical Science*, 12(3), 603–613.

Ming, L.C., Hameed, M.A., Lee, D.D., Apidi, N.A., Lai, P.S.M., Hadi, M.A., Al-Worafi, Y.M.A., & Khan, T.M., (2016). Use of medical mobile applications among hospital pharmacists in Malaysia. *Therapeutic innovation & regulatory science*, 50(4), pp. 419–426.

Ming, L.C., Untong, N., Aliudin, N.A., Osili, N., Kifli, N., Tan, C.S., ... & Goh, H.P. (2020). Mobile health apps on COVID-19 launched in the early days of the pandemic: content analysis and review. *JMIR mHealth and uHealth*, 8(9), e19796.

Othman, G., Ali, F., Ibrahim, M.I.M., Al-Worafi, Y.M., Ansari, M., & Halboup, A.M. (2020). Assessment of Anti-Diabetic Medications Adherence among Diabetic Patients in Sana'a City, Yemen: A Cross Sectional Study. *Journal of Pharmaceutical Research International*, 32(21), 114–122.

Polgar, S., & Thomas, S.A. (2011). *Introduction to research in the health sciences E-Book*. Elsevier Health Sciences.

Saeed, M.S., Alkhoshaiban, A.S., Al-Worafi, Y.M.A., & Long, C.M., (2014). Perception of self-medication among university students in Saudi Arabia. *Archives of Pharmacy Practice*, 5(4), p. 149.

44 Patient Safety Research
Mixed Methods

44.1 BACKGROUND

Mixed methods research is a type of research design that involves combining qualitative and quantitative research methods in a single study. The purpose of using mixed methods is to provide a more comprehensive understanding of a research problem by incorporating both numerical data and subjective insights.

Mixed methods research typically involves three main phases:

1. The first phase involves collecting quantitative data through surveys, experiments, or other numerical methods.

2. The second phase involves collecting qualitative data through interviews, focus groups, or observations.

3. The third phase involves analyzing and integrating both quantitative and qualitative data to draw conclusions and insights.

Mixed methods research has become increasingly popular in social sciences and healthcare research, as it allows researchers to combine the strengths of both qualitative and quantitative research methods. For example, it can provide a better understanding of complex social phenomena that cannot be fully captured by numerical data alone, while also providing statistical evidence to support the findings. Mixed-methods research is an approach that combines both qualitative and quantitative research methods to gain a better understanding of a research question. In the context of patient care and safety, mixed-methods research can be used to explore a range of topics, including patient experiences, healthcare provider attitudes, and the effectiveness of interventions. For example, a mixed-methods study on patient care and safety might begin with a survey to quantify the prevalence of a particular safety concern, such as medication errors. Researchers might then conduct focus groups or interviews with patients, caregivers, and healthcare providers to explore the factors contributing to medication errors and to better understand the impact of these errors on patient outcomes. By combining both quantitative and qualitative data, mixed-methods research can provide a more comprehensive and nuanced understanding of complex healthcare issues. This can be particularly valuable in patient care and safety research, where the experiences and perspectives of patients, caregivers, and healthcare providers can be central to understanding the impact of safety interventions (Polgar & Thomas, 2011; Watkins & Gioia, 2015).

44.2 RATIONALITY OF MIXED METHOD RESEARCH

Mixed-methods research is a rational approach to research because it allows researchers to combine the strengths of both quantitative and qualitative research methods, while also addressing their respective limitations. Quantitative research methods, such as surveys and experiments, can provide precise and objective data that can be analyzed statistically to identify patterns and relationships between variables. However, they may not provide a complete understanding of the complex and subjective experiences of individuals. Qualitative research methods, such as interviews and focus groups, can provide rich and detailed data on individuals' experiences, attitudes, and behaviors. However, the data collected through qualitative research methods may not be generalizable to larger populations, and may be subject to researcher bias and interpretation. Mixed-methods research allows researchers to overcome these limitations by using both quantitative and qualitative data to provide a more complete and accurate understanding of the research question. For example, a mixed-methods study on patient satisfaction with healthcare services might begin with a quantitative survey to gather data on patient satisfaction scores. The survey could be followed up with qualitative interviews or focus groups to provide more in-depth insights into the factors that contribute to patient satisfaction. Overall, the rationality of mixed-methods research lies in its ability to provide a more comprehensive and holistic understanding of complex phenomena, and to produce findings that are both rigorous and meaningful. The rationality of using mixed-methods research in patient safety is evident in its ability to provide a comprehensive understanding of the complex factors that contribute to patient safety incidents, as well as the effectiveness of interventions aimed at improving patient safety. Quantitative research methods are

DOI: 10.1201/9781003230465-47

useful for providing statistical data on the prevalence and severity of patient safety incidents, as well as the impact of interventions on patient outcomes. However, these methods may not capture the subjective experiences of patients and healthcare providers, or the underlying causes of safety incidents. Qualitative research methods, on the other hand, can provide in-depth insights into the experiences, attitudes, and behaviors of patients and healthcare providers, as well as the underlying causes of safety incidents. However, these methods may not provide the statistical data needed to make generalizations about larger populations or the effectiveness of interventions. Mixed-methods research combines both quantitative and qualitative data, allowing researchers to triangulate their findings and provide a more complete understanding of patient safety. For example, a mixed-methods study on medication errors might begin with a quantitative analysis of medication error rates, followed by qualitative interviews with patients, caregivers, and healthcare providers to explore the causes and consequences of medication errors. By using mixed-methods research, researchers can provide more robust and valid evidence to support the development and implementation of interventions aimed at improving patient safety. This can ultimately lead to better outcomes for patients and a safer healthcare system overall.

44.3 IMPORTANCE OF MIXED METHOD RESEARCH

Mixed-method research is important because it offers several advantages ovr using a single research method, including:

1. Comprehensive understanding: Mixed-method research allows researchers to gain a comprehensive understanding of the research question or phenomenon being studied. By combining both quantitative and qualitative data, researchers can provide a more complete picture of the issue at hand.

2. Increased validity and reliability: Using multiple methods to collect data can increase the validity and reliability of research findings. Triangulating data from different sources and using different methods can help to confirm or refute findings, leading to more trustworthy conclusions.

3. Improved generalizability: Quantitative data can be used to make generalizations about larger populations, while qualitative data can provide a rich understanding of individual experiences. Combining both methods can improve the generalizability of findings while also capturing the nuances of individual experiences.

4. Better understanding of complex phenomena: Mixed-method research is particularly useful for studying complex phenomena that cannot be fully understood using a single method. For example, studying patient safety may require both quantitative data on error rates and qualitative data on the experiences of patients and healthcare providers.

5. More impactful research: By providing a more comprehensive and nuanced understanding of the research question, mixed-method research can lead to more impactful research findings. This can ultimately lead to better-informed policies and interventions aimed at addressing social and health-related problems.

Overall, mixed-method research is an important approach to research that can provide researchers with a deeper understanding of the complex issues they are studying, leading to more impactful research findings and better outcomes for individuals and society as a whole. Mixed methods research in patient safety is important because it allows researchers to collect and analyze both qualitative and quantitative data, providing a more comprehensive understanding of the issues related to patient safety. Patient safety is a complex and multifaceted issue that involves both technical and human factors, and a mixed methods approach can help capture this complexity. Quantitative research can provide statistical evidence of the prevalence and severity of patient safety issues, such as adverse events or near misses. However, it may not capture the underlying factors that contribute to these events or the experiences of patients and healthcare providers. Qualitative research can help fill this gap by exploring the perspectives, attitudes, and experiences of patients and healthcare providers, as well as the contextual factors that contribute to patient safety events. By using both qualitative and quantitative methods, researchers can triangulate data from different sources to gain a more comprehensive understanding of patient safety issues. This can help identify potential interventions and solutions that are more likely to be effective in addressing patient safety concerns. Overall, mixed methods research in patient safety is important for advancing our understanding of patient safety issues, identifying potential interventions, and improving the quality of care and outcomes for patients.

44.4 ADVANTAGES OF MIXED METHOD RESEARCH

Mixed method research offers several advantages over using only quantitative or qualitative research methods:

1. Comprehensiveness: Mixed method research can provide a more comprehensive understanding of a research question by combining quantitative and qualitative data. This can help researchers to gain a more complete picture of the phenomenon being studied.

2. Validity: By triangulating data from different sources, mixed method research can enhance the validity of the findings. The use of multiple methods can help to reduce bias and increase the reliability of the results.

3. Flexibility: Mixed method research allows for flexibility in data collection and analysis. Researchers can adapt their approach as needed to address unexpected findings or changes in the research context.

4. Convergence: By combining quantitative and qualitative data, mixed method research can help to identify areas of convergence between the different types of data. This can help to provide a more nuanced and in-depth understanding of the research question.

5. Completeness: Mixed method research can help to provide a more complete understanding of a research question by addressing both the what (quantitative) and the why (qualitative) aspects of the phenomenon being studied.

6. Practicality: Mixed method research can be a practical approach in situations where one method alone may not be sufficient. For example, it may be more feasible to use a mixed method approach in a complex research question that requires both quantitative and qualitative data.

Overall, mixed method research can provide a more comprehensive and valid understanding of a research question by combining the strengths of both quantitative and qualitative methods.

44.5 DISADVANTAGES OF MIXED METHOD RESEARCH

Mixed method research also has some potential disadvantages that researchers need to consider:

1. Complexity: Mixed method research can be complex and time-consuming due to the need to use multiple methods and analyze different types of data. This can increase the cost of the research and make it more difficult to manage.

2. Integration: Integrating different types of data and methods can be challenging. Researchers need to carefully consider how to integrate the quantitative and qualitative data to ensure that the findings are valid and reliable.

3. Expertise: Mixed method research requires expertise in both quantitative and qualitative methods. Researchers need to have a strong understanding of both approaches to effectively design and implement a mixed method study.

4. Bias: Bias can be introduced if the data from one method is given more weight than the other. Researchers need to be careful to give equal weight to both the quantitative and qualitative data to ensure that the findings are balanced.

5. Resource Intensive: Mixed method research can be resource-intensive in terms of time, personnel, and budget. Conducting a mixed method study can be more expensive than using only one method, and may require a larger team of researchers.

6. Generalizability: Mixed method research may have limitations in terms of generalizability. The findings may be specific to the context in which the study was conducted, and may not be applicable to other contexts or populations.

Overall, while mixed method research offers several advantages, researchers need to be aware of the potential disadvantages and carefully consider whether a mixed method approach is appropriate for their research question and resources.

44.6 FACILITATORS OF MIXED METHOD RESEARCH

There are several factors that can facilitate the successful implementation of mixed method research:

1. Clear research question: A clear research question that requires both quantitative and qualitative data is essential for a successful mixed method study. The research question should be well-defined, relevant, and feasible to address using a mixed method approach.

2. Collaboration: Collaboration between researchers with expertise in both quantitative and qualitative methods can facilitate the design and implementation of a mixed method study. Collaboration can also help to ensure that the study design is appropriate, and that the data analysis and interpretation are well-rounded.

3. Adequate resources: Adequate resources, including time, funding, and personnel, are essential for a successful mixed method study. Researchers need to have enough resources to design, implement, and analyze the data from both the quantitative and qualitative components of the study.

4. Methodological expertise: Methodological expertise in both quantitative and qualitative methods is important for a successful mixed method study. Researchers should have a deep understanding of both methods and be able to integrate the data appropriately to ensure that the study findings are valid and reliable.

5. Integration plan: A clear plan for integrating the quantitative and qualitative data is essential for a successful mixed method study. The plan should outline how the data will be collected, analyzed, and integrated to ensure that the findings are balanced and comprehensive.

6. Flexibility: Flexibility is important in a mixed method study. Researchers may need to adapt their approach as they collect and analyze the data to ensure that the study remains relevant and feasible.

Overall, a successful mixed method study requires a clear research question, collaboration between researchers with expertise in both quantitative and qualitative methods, adequate resources, methodological expertise, a clear integration plan, and flexibility.

44.7 BARRIERS OF MIXED METHOD RESEARCH

There are several potential barriers to conducting mixed method research:

1. Limited resources: Conducting mixed method research can be resource-intensive, requiring more time, funding, and personnel than using only one research method. This can be a significant barrier, particularly for researchers with limited resources.

2. Lack of expertise: Conducting mixed method research requires expertise in both quantitative and qualitative methods. Researchers who lack this expertise may struggle to design and implement a mixed method study effectively.

3. Data integration: Integrating data from different sources can be challenging, particularly if the data are collected at different times or using different methods. Researchers need to carefully consider how to integrate the data to ensure that the findings are valid and reliable.

4. Epistemological differences: Quantitative and qualitative methods are based on different epistemological assumptions and ways of knowing. These differences can create challenges when integrating data from the two methods, and researchers need to carefully consider how to reconcile these differences.

5. Time constraints: Conducting a mixed method study can take longer than using only one research method, particularly if the study requires data collection at multiple time points or using multiple methods. Time constraints can be a significant barrier, particularly for researchers working in fast-paced environments such as healthcare.

6. Ethics considerations: Mixed method research can raise unique ethical considerations, particularly when working with vulnerable populations or collecting sensitive data. Researchers need to carefully consider the ethical implications of their study design and ensure that they comply with relevant ethical guidelines.

Overall, mixed method research can face several barriers, including limited resources, lack of expertise, data integration challenges, epistemological differences, time constraints, and ethics considerations. Researchers need to be aware of these potential barriers and carefully consider whether a mixed method approach is appropriate for their research question and resources.

44.8 QUALITY OF MIXED METHOD RESEARCH

The quality of mixed method research depends on several factors, including:

1. Clarity of research question: The research question should be well-defined, relevant, and feasible to address using a mixed method approach.

2. Adequacy of sample size: The sample size should be adequate for both the quantitative and qualitative components of the study to ensure that the findings are representative and reliable.

3. Quality of data collection: Both quantitative and qualitative data collection should be rigorous and use appropriate methods to ensure that the data are valid and reliable.

4. Quality of data analysis: Both quantitative and qualitative data analysis should be rigorous and use appropriate methods to ensure that the findings are valid and reliable.

5. Integration of data: The integration of quantitative and qualitative data should be appropriate and well-supported by the research question and methods used.

6. Transparency: Mixed method research should be transparent and clearly report the methods used, the data collected, and the findings.

7. Validity and reliability: Mixed method research should use appropriate methods to ensure the validity and reliability of the findings.

8. Generalizability: The generalizability of the findings should be carefully considered and reported, taking into account the specific context and population studied.

Overall, the quality of mixed method research depends on careful consideration of the research question, rigorous data collection and analysis, appropriate integration of quantitative and qualitative data, transparency in reporting, and attention to validity, reliability, and generalizability of the findings.

44.9 ONLINE MIXED METHOD RESEARCH

Online mixed method research refers to studies that use both quantitative and qualitative research methods and are conducted online. With the growth of the internet and advances in technology, online mixed method research has become increasingly common and offers several advantages over traditional research methods. Some examples of online mixed method research include online surveys with open-ended questions, online focus groups, and online interviews.

Advantages of online mixed method research include:

1. Increased access to participants: Conducting research online can make it easier to access participants who may be difficult to reach using traditional research methods, such as those who live in remote areas or have limited mobility.

2. Convenience for participants: Participants can complete online surveys or participate in online focus groups from the comfort of their own homes, which can be more convenient and reduce the burden of participation.

3. Cost-effectiveness: Conducting research online can be more cost-effective than traditional research methods, as it eliminates the need for physical space, equipment, and travel expenses.

4. Rapid data collection: Online mixed method research can allow for rapid data collection, as participants can complete surveys or participate in focus groups in a relatively short amount of time.

5. Anonymity: Participants may feel more comfortable sharing sensitive information online, as they can remain anonymous and may feel less self-conscious than in face-to-face interviews.

However, online mixed method research also presents some challenges and limitations, such as:

1. Sampling bias: Online samples may not be representative of the broader population, as access to the internet and technology may vary across different demographics.

2. Technical issues: Online research is subject to technical issues such as internet connectivity, server crashes, and software bugs that can disrupt data collection and analysis.

3. Data quality: Online research may be subject to low response rates, incomplete responses, or inaccurate responses, which can compromise the quality of the data collected.

4. Ethical considerations: Online research raises ethical considerations related to data privacy, informed consent, and confidentiality that need to be carefully considered and addressed.

Overall, online mixed method research offers several advantages and presents some unique challenges and limitations that need to be carefully considered and addressed to ensure the validity and reliability of the findings.

44.10 MIXED METHOD RESEARCH IN DEVELOPING COUNTRIES: Challenges and Recommendations

Patient safety research in developing countries has made significant achievements in recent years. Many developing countries have conducted many researches about the various issues of patient safety and care research (Alshahrani et al., 2019a,b; Al-Qahtani et al., 2015; Alshahrani et al., 2020a,b; Al-Worafi, 2014; Al-Worafi, 2015; Al-Worafi, 2016; Al-Worafi et al., 2017; Al-Worafi, 2018a-d; Al-Worafi et al., 2018a-b; Al-Worafi et al., 2019; Al-Worafi, 2020a-z; Al-Worafi et al., 2020a-b; Al-Worafi et al., 2021a,b; Al-Worafi, 2022a-e; Al-Worafi, 2023; Baig et al., 2020; Elkalmi et al., 2020; Elsayed & Al-Worafi, 2020; Hasan et al., 2019; Hassan et al., 2014; Izahar et al., 2017; Lee et al., 2017; Mahmoud et al., 2020; Manan et al., 2014; Manan et al., 2016; Ming et al., 2016; Ming et al., 2020; Othman et al., 2020; Saeed et al., 2014), however, there are many however, there are many challenges and recommendations for conducting mixed methods studies in developing countries such as:
   Challenges:

1. Limited resources: Developing countries may have limited resources for research, including funding, equipment, and personnel.

2. Cultural differences: Cultural differences can pose challenges for research design, data collection, and interpretation of findings.

3. Language barriers: Language barriers can pose challenges for data collection, as researchers may need to work with interpreters or translate survey instruments.

4. Lack of expertise: Developing countries may have limited expertise in mixed method research, which can limit the quality of the research conducted.

5. Ethical considerations: Conducting research in developing countries raises ethical considerations related to informed consent, data privacy, and confidentiality.

Recommendations:

1. Build local research capacity: Developing local research capacity can help overcome the lack of expertise and resources in mixed method research. This can include providing training and resources for local researchers, building partnerships with local institutions, and involving local communities in the research process.

2. Adapt research methods to the local context: Researchers should consider the local context when designing research methods, including language, cultural norms, and literacy levels.

3. Use mixed method research to address complex issues: Mixed method research can provide valuable insights into complex issues facing developing countries, including healthcare, poverty, education, and social inequality.

4. Work with local communities: Working with local communities can help ensure that research is relevant, ethical, and respectful of local norms and values.

5. Address ethical considerations: Researchers should carefully consider ethical considerations related to informed consent, data privacy, and confidentiality, and take steps to ensure that research is conducted ethically and with respect for the rights of research participants.

6. Access to data: In some developing countries, there may be limited access to data, such as health records or government statistics, which can make it difficult to conduct research.

7. Political instability: Political instability can pose challenges for research, as researchers may face safety concerns or restrictions on their ability to conduct research.

8. Limited infrastructure: Limited infrastructure, such as unreliable electricity or limited internet access, can make it difficult to conduct online surveys or access research data.

9. Limited funding: Funding for research in developing countries may be limited, which can pose challenges for conducting comprehensive mixed method research studies.

10. Data quality: Data quality can be a challenge in developing countries, as data may be incomplete or inaccurate, making it difficult to draw meaningful conclusions from the data.

11. Limited research collaborations: Developing countries may have limited research collaborations, which can limit the opportunities for researchers to work together and share knowledge and resources.

12. Limited participant engagement: Engaging participants in research can be a challenge in developing countries due to factors such as language barriers, low literacy rates, and cultural beliefs.

13. Limited access to technology: Limited access to technology, such as computers or smartphones, can make it difficult to conduct online surveys or use digital data collection tools.

14. Limited representation: Developing countries are diverse, and it can be challenging to ensure that research samples are representative of the population of interest.

15. Limited dissemination: Disseminating research findings can be a challenge in developing countries due to limited access to academic journals, language barriers, and limited resources for dissemination.

44.11 CONCLUSION

This chapter has discussed the patient safety research issues related to the mixed methods studies, importance, facilitators, barriers, challenges and recommendations for the best practice in developing countries. mixed method research in developing countries can provide valuable insights into complex issues facing these countries, including healthcare, poverty, education, and social inequality. However, conducting mixed method research in developing countries presents several challenges, including limited resources, cultural differences, language barriers, lack of expertise, and ethical considerations. To overcome these challenges, researchers can build local research capacity, adapt research methods to the local context, use mixed method research to address complex issues, work with local communities, and address ethical considerations. Additional strategies include leveraging existing data sources, using community-based participatory research methods, and prioritizing diverse and representative recruitment strategies. By addressing these challenges, researchers can conduct valuable mixed method research that contributes to the development of these countries while ensuring that the research is ethical and respectful of local norms and values.

REFERENCES

Al-Qahtani, I., Almoteb, T.M., & Al-Warafi, Y. (2015). Competency of metered-dose inhaler use among Saudi community pharmacists: A Simulation method study. *RRJPPS*, 4(2), 37–31.

Alshahrani, S.M., Alakhali, K.M., & Al-Worafi, Y.M., (2019a). Medication errors in a health care facility in southern Saudi Arabia. *Tropical Journal of Pharmaceutical Research*, 18(5), pp. 1119–1122.

Alshahrani, S.M., Alavudeen, S.S., Alakhali, K.M., Al-Worafi, Y.M., Bahamdan, A.K., & Vigneshwaran, E., (2019b). Self-Medication Among King Khalid University Students, Saudi Arabia. *Risk Management and Healthcare Policy*, 12, pp. 243–249.

Alshahrani, S.M., Alakhali, K.M., Al-Worafi, Y.M., & Alshahrani, N.Z. (2020a). Awareness and use of over the counter analgesic medication: a survey in the Aseer region population, Saudi Arabia. *Int J Advan Appl Sci*, 7(3), 130–134.

Alshahrani, S.M., Alzahran, M., Alakhali, K., Vigneshwaran, E., Iqbal, M.J., Khan, N.A., … & Alavudeen, S.S. (2020b). Association Between Diabetes Consequences and Quality of Life Among Patients With Diabetes Mellitus in the Aseer Province of Saudi Arabia. *Open Access Macedonian Journal of Medical Sciences*, 8(E), 325–330.

Al-Worafi, Y.M. (2014). Prescription writing errors at a tertiary care hospital in Yemen: prevalence, types, causes and recommendations. *Am J Pharm Health Res*, 2, 134–140.

Al-Worafi, Y.M.A. (2015). Appropriateness of metered-dose inhaler use in the Yemeni community pharmacies. *Journal of Taibah University Medical Sciences*, 10(3), 353–358.

Al-Worafi, Y.M.A., (2016). Pharmacy practice in Yemen. In *Pharmacy Practice in Developing Countries* (pp. 267–287). Academic Press.

Al-Worafi, Y.M., Kassab, Y.W., Alseragi, W.M., Almutairi, M.S., Ahmed, A., Ming, L.C., Alkhoshaiban, A.S., & Hadi, M.A., (2017). Pharmacovigilance and adverse drg reaction reporting: a perspective of community pharmacists and pharmacy technicians in Sana'a, Yemen. *Therapeutics and clinical risk management*, 13, p. 1175.

Al-Worafi, Y.M., (2018a). Knowledge, Attitude and Practice of Yemeni Physicians Toward Pharmacovigilance: A Mixed Method Study. *International Journal of Pharmacy and Pharmaceutical Sciences*, 10(10), 74–77.

Al-Worafi, Y. (2018b). Knowledge, attitude and practice of Yemeni physicians toward pharmacovigilance: A mixed method study. *Int. J. Pharm. Pharm. Sci*, 10, 74–77.

Al-Worafi, Y.M. (2018c). Dispensing errors observed by community pharmacy dispensers in IBB–YEMEN. *Asian J. Pharm. Clin. Res*, 11(11).

Al-Worafi, Y.M. (2018d). Evauation of inhaler technique among patients with asthma and COPD in Yemen. *Journal of Taibah University medical sciences*, 13(5), 488–490.

Al-Worafi, Y.M., Patel, R.P., Zaidi, S.T.R., Alseragi, W.M., Almutairi, M.S., Alkhoshaiban, A.S., & Ming, L.C. (2018a). Completeness and legibility of handwritten prescriptions in Sana'a, Yemen. *Medical Principles and Practice*, 27, 290–292.

Al-Worafi, Y.M., Alseragi, W.M., Seng, L.K., Kassab, Y.W., Yeoh, S.F., Chiau, L., … & Husain, K. (2018b). Dispensing errors in community pharmacies: a prospective study in Sana'a, Yemen. *Arch Pharm Pract*, 9(4), 1–3.

Al-Worafi, Y.M., Alseragi, W.M., & Mahmoud, M.A. (2019). Competency of metered-dose inhaler use among community pharmacy dispensers in Ibb, Yemen: A simulation method study. *Latin American Journal of Pharmacy*, 38(3), 489–494.

Al-Worafi, Y.M. (Ed.). (2020a). *Drug Safety in Developing Countries: Achievements and Challenges*.

Al-Worafi, Y.M. (2020b). Medication errors. In *Drug Safety in Developing Countries* (pp. 105–117). Academic Press.

Al-Worafi, Y.M. (2020c). Adverse drug reactions. In *Drug Safety in Developing Countries* (pp. 39–57). Academic Press.

Al-Worafi, Y.M. (2020d). Medications registration and marketing: safety-related issues. In *Drug Safety in Developing Countries* (pp. 21–28). Academic Press.

Al-Worafi, Y.M. (2020e). Pharmacovigilance. In *Drug Safety in Developing Countries* (pp. 29–38). Academic Press.

Al-Worafi, Y.M. (2020f). Drug-related problems. In *Drug safety in developing countries* (pp. 59–71). Academic Press.

Al-Worafi, Y.M. (2020g). Medications safety-related terminology. In *Drug safety in developing countries* (pp. 7–19). Academic Press.

Al-Worafi, Y.M. (2020h). Self-medication. In *Drug Safety in Developing Countries* (pp. 73–86). Academic Press.

Al-Worafi, Y.M. (2020j). Antibiotics safety issues. In *Drug Safety in Developing Countries* (pp. 87–103). Academic Press.

Al-Worafi, Y.M. (2020k). Medications safety research issues. In *Drug Safety in Developing Countries* (pp. 213–227). Academic Press.

Al-Worafi, Y.M. (2020l). Counterfeit and substandard medications. In *Drug safety in developing countries* (pp. 119–126). Academic Press.

Al-Worafi, Y.M. (2020m). Medication abuse and misuse. In *Drug safety in developing countries* (pp. 127–135). Academic Press.

Al-Worafi, Y.M. (2020n). Storage and disposal of medications. In *Drug Safety in Developing Countries* (pp. 137–142). Academic Press.

Al-Worafi, Y.M. (2020o). Safety of medications in special population. In *Drug safety in developing countries* (pp. 143–162). Academic Press.

Al-Worafi, Y.M. (2020p). Herbal medicines safety issues. In *Drug Safety in developing countries* (pp. 163–178). Academic Press.

Al-Worafi, Y.M. (2020q). Medications safety pharmacoeconomics-related issues. In *Drug Safety in Developing Countries* (pp. 187–195). Academic Press.

Al-Worafi, Y.M. (2020r). Evidence-based medications safety practice. In *Drug Safety in Developing Countries* (pp. 197–201). Academic Press.

Al-Worafi, Y.M. (2020s). Quality indicators for medications safety. In *Drug safety in developing countries* (pp. 229–242). Academic Press.

Al-Worafi, Y.M. (2020t). Drug safety in Yemen. In *Drug Safety in Developing Countries* (pp. 391–405). Academic Press.

Al-Worafi, Y.M. (2020u). Drug safety in Saudi Arabia. In *Drug Safety in Developing Countries* (pp. 407–417). Academic Press.

Al-Worafi, Y.M. (2020v). Drug safety in United Arab Emirates. In *Drug Safety in Developing Countries* (pp. 419–428). Academic Press.

Al-Worafi, Y.M. (2020w). Drug safety in Indonesia. In *Drug Safety in Developing Countries* (pp. 279–285). Academic Press.

Al-Worafi, Y.M. (2020x). Drug safety in Palestine. In *Drug Safety in Developing Countries* (pp. 471–480). Academic Press.

Al-Worafi, Y.M. (2020y). Drug safety: comparison between developing countries. In *Drug Safety in Developing Countries* (pp. 603–611). Academic Press.

Al-Worafi, Y.M. (2020z). Drug safety in developing versus developed countries. In *Drug Safety in Developing Countries* (pp. 613–615). Academic Press.

Al-Worafi, Y.M., Alseragi, W.M., Ming, L.C., & Alakhali, K.M. (2020a). Drug safety in China. In *Drug Safety in Developing Countries* (pp. 381–388). Academic Press.

Al-Worafi, Y.M., Alseragi, W.M., Alakhali, K.M., Ming, L.C., Othman, G., Halboup, A.M., … & Elkalmi, R.M. (2020b). Knowledge, beliefs and factors affecting the use of generic medicines among patients in Ibb, Yemen: a mixed-method study. *Journal of Pharmacy Practice and Community Medicine*, 6(4).

Al-Worafi, Y.M., Elkalmi, R.M., Ming, L.C., Othman, G., Halboup, A.M., Battah, M.M., … & Mani, V. (2021a). Dispensing errors in hospital pharmacies: A prospective study in Yemen.

Al-Worafi, Y.M., Hasan, S., Hassan, N.M., & Gaili, A.A. (2021b). Knowledge, Attitude and Experience of Pharmacist in the UAE towards Pharmacovigilance. *Research Journal of Pharmacy and Technology*, 14(1), 265–269.

Al-Worafi, Y. (2022a). *A Guide to Online Pharmacy Education: Teaching Strategies and Assessment Methods*. CRC Press.

Al-Worafi, Y. (2022b). History and Importance. In *A Guide to Online Pharmacy Education: Teaching Strategies and Assessment Methods*. CRC Press.

Al-Worafi, Y. (2022c). Terminologies. In *A Guide to Online Pharmacy Education: Teaching Strategies and Assessment Methods*. CRC Press.

Al-Worafi, Y. (2022d). Research Methods and Methodology. In *A Guide to Online Pharmacy Education: Teaching Strategies and Assessment Methods*. CRC Press.

Al-Worafi, Y.M. (2022e). Patient care errors and related problems (part I): development and validation of the model. 0000-0002-5752-2913

Al-Worafi, Y.M. (Ed.). (2023). *Clinical Case Studies on medication Safety*. Academic Press.

Baig, M.R., Al-Worafi, Y.M., Alseragi, W.M., Ming, L.C., & Siddique, A. (2020). Drug safety in India. In *Drug Safety in Developing Countries* (pp. 327–334). Academic Press.

Elkalmi, R.M., Al-Worafi, Y.M., Alseragi, W.M., Ming, L.C., & Siddique, A. (2020). Drug safety in Malaysia. In *Drug Safety in Developing Countries* (pp. 245–253). Academic Press.

Elsayed, T., & Al-Worafi, Y.M. (2020). Drug safety in Egypt. In *Drug Safety in Developing Countries* (pp. 511–523). Academic Press.

Hasan, S., Al-Omar, M.J., AlZubaidy, H., & Al-Worafi, Y.M. (2019). Use of medications in Arab Countries. *Handbook of Healthcare in the Arab World*. Cham: Springer, 42.

Hassan, Y., Abd Aziz, N., Kassab, Y.W., Elgasim, I., Shaharuddin, S., Al-Worafi, Y.M.A., … & Ming, L.C. (2014). How to help patients to control their blood pressure? Blood pressure control and its predictor. *Archives of Pharmacy Practice*, 5(4).

Izahar, S., Lean, Q.Y., Hameed, M.A., Murugiah, M.K., Patel, R.P., Al-Worafi, Y.M., ... & Ming, L.C. (2017). Content analysis of mobile health applications on diabetes mellitus. *Frontiers in Endocrinology*, 8, 318.

Lee, K.S., Yee, S.M., Zaidi, S.T.R., Patel, R.P., Yang, Q., Al-Worafi, Y.M., & Ming, L.C., 2017. Combating sale of counterfeit and falsified medicines online: a losing battle. *Frontiers in pharmacology*, 8, p. 268.

Mahmoud, M.A., Wajid, S., Naqvi, A.A., Samreen, S., Althagfan, S.S., & Al-Worafi, Y. (2020). Self-medication with antibiotics: A cross-sectional community-based study. *Latin american journal of pharmacy*, 39(2), 348–353.

Manan, M.M., Rusli, R.A., Ang, W.C., Al-Worafi, Y.M., & Ming, L.C. (2014). Assessing the pharmaceutical care issues of antiepileptic drug therapy in hospitalised epileptic patients. *Journal of Pharmacy Practice and Research*, 44(3), 83–88.

Manan, M.M., Ibrahim, N.A., Aziz, N.A., Zulkifly, H.H., Al-Worafi, Y.M.A., & Long, C.M. (2016). Empirical use of antibiotic therapy in the prevention of early onset sepsis in neonates: a pilot study. *Archives of Medical Science*, 12(3), 603–613.

Ming, L.C., Hameed, M.A., Lee, D.D., Apidi, N.A., Lai, P.S.M., Hadi, M.A., Al-Worafi, Y.M.A., & Khan, T.M., (2016). Use of medical mobile applications among hospital pharmacists in Malaysia. *Therapeutic innovation & regulatory science*, 50(4), pp. 419–426.

Ming, L.C., Untong, N., Aliudin, N.A., Osili, N., Kifli, N., Tan, C.S., ... & Goh, H.P. (2020). Mobile health apps on COVID-19 launched in the early days of the pandemic: content analysis and review. *JMIR mHealth and uHealth*, 8(9), e19796.

Othman, G., Ali, F., Ibrahim, M.I.M., Al-Worafi, Y.M., Ansari, M., & Halboup, A.M. (2020). Assessment of Anti-Diabetic Medications Adherence among Diabetic Patients in Sana'a City, Yemen: A Cross Sectional Study. *Journal of Pharmaceutical Research International*, 32(21), 114–122.

Polgar, S., & Thomas, S.A. (2011). Introduction to research in the health sciences E-Book. *Elsevier Health Sciences*.

Saeed, M.S., Alkhoshaiban, A.S., Al-Worafi, Y.M.A., & Long, C.M., (2014). Perception of self-medication among university students in Saudi Arabia. *Archives of Pharmacy Practice*, 5(4), p. 149.

Watkins, D., & Gioia, D. (2015). Mixed methods research. *Pocket Guide to Social Work Re.*

45 Patient Safety Research

Clinical Trials

45.1 BACKGROUND

Clinical trials are scientific studies that involve human participants to test the safety and effectiveness of new medical treatments, interventions, and procedures. Clinical trials are designed to answer specific research questions and to determine whether a new intervention is safe, effective, and better than existing treatments or placebo. Clinical trials are crucial for advancing medical knowledge and developing new treatments for various diseases. Patient safety is a critical aspect of clinical trials, and ensuring the safety of study participants is of utmost importance. Clinical trials present unique challenges related to patient safety, including adverse events, study design, participant selection, and data management. Researchers must take steps to minimize risks to study participants and ensure that any adverse events are promptly addressed. Additionally, regulatory bodies and ethics committees play a vital role in ensuring that clinical trials are conducted ethically and in compliance with international standards. Patient safety monitoring is an ongoing process that involves close monitoring of study participants, data collection, analysis, and dissemination. To ensure patient safety in clinical trials, it is essential to have robust safety planning, clear communication, and transparent reporting of adverse events. Ultimately, the goal of clinical trials is to advance medical knowledge and develop safe and effective treatments for patients, and ensuring patient safety is a critical component of achieving this goal. Clinical trials are usually conducted in phases, with each phase serving a specific purpose. Phase I trials involve a small number of healthy volunteers to determine the safety and dosage of the intervention. Phase II trials involve a larger number of participants who have the condition or disease the intervention is designed to treat, and the goal is to determine whether the intervention is effective and safe. Phase III trials involve an even larger number of participants and are designed to confirm the effectiveness and safety of the intervention. Clinical trials are usually conducted under strict ethical and regulatory guidelines to ensure that the rights and welfare of the participants are protected. The results of clinical trials are used to obtain regulatory approval for the intervention and to guide medical practice Bhatt, 2010; Jenkins & Hubbard, 1991; Polgar & Thomas, 2011; GSU Library Research Guides, 2020).

45.2 HISTORY OF CLINICAL TRIALS

The history of clinical trials dates back to ancient times when early physicians and healers experimented with various treatments and remedies to cure illnesses. However, the first recorded clinical trial was conducted by James Lind, a British naval surgeon, in 1747. Lind conducted a trial on 12 sailors who were suffering from scurvy, a disease caused by a deficiency of vitamin C. He divided the sailors into six groups and treated each group with a different remedy. The group that received citrus fruits, which are rich in vitamin C, showed the most improvement, and thus Lind concluded that citrus fruits were an effective treatment for scurvy.

Here is a timeline of some of the key events in the history of clinical trials Bhatt, 2010; Jenkins & Hubbard, 1991; Polgar & Thomas, 2011).

- 1747: James Lind conducts the first recorded clinical trial, testing different treatments for scurvy on sailors.

- 1863: Louis Pasteur conducts the first human vaccine trial, testing a vaccine for anthrax.

- 1906: The Pure Food and Drug Act is passed in the United States, requiring pharmaceutical companies to prove the safety of their products.

- 1926: The randomized controlled trial (RCT) is introduced by Ronald A. Fisher, a British statistician.

- 1946: The first double-blind trial is conducted by Austin Bradford Hill, a British epidemiologist.

- 1962: The Kefauver-Harris Amendment to the Federal Food, Drug, and Cosmetic Act is passed in the United States, requiring pharmaceutical companies to demonstrate the efficacy of their products as well as their safety.

- 1975: The Declaration of Helsinki is adopted by the World Medical Association, providing ethical guidelines for medical research involving human subjects.

- 1986: The International Conference on Harmonisation (ICH) is established to develop guidelines for the conduct of clinical trials.

- 1996: The first clinical trial registry is established by the National Institutes of Health in the United States.

- 2005: The Clinical Trials Directive is introduced by the European Union, harmonizing regulations for clinical trials across member states.

- 2007: The Food and Drug Administration Amendments Act (FDAAA) is passed in the United States, requiring pharmaceutical companies to register clinical trials and report their results on ClinicalTrials.gov.

- 2020: The COVID-19 pandemic leads to a surge in clinical trials testing treatments and vaccines for the virus, highlighting the importance of clinical trials in advancing medical science and improving patient outcomes.

45.3 RATIONALITY OF CLINICAL TRIALS

Clinical trials are scientific studies that evaluate the effectiveness, safety, and tolerability of new medications, medical devices, and treatments in humans. These trials are an essential part of the drug development process and play a critical role in advancing medical knowledge and improving patient outcomes. The rationality of clinical trials lies in the following:

1. Controlled environment: Clinical trials are conducted in a controlled environment, which allows researchers to observe and analyze the effects of a treatment on a specific population. This helps to minimize the influence of confounding factors and ensure that the results are reliable and accurate.

2. Objectivity: Clinical trials are designed to be objective, which means that they are conducted without any bias or preconceived notions about the treatment being studied. This helps to ensure that the results are based on scientific evidence and not on subjective opinions.

3. Randomization: Clinical trials use randomization to ensure that the study groups are similar in terms of age, gender, health status, and other relevant factors. This helps to ensure that the results are not influenced by differences between the study groups.

4. Blinding: Clinical trials often use blinding to prevent bias. Blinding can be single-blind (where either the patient or the researcher is blinded) or double-blind (where both the patient and the researcher are blinded). This helps to ensure that the results are not influenced by the expectations or opinions of the patient or the researcher.

5. Ethical considerations: Clinical trials are conducted with strict adherence to ethical guidelines and regulations. This helps to protect the rights and welfare of the study participants and ensure that the study is conducted in a responsible and ethical manner.

Overall, the rationality of clinical trials lies in their ability to provide reliable, objective, and scientifically valid information about the safety and effectiveness of new treatments. This information is critical for healthcare professionals, regulators, and patients to make informed decisions about the best course of treatment for a particular condition.

45.4 IMPORTANCE OF CLINICAL TRIALS

Clinical trials are critical to advancing medical knowledge and improving patient care. Here are some of the key reasons why clinical trials are important:

1. Developing new treatments: Clinical trials are essential for developing new treatments for a wide range of diseases and conditions. They help researchers test the safety and effectiveness of new medications, medical devices, and other interventions before they can be approved for widespread use.

2. Improving existing treatments: Clinical trials can also help to improve existing treatments by testing new formulations or dosages, or by comparing different treatment approaches to determine which is most effective.

3. Understanding disease mechanisms: Clinical trials can help researchers better understand the underlying mechanisms of diseases and conditions, which can lead to new insights and potential new treatments.

4. Ensuring safety: Clinical trials are designed to ensure that new treatments are safe for patients. They help to identify potential side effects and risks, and ensure that the benefits of a treatment outweigh any potential harms.

5. Personalized medicine: Clinical trials can help to identify which treatments are most effective for specific patient populations, based on factors such as age, gender, genetics, and other health conditions.

6. Regulatory approval: Clinical trial data is used by regulatory agencies such as the FDA to determine whether a new treatment should be approved for widespread use. Without clinical trials, it would be difficult to ensure that new treatments are safe and effective for patients.

7. Evidence-based medicine: Clinical trial data is also used by healthcare professionals to make evidence-based decisions about the best course of treatment for their patients.

In summary, clinical trials are critical to advancing medical knowledge and improving patient care. They are essential for developing new treatments, improving existing treatments, ensuring safety, and advancing personalized medicine. Without clinical trials, medical progress would be severely limited, and patients would be left without many of the lifesaving treatments and therapies that are available today.

45.5 CLINICAL TRIALS PHASES

Clinical trials are conducted in a series of phases, each designed to answer specific questions about the safety, efficacy, and optimal dosing of a new drug or treatment. Here are the four main phases of clinical trials:

1. Phase 1: Phase 1 trials are usually the first step in testing a new drug or treatment in humans. They are typically small studies that involve healthy volunteers and are designed to assess the safety and tolerability of the treatment, as well as the optimal dosage and method of administration. Phase 1 trials may also provide some initial information about the drug's pharmacokinetics (how the drug is absorbed, metabolized, and eliminated by the body) and pharmacodynamics (how the drug interacts with the body's systems).

2. Phase 2: Phase 2 trials are larger studies that involve patients with the disease or condition that the treatment is intended to treat. The main goal of phase 2 trials is to determine the efficacy of the treatment, as well as the optimal dosage and treatment regimen. Phase 2 trials may also provide additional safety data and help to identify any potential side effects.

3. Phase 3: Phase 3 trials are large-scale studies that are designed to confirm the efficacy and safety of the treatment in a much larger population of patients. Phase 3 trials typically involve hundreds or thousands of patients and may be conducted at multiple sites around the world. The results of phase 3 trials are used to support regulatory approval of the treatment.

4. Phase 4: Phase 4 trials are post-marketing studies that are conducted after a treatment has been approved and is available for widespread use. Phase 4 trials are designed to monitor the long-term safety and effectiveness of the treatment, as well as to identify any rare or unexpected side effects.

Overall, the phases of clinical trials are designed to ensure that new treatments are safe, effective, and appropriate for use in humans. The results of clinical trials are used to support regulatory approval, guide clinical practice, and improve patient outcomes.

45.6 ADVANTAGES OF CLINICAL TRIALS

Clinical trials have several advantages that make them an essential part of advancing medical knowledge and improving patient care. Here are some of the key advantages of clinical trials:

1. Scientific rigor: Clinical trials are designed to be scientifically rigorous, which means that they are conducted using standardized methods and protocols. This helps to ensure that the results are reliable and accurate.

2. Controlled environment: Clinical trials are conducted in a controlled environment, which allows researchers to observe and analyze the effects of a treatment on a specific population. This helps to minimize the influence of confounding factors and ensure that the results are valid.

3. Objectivity: Clinical trials are designed to be objective, which means that they are conducted without any bias or preconceived notions about the treatment being studied. This helps to ensure that the results are based on scientific evidence and not on subjective opinions.

4. Safety: Clinical trials are designed to ensure that new treatments are safe for patients. They help to identify potential side effects and risks, and ensure that the benefits of a treatment outweigh any potential harms.

5. Efficacy: Clinical trials are designed to determine whether a treatment is effective in treating a specific condition or disease. This helps to ensure that patients receive the most appropriate and effective treatment for their condition.

6. Innovation: Clinical trials are essential for advancing medical knowledge and developing new treatments. They help to identify new treatment options and improve existing treatments, which can lead to better patient outcomes and quality of life.

7. Personalized medicine: Clinical trials can help to identify which treatments are most effective for specific patient populations, based on factors such as age, gender, genetics, and other health conditions.

8. Regulatory approval: Clinical trial data is used by regulatory agencies such as the FDA to determine whether a new treatment should be approved for widespread use. Without clinical trials, it would be difficult to ensure that new treatments are safe and effective for patients.

Overall, the advantages of clinical trials are numerous and significant. They play a critical role in advancing medical knowledge, improving patient care, and ensuring that new treatments are safe and effective for patients.

45.7 DISADVANTAGES OF CLINICAL TRIALS

While clinical trials have many advantages, they also have some disadvantages and potential drawbacks that must be considered. Here are some of the main disadvantages of clinical trials:

1. Potential risks: Clinical trials involve testing new treatments and drugs, which can pose potential risks and side effects to participants. While measures are taken to minimize these risks, they can still occur, and participants must be fully informed of the potential risks and benefits before consenting to participate.

2. Ethical concerns: There are several ethical concerns associated with clinical trials, such as ensuring that participants are fully informed about the potential risks and benefits, and that they are treated fairly and respectfully throughout the trial.

3. Cost: Clinical trials can be expensive to conduct, which can limit the number of trials that can be performed and may lead to higher drug prices to recoup the costs of research and development.

4. Lengthy process: Clinical trials can take several years to complete, which can delay the availability of new treatments and drugs to patients who need them.

5. Limited sample size: Clinical trials often involve a relatively small sample size of participants, which can limit the generalizability of the results to a larger population.

6. Bias: Despite efforts to minimize bias, clinical trials may still be influenced by various sources of bias, such as selection bias, measurement bias, or publication bias.

7. Inconclusive results: Clinical trials may sometimes produce inconclusive or conflicting results, which can make it difficult to determine the safety and efficacy of a treatment.

Overall, clinical trials are an essential part of advancing medical knowledge and improving patient care. While they have some disadvantages, the benefits of clinical trials generally outweigh the potential risks and drawbacks. It is important to carefully consider these issues and ensure that clinical trials are conducted in an ethical, safe, and effective manner.

45.8 FACILITATORS OF CLINICAL TRIALS

Clinical trials are an essential part of the drug development process, and they require significant resources, expertise, and coordination to carry out successfully. Clinical trials facilitators play a crucial role in overseeing and managing the various aspects of a clinical trial. Here are some of the key roles and responsibilities of clinical trial facilitators:

1. Protocol development: Clinical trials facilitators work closely with medical professionals to develop study protocols, which are detailed plans that outline the objectives, procedures, and eligibility criteria for the trial.

2. Participant recruitment: Clinical trials facilitators help recruit participants for the trial by developing advertising and outreach strategies and working with medical professionals to identify potential participants.

3. Data collection and analysis: Clinical trials facilitators oversee data collection and analysis throughout the trial, ensuring that all information is recorded accurately and efficiently.

4. Regulatory compliance: Clinical trials facilitators ensure that all aspects of the trial comply with local, state, and federal regulations, including obtaining necessary approvals and permissions.

5. Budget management: Clinical trials facilitators manage the budget for the trial, including allocating resources, negotiating contracts, and ensuring that expenses are within the approved budget.

6. Project management: Clinical trials facilitators oversee the overall management of the trial, including coordinating with various stakeholders, managing timelines, and ensuring that all aspects of the trial are on track.

7. Risk management: Clinical trials facilitators identify potential risks and develop risk mitigation strategies to minimize the impact on the trial.

Overall, clinical trials facilitators play a critical role in ensuring the success of clinical trials, from developing study protocols to overseeing data collection and analysis to managing budgets and timelines. They work closely with medical professionals, regulatory agencies, and other stakeholders to ensure that the trial is conducted safely, efficiently, and effectively.

45.9 BARRIERS OF CLINICAL TRIALS

Clinical trials are research studies conducted to evaluate the safety and effectiveness of new drugs, devices, or treatments on human subjects. While clinical trials are essential in advancing medical knowledge and improving patient outcomes, there are several barriers that can make it challenging to conduct them effectively. Some of these barriers include:

1. Patient recruitment: Finding and enrolling enough eligible participants can be a significant challenge for clinical trial researchers. Some patients may not be aware of clinical trials or may be hesitant to participate due to concerns about safety or potential side effects.

2. Cost: Clinical trials can be expensive, and funding is often limited. Researchers must secure funding from various sources, including government grants and private organizations, to cover the costs of the trial.

3. Regulatory hurdles: Clinical trials are heavily regulated, and researchers must navigate complex rules and guidelines to ensure that their study is compliant. These regulations can create significant delays and additional costs for researchers.

4. Access to technology: Clinical trials often require the use of advanced technology and equipment, which may not be readily available in all locations. This can make it difficult for researchers to conduct trials in certain areas.

5. Time constraints: Clinical trials can take years to complete, which can be a significant barrier for researchers who need to meet deadlines or obtain results quickly.

6. Ethics and patient safety: Researchers must ensure that the clinical trial is conducted ethically and that patient safety is always a top priority. This can create additional challenges, such as the need for informed consent and monitoring of adverse events.

7. Diversity: Ensuring that clinical trials include a diverse range of participants is essential to ensure that the results are applicable to a broader population. However, recruiting a diverse range of participants can be challenging, particularly for rare diseases or conditions.

These barriers can make it challenging to conduct clinical trials effectively, but researchers must work to overcome them to advance medical knowledge and improve patient outcomes.

45.10 QUALITY OF CLINICAL TRIALS

The quality of clinical trials is critical for ensuring that the results are reliable and accurate. Poor quality trials can lead to incorrect conclusions, wasted resources, and potential harm to patients. Here are some factors that contribute to the quality of clinical trials:

1. Study design: The study design should be appropriate to answer the research question effectively. The study design should consider factors such as the sample size, the choice of control group, the randomization process, and the blinding process.

2. Participant selection: Participants should be selected based on strict inclusion and exclusion criteria to ensure that the study population is appropriate for the research question. Participants should also be representative of the population to which the study findings will be applied.

3. Intervention: The intervention or treatment being studied should be clearly defined and standardized to ensure consistency across participants and sites.

4. Data collection: Data collection methods should be rigorous and reliable, with standardized procedures in place to ensure consistency across participants and sites. Data should be collected in a timely manner and checked for completeness and accuracy.

5. Statistical analysis: Statistical analysis should be appropriate for the study design and the research question. The analysis should be conducted in a blinded manner to avoid bias.

6. Ethical considerations: Ethical considerations are critical in ensuring that the study is conducted in a manner that protects the welfare and rights of participants. Ethical considerations include obtaining informed consent from participants, monitoring adverse events, and ensuring participant confidentiality.

7. Study reporting: Study reporting should be transparent and complete, with all study results reported, including negative findings. Reporting should follow established guidelines, such as the Consolidated Standards of Reporting Trials (CONSORT) statement.

In summary, the quality of clinical trials is critical for ensuring that the results are reliable and accurate. To ensure quality, researchers should carefully consider study design, participant selection, intervention, data collection, statistical analysis, ethical considerations, and study reporting.

45.11 CLINICAL TRIALS IN DEVELOPING COUNTRIES: Challenges and Recommendations

Clinical trials are essential for advancing medical knowledge and improving patient outcomes, but conducting clinical trials in developing countries can present unique challenges. Patient safety research in developing countries has made significant achievements in recent years. Many developing countries have conducted many researches about the various issues of patient safety and care research (Alshahrani et al., 2019a,b; Al-Qahtani et al., 2015; Alshahrani et al., 2020a,b; Al-Worafi, 2014; Al-Worafi, 2015; Al-Worafi, 2016; Al-Worafi et al., 2017; Al-Worafi, 2018a-d; Al-Worafi et al., 2018a-b; Al-Worafi et al., 2019; Al-Worafi, 2020a-z; Al-Worafi et al., 2020a-b; Al-Worafi et al., 2021a,b; Al-Worafi, 2022a-e; Al-Worafi, 2023; Baig et al., 2020; Elkalmi et al., 2020; Elsayed and Al-Worafi, 2020; Hasan et al., 2019; Hassan et al., 2014; Izahar et al., 2017; Lee et al., 2017; Mahmoud et al., 2020; Manan et al., 2014; Manan et al., 2016; Ming et al., 2016; Ming et al., 2020; Othman et al., 2020; Saeed et al., 2014), however, there are many however, there are many challenges and recommendations for conducting literature reviews in developing countries such as:
 Challenges:

1. Limited resources: Developing countries may have limited resources for conducting clinical trials, such as funding, infrastructure, and trained personnel.

2. Ethical concerns: There may be ethical concerns regarding informed consent and vulnerability of participants in developing countries.

3. Limited access to technology: Developing countries may have limited access to technology required for clinical trials, such as advanced medical devices and electronic data management systems.

4. Regulatory issues: Regulatory frameworks for clinical trials in developing countries may not be as well established as in developed countries, which may lead to delays or inconsistencies in approval processes.

5. Language barriers: Language barriers can make it difficult to communicate effectively with participants and can lead to misunderstandings and incorrect data collection.

6. Cultural differences: Cultural differences can impact the way participants perceive and respond to medical interventions, leading to variations in outcomes.

7. Health system challenges: Developing countries may have limited access to healthcare and may lack the necessary infrastructure to support clinical trials, such as reliable electricity, clean water, and appropriate storage facilities.

8. Political instability: Political instability and conflicts in developing countries can disrupt clinical trials and make it difficult to ensure participant safety.

9. Limited patient awareness and education: Patients in developing countries may have limited awareness and education regarding clinical trials, which can make it difficult to recruit and retain participants.

10. Access to standard care: Patients in developing countries may have limited access to standard care, which can impact the control group in clinical trials.

11. Intellectual property rights: Intellectual property rights may not be as well protected in developing countries, which can make it difficult to ensure that the results of clinical trials are properly utilized and disseminated.

12. Data security: Data security can be a concern in developing countries, particularly in areas where there are political or social tensions, which can lead to issues with data privacy and security.

Recommendations:

1. Collaborative partnerships: Collaborative partnerships between academic institutions, non-governmental organizations, and local communities can help to address limited resources and infrastructure challenges.

2. Capacity building: Capacity building efforts can help to address the limited availability of trained personnel in developing countries. This includes training programs for local researchers, healthcare professionals, and regulatory authorities.

3. Ethical considerations: Ethical considerations must be given utmost importance in clinical trials, particularly in developing countries. It is important to ensure that participants are fully informed about the risks and benefits of participating in the study and that their rights and welfare are protected.

4. Technology solutions: Technology solutions such as mobile health (mHealth) and electronic data capture systems can be utilized to overcome challenges in data management and trial monitoring.

5. Regulatory harmonization: Developing countries can work towards harmonization of their regulatory frameworks with international standards to ensure consistency in approval processes.

6. Translation services: Providing translation services for participants and study staff can help to overcome language barriers and improve communication.

7. Cultural sensitivity: Study staff should receive cultural sensitivity training to ensure that they understand the cultural norms and beliefs of participants, and to tailor the study approach accordingly.

8. Strengthen health systems: Investment in healthcare infrastructure can improve access to healthcare and support the conduct of clinical trials in developing countries.

9. Safety planning: Robust safety planning, including contingency plans for political instability, is critical to ensuring the safety of participants and study staff.

10. Education and awareness campaigns: Education and awareness campaigns can help to increase patient awareness of clinical trials and their potential benefits.

11. Access to standard care: Researchers should work to ensure that participants have access to standard care, even if it is not directly related to the study intervention.

12. Intellectual property protections: Researchers and sponsors should work to ensure that intellectual property rights are protected in developing countries, and that the results of clinical trials are disseminated in a way that benefits the local community.

13. Data security measures: Researchers should implement robust data security measures to protect the privacy and security of study participants and their data.

45.12 CONCLUSION

This chapter has discussed the patient safety research issues related to the clinical trials, importance, facilitators, barriers, challenges and recommendations for the best practice in developing countries.

conducting clinical trials in developing countries can present a range of challenges, but it is essential for advancing medical knowledge and improving patient outcomes. Some of the challenges include limited resources, ethical concerns, limited access to technology, regulatory issues, language barriers, cultural differences, health system challenges, political instability, limited patient awareness and education, access to standard care, intellectual property rights, and data security. To address these challenges, collaborative partnerships, capacity building, ethical considerations, technology solutions, regulatory harmonization, translation services, cultural sensitivity, healthcare infrastructure investment, safety planning, education and awareness campaigns, access to standard care, intellectual property protections, and data security measures can be implemented. By overcoming these challenges, we can ensure that clinical trials are conducted ethically, generate high-quality data, and advance medical knowledge to improve patient outcomes in both developing and developed countries.

REFERENCES

Al-Qahtani, I., Almoteb, T.M., & Al-Warafi, Y. (2015). Competency of metered-dose inhaler use among Saudi community pharmacists: A Simulation method study. *RRJPPS*, 4(2), 37–31.

Al-Worafi, Y. (2018b). Knowledge, attitude and practice of Yemeni physicians toward pharmacovigilance: A mixed method study. *Int. J. Pharm. Pharm. Sci*, 10, 74–77.

Al-Worafi, Y. (2022a). *A Guide to Online Pharmacy Education: Teaching Strategies and Assessment Methods*. CRC Press.

Al-Worafi, Y. (2022b). History and Importance. In *A Guide to Online Pharmacy Education: Teaching Strategies and Assessment Methods*. CRC Press.

Al-Worafi, Y. (2022c). Terminologies. In *A Guide to Online Pharmacy Education: Teaching Strategies and Assessment Methods*. CRC Press.

Al-Worafi, Y. (2022d). Research Methods and Methodology. In *A Guide to Online Pharmacy Education: Teaching Strategies and Assessment Methods*. CRC Press.

Al-Worafi, Y.M. (2020y). Drug safety: comparison between developing countries. In *Drug Safety in Developing Countries* (pp. 603–611). Academic Press.

Al-Worafi, Y.M. (2014). Prescription writing errors at a tertiary care hospital in Yemen: prevalence, types, causes and recommendations. *Am J Pharm Health Res*, 2, 134–140.

Al-Worafi, Y.M., (2018a). Knowledge, Attitude and Practice of Yemeni Physicians Toward Pharmacovigilance: A Mixed Method Study. *International Journal of Pharmacy and Pharmaceutical Sciences*. 10 (10), 74–77.

Al-Worafi, Y.M. (2018d). Evauation of inhaler technique among patients with asthma and COPD in Yemen. *Journal of Taibah University Medical Sciences*, 13(5), 488–490.

Al-Worafi, Y.M. (Ed.). (2020a). Drug Safety in Developing Countries: Achievements and Challenges.

Al-Worafi, Y.M. (2020b). Medication errors. In *Drug Safety in Developing Countries* (pp. 105–117). Academic Press.

Al-Worafi, Y.M. (2020c). Adverse drug reactions. In *Drug Safety in Developing Countries* (pp. 39–57). Academic Press.

Al-Worafi, Y.M. (2020d). Medications registration and marketing: safety-related issues. In *Drug Safety in Developing Countries* (pp. 21–28). Academic Press.

Al-Worafi, Y.M. (2020e). Pharmacovigilance. In *Drug Safety in Developing Countries* (pp. 29–38). Academic Press.

Al-Worafi, Y.M. (2020f). Drug-related problems. In *Drug safety in developing countries* (pp. 59–71). Academic Press.

Al-Worafi, Y.M. (2020g). Medications safety-related terminology. In *Drug safety in developing countries* (pp. 7–19). Academic Press.

Al-Worafi, Y.M. (2020h). Self-medication. In *Drug Safety in Developing Countries* (pp. 73–86). Academic Press.

Al-Worafi, Y.M. (2020j). Antibiotics safety issues. In *Drug Safety in Developing Countries* (pp. 87–103). Academic Press.

Al-Worafi, Y.M. (2020k). Medications safety research issues. In *Drug Safety in Developing Countries* (pp. 213–227). Academic Press.

Al-Worafi, Y.M. (2020l). Counterfeit and substandard medications. In *Drug safety in developing countries* (pp. 119–126). Academic Press.

Al-Worafi, Y.M. (2020m). Medication abuse and misuse. In *Drug safety in developing countries* (pp. 127–135). Academic Press.

Al-Worafi, Y.M. (2020n). Storage and disposal of medications. In *Drug Safety in Developing Countries* (pp. 137–142). Academic Press.

Al-Worafi, Y.M. (2020o). Safety of medications in special population. In *Drug safety in developing countries* (pp. 143–162). Academic Press.

Al-Worafi, Y.M. (2020p). Herbal medicines safety issues. In *Drug Safety in developing countries* (pp. 163–178). Academic Press.

Al-Worafi, Y.M. (2020q). Medications safety pharmacoeconomics-related issues. In *Drug Safety in Developing Countries* (pp. 187–195). Academic Press.

Al-Worafi, Y.M. (2020r). Evidence-based medications safety practice. In *Drug Safety in Developing Countries* (pp. 197–201). Academic Press.

Al-Worafi, Y.M. (2020s). Quality indicators for medications safety. In *Drug safety in developing countries* (pp. 229–242). Academic Press.

Al-Worafi, Y.M. (2020t). Drug safety in Yemen. In *Drug Safety in Developing Countries* (pp. 391–405). Academic Press.

Al-Worafi, Y.M. (2020u). Drug safety in Saudi Arabia. In *Drug Safety in Developing Countries* (pp. 407–417). Academic Press.

Al-Worafi, Y.M. (2020v). Drug safety in United Arab Emirates. In *Drug Safety in Developing Countries* (pp. 419–428). Academic Press.

Al-Worafi, Y.M. (2020w). Drug safety in Indonesia. In *Drug Safety in Developing Countries* (pp. 279–285). Academic Press.

Al-Worafi, Y.M. (2020x). Drug safety in Palestine. In *Drug Safety in Developing Countries* (pp. 471–480). Academic Press.

Al-Worafi, Y.M. (2020z). Drug safety in developing versus developed countries. In *Drug Safety in Developing Countries* (pp. 613–615). Academic Press.

Al-Worafi, Y.M. (2022e). Patient care errors and related problems (part I): development and validation of the model. https://orcid.org/0000-0002-5752-2913

Al-Worafi, Y.M. (Ed.). (2023). *Clinical Case Studies on medication Safety*. Academic Press.

Al-Worafi, Y.M., Kassab, Y.W., Alseragi, W.M., Almutairi, M.S., Ahmed, A., Ming, L.C., Alkhoshaiban, A.S., & Hadi, M.A., (2017). Pharmacovigilance and adverse drg reaction reporting: a perspective of community pharmacists and pharmacy technicians in Sana'a, Yemen. *Therapeutics and Clinical Risk Management*, 13, p. 1175.

Al-Worafi, Y.M., Patel, R.P., Zaidi, S.T.R., Alseragi, W.M., Almutairi, M.S., Alkhoshaiban, A.S., & Ming, L.C. (2018a). Completeness and legibility of handwritten prescriptions in Sana'a, Yemen. *Medical Principles and Practice*, 27, 290–292.

Al-Worafi, Y.M., Alseragi, W.M., Seng, L.K., Kassab, Y.W., Yeoh, S.F., Chiau, L., ... & Husain, K. (2018b). Dispensing errors in community pharmacies: a prospective study in Sana'a, Yemen. *Arch Pharm Pract*, 9(4), 1–3.

Al-Worafi, Y.M., Alseragi, W.M., & Mahmoud, M.A. (2019). Competency of metered-dose inhaler use among community pharmacy dispensers in Ibb, Yemen: A simulation method study. *Latin American Journal of Pharmacy*, 38(3), 489–494.

Al-Worafi, Y.M., Alseragi, W.M., Ming, L.C., & Alakhali, K.M. (2020a). Drug safety in China. In *Drug Safety in Developing Countries* (pp. 381–388). Academic Press.

Al-Worafi, Y.M., Alseragi, W.M., Alakhali, K.M., Ming, L.C., Othman, G., Halboup, A.M., ... & Elkalmi, R.M. (2020b). Knowledge, beliefs and factors affecting the use of generic medicines among patients in Ibb, Yemen: a mixed-method study. *Journal of Pharmacy Practice and Community Medicine*, 6(4), 53–56.

Al-Worafi, Y.M., Elkalmi, R.M., Ming, L.C., Othman, G., Halboup, A.M., Battah, M.M., ... & Mani, V. (2021a). Dispensing errors in hospital pharmacies: A prospective study in Yemen.

Al-Worafi, Y.M.A. (2015). Appropriateness of metered-dose inhaler use in the Yemeni community pharmacies. *Journal of Taibah University Medical Sciences*, 10(3), 353–358.

Al-Worafi, Y.M.A. (2016). Pharmacy practice in Yemen. In *Pharmacy Practice in Developing Countries* (pp. 267–287). Academic Press.

Al-Worafi, Y.M. (2018c). Dispensing errors observed by community pharmacy dispensers in IBB–YEMEN. *Asian J. Pharm. Clin. Res*, 11(11), 478–481.

Al-Worafi, Y.M., Hasan, S., Hassan, N.M., & Gaili, A.A. (2021b). Knowledge, Attitude and Experience of Pharmacist in the UAE towards Pharmacovigilance. *Research Journal of Pharmacy and Technology*, 14(1), 265–269.

Alshahrani, S.M., Alakhali, K.M., & Al-Worafi, Y.M., (2019a). Medication errors in a health care facility in southern Saudi Arabia. *Tropical Journal of Pharmaceutical Research*, 18(5), 1119–1122.

Alshahrani, S.M., Alavudeen, S.S., Alakhali, K.M., Al-Worafi, Y.M., Bahamdan, A.K., & Vigneshwaran, E., (2019b). Self-Medication Among King Khalid University Students, *Saudi Arabia. Risk Management and Healthcare Policy*, 12, 243–249.

Alshahrani, S.M., Alakhali, K.M., Al-Worafi, Y.M., & Alshahrani, N.Z. (2020b). Awareness and use of over the counter analgesic medication: a survey in the Aseer region population, *Saudi Arabia. Int J Advan Appl Sci*, 7(3), 130–134.

Alshahrani, S.M., Alzahran, M., Alakhali, K., Vigneshwaran, E., Iqbal, M.J., Khan, N.A., … & Alavudeen, S.S. (2020a). Association Between Diabetes Consequences and Quality of Life Among Patients With Diabetes Mellitus in the Aseer Province of Saudi Arabia. *Open Access Macedonian Journal of Medical Sciences*, 8(E), 325–330.

Baig, M.R., Al-Worafi, Y.M., Alseragi, W.M., Ming, L.C., & Siddique, A. (2020). Drug safety in India. In *Drug Safety in Developing Countries* (pp. 327–334). Academic Press.

Bhatt, A. (2010). Evolution of clinical research: a history before and beyond James Lind. *Perspectives in Clinical Research*, 1(1), p. 6.

Elkalmi, R.M., Al-Worafi, Y.M., Alseragi, W.M., Ming, L.C., & Siddique, A. (2020). Drug safety in Malaysia. In *Drug Safety in Developing Countries* (pp. 245–253). Academic Press.

Elsayed, T., & Al-Worafi, Y.M. (2020). Drug safety in Egypt. In *Drug Safety in Developing Countries* (pp. 511–523). Academic Press.

Hasan, S., Al-Omar, M.J., AlZubaidy, H., & Al-Worafi, Y.M. (2019). Use of medications in Arab Countries. In *Handbook of Healthcare in the Arab World*. Cham: Springer, 42.

Hassan, Y., Abd Aziz, N., Kassab, Y.W., Elgasim, I., Shaharuddin, S., Al-Worafi, Y. M. A., … & Ming, L.C. (2014). How to help patients to control their blood pressure? Blood pressure control and its predictor. *Archives of Pharmacy Practice*, 5(4), 153–161.

Izahar, S., Lean, Q.Y., Hameed, M.A., Murugiah, M.K., Patel, R.P., Al-Worafi, Y.M., … & Ming, L.C. (2017). Content analysis of mobile health applications on diabetes mellitus. *Frontiers in Endocrinology*, 8, p. 318.

Jenkins, J., & Hubbard, S. (1991). History of clinical trials. In *Seminars in oncology nursing*. 7(4), 228–234.

Lee, K.S., Yee, S.M., Zaidi, S.T.R., Patel, R.P., Yang, Q., Al-Worafi, Y.M., & Ming, L.C., 2017. Combating sale of counterfeit and falsified medicines online: a losing battle. *Frontiers in pharmacology*, 8, p. 268.

Mahmoud, M.A., Wajid, S., Naqvi, A.A., Samreen, S., Althagfan, S.S., & Al-Worafi, Y. (2020). Self-medication with antibiotics: A cross-sectional community-based study. *Latin American Journal of Pharmacy*, 39(2), 348–353.

Manan, M.M., Rusli, R.A., Ang, W.C., Al-Worafi, Y.M., & Ming, L.C. (2014). Assessing the pharmaceutical care issues of antiepileptic drug therapy in hospitalised epileptic patients. *Journal of Pharmacy Practice and Research*, 44(3), 83–88.

Manan, M.M., Ibrahim, N.A., Aziz, N.A., Zulkifly, H.H., Al-Worafi, Y.M.A., & Long, C.M. (2016). Empirical use of antibiotic therapy in the prevention of early onset sepsis in neonates: a pilot study. *Archives of Medical Science*, 12(3), 603–613.

Ming, L.C., Hameed, M.A., Lee, D.D., Apidi, N.A., Lai, P.S.M., Hadi, M.A., Al-Worafi, Y.M.A., & Khan, T.M., (2016). Use of medical mobile applications among hospital pharmacists in Malaysia. *Therapeutic innovation & regulatory science*, 50(4), 419–426.

Ming, L.C., Untong, N., Aliudin, N.A., Osili, N., Kifli, N., Tan, C.S., … & Goh, H.P. (2020). Mobile health apps on COVID-19 launched in the early days of the pandemic: content analysis and review. *JMIR mHealth and uHealth*, 8(9), p. e19796.

Othman, G., Ali, F., Ibrahim, M.I.M., Al-Worafi, Y.M., Ansari, M., & Halboup, A.M. (2020). Assessment of Anti-Diabetic Medications Adherence among Diabetic Patients in Sana'a City, Yemen: A Cross Sectional Study. *Journal of Pharmaceutical Research International*, 32(21), 114–122.

Polgar, S., & Thomas, S.A. (2011). *Introduction to research in the health sciences E-Book*. Elsevier Health Sciences.

Saeed, M.S., Alkhoshaiban, A.S., Al-Worafi, Y.M.A., & Long, C.M., (2014). Perception of self-medication among university students in Saudi Arabia. *Archives of Pharmacy Practice*, 5(4), p. 149.

46 Patient Safety Research

Epidemiology and Pharmacoepidemiology

46.1 BACKGROUND

Epidemiology is the study of the distribution and determinants of health and disease in human populations. It involves the collection, analysis, and interpretation of data to identify patterns and trends in health outcomes and their potential risk factors. Epidemiology is essential for understanding the burden of disease, identifying populations at risk, and developing strategies for disease prevention and control. Pharmacoepidemiology is a specialized field within epidemiology that focuses on the study of the use, effects, and outcomes of medications in populations. It involves the application of epidemiological methods to assess the safety and effectiveness of drugs, as well as to identify and quantify the risks associated with their use. Pharmacoepidemiology research is critical for evaluating the benefits and risks of drugs, determining appropriate dosages, and identifying potential drug interactions or adverse effects. Both epidemiology and pharmacoepidemiology research are essential for improving public health and informing healthcare policy and decision-making. They are multidisciplinary fields that involve collaboration between epidemiologists, healthcare providers, pharmacists, statisticians, and other experts. By conducting rigorous and well-designed studies, epidemiologists and pharmacoepidemiologists can provide important insights into the causes, prevention, and treatment of diseases, as well as help to ensure the safety and effectiveness of medications. Epidemiology and pharmacoepidemiology are important fields of study in patient safety research. These disciplines are concerned with studying the distribution and determinants of diseases and adverse health events in populations. Epidemiology research in patient safety aims to identify factors that contribute to the occurrence of adverse events in healthcare settings. This may involve studying the prevalence and incidence of adverse events, the risk factors associated with their occurrence, and the impact of interventions aimed at preventing or reducing their occurrence. Examples of adverse events that may be studied include healthcare-associated infections, medication errors, falls, and pressure ulcers. Pharmacoepidemiology research focuses specifically on the study of medication use and its effects on health outcomes. This may involve investigating the safety and effectiveness of medications, as well as identifying risk factors for adverse drug reactions and drug interactions. Pharmacoepidemiology research may also evaluate the impact of medication-related interventions, such as drug utilization reviews or medication reconciliation programs. Together, epidemiology and pharmacoepidemiology research provide valuable insights into the causes and consequences of adverse events in healthcare settings. This information can be used to develop and implement strategies to improve patient safety, reduce healthcare costs, and improve the quality of care delivered to patients (Ahrens & Pigeot, 2014; Polgar & Thomas, 2011; Strom et al., 2013; Waning et al., 2001).

46.2 RATIONALITY OF EPIDEMIOLOGY AND PHARMACOEPIDEMIOLOGY RESEARCH

Epidemiology and pharmacoepidemiology are both highly rational fields of research that aim to systematically study the occurrence and distribution of health and disease in populations, as well as the effects of medications on health outcomes.

Epidemiology involves the study of the distribution and determinants of health and disease in populations. This includes identifying risk factors for various diseases, understanding the patterns and trends of diseases over time and across different populations, and evaluating the effectiveness of interventions aimed at preventing or treating diseases. Epidemiologists use a variety of research methods, including observational studies, randomized controlled trials, and meta-analyses, to collect and analyze data on health outcomes. Pharmacoepidemiology is a specialized field of epidemiology that focuses specifically on the study of the effects of medications on health outcomes in populations. This includes evaluating the safety and effectiveness of medications, identifying adverse drug reactions, and assessing the impact of medication use on healthcare utilization and costs. Like epidemiologists, pharmacoepidemiologists use a range of research methods to gather and analyze data on medication use and health outcomes. Both epidemiology and pharmacoepidemiology are highly rational fields of research because they rely on rigorous scientific methods to systematically study health and disease in populations. Researchers in these fields carefully design studies to minimize bias and confounding, use appropriate statistical analyses to draw valid conclusions from

DOI: 10.1201/9781003230465-49

their data, and communicate their findings in a transparent and reproducible manner. This approach helps to ensure that the results of epidemiology and pharmacoepidemiology research are reliable, accurate, and useful for informing public health policy and clinical practice.

46.3 IMPORTANCE OF EPIDEMIOLOGY AND PHARMACOEPIDEMIOLOGY RESEARCH

Epidemiology and pharmacoepidemiology research play crucial roles in improving public health and informing clinical practice. Here are some of the key reasons why these fields of research are important:

1. Understanding the distribution and determinants of health and disease: Epidemiology helps us to identify patterns and trends in the occurrence of various diseases across different populations, and to understand the factors that contribute to these differences. This knowledge is essential for developing targeted interventions to prevent or control diseases.

2. Identifying risk factors for diseases: By studying the factors that increase the risk of developing certain diseases, epidemiologists can help to identify strategies for preventing or reducing the incidence of these diseases.

3. Evaluating the safety and effectiveness of medications: Pharmacoepidemiology research is essential for identifying adverse drug reactions and evaluating the safety and effectiveness of medications in real-world settings. This information is critical for ensuring that medications are used safely and effectively in clinical practice.

4. Informing public health policy: The findings from epidemiology and pharmacoepidemiology research can help to inform public health policies and guidelines related to disease prevention, screening, and treatment.

5. Improving clinical practice: By providing clinicians with evidence-based information on the safety and effectiveness of medications, epidemiology and pharmacoepidemiology research can help to improve clinical decision-making and optimize patient outcomes.

Overall, epidemiology and pharmacoepidemiology research are essential for improving public health and advancing our understanding of the factors that contribute to health and disease in populations.

46.4 ADVANTAGES OF EPIDEMIOLOGY AND PHARMACOEPIDEMIOLOGY RESEARCH

Epidemiology and pharmacoepidemiology research offer several advantages that are crucial for advancing our understanding of health and disease in populations. Here are some of the key advantages of these fields of research:

1. Systematic and rigorous approach: Epidemiology and pharmacoepidemiology research use systematic and rigorous scientific methods to collect and analyze data on health outcomes. This approach helps to ensure that the results of these studies are reliable, accurate, and unbiased.

2. Large sample sizes: Epidemiology and pharmacoepidemiology research often involve large sample sizes, which can provide more robust and statistically significant findings than smaller studies.

3. Real-world setting: Pharmacoepidemiology research is often conducted in real-world settings, which provides important insights into how medications are used in clinical practice and how they impact patient outcomes.

4. Population-based approach: Epidemiology research focuses on the health of populations, rather than individual patients. This approach allows researchers to identify patterns and trends in disease occurrence across different populations, and to develop targeted interventions to prevent or control diseases.

5. Longitudinal studies: Epidemiology and pharmacoepidemiology research often involve longitudinal studies, which track health outcomes over time. This allows researchers to study the long-term effects of medications and to identify risk factors for disease development.

6. Multi-disciplinary approach: Epidemiology and pharmacoepidemiology research often involve collaboration between researchers from different disciplines, such as medicine, statistics, and epidemiology. This multi-disciplinary approach can lead to a more comprehensive understanding of health and disease in populations.

Overall, the advantages of epidemiology and pharmacoepidemiology research make them essential tools for advancing our understanding of health and disease and for informing public health policies and clinical practice.

46.5 DISADVANTAGES OF EPIDEMIOLOGY AND PHARMACOEPIDEMIOLOGY RESEARCH

While epidemiology and pharmacoepidemiology research offer many advantages, there are also some potential disadvantages to consider. Here are some of the key disadvantages of these fields of research:

1. Observational studies: Many epidemiology and pharmacoepidemiology studies are observational, rather than randomized controlled trials. This can make it more difficult to establish causality, as there may be confounding factors that influence the relationship between exposure and outcome.

2. Bias: Epidemiology and pharmacoepidemiology studies are vulnerable to various sources of bias, such as selection bias, recall bias, and publication bias. Researchers need to carefully design studies and use appropriate statistical methods to minimize these biases.

3. Generalizability: Epidemiology and pharmacoepidemiology studies often focus on specific populations, which may limit the generalizability of their findings to other populations. Researchers need to carefully consider the representativeness of their sample when interpreting their results.

4. Ethics: Epidemiology and pharmacoepidemiology studies may involve collecting sensitive or personal information from participants, which raises ethical concerns around confidentiality and privacy. Researchers need to obtain informed consent from participants and follow ethical guidelines to ensure the protection of human subjects.

5. Cost: Epidemiology and pharmacoepidemiology studies can be costly and time-consuming.

6. Study design limitations: Epidemiology and pharmacoepidemiology studies are often observational in nature, meaning they rely on data collected from existing patient records rather than from randomized controlled trials. This can limit the ability of researchers to establish causal relationships between exposures and outcomes.

7. Bias and confounding: Observational studies are also vulnerable to bias and confounding, which can distort the results of the study. For example, selection bias may occur if patients who receive certain treatments or are at higher risk for adverse events are more likely to be included in the study, leading to inaccurate results.

8. Data limitations: Epidemiology and pharmacoepidemiology studies rely on accurate and comprehensive data, which may be challenging to obtain. Electronic health records may contain incomplete or inaccurate information, and patients may be unaware of adverse events or hesitant to report them.

9. Generalizability: Epidemiology and pharmacoepidemiology studies are often conducted in specific populations, which may limit their generalizability to other settings or populations.

10. Ethical considerations: Some epidemiology and pharmacoepidemiology studies may involve the use of patient data without explicit consent, raising ethical concerns around patient privacy and autonomy.

Despite these potential disadvantages, epidemiology and pharmacoepidemiology research remain important tools for advancing patient safety research and improving the quality of care delivered to patients. By carefully considering the limitations of these research methods, researchers can develop rigorous and informative studies that contribute to our understanding of patient safety.

46.6 FACILITATORS OF EPIDEMIOLOGY AND PHARMACOEPIDEMIOLOGY RESEARCH

There are several facilitators of epidemiology and pharmacoepidemiology research that can contribute to successful studies and reliable findings. Here are some of the key facilitators:

1. Robust study design: A well-designed study with a clear research question and appropriate methodology can increase the validity and reliability of the study findings.

2. High-quality data sources: Access to high-quality data sources such as electronic health records, disease registries, and administrative databases can enhance the accuracy and completeness of the data collected.

3. Adequate sample size: Adequate sample size is crucial for the statistical power of the study and can increase the precision of the estimates.

4. Collaborative research teams: Collaboration between researchers from different disciplines, such as epidemiologists, biostatisticians, clinicians, and pharmacists, can bring diverse perspectives and expertise to the research project.

5. Good communication and dissemination strategies: Effective communication and dissemination strategies, such as peer-reviewed publications, presentations at scientific conferences, and media outreach, can ensure that the research findings reach the intended audiences and have a positive impact on public health.

6. Funding support: Adequate funding is essential for conducting high-quality epidemiology and pharmacoepidemiology research. Funding can support the collection and analysis of data, the development of innovative research methods, and the dissemination of findings.

46.7 BARRIERS OF EPIDEMIOLOGY AND PHARMACOEPIDEMIOLOGY RESEARCH

There are several barriers that can hinder the progress and success of epidemiology and pharmacoepidemiology research. Here are some of the common barriers:

1. Limited funding: Lack of funding can restrict the scope of the research, limit the sample size, and reduce the quality of data collected.

2. Access to data: Access to high-quality data sources can be a major barrier, especially when data is fragmented, incomplete, or inaccessible due to privacy concerns.

3. Regulatory hurdles: Regulations around data privacy, informed consent, and ethical considerations can pose a significant challenge to conducting epidemiological and pharmacoepidemiological research.

4. Recruitment and retention: Recruiting participants and retaining them over the course of the study can be difficult, particularly in populations that are hard to reach, have low levels of health literacy, or are wary of participating in research.

5. Confounding factors: Epidemiological and pharmacoepidemiological research often involves studying complex relationships between variables that can be influenced by numerous confounding factors, such as lifestyle, genetic predisposition, and environmental exposures.

6. Bias and measurement errors: Bias and measurement errors can occur in the collection and analysis of data, leading to incorrect conclusions and inaccurate estimates.

7. Limited generalizability: The findings of epidemiological and pharmacoepidemiologic studies may not be generalizable to other populations or settings, making it challenging to apply the findings to public health policy and practice.

46.8 QUALITY OF EPIDEMIOLOGY AND PHARMACOEPIDEMIOLOGY RESEARCH

The quality of epidemiology and pharmacoepidemiology research is determined by the rigor and validity of the study design, the accuracy and completeness of the data collected, the appropriateness of the statistical analysis, and the generalizability of the findings. Here are some factors that contribute to high-quality research:

1. Study design: A well-designed study with a clear research question, appropriate selection of participants, and appropriate methodology can enhance the validity and reliability of the findings.

2. Data quality: The accuracy, completeness, and reliability of the data collected are crucial to ensuring the validity of the research. Quality assurance measures, such as validation checks and data cleaning, can help to reduce errors and increase the accuracy of the data.

3. Statistical analysis: The appropriate use of statistical methods, including appropriate adjustment for confounding factors, can ensure that the findings are valid and reliable.

4. Transparency and reproducibility: A transparent reporting of study methods and results, along with open access to data and analysis code, can enhance the reproducibility of the findings and improve the confidence in the results.

5. Peer review: Peer review by experts in the field can provide critical feedback and ensure that the study adheres to the highest standards of research quality.

6. Ethical considerations: Ethical considerations, including informed consent, privacy protections, and adherence to ethical guidelines, can enhance the credibility and trustworthiness of the research.

Overall, high-quality epidemiology and pharmacoepidemiology research can provide critical insights into the relationships between exposures, treatments, and health outcomes, and inform public health policy and practice.

46.9 EPIDEMIOLOGY AND PHARMACOEPIDEMIOLOGY RESEARCH IN DEVELOPING COUNTRIES: Challenges and Recommendations

Patient safety research in developing countries has made significant achievements in recent years. Many developing countries have conducted many researches about the various issues of patient safety and care research (Alshahrani et al., 2019a,b; Al-Qahtani et al., 2015; Alshahrani et al., 2020a,b; Al-Worafi, 2014; Al-Worafi, 2015; Al-Worafi, 2016; Al-Worafi et al., 2017; Al-Worafi, 2018a-d;Al-Worafi et al., 2018a-b; Al-Worafi et al., 2019; Al-Worafi, 2020a-z; Al-Worafi et al., 2020a-b; Al-Worafi et al., 2021a,b; Al-Worafi, 2022a-e; Al-Worafi, 2023; Baig et al., 2020; Elkalmi et al., 2020; Elsayed & Al-Worafi, 2020; Hasan et al., 2019; Hassan et al., 2014; Izahar et al., 2017; Lee et al., 2017; Mahmoud et al., 2020; Manan et al., 2014; Manan et al., 2016; Ming et al., 2016; Ming et al., 2020; Othman et al., 2020; Saeed et al., 2014), however, there are many however, there are many challenges and recommendations for conducting epidemiology and pharmacoepidemiology in developing countries such as:

1. Increase funding: Increased funding from both public and private sources can help to support the development of research infrastructure and improve the quality of data collection and analysis.

2. Strengthen data systems: Improving the quality and accessibility of data sources, such as electronic health records, disease registries, and administrative databases, can enhance the accuracy and completeness of the data collected.

3. Capacity building: Developing the research skills of local researchers, clinicians, and other stakeholders can help to build local capacity for conducting high-quality epidemiological and pharmacoepidemiological research.

4. Collaborative research partnerships: Collaboration between researchers from different countries and disciplines can bring diverse perspectives and expertise to the research project, leading to more innovative and impactful research.

5. Address ethical considerations: Ensuring that ethical considerations are addressed in a culturally sensitive manner can improve the trustworthiness of the research and reduce potential harm to study participants.

6. Address healthcare access disparities: Consideration of healthcare access disparities can aid in the development of targeted strategies for disease prevention and treatment.

7. Open access publishing: Open access publishing can increase the visibility and impact of research findings and enable researchers from developing countries to contribute to global research efforts.

8. Lack of infrastructure: Developing countries may have inadequate research infrastructure, including laboratory facilities, electronic health records, and computer systems. This can limit the scope of research and make it difficult to collect and analyze data.

9. Limited availability of research tools and resources: Access to research tools and resources, such as software, databases, and research instruments, may be limited in developing countries. This can affect the quality of research and make it difficult to replicate studies.

10. Limited research culture: Developing countries may lack a strong research culture, which can make it difficult to attract and retain researchers, and limit the scope of research projects.

11. Political instability: Political instability, including conflicts and civil unrest, can disrupt research projects, limit the availability of funding, and hinder collaboration between researchers from different countries.

12. Limited access to healthcare: Developing countries may have limited access to healthcare, which can make it difficult to recruit participants for research studies and limit the generalizability of the findings.

13. Language barriers: Language barriers can make it difficult for researchers from different countries to collaborate and share information, which can limit the scope and impact of research projects.

Overall, addressing the challenges facing epidemiology and pharmacoepidemiology research in developing countries requires a multifaceted approach that involves collaboration between different stakeholders, building local capacity, and addressing ethical considerations in a culturally sensitive manner. With the right investments and partnerships, it is possible to improve the quality and impact of research in developing countries and contribute to improved public health outcomes.

46.10 CONCLUSION

This chapter has discussed the patient safety research issues related to the epidemiology and pharmacoepidemiology, importance, facilitators, barriers, challenges and recommendations for the best practice in developing countries. Epidemiology and pharmacoepidemiology research play a critical role in informing public health policy and practice and improving health outcomes. However, conducting high-quality research in developing countries can be challenging due to limited funding, limited access to high-quality data sources, inadequate infrastructure, and ethical considerations. To overcome these challenges, it is necessary to increase funding, strengthen data systems, build local capacity, address ethical considerations, and collaborate between different stakeholders. Additionally, it is essential to address issues such as limited availability of research tools and resources, limited research culture, political instability, limited access to healthcare, and language barriers. By addressing these challenges and issues, it is possible to improve the quality and impact of epidemiology and pharmacoepidemiology research in developing countries, contributing to improved public health outcomes and better health equity. Ultimately, investing in research in developing countries is critical for improving the health and well-being of populations around the world.

REFERENCES

Ahrens, W., & Pigeot, I. (Eds.). (2014). *Handbook of epidemiology* (Vol. 451). New York: Springer.

Al-Qahtani, I., Almoteb, T.M., & Al-Warafi, Y. (2015). Competency of metered-dose inhaler use among Saudi community pharmacists: A Simulation method study. *RRJPPS*, 4(2), 37–31.

Alshahrani, S.M., Alakhali, K.M., & Al-Worafi, Y.M., (2019a). Medication errors in a health care facility in southern Saudi Arabia. *Tropical Journal of Pharmaceutical Research*, 18(5), 1119–1122.

Alshahrani, S.M., Alavudeen, S.S., Alakhali, K.M., Al-Worafi, Y.M., Bahamdan, A.K., & Vigneshwaran, E., (2019b). Self-Medication Among King Khalid University Students, Saudi Arabia. *Risk Management and Healthcare Policy*, 12, 243–249.

Alshahrani, S.M., Alakhali, K.M., Al-Worafi, Y.M., & Alshahrani, N.Z. (2020b). Awareness and use of over the counter analgesic medication: a survey in the Aseer region population, Saudi Arabia. *Int J Advan Appl Sci*, 7(3), 130–134.

Alshahrani, S.M., Alzahran, M., Alakhali, K., Vigneshwaran, E., Iqbal, M.J., Khan, N.A., … & Alavudeen, S.S. (2020b). Association Between Diabetes Consequences and Quality of Life Among Patients With Diabetes Mellitus in the Aseer Province of Saudi Arabia. *Open Access Macedonian Journal of Medical Sciences*, 8(E), 325–330.

Al-Worafi, Y.M. (2014). Prescription writing errors at a tertiary care hospital in Yemen: prevalence, types, causes and recommendations. *Am J Pharm Health Res*, 2, 134–140.

Al-Worafi, Y.M.A. (2015). Appropriateness of metered-dose inhaler use in the Yemeni community pharmacies. *Journal of Taibah University Medical Sciences*, 10(3), 353–358.

Al-Worafi, Y.M.A., (2016). Pharmacy practice in Yemen. In *Pharmacy Practice in Developing Countries* (pp. 267–287). Academic Press.

Al-Worafi, Y.M., Kassab, Y.W., Alseragi, W.M., Almutairi, M.S., Ahmed, A., Ming, L.C., Alkhoshaiban, A.S., & Hadi, M.A., (2017). Pharmacovigilance and adverse drg reaction reporting: a perspective of community pharmacists and pharmacy technicians in Sana'a, Yemen. *Therapeutics and Clinical Risk Management*, 13, p. 1175.

Al-Worafi, Y.M., (2018a). Knowledge, Attitude and Practice of Yemeni Physicians Toward Pharmacovigilance: A Mixed Method Study. *International Journal of Pharmacy and Pharmaceutical Sciences*. 10 (10), 74–77.

Al-Worafi, Y. (2018b). Knowledge, attitude and practice of Yemeni physicians toward pharmacovigilance: A mixed method study. *Int. J. Pharm. Pharm. Sci*, 10, 74–77.

Al-Worafi, Y.M. (2018c). Dispensing errors observed by community pharmacy dispensers in IBB–YEMEN. *Asian J. Pharm. Clin. Res*, 11(11), 478–482.

Al-Worafi, Y.M. (2018d). Evauation of inhaler technique among patients with asthma and COPD in Yemen. *Journal of Taibah University Medical Sciences*, 13(5), 488–490.

Al-Worafi, Y.M., Patel, R.P., Zaidi, S.T.R., Alseragi, W.M., Almutairi, M.S., Alkhoshaiban, A.S., & Ming, L.C. (2018a). Completeness and legibility of handwritten prescriptions in Sana'a, Yemen. *Medical Principles and Practice*, 27, 290–292.

Al-Worafi, Y.M., Alseragi, W.M., Seng, L.K., Kassab, Y.W., Yeoh, S.F., Chiau, L., … & Husain, K. (2018b). Dispensing errors in community pharmacies: a prospective study in Sana'a, Yemen. Arch *Pharm Pract*, 9(4), 1–3.

Al-Worafi, Y.M., Alseragi, W.M., & Mahmoud, M.A. (2019). Competency of metered-dose inhaler use among community pharmacy dispensers in Ibb, Yemen: A simulation method study. *Latin American Journal of Pharmacy*, 38(3), 489–494.

Al-Worafi, Y.M. (Ed.). (2020a). Drug Safety in Developing Countries: Achievements and Challenges.

Al-Worafi, Y.M. (2020b). Medication errors. In *Drug Safety in Developing Countries* (pp. 105–117). Academic Press.

Al-Worafi, Y.M. (2020c). Adverse drug reactions. In *Drug Safety in Developing Countries* (pp. 39–57). Academic Press.

Al-Worafi, Y.M. (2020d). Medications registration and marketing: safety-related issues. In *Drug Safety in Developing Countries* (pp. 21–28). Academic Press.

Al-Worafi, Y.M. (2020e). Pharmacovigilance. In *Drug Safety in Developing Countries* (pp. 29–38). Academic Press.

Al-Worafi, Y.M. (2020f). Drug-related problems. In *Drug Safety in Developing Countries* (pp. 59–71). Academic Press.

Al-Worafi, Y.M. (2020g). Medications safety-related terminology. In *Drug safety in developing countries* (pp. 7–19). Academic Press.

Al-Worafi, Y.M. (2020h). Self-medication. In *Drug Safety in Developing Countries* (pp. 73–86). Academic Press.

Al-Worafi, Y.M. (2020j). Antibiotics safety issues. In *Drug Safety in Developing Countries* (pp. 87–103). Academic Press.

Al-Worafi, Y.M. (2020k). Medications safety research issues. In *Drug Safety in Developing Countries* (pp. 213–227). Academic Press.

Al-Worafi, Y.M. (2020l). Counterfeit and substandard medications. In *Drug Safety in Developing Countries* (pp. 119–126). Academic Press.

Al-Worafi, Y.M. (2020m). Medication abuse and misuse. In *Drug safety in developing countries* (pp. 127–135). Academic Press.

Al-Worafi, Y.M. (2020n). Storage and disposal of medications. In *Drug Safety in Developing Countries* (pp. 137–142). Academic Press.

Al-Worafi, Y.M. (2020o). Safety of medications in special population. In *Drug safety in developing countries* (pp. 143–162). Academic Press.

Al-Worafi, Y.M. (2020p). Herbal medicines safety issues. In *Drug Safety in Developing Countries* (pp. 163–178). Academic Press.

Al-Worafi, Y.M. (2020q). Medications safety pharmacoeconomics-related issues. In *Drug Safety in Developing Countries* (pp. 187–195). Academic Press.

Al-Worafi, Y.M. (2020r). Evidence-based medications safety practice. In *Drug Safety in Developing Countries* (pp. 197–201). Academic Press.

Al-Worafi, Y.M. (2020s). Quality indicators for medications safety. In *Drug safety in developing countries* (pp. 229–242). Academic Press.

Al-Worafi, Y.M. (2020t). Drug safety in Yemen. In *Drug Safety in Developing Countries* (pp. 391–405). Academic Press.

Al-Worafi, Y.M. (2020u). Drug safety in Saudi Arabia. In *Drug Safety in Developing Countries* (pp. 407–417). Academic Press.

Al-Worafi, Y.M. (2020v). Drug safety in United Arab Emirates. In *Drug Safety in Developing Countries* (pp. 419–428). Academic Press.

Al-Worafi, Y.M. (2020w). Drug safety in Indonesia. In *Drug Safety in Developing Countries* (pp. 279–285). Academic Press.

Al-Worafi, Y.M. (2020x). Drug safety in Palestine. In *Drug Safety in Developing Countries* (pp. 471–480). Academic Press.

Al-Worafi, Y.M. (2020y). Drug safety: comparison between developing countries. In *Drug Safety in Developing Countries* (pp. 603–611). Academic Press.

Al-Worafi, Y.M. (2020z). Drug safety in developing versus developed countries. In *Drug Safety in Developing Countries* (pp. 613–615). Academic Press.

Al-Worafi, Y.M., Alseragi, W.M., Ming, L.C., & Alakhali, K.M. (2020a). Drug safety in China. In *Drug Safety in Developing Countries* (pp. 381–388). Academic Press.

Al-Worafi, Y.M., Alseragi, W.M., Alakhali, K.M., Ming, L.C., Othman, G., Halboup, A.M., ... & Elkalmi, R.M. (2020b). Knowledge, beliefs and factors affecting the use of generic medicines among patients in Ibb, Yemen: a mixed-method study. *Journal of Pharmacy Practice and Community Medicine,* 6(4), 53–56.

Al-Worafi, Y.M., Elkalmi, R.M., Ming, L.C., Othman, G., Halboup, A.M., Battah, M.M., ... & Mani, V. (2021a). Dispensing errors in hospital pharmacies: A prospective study in Yemen.

Al-Worafi, Y.M., Hasan, S., Hassan, N.M., & Gaili, A.A. (2021b). Knowledge, Attitude and Experience of Pharmacist in the UAE towards Pharmacovigilance. *Research Journal of Pharmacy and Technology,* 14(1), 265–269.

Al-Worafi, Y. (2022a). *A Guide to Online Pharmacy Education: Teaching Strategies and Assessment Methods.* CRC Press.

Al-Worafi, Y. (2022b). History and Importance. In *A Guide to Online Pharmacy Education: Teaching Strategies and Assessment Methods.* CRC Press.

Al-Worafi, Y. (2022c). Terminologies. In *A Guide to Online Pharmacy Education: Teaching Strategies and Assessment Methods.* CRC Press.

Al-Worafi, Y. (2022d). Research Methods and Methodology. In *A Guide to Online Pharmacy Education: Teaching Strategies and Assessment Methods.* CRC Press.

Al-Worafi, Y.M. (2022e). Patient care errors and related problems (part I): development and validation of the model. https://orcid.org/0000–0002-5752-2913

Al-Worafi, Y.M. (Ed.). (2023). *Clinical Case Studies on medication Safety.* Academic Press.

Baig, M.R., Al-Worafi, Y.M., Alseragi, W.M., Ming, L.C., & Siddique, A. (2020). Drug safety in India. In *Drug Safety in Developing Countries* (pp. 327–334). Academic Press.

Elkalmi, R.M., Al-Worafi, Y.M., Alseragi, W.M., Ming, L.C., & Siddique, A. (2020). Drug safety in Malaysia. In *Drug Safety in Developing Countries* (pp. 245–253). Academic Press.

Elsayed, T., & Al-Worafi, Y.M. (2020). Drug safety in Egypt. In *Drug Safety in Developing Countries* (pp. 511–523). Academic Press.

Hasan, S., Al-Omar, M.J., AlZubaidy, H., & Al-Worafi, Y.M. (2019). Use of medications in Arab Countries. In *Handbook of Healthcare in the Arab World.* Cham: Springer, 42.

Hassan, Y., Abd Aziz, N., Kassab, Y.W., Elgasim, I., Shaharuddin, S., Al-Worafi, Y.M.A., ... & Ming, L.C. (2014). How to help patients to control their blood pressure? Blood pressure control and its predictor. *Archives of Pharmacy Practice.* 5(4), 153–161.

Izahar, S., Lean, Q.Y., Hameed, M.A., Murugiah, M.K., Patel, R.P., Al-Worafi, Y.M., ... & Ming, L.C. (2017). Content analysis of mobile health applications on diabetes mellitus. *Frontiers in Endocrinology,* 8, p. 318.

Lee, K.S., Yee, S.M., Zaidi, S.T.R., Patel, R.P., Yang, Q., Al-Worafi, Y.M., & Ming, L.C., 2017. Combating sale of counterfeit and falsified medicines online: a losing battle. *Frontiers in pharmacology,* 8, p. 268.

Mahmoud, M.A., Wajid, S., Naqvi, A.A., Samreen, S., Althagfan, S.S., & Al-Worafi, Y. (2020). Self-medication with antibiotics: A cross-sectional community-based study. *Latin American Journal of Pharmacy*, 39(2), 348–353.

Manan, M.M., Rusli, R.A., Ang, W.C., Al-Worafi, Y.M., & Ming, L.C. (2014). Assessing the pharmaceutical care issues of antiepileptic drug therapy in hospitalised epileptic patients. *Journal of Pharmacy Practice and Research*, 44(3), 83–88.

Manan, M.M., Ibrahim, N.A., Aziz, N.A., Zulkifly, H.H., Al-Worafi, Y.M.A., & Long, C.M. (2016). Empirical use of antibiotic therapy in the prevention of early onset sepsis in neonates: a pilot study. *Archives of Medical Science*, 12(3), 603–613.

Ming, L.C., Hameed, M.A., Lee, D.D., Apidi, N.A., Lai, P.S.M., Hadi, M.A., Al-Worafi, Y.M.A., & Khan, T.M., (2016). Use of medical mobile applications among hospital pharmacists in Malaysia. *Therapeutic innovation & regulatory science*, 50(4), 419–426.

Ming, L.C., Untong, N., Aliudin, N.A., Osili, N., Kifli, N., Tan, C.S., ... & Goh, H.P. (2020). Mobile health apps on COVID-19 launched in the early days of the pandemic: content analysis and review. *JMIR mHealth and uHealth*, 8(9), p. e19796.

Othman, G., Ali, F., Ibrahim, M.I.M., Al-Worafi, Y.M., Ansari, M., & Halboup, A.M. (2020). Assessment of Anti-Diabetic Medications Adherence among Diabetic Patients in Sana'a City, Yemen: A Cross Sectional Study. *Journal of Pharmaceutical Research International*, 32(21), 114–122.

Polgar, S., & Thomas, S.A. (2011). *Introduction to Research in the Health Sciences E-Book*. Elsevier Health Sciences.

Saeed, M.S., Alkhoshaiban, A.S., Al-Worafi, Y.M.A., & Long, C.M., (2014). Perception of self-medication among university students in Saudi Arabia. *Archives of Pharmacy Practice*, 5(4), p. 149.

Strom, B.L., Kimmel, S.E., & Hennessy, S. (Eds.). (2013). *Textbook of Pharmacoepidemiology* (pp. 447–454). John Wiley & Sons.

Waning, B., Montagne, M., & McCloskey, W.W. (2001). *Pharmacoepidemiology: Principles and Practice*. New York: McGraw-Hill.

47 Patient Safety Research in Developing Countries

Achievements, Challenges, and Recommendations

47.1 PATIENT SAFETY RESEARCH IN DEVELOPING COUNTRIES: Achievements

Despite facing many challenges, including limited resources and research capacity, there have been notable achievements in this field. These include the development of innovative patient safety interventions, the promotion of patient engagement and empowerment, and the integration of patient safety into healthcare policy and practice. In addition, there has been progress in addressing healthcare disparities, improving healthcare quality, and promoting interdisciplinary collaboration. These achievements demonstrate the potential for patient safety research to have a positive impact on healthcare outcomes in developing countries. However, there is still much work to be done to ensure that all patients receive safe and effective healthcare. It is important to continue investing in patient safety research in developing countries and promoting global partnerships and knowledge-sharing to build on these achievements and improve patient safety around the world. There have been significant achievements in patient safety research in developing countries in recent years. Some of the notable achievements are:

1. Establishing national patient safety programs: Many developing countries have established national patient safety programs to improve the quality of care and reduce medical errors. These programs focus on improving communication, identifying and reporting adverse events, and implementing best practices in patient safety.

2. Implementation of patient safety guidelines: Developing countries have made significant progress in implementing evidence-based guidelines for patient safety. These guidelines address issues such as hand hygiene, medication safety, surgical safety, and infection control.

3. Building capacity for patient safety: Developing countries have invested in building the capacity of healthcare providers to ensure patient safety. This includes training programs for healthcare workers, strengthening regulatory frameworks, and developing systems for monitoring and reporting adverse events.

4. Collaborative efforts: Many developing countries have formed collaborations with international organizations to improve patient safety. These collaborations provide technical assistance, funding, and expertise to support patient safety initiatives.

5. Technology-based solutions: Technology-based solutions, such as electronic medical records, telemedicine, and clinical decision support systems, have been developed and implemented to improve patient safety in developing countries. These solutions help to reduce errors, improve communication, and enhance the overall quality of care.

6. Patient engagement: There has been increasing recognition of the importance of engaging patients and their families in patient safety efforts in developing countries. This includes educating patients on how to participate in their care, empowering them to ask questions and raise concerns, and involving them in the development of patient safety policies and programs.

7. Improving medication safety: Developing countries have made significant strides in improving medication safety, such as implementing medication reconciliation processes and promoting the use of standardized medication labeling and packaging.

8. Addressing healthcare-associated infections (HAIs): HAIs remain a significant problem in developing countries, but there have been efforts to address this issue. These efforts include implementing infection prevention and control measures, improving hand hygiene practices, and promoting the appropriate use of antibiotics.

9. Addressing workforce challenges: Developing countries often face challenges in recruiting and retaining qualified healthcare workers, which can impact patient safety. Efforts have been made to address this issue, such as investing in training and education programs, implementing workforce retention strategies, and improving working conditions.

10. Addressing resource constraints: Many developing countries face resource constraints that can impact patient safety. Efforts have been made to address this issue, such as promoting the use

DOI: 10.1201/9781003230465-50

of low-cost, high-impact interventions, leveraging technology to improve efficiency, and developing innovative financing models.

11. Improving maternal and child health: Developing countries have made progress in improving maternal and child health, which is an important aspect of patient safety. This includes initiatives to improve access to maternal and child healthcare services, promoting evidence-based practices for safe childbirth, and addressing the underlying social and economic determinants of maternal and child health.

12. Addressing cultural and linguistic barriers: Developing countries often have diverse populations with varying cultural and linguistic backgrounds. This can create communication barriers that impact patient safety. Efforts are needed to promote culturally competent care and to ensure that patients have access to language services and support.

13. Addressing the social determinants of health: The social determinants of health, such as poverty, education, and access to clean water and sanitation, can have a significant impact on patient safety. Efforts are needed to address these underlying factors to improve patient outcomes.

14. Addressing the impact of conflict and disasters: Developing countries are often affected by conflict and natural disasters, which can impact patient safety. Efforts are needed to build resilient healthcare systems that can respond to emergencies and provide care in challenging environments.

15. Improving data collection and analysis: Developing countries often lack comprehensive data on patient safety, which can make it difficult to identify and address problems. Efforts are needed to improve data collection and analysis systems to support evidence-based decision-making.

16. Promoting accountability and transparency: Ensuring accountability and transparency is critical to improving patient safety. Developing countries need to establish regulatory frameworks and mechanisms to promote transparency and accountability across the healthcare system.

17. Promoting patient safety culture: Promoting a culture of safety is essential to improving patient safety. Developing countries need to foster a culture that prioritizes patient safety and encourages healthcare workers to speak up and report safety concerns (Alshahrani et al., 2019a,b; Al-Qahtani et al., 2015; Alshahrani et al., 2020a,b; Al-Worafi, 2014; Al-Worafi, 2015; Al-Worafi, 2016; Al-Worafi et al., 2017; Al-Worafi, 2018a-d;Al-Worafi et al., 2018a-b; Al-Worafi et al., 2019; Al-Worafi, 2020a-z; Al-Worafi et al., 2020a-b; Al-Worafi et al., 2021a,b; Al-Worafi, 2022a-d; Al-Worafi, 2023; Baig et al., 2020; Elkalmi et al., 2020; Elsayed & Al-Worafi, 2020; Hasan et al., 2019; Hassan et al., 2014; Izahar et al., 2017; Lee et al., 2017; Mahmoud et al., 2020; Manan et al., 2014; Manan et al., 2016; Ming et al., 2016; Ming et al., 2020; Othman et al., 2020; Saeed et al., 2014).

In conclusion, patient safety research in developing countries has made significant progress in recent years. National patient safety programs, evidence-based guidelines, technology-based solutions, capacity building, and collaborative efforts are just a few examples of the achievements made in this area. However, there are still many challenges to be addressed, including cultural and linguistic barriers, social determinants of health, conflict and disasters, data collection and analysis, accountability and transparency, and promoting a patient safety culture. Addressing these issues will require ongoing efforts and investment in patient safety research and interventions in developing countries. By promoting a culture of safety, improving access to quality care, addressing social determinants of health, and investing in workforce development, we can work towards ensuring that patients in developing countries receive safe and effective healthcare. Overall, patient safety research in developing countries has the potential to make a significant impact on global health and well-being, and should be a priority for policymakers, healthcare providers, and researchers around the world.

47.2 PATIENT SAFETY RESEARCH IN DEVELOPING COUNTRIES: Challenges

Research on patient safety in developing countries faces several challenges, including:

1. Lack of resources: Developing countries often have limited resources for healthcare, which can make it difficult to conduct patient safety research. There may be a shortage of trained personnel, equipment, and funding for research studies.

2. Limited data: Patient safety data may not be readily available in developing countries, making it difficult to establish a baseline for safety practices and measure improvement.

3. Cultural differences: Healthcare practices and beliefs can vary widely across different cultures and regions, making it challenging to design interventions that are effective in all settings.

4. Language barriers: Many developing countries have multiple official languages or dialects, which can make it difficult to communicate with patients and gather accurate data.

5. Political instability: Political instability, conflict, and economic instability can disrupt healthcare systems and make it difficult to conduct patient safety research.

6. Lack of infrastructure: Developing countries may have limited infrastructure for healthcare, such as hospitals, clinics, and laboratories, which can make it difficult to conduct research studies.

7. Limited access to technology: Limited access to technology, such as electronic health records or telemedicine, can make it difficult to collect and analyze patient safety data.

8. Limited training: Healthcare professionals in developing countries may have limited training in patient safety practices, which can make it difficult to implement and evaluate interventions.

9. Lack of regulatory frameworks: Many developing countries have weak or nonexistent regulatory frameworks for healthcare, making it difficult to enforce patient safety standards and ensure accountability.

10. Stigma and discrimination: Patients in developing countries may face stigma and discrimination based on factors such as their gender, sexual orientation, or socioeconomic status, which can affect their willingness to report safety incidents or seek care.

11. Limited public awareness: Patients in developing countries may not be aware of their rights or understand the importance of reporting safety incidents, making it difficult to identify and address safety issues.

12. Limited engagement with communities: Healthcare providers and researchers may not have strong relationships with the communities they serve, which can limit their ability to gather accurate data or implement effective interventions.

13. Lack of collaboration: Healthcare providers, researchers, and policymakers may not have strong collaborations with one another, making it difficult to coordinate efforts to improve patient safety.

14. Limited access to quality medicines and medical products: Many developing countries have limited access to quality medicines and medical products, which can put patients at risk of harm.

15. Inadequate monitoring and evaluation: Healthcare providers and researchers may not have adequate monitoring and evaluation systems in place to track progress and measure the impact of patient safety interventions.

16. Lack of standardization: There may be a lack of standardization in healthcare practices and protocols across different regions, making it difficult to implement and evaluate patient safety interventions.

17. Limited understanding of root causes: Healthcare providers and researchers may have a limited understanding of the root causes of patient safety incidents in developing countries, making it difficult to develop effective interventions.

18. Limited use of evidence-based practices: Healthcare providers in developing countries may not have access to or may not be using evidence-based practices for patient safety, which can put patients at risk of harm.

19. Limited patient engagement: Patients in developing countries may not be actively engaged in their healthcare, making it difficult to identify and address safety issues.

20. Limited research capacity: Developing countries may have limited research capacity, including a shortage of trained researchers and limited funding for research studies.

21. Limited dissemination of findings: There may be limited dissemination of research findings on patient safety in developing countries, making it difficult for healthcare providers, policy-makers, and the public to learn about effective interventions.

22. Limited integration with existing systems: Patient safety interventions may not be well-integrated with existing healthcare systems in developing countries, making it difficult to sustain improvements over time.

23. Lack of political will: Policymakers in developing countries may not prioritize patient safety or may not allocate adequate resources for patient safety research and interventions.

47.3 PATIENT SAFETY RESEARCH IN DEVELOPING COUNTRIES: Recommendations

Patient safety research in developing countries has made significant achievements in recent years. Many developing countries have conducted many researches about the various issues of patient safety and care research (Alshahrani et al., 2019a,b; Al-Qahtani et al., 2015;Alshahrani et al., 2020a,b; Al-Worafi, 2014; Al-Worafi, 2015; Al-Worafi, 2016; Al-Worafi et al., 2017; Al-Worafi, 2018a-d; Al-Worafi et al., 2018a-b; Al-Worafi et al., 2019; Al-Worafi, 2020a-z; Al-Worafi et al., 2020a-b; Al-Worafi et al., 2021a,b; Al-Worafi, 2022a-d; Al-Worafi, 2023a; Baig et al., 2020; Elkalmi et al., 2020; Elsayed & Al-Worafi, 2020; Hasan et al., 2019; Hassan et al., 2014; Izahar et al., 2017; Lee et al., 2017; Mahmoud et al., 2020; Manan et al., 2014; Manan et al., 2016; Ming et al., 2016; Ming et al., 2020; Othman et al., 2020; Saeed et al., 2014), however, there are many recommendations to improve the patient safety research such as:

1. Collaborate with local stakeholders: Work closely with local healthcare providers, policy-makers, and communities to develop interventions that are culturally appropriate and relevant to local needs.

2. Build research capacity: Invest in building research capacity in developing countries by providing training and resources for researchers, and supporting the development of local research networks.

3. Use mixed methods: Use a combination of quantitative and qualitative research methods to gain a comprehensive understanding of patient safety issues in developing countries.

4. Prioritize patient engagement: Involve patients in the design, implementation, and evaluation of patient safety interventions to ensure that their perspectives and needs are addressed.

5. Address root causes: Conduct research to identify the underlying causes of patient safety incidents in developing countries, and develop interventions that address these root causes.

6. Promote evidence-based practices: Promote the use of evidence-based practices for patient safety in developing countries, and invest in research to develop and test new interventions.

7. Foster collaboration: Foster collaboration between healthcare providers, researchers, policymakers, and other stakeholders to ensure that patient safety research is well-coordinated and effective.

8. Advocate for policy change: Advocate for policy change to promote patient safety in developing countries, and work with policymakers to ensure that patient safety is a priority in national health strategies.

9. Share findings: Share research findings and best practices with healthcare providers, policy-makers, and the public in developing countries, and support efforts to disseminate this information widely.

10. Monitor and evaluate: Develop monitoring and evaluation systems to track the effectiveness of patient safety interventions in developing countries, and use this information to make improvements over time.

11. Use technology: Use technology, such as electronic health records and telemedicine, to improve patient safety in developing countries, and invest in research to identify the most effective uses of these technologies.

12. Address social determinants of health: Address social determinants of health, such as poverty, gender inequality, and lack of access to education, that can contribute to patient safety issues in developing countries.

13. Support community-based interventions: Support the development of community-based interventions to improve patient safety in developing countries, and work with community leaders to ensure that these interventions are well-received and effective.

14. Build public awareness: Build public awareness of patient safety issues in developing countries, and work with communities to promote patient empowerment and engagement in healthcare.

15. Promote interdisciplinary collaboration: Promote collaboration between healthcare providers, researchers, and other professionals from different disciplines, such as public health, engineering, and psychology, to develop comprehensive and effective patient safety interventions.

16. Develop sustainable solutions: Develop sustainable solutions for patient safety in developing countries that are feasible and affordable in local contexts, and work with policymakers to ensure that these solutions are well-integrated into existing healthcare systems.

17. Build global partnerships: Build global partnerships between developed and developing countries to promote knowledge-sharing and collaboration on patient safety research and interventions.

18. Support advocacy efforts: Support advocacy efforts to promote patient safety in developing countries, and work with local organizations and international agencies to advance this agenda.

19. Foster ethical research: Foster ethical research practices in patient safety research in developing countries, and ensure that research is conducted in a way that respects the rights and dignity of patients and communities.

20. Promote accountability: Promote accountability for patient safety in developing countries by encouraging the use of incident reporting systems, establishing clear standards and guidelines for healthcare providers, and enforcing regulations and policies that promote patient safety.

21. Involve policymakers: Involve policymakers in the design and implementation of patient safety research in developing countries, and ensure that their perspectives and priorities are incorporated into research agendas.

22. Address healthcare disparities: Address healthcare disparities in developing countries by conducting research to identify the causes and consequences of these disparities, and developing interventions to address them.

23. Build trust: Build trust with patients, communities, and healthcare providers in developing countries by engaging in transparent and ethical research practices, and by communicating research findings clearly and effectively.

24. Promote education and training: Promote education and training in patient safety for healthcare providers in developing countries, and invest in the development of training materials and curricula that are tailored to local contexts.

25. Foster innovation: Foster innovation in patient safety research in developing countries by supporting the development of new tools, technologies, and approaches to improve patient safety.

26. Address resource constraints: Address resource constraints in developing countries by developing interventions that are cost-effective and scalable, and by working with policymakers to secure funding and resources for patient safety research and interventions.

27. Address data limitations: Address data limitations in developing countries by investing in the development of robust data collection and analysis systems, and by using innovative approaches to gather and analyze data on patient safety incidents.

28. Promote advocacy and activism: Promote advocacy and activism for patient safety in developing countries by working with patient and community organizations, and by supporting the development of patient-led initiatives to promote patient safety.

29. Foster cultural sensitivity: Foster cultural sensitivity in patient safety research in developing countries by working with local communities to understand their beliefs, values, and practices related to healthcare, and by incorporating these perspectives into research and interventions.

30. Promote collaboration with industry: Promote collaboration with industry to develop and implement patient safety interventions in developing countries, and ensure that these collaborations are transparent, ethical, and aligned with the needs and priorities of local communities.

47.4 CONCLUSION

This chapter has discussed the patient safety research in developing countries in terms of achievement, challenges and recommendations. Patient safety research in developing countries faces many challenges, including limited resources, infrastructure, and research capacity. However, by collaborating with local stakeholders, prioritizing patient engagement, addressing root causes of patient safety incidents, and fostering interdisciplinary collaboration, we can overcome these challenges and develop effective interventions to improve patient safety. It is also important to address social determinants of health, healthcare disparities, and resource constraints, and to promote education, innovation, and advocacy for patient safety in developing countries. By investing in patient safety research in developing countries and promoting global partnerships and knowledge-sharing, we can help ensure that patients around the world receive safe and effective healthcare.

REFERENCES

Al-Qahtani, I., Almoteb, T.M., & Al-Warafi, Y. (2015). Competency of metered-dose inhaler use among Saudi community pharmacists: A Simulation method study. *RRJPPS*, 4(2), 37–31.

Alshahrani, S.M., Alakhali, K.M., &Al-Worafi, Y.M., (2019a). Medication errors in a health care facility in southern Saudi Arabia. *Tropical Journal of Pharmaceutical Research*, 18(5), pp. 1119–1122.

Alshahrani, S.M., Alavudeen, S.S., Alakhali, K.M., Al-Worafi, Y.M., Bahamdan, A.K., & Vigneshwaran, E., (2019b). Self-Medication Among King Khalid University Students, *Saudi Arabia. Risk Management and Healthcare Policy*, 12, pp. 243–249.

Alshahrani, S.M., Alakhali, K.M., Al-Worafi, Y.M., & Alshahrani, N.Z. (2020b). Awareness and use of over the counter analgesic medication: a survey in the Aseer region population, *Saudi Arabia. Int J Advan Appl Sci*, 7(3), 130–134.

Alshahrani, S.M., Alzahran, M., Alakhali, K., Vigneshwaran, E., Iqbal, M.J., Khan, N.A., … & Alavudeen, S.S. (2020b). Association Between Diabetes Consequences and Quality of Life Among Patients With Diabetes Mellitus in the Aseer Province of Saudi Arabia. *Open Access Macedonian Journal of Medical Sciences*, 8(E), 325–330.

Al-Worafi, Y.M. (2014). Prescription writing errors at a tertiary care hospital in Yemen: prevalence, types, causes and recommendations. *Am J Pharm Health Res*, 2, 134–140.

Al-Worafi, Y.M.A. (2015). Appropriateness of metered-dose inhaler use in the Yemeni community pharmacies. *Journal of Taibah University Medical Sciences*, 10(3), 353–358.

Al-Worafi, Y.M.A. (2016). Pharmacy practice in Yemen. In *Pharmacy Practice in Developing Countries* (pp. 267–287). Academic Press.

Al-Worafi, Y.M., Kassab, Y.W., Alseragi, W.M., Almutairi, M.S., Ahmed, A., Ming, L.C., Alkhoshaiban, A.S., & Hadi, M.A., (2017). Pharmacovigilance and adverse drg reaction reporting: a perspective of community pharmacists and pharmacy technicians in Sana'a, Yemen. *Therapeutics and clinical risk management*, 13, p. 1175.

Al-Worafi, Y.M. (2018a). Knowledge, Attitude and Practice of Yemeni Physicians Toward Pharmacovigilance: A Mixed Method Study. *International Journal of Pharmacy and Pharmaceutical Sciences*. 10 (10), 74–77.

Al-Worafi, Y. (2018b). Knowledge, attitude and practice of Yemeni physicians toward pharmacovigilance: A mixed method study. *Int. J. Pharm. Pharm. Sci*, 10, 74–77.

Al-Worafi, Y.M. (2018c). Dispensing errors observed by community pharmacy dispensers in IBB–YEMEN. *Asian J. Pharm. Clin. Res*, 11(11), 478–481.

Al-Worafi, Y.M. (2018d). Evauation of inhaler technique among patients with asthma and COPD in Yemen. *Journal of Taibah University medical sciences*, 13(5), 488–490.

Al-Worafi, Y.M., Patel, R.P., Zaidi, S.T.R., Alseragi, W.M., Almutairi, M.S., Alkhoshaiban, A.S., & Ming, L.C. (2018a). Completeness and legibility of handwritten prescriptions in Sana'a, Yemen. *Medical Principles and Practice*, 27, 290–292.

Al-Worafi, Y.M., Alseragi, W.M., Seng, L.K., Kassab, Y.W., Yeoh, S.F., Chiau, L., ... & Husain, K. (2018b). Dispensing errors in community pharmacies: a prospective study in Sana'a, Yemen. *Arch Pharm Pract*, 9(4), 1–3.

Al-Worafi, Y.M., Alseragi, W.M., & Mahmoud, M.A. (2019). Competency of metered-dose inhaler use among community pharmacy dispensers in Ibb, Yemen: A simulation method study. *Latin American Journal of Pharmacy*, 38(3), 489–494.

Al-Worafi, Y.M. (Ed.). (2020a). Drug Safety in Developing Countries: Achievements and Challenges.

Al-Worafi, Y.M. (2020b). Medication errors. In *Drug Safety in Developing Countries* (pp. 105–117). Academic Press.

Al-Worafi, Y.M. (2020c). Adverse drug reactions. In *Drug Safety in Developing Countries* (pp. 39–57). Academic Press.

Al-Worafi, Y.M. (2020d). Medications registration and marketing: safety-related issues. In *Drug Safety in Developing Countries* (pp. 21–28). Academic Press.

Al-Worafi, Y.M. (2020e). Pharmacovigilance. In *Drug Safety in Developing Countries* (pp. 29–38). Academic Press.

Al-Worafi, Y.M. (2020f). Drug-related problems. In *Drug safety in developing countries* (pp. 59–71). Academic Press.

Al-Worafi, Y.M. (2020g). Medications safety-related terminology. In *Drug safety in developing countries* (pp. 7–19). Academic Press.

Al-Worafi, Y.M. (2020h). Self-medication. In *Drug Safety in Developing Countries* (pp. 73–86). Academic Press.

Al-Worafi, Y.M. (2020j). Antibiotics safety issues. In *Drug Safety in Developing Countries* (pp. 87–103). Academic Press.

Al-Worafi, Y.M. (2020k). Medications safety research issues. In *Drug Safety in Developing Countries* (pp. 213–227). Academic Press.

Al-Worafi, Y.M. (2020l). Counterfeit and substandard medications. In *Drug safety in developing countries* (pp. 119–126). Academic Press.

Al-Worafi, Y.M. (2020m). Medication abuse and misuse. In *Drug safety in developing countries* (pp. 127–135). Academic Press.

Al-Worafi, Y.M. (2020n). Storage and disposal of medications. In *Drug Safety in Developing Countries* (pp. 137–142). Academic Press.

Al-Worafi, Y.M. (2020o). Safety of medications in special population. In *Drug safety in developing countries* (pp. 143–162). Academic Press.

Al-Worafi, Y.M. (2020p). Herbal medicines safety issues. In *Drug Safety in developing countries* (pp. 163–178). Academic Press.

Al-Worafi, Y.M. (2020q). Medications safety pharmacoeconomics-related issues. In *Drug Safety in Developing Countries* (pp. 187–195). Academic Press.

Al-Worafi, Y.M. (2020r). Evidence-based medications safety practice. In *Drug Safety in Developing Countries* (pp. 197–201). Academic Press.

Al-Worafi, Y.M. (2020s). Quality indicators for medications safety. In *Drug safety in developing countries* (pp. 229–242). Academic Press.

Al-Worafi, Y.M. (2020t). Drug safety in Yemen. In *Drug Safety in Developing Countries* (pp. 391–405). Academic Press.

Al-Worafi, Y.M. (2020u). Drug safety in Saudi Arabia. In *Drug Safety in Developing Countries* (pp. 407–417). Academic Press.

Al-Worafi, Y.M. (2020v). Drug safety in United Arab Emirates. In *Drug Safety in Developing Countries* (pp. 419–428). Academic Press.

Al-Worafi, Y.M. (2020w). Drug safety in Indonesia. In *Drug Safety in Developing Countries* (pp. 279–285). Academic Press.

Al-Worafi, Y.M. (2020x). Drug safety in Palestine. In *Drug Safety in Developing Countries* (pp. 471–480). Academic Press.

Al-Worafi, Y.M. (2020y). Drug safety: comparison between developing countries. In *Drug Safety in Developing Countries* (pp. 603–611). Academic Press.

Al-Worafi, Y.M. (2020z). Drug safety in developing versus developed countries. In *Drug Safety in Developing Countries* (pp. 613–615). Academic Press.

Al-Worafi, Y.M., Alseragi, W.M., Ming, L.C., & Alakhali, K.M. (2020a). Drug safety in China. In *Drug Safety in Developing Countries* (pp. 381–388). Academic Press.

Al-Worafi, Y.M., Alseragi, W.M., Alakhali, K.M., Ming, L.C., Othman, G., Halboup, A.M., … & Elkalmi, R.M. (2020b). Knowledge, beliefs and factors affecting the use of generic medicines among patients in Ibb, Yemen: a mixed-method study. *Journal of Pharmacy Practice and Community Medicine*, 6(4), 53–56.

Al-Worafi, Y.M., Elkalmi, R.M., Ming, L.C., Othman, G., Halboup, A.M., Battah, M.M., … & Mani, V. (2021a). Dispensing errors in hospital pharmacies: A prospective study in Yemen.

Al-Worafi, Y.M., Hasan, S., Hassan, N.M., & Gaili, A.A. (2021b). Knowledge, Attitude and Experience of Pharmacist in the UAE towards Pharmacovigilance. *Research Journal of Pharmacy and Technology*, 14(1), 265–269.

Al-Worafi, Y. (2022a). *A Guide to Online Pharmacy Education: Teaching Strategies and Assessment Methods*. CRC Press.

Al-Worafi, Y. (2022b). History and Importance. In *A Guide to Online Pharmacy Education: Teaching Strategies and Assessment Methods*. CRC Press.

Al-Worafi, Y. (2022c). Terminologies. In *A Guide to Online Pharmacy Education: Teaching Strategies and Assessment Methods*. CRC Press.

Al-Worafi, Y. (2022d). Research Methods and Methodology. In *A Guide to Online Pharmacy Education: Teaching Strategies and Assessment Methods*. CRC Press.

Al-Worafi, Y.M. (Ed.). (2023). *Clinical Case Studies on medication Safety*. Academic Press.

Baig, M.R., Al-Worafi, Y.M., Alseragi, W.M., Ming, L.C., & Siddique, A. (2020). Drug safety in India. In *Drug Safety in Developing Countries* (pp. 327–334). Academic Press.

Elkalmi, R.M., Al-Worafi, Y.M., Alseragi, W.M., Ming, L.C., & Siddique, A. (2020). Drug safety in Malaysia. In *Drug Safety in Developing Countries* (pp. 245–253). Academic Press.

Elsayed, T., & Al-Worafi, Y.M. (2020). Drug safety in Egypt. In *Drug Safety in Developing Countries* (pp. 511–523). Academic Press.

Hasan, S., Al-Omar, M.J., AlZubaidy, H., & Al-Worafi, Y.M. (2019). Use of medications in Arab Countries. In *Handbook of Healthcare in the Arab World*. Cham: Springer, 42.

Hassan, Y., Abd Aziz, N., Kassab, Y.W., Elgasim, I., Shaharuddin, S., Al-Worafi, Y.M.A., ... & Ming, L.C. (2014). How to help patients to control their blood pressure? Blood pressure control and its predictor. *Archives of Pharmacy Practice*. 5(4), 153–161.

Izahar, S., Lean, Q.Y., Hameed, M.A., Murugiah, M.K., Patel, R.P., Al-Worafi, Y.M., ... & Ming, L.C. (2017). Content analysis of mobile health applications on diabetes mellitus. *Frontiers in Endocrinology*, 8, p. 318.

Lee, K.S., Yee, S.M., Zaidi, S.T.R., Patel, R.P., Yang, Q., Al-Worafi, Y.M., & Ming, L.C., 2017. Combating sale of counterfeit and falsified medicines online: a losing battle. *Frontiers in pharmacology*, 8, p. 268.

Mahmoud, M.A., Wajid, S., Naqvi, A.A., Samreen, S., Althagfan, S.S., & Al-Worafi, Y. (2020). Self-medication with antibiotics: A cross-sectional community-based study. *Latin American Journal Of Pharmacy*, 39(2), 348–353.

Manan, M.M., Rusli, R.A., Ang, W.C., Al-Worafi, Y.M., & Ming, L.C. (2014). Assessing the pharmaceutical care issues of antiepileptic drug therapy in hospitalised epileptic patients. *Journal of Pharmacy Practice and Research*, 44(3), 83–88.

Manan, M.M., Ibrahim, N.A., Aziz, N.A., Zulkifly, H.H., Al-Worafi, Y.M.A., & Long, C.M. (2016). Empirical use of antibiotic therapy in the prevention of early onset sepsis in neonates: a pilot study. *Archives of Medical Science*, 12(3), 603–613.

Ming, L.C., Hameed, M.A., Lee, D.D., Apidi, N.A., Lai, P.S.M., Hadi, M.A., Al-Worafi, Y.M.A., & Khan, T.M., (2016). Use of medical mobile applications among hospital pharmacists in Malaysia. *Therapeutic innovation & regulatory science*, 50(4), pp. 419–426.

Ming, L.C., Untong, N., Aliudin, N.A., Osili, N., Kifli, N., Tan, C.S., … & Goh, H.P. (2020). Mobile health apps on COVID-19 launched in the early days of the pandemic: content analysis and review. *JMIR mHealth and uHealth*, 8(9), e19796.

Othman, G., Ali, F., Ibrahim, M.I.M., Al-Worafi, Y.M., Ansari, M., & Halboup, A.M. (2020). Assessment of Anti-Diabetic Medications Adherence among Diabetic Patients in Sana'a City, Yemen: A Cross Sectional Study. *Journal of Pharmaceutical Research International*, 32(21), 114–122.

Saeed, M.S., Alkhoshaiban, A.S., Al-Worafi, Y.M.A., & Long, C.M., (2014). Perception of self-medication among university students in Saudi Arabia. *Archives of Pharmacy Practice*, 5(4), p. 149.

SECTION 4

PATIENT SAFETY CASE STUDIES

48 Patient Safety Case Studies

Patient Care Plan Errors and Related Problems (Part I)

48.1 IMPORTANCE OF PATIENT SAFETY & PATIENT CARE PLAN ERRORS AND RELATED PROBLEMS CASE STUDIES

Patient safety case studies are an essential tool for improving healthcare quality and safety. Prepare the future healthcare professionals with the necessary competencies related to the patient safety-related issues are the key to success in medication safety practice in the future, however, improving the current healthcare professionals' medication safety competencies is very important in order to improve the patients' treating outcomes in terms of efficacy and safety. They provide a detailed analysis of a specific patient safety incident or event, which can help identify the root causes, contributing factors, and possible solutions to prevent similar incidents from occurring in the future. Here are some of the key reasons why patient safety case studies are important:

1. Learning from mistakes: Patient safety case studies highlight the mistakes that were made in a specific incident, providing an opportunity for healthcare providers to learn from those mistakes and prevent them from happening again in the future.

2. Improving safety culture: By sharing patient safety case studies across healthcare organizations, staff can become more aware of the importance of safety culture, and how their actions and decisions can impact patient safety.

3. Identifying systemic issues: Patient safety case studies can reveal patterns or trends in safety incidents, which can help identify systemic issues that need to be addressed to improve patient safety.

4. Developing best practices: By analyzing patient safety case studies, healthcare providers can develop best practices for preventing similar incidents from occurring in the future. This can include changes to policies, procedures, or training programs.

5. Enhancing communication: Patient safety case studies can be used as a tool to enhance communication between healthcare providers, patients, and their families. Sharing these stories can help to build trust, foster transparency, and encourage open communication.

Overall, patient safety case studies are a critical component of any patient safety program. By examining specific incidents in detail, healthcare providers can learn from mistakes, improve safety culture, and ultimately improve patient outcomes (Al-Worafi et al., 2020a–e; Al-Worafi, 2022a,b; Al-Worafi, 2023; Vincent, 2011).

48.2 CASE 1. PREVENTIVE MEDICINE ERRORS

Patient data
Age: 46 years. **Gender:** Feale. **Weight:** 76 kg, **Height:** 1.65 m

Chief Complaint
The patient presented to a primary care clinic for a routine check-up and to receive preventive medicine.

History of Present Illness
NA

Past Medical History
Not significant for any disease.

Past Medications History
NA

Family History
Father with diabetes mellitus and hypertension

Social History

■ Married

DOI: 10.1201/9781003230465-52

- Non-Smoker

- Lack of exercise

Allergies
NKDA

Physical Examination
Vital Signs: Blood pressure: 120/80 mmHg Heart rate: 76 bpm Respiratory rate: 18 breaths per minute Temperature: 98.6 °F
General: The patient appeared healthy and in no acute distress.
Skin: No lesions or abnormalities were noted.
Head, Eyes, Ears, Nose, and Throat (HEENT): No abnormalities were noted.
Chest: Lungs were clear to auscultation.
Cardiovascular: Heart sounds were regular and without murmurs or gallops.
Abdomen: No tenderness, distention, or masses were noted.
Genitourinary: Normal female external genitalia without discharge or lesions.
Extremities: No swelling, deformity, or tenderness were noted.
Neurological: Cranial nerves were intact. Muscle strength, tone, and reflexes were normal.
Laboratory Findings: None ordered.

Medication safety issue analysis
Diagnosis and Management: The patient was due for a Tdap vaccine and HPV vaccine as part of her routine preventive medicine. The healthcare provider mistakenly administered the Tdap vaccine twice, instead of administering the HPV vaccine. The patient was not informed of the error at the time of administration.

Preventive Medicine Errors: Preventive medicine errors can occur when healthcare providers do not follow proper protocols or when there is a lack of communication or documentation. In this case, the healthcare provider mistakenly administered the wrong vaccine, which could have potentially harmful consequences. It is important for healthcare providers to follow protocols and double-check medications and vaccines to prevent errors from occurring. Additionally, patients should be informed of any errors that occur, so they can receive appropriate care and monitoring.

Follow-Up: The patient should be informed of the error and should receive appropriate monitoring for any adverse effects. The correct HPV vaccine should be administered at the next visit, and the healthcare provider should take steps to prevent future errors. The incident should be reported to the appropriate governing body and documented in the patient's medical record.

48.3 CASE 2. HEALTH EDUCATION ERROR

A 37-year-old male who presented to his primary care physician with a complaint of chronic cough, which has been persistent for the last six months. Upon further evaluation, it was revealed that this patient has a history of asthma, which he was diagnosed with during childhood. His asthma has been well-controlled over the years, but he has been experiencing more frequent exacerbations in the last six months.

During the consultation, the physician prescribed a combination inhaler containing both a bronchodilator and an inhaled corticosteroid, as well as provided Patient X with health education on how to use the inhaler correctly. The physician demonstrated how to use the inhaler, and the patient was asked to demonstrate the technique back to the physician to ensure that he understood how to use it correctly. A few weeks later, the patient returned to the clinic with no improvement in his symptoms. Upon further inquiry, it was discovered that the patient had not been using the inhaler as prescribed. The patient reported that he found the inhaler too complicated to use and had not been using it regularly. Upon further discussion, it became clear that the patient had misunderstood the health education provided to him during his initial consultation.

Root Cause Analysis:
The root cause of this error was a breakdown in communication during the health education process. Although the physician had demonstrated the correct technique for using the inhaler, the patient had not fully understood the instructions provided to him. The physician had assumed that the patient had understood the instructions and had not taken the time to confirm that he had

understood them correctly. Additionally, Patient X had not been provided with written instructions or other resources that could have helped him to better understand how to use the inhaler.

Lessons Learned:
This case highlights the importance of effective health education and communication in ensuring that patients understand how to manage their conditions effectively. Physicians and other healthcare professionals should take the time to ensure that patients understand their instructions and are comfortable with the techniques and devices they need to use to manage their conditions. Written instructions and other resources, such as videos or online tutorials, can be helpful in reinforcing health education and ensuring that patients are able to manage their conditions effectively. Additionally, follow-up appointments and check-ins can help to ensure that patients are adhering to their treatment plans and using medications and devices correctly.

48.4 CASE 3. HEALTH SCREENING ERROR

Patient Data: A 52-year-old woman, presented to a primary care clinic for her routine annual health screening. She had no significant medical history and no current complaints or symptoms. Her family history was significant for hypertension and heart disease.

Medical History: She had a history of smoking 10 cigarettes per day for the past 20 years. She had never had a mammogram or colonoscopy.

Physical Examination: vital signs were within normal limits. Her physical examination was unremarkable.

Screening Tests: She was scheduled for a mammogram and colonoscopy as part of her routine health screening.

Case Discussion: The patient returned to the clinic two weeks later for a follow-up visit to discuss the results of her health screening tests. The mammogram results were normal. However, the colonoscopy report indicated the presence of a large polyp in her colon. The polyp was removed during the procedure, and subsequent biopsy results confirmed it was cancerous.
The clinic staff reviewed her chart and discovered that they had failed to order a fecal occult blood test (FOBT) as part of her health screening. FOBT is a non-invasive test that can detect the presence of blood in the stool, which can be an early sign of colon cancer.
It was determined that the error occurred because the staff member who entered the screening order into the electronic medical record system did not include the FOBT test. Instead, they only ordered the colonoscopy.
Recommendations: Health screening errors can have serious consequences for patients. To prevent such errors, clinics and healthcare providers must have a robust system in place for ordering and tracking screening tests. It is essential to ensure that all recommended screening tests are ordered, and the results are appropriately reviewed and communicated to the patient.
Clinics should also consider using electronic health records and decision support systems to help ensure that all recommended screening tests are ordered for patients based on their age, gender, medical history, and other risk factors.
In this case, it is crucial to inform the patient about the missed test and the need for regular follow-up screening. The clinic staff should also offer counseling and support for the patient to help her cope with the diagnosis and provide appropriate treatment referrals.

48.5 CASE 4. CASE OF PATIENT EDUCATION ERROR

A 41 year old male patient presented at the local community pharmacy with a new prescription containing asthma related medications.
Medication safety name
Education and counseling errors

Medication safety issue analysis
The patient received the prescribed medications from the pharmacy without any education and counseling.

Recommendations
The appropriate management should include the appropriate patient education and counseling about the management plan, adherence towards the management plan (non-pharmacological,

pharmacological therapies and monitoring parameters), self-management, potential adverse drug effects & reactions, possible interactions, cautions & precautions, contraindications & warning, proper storage, disposal of medications and other related information about medications. Improving the knowledge of health care professionals towards the recent treatment guidelines are very important and can be done through workshops and training courses.

48.6 CASE 5. CASE OF PRESCRIBING ERROR

Patient data
Age: 49 years. **Gender:** Male. **Weight:** 96 kg **Height:** 1.77 m

Chief Complaint
Headache

History of Present Illness
A 49-year-old man visited the local hospital suffering from headache during the last two weeks and not improved with analgesics

Past Medical History
Not significant for any disease

Past Medications History
NA

Family History
Not significant

Social History

■ Married

■ Smoker

Allergies
NKDA

Physical Examination

General	The patient appeared well
BP	145/90 mmHg
HR	98 bpm
RR	20 bpm
Temperature	°C 37
Skin	Normal
HEENT	Normal
Chest	Normal
Heart	Normal
Abd	Normal
Genit/Rect	Normal
Ext	Normal
Neuro	Normal

Laboratory findings
Complete blood count
Within normal limits

Kidney function and electrolyte tests
Within normal limits

Liver function tests
Within normal limits

Lipid profile
Significant for increasing total cholesterol and low-density lipoprotein, the increase were low.

Cardio enzymes tests
Within normal limits

Endocrine tests
HbA1c was 6.5

Other investigations
None.

Diagnosis
Hypertension and dyslipidemia

Case discussion and Medication safety issue analysis
Medication safety name
Prescribing errors

Medication safety issue analysis
A man aged 49 presented himself at the nearby hospital due to persistent headaches for the past two weeks, which did not subside despite taking painkillers. Following examination, the patient was found to be suffering from hypertension and dyslipidemia. As a treatment plan, the doctor prescribed simvastatin and perindopril. This was the first time that the patient had been diagnosed with hypertension and dyslipidemia, and the results of his medical tests were generally within normal ranges, except for slightly elevated lipid profile and blood pressure readings. Statin could be delay to another follow-up if the patient lipid profile will not improv with the non-pharmacological interventions. Another related problem, the patient hbA1c level was above the normal range, therefore, educate patient about the importance of weight control and other lfe-style changes could help patient.

Recommendations
It is crucial to choose the appropriate treatment plan in order to achieve desired outcomes, prevent complications, and improve the overall health and well-being of patients. To determine the best course of drug therapy, prescribers should remain informed about the latest research through various means, such as reviewing literature, consulting with pharmacists and other physicians, participating in continuing education programs, and other similar methods. Healthcare professionals have a responsibility to ensure patient safety, including the safety of the medications prescribed and dispensed. Effective communication among healthcare professionals during the management process is vital to achieving desired outcomes. Enhancing the knowledge of healthcare professionals regarding prescription errors and ways to avoid them is critical to minimizing their occurrence and treating them when they do occur. Identifying potential causes and reasons for prescription errors is crucial in designing necessary interventions to prevent them. Staying up-to-date with recent guidelines is essential for the best practices.

48.7 CASE 6. CASE OF PATIENT EDUCATION ERROR

Case summary
Patient data
Age: 22 years. **Gender:** Female. **Weight:** 70 kg, **Height:** 1.61 m

Chief Complaint
Acne

History of Present Illness
A 22-year-old woman taking isotretinoin tablets for her acne.

Past Medical History
Not significant for any disease

Past Medications History
NA

Family History
Not significant for any disease

Social History

■ Single

■ Non smoker

Allergies
NKDA

Physical Examination

General	The patient appeared generally well
BP	130/80 mmHg
HR	84 bpm
RR	19
Temperature	°C 37
Skin	Dry
HEENT	Normal
Chest	Normal
Heart	Normal
Abd	Normal
Genit/Rect	Normal
Ext	Normal
Neuro	Normal

Laboratory findings
Complete blood count
NA

Kidney function and electrolyte tests
NA

Liver function tests
NA

Lipid profile
NA

Cardio enzymes tests
NA

Endocrine tests
NA

Other investigations
None.

Case discussion and Medication safety issue analysis
Medication safety name
Education and counseling errors

Medication safety issue analysis
The patient takes isotretinoin for her acne. However, there were many essential monitoring parameters to evaluate the treating outcomes not requested for her such as liver function tests.

Recommendations
The appropriate management should include the appropriate patient education and counseling about the management plan, adherence towards the management plan (non-pharmacological,

pharmacological therapies and monitoring parameters), self-management, potential adverse drug effects & reactions, possible interactions, cautions & precautions, contraindications & warning, proper storage, disposal of medications and other related information about medications. Improving the knowledge of health care professionals towards the recent treatment guidelines are very important and can be done through workshops and training courses.

48.8 CONCLUSION

This chapter has discussed the real cases of patient care errors and problems. Patient safety case studies are an essential tool for improving healthcare quality and safety. They provide a detailed analysis of a specific patient safety incident or event, which can help identify the root causes, contributing factors, and possible solutions to prevent similar incidents from occurring in the future.

REFERENCES

Al-Worafi, Y. M. (Ed.). (2020a). Drug Safety in Developing Countries: Achievements and Challenges.

Al-Worafi, Y. M. (2020b). Evidence-based medications safety practice. In *Drug Safety in Developing Countries* (pp. 197–201). Academic Press

Al-Worafi, Y. M. (2020c). Quality indicators for medications safety. In *Drug safety in developing countries* (pp. 229–242). Academic Press.

Al-Worafi, Y. M. (2020d). Drug safety: comparison between developing countries. In *Drug Safety in Developing Countries* (pp. 603–611). Academic Press.

Al-Worafi, Y. M. (2020e). Drug safety in developing versus developed countries. In *Drug Safety in Developing Countries* (pp. 613–615). Academic Press.

Al-Worafi, Y.M. (2022a). *A Guide to Online Pharmacy Education: Teaching Strategies and Assessment Methods*. CRC Press.

Al-Worafi, Y. M. (2022b). Patient care errors and related problems (part I): development and validation of the model. https://orcid.org/0000-0002-5752-2913

Al-Worafi, Y. M. (Ed.). (2023). *Clinical Case Studies on medication Safety*. Academic Press.

Vincent, C. (2011). *Patient safety*. John Wiley & Sons.

49 Patient Safety Case Studies

Patient Care Plan Errors and Related Problems (Part II)

49.1 IMPORTANCE OF PATIENT SAFETY & PATIENT CARE PLAN ERRORS AND RELATED PROBLEMS CASE STUDIES

Patient care case studies are important for healthcare professionals, including doctors, nurses, and pharmacists, for several reasons: Improving diagnostic and clinical skills: Patient care case studies provide healthcare professionals with real-world examples of patients with a variety of medical conditions. Analyzing case studies can improve diagnostic and clinical skills by exposing healthcare professionals to a range of presentations and challenging them to identify and treat the underlying conditions. Enhancing problem-solving abilities: Patient care case studies often involve complex medical issues that require critical thinking and problem-solving skills. Healthcare professionals can benefit from analyzing and discussing case studies to develop their ability to address complex medical issues. Promoting evidence-based practice: Patient care case studies can highlight best practices and provide examples of how to apply evidence-based medicine in clinical settings. Reviewing and analyzing case studies can promote adherence to evidence-based guidelines and improve patient outcomes. Fostering teamwork and communication skills: Patient care often involves a multidisciplinary team of healthcare professionals. Case studies provide an opportunity for healthcare professionals to collaborate and communicate with each other, developing their teamwork and communication skills. Improving patient care: Ultimately, patient care case studies can help healthcare professionals provide better care to their patients. Analyzing and discussing real-world examples can help healthcare professionals identify gaps in their knowledge and skills, improve their clinical decision-making, and ultimately provide better care to their patients Patient safety case studies are an essential tool for improving healthcare quality and safety. Prepare the future healthcare professionals with the necessary competencies related to the patient safety-related issues are the key to success in medication safety practice in the future, however, improving the current healthcare professionals' medication safety competencies is very important in order to improve the patients' treating outcomes in terms of efficacy and safety. They provide a detailed analysis of a specific patient safety incident or event, which can help identify the root causes, contributing factors, and possible solutions to prevent similar incidents from occurring in the future. Here are some of the key reasons why patient safety case studies are important:

1. Learning from mistakes: Patient safety case studies highlight the mistakes that were made in a specific incident, providing an opportunity for healthcare providers to learn from those mistakes and prevent them from happening again in the future.

2. Improving safety culture: By sharing patient safety case studies across healthcare organizations, staff can become more aware of the importance of safety culture, and how their actions and decisions can impact patient safety.

3. Identifying systemic issues: Patient safety case studies can reveal patterns or trends in safety incidents, which can help identify systemic issues that need to be addressed to improve patient safety.

4. Developing best practices: By analyzing patient safety case studies, healthcare providers can develop best practices for preventing similar incidents from occurring in the future. This can include changes to policies, procedures, or training programs.

5. Enhancing communication: Patient safety case studies can be used as a tool to enhance communication between healthcare providers, patients, and their families. Sharing these stories can help to build trust, foster transparency, and encourage open communication.

Overall, patient safety case studies are a critical component of any patient safety program. By examining specific incidents in detail, healthcare providers can learn from mistakes, improve safety culture, and ultimately improve patient outcomes (Al-Worafi et al., 2020a-e; Al-Worafi, 2022a,b; Al-Worafi, 2023; Vincent, 2011).

49.2 CASE 1. CASE OF MILD ADVERSE DRUG REACTION

Patient data

Age: 7 years. **Gender:** Female. **Weight:** 22 kg **Height:** 1.11 m

Chief Complaint

Vomiting

History of Present Illness

A 7-year-old girl accompanied by her mother visited a community pharmacy complaining of vomiting that had started a day ago. The mother reported that the vomiting began after administering amoxicillin/clavulanate suspension for her daughter's otitis media. The mother also mentioned that her child was unable to tolerate the medication and vomited it out.

Past Medical History

Not significant for any disease

Past Medications History

None

Family History

Not significant for any disease

Social History

Both parents are in good health. She is living with one brother, and they are in good health.

Allergies

NKDA

Physical Examination

General	Pale
BP	NA
HR	NA
RR	NA
Temperature	°C 38
Skin	NA
HEENT	NA
Chest	NA
Heart	NA
Abd	NA
Genit/Rect	NA
Ext	NA
Neuro	NA

Laboratory findings

Complete blood count

Significant for high white blood cells.

Kidney function and electrolyte tests

NA

Liver function tests

NA

Lipid profile

NA

Cardio enzymes tests

NA

Endocrine tests
NA

Other investigations
NA

Case discussion and Medication safety issue analysis
The patient was diagnosed with otitis media. She had vomiting occurred after taking amoxicillin-clavulanate.

Medication safety name	Mild adverse drug reactions
Medication safety potential causes	amoxicillin-clavulanate.
Management	Stop amoxicillin-clavulanate. Change amoxicillin-clavulanate to ceftriaxone intramuscular injection.
Recommendations	Adherence to prescribed regimens may be affected by various reasons, one of which is vomiting. Pharmacists can play a vital role in ensuring medication safety by improving adherence to both non-pharmacological and pharmacological interventions, thereby preventing or minimizing potential drug-related problems, including adverse drug reactions. Effective patient education and counseling by pharmacists are essential for achieving the desired outcomes for treating patients, including clinical, economical, and humanistic outcomes. By educating patients about adverse drug reactions and how to minimize or prevent them, especially mild ADRs, pharmacists can prevent or minimize them at the time of dispensing medications. If adverse drug reactions occur due to any reason, pharmacists can manage them, as in this case, by stopping the medication and changing it to another medication that will not cause vomiting.

49.3 CASE 2. CASE OF THERAPEUTIC EVALUATION ERROR (MONITORING PARAMETERS ERRORS)

Patient data
Age: 55 years. **Gender:** Male. **Weight:** 80 kg **Height:** 1.72 m

Chief Complaint
Chest pain

History of Present Illness
A 55-year-old man visited the hospital with chest pain

Past Medical History
Not significant for any disease

Past Medications History
NA

Family History
Father with hypertension and diabetes mellitus

Social History
Married
Smoker for 25 years

Allergies
NKDA

Physical Examination

General	The patient appeared well
BP	145/90
HR	102
RR	20
Temperature	°C 37
Skin	Normal
HEENT	Normal
Chest	Chest pain
Heart	Normal
Abd	Normal
Genit/Rect	Normal
Ext	Normal
Neuro	Normal

Laboratory findings
Complete blood count
Within normal limits

Kidney function and electrolyte tests
Within normal limits

Liver function tests
Within normal limits

Lipid profile
Significant for increased low-density lipoprotein, triglycerides and total cholesterol

Cardio enzymes tests
Within normal limits

Endocrine tests
Within normal limits

Other investigations
NA

Diagnosis
Hypertension
Dyslipidemia

Case discussion and Medication safety issue analysis
A 55-year-old man visited the hospital with chest pain.

Medication safety name
Monitoring errors

Medication safety issue analysis
The patient left the hospital with a prescription of medications for his hypertension and dyslipidemia. The patient was discharged from the hospital with a scheduled appointment three months later. Unfortunately, there were critical monitoring parameters that were not requested, including daily blood pressure measurements at home and recording the readings for the upcoming visit. It's crucial to follow up with newly diagnosed patients during the first two weeks and first month to assess their adherence to non-pharmacological and pharmacological interventions.

Recommendations
The appropriate management should include the recommended monitoring parameters to evaluate the therapeutic outcomes. Evaluate the efficacy, safety of medications, adherence to the non-pharmacological and pharmacological interventions, the absence of adverse drug reactions and the

potential complications are the keys of success in the treatment. Improving the knowledge of health care professionals towards the recent treatment guidelines are very important and can be done through workshops and training courses.

49.4 CASE 3. CASE OF PRESCRIBING ERRORS

Patient data
Age: 43 years. **Gender:** Male. **Weight:** 94 kg, **Height:** 1.76 m

Chief Complaint
Headache

History of Present Illness
A 43-year-old man presented to the local hospital suffering from recurrent headache

Past Medical History
Not significant for any disease.

Past Medications History
NA

Family History
Father & mother with diabetes mellitus and hypertension

Social History
Married
Smoker

Allergies
NKDA

Physical Examination
Vital signs

General	The patient appeared generally well
BP	150/90 mmHg
HR	101 bpm
RR	17
Temperature	°C 37
Skin	Normal
HEENT	Normal
Chest	Normal
Heart	Normal
Abd	Normal
Genit/Rect	Normal
Ext	Normal
Neuro	Normal

Laboratory findings
Complete blood count
Within normal limits

Kidney function and electrolyte tests
Within normal limits

Liver function tests
Within normal limits

Lipid profile
Significant for high total cholesterol, low-density lipoprotein and triglycerides

Cardio enzymes tests
Within normal limits

Endocrine tests
Significant for high fasting blood glucose level (220 mg/dl) and HbA1c (13%)

Other investigations
NA

Diagnosis
Dyslipidemia
Hypertension
Diabetes mellitus type 2

Case discussion and Medication safety issue analysis
A 43-year-old man presented to the local hospital suffering from recurrent headache

Medication safety name
Prescribing errors

Medication safety issue analysis
Upon arrival at the local hospital, a man who is 43 years old complained of recurrent headaches. He was subsequently diagnosed with Dyslipidemia, Hypertension, and Diabetes mellitus type 2. His prescribed medications include Metformin, Captopril, and Atorvastatin. When a patient's HbA1c level exceeds 9%, combination therapy is required to manage diabetes mellitus type 2. The patient's HbA1c level is 11%, indicating that the addition of Glibenclamide is necessary.

Recommendations
It is crucial to select the appropriate treatment regimen in order to achieve desired outcomes, prevent complications, and enhance the health and well-being of patients. To determine the most appropriate drug therapy, prescribers should remain up-to-date with the latest research by conducting literature reviews, consulting with pharmacists and other physicians, participating in continuing professional education programs, and utilizing other relevant resources. Healthcare professionals have a responsibility to ensure the safety of their patients by prescribing and dispensing medications in a safe manner. Communication between healthcare professionals during the management cycle is paramount in achieving the desired outcomes. To prevent and minimize prescribing errors, healthcare professionals should increase their knowledge of such errors and learn how to avoid them. Identifying the potential causes and reasons for prescribing errors is essential to implementing necessary interventions. Keeping up-to-date with recent guidelines is crucial to ensuring best practices.

49.5 CASE 4. CASE OF DISPENSING ERROR

A male patient of 52 years of age visited the local pharmacy with a prescription for metformin 750 mg XR twice daily and Glibenclamide 5 mg once daily. However, the pharmacy provided him with metformin 500 mg/Glibenclamide 2.5 mg instead.

Medication safety name
Dispensing errors

Medication safety issue analysis
The patient received the medication with different dosage regimen, which could affect the efficacy of regimen as well as increase the risk of gastrointestinal tract adverse effects.

Recommendations
Following good dispensing practices has a positive impact on both the patient's health and the healthcare system. It can lead to improved treatment outcomes, decreased hospital admissions, reduced morbidity and mortality, lower therapy costs, enhanced quality of life, increased patient satisfaction with healthcare, and a reduced burden on hospitals. Dispensing quality indicators are crucial for evaluating dispensing practices, identifying challenges and problems, and developing and implementing action plans to improve the practice (Al-Worafi, 2020a-c). Accurate medication dispensing is vital, and healthcare professionals, including pharmacists, have a responsibility to ensure the safety of prescribed and dispensed medications. Effective communication among healthcare

professionals during the management cycle is crucial to achieve desired treatment outcomes. Improving healthcare professionals' knowledge of dispensing errors and how to prevent them can help avoid/minimize prescribing errors and manage them when they occur. Identifying potential causes and reasons for dispensing errors is critical in designing necessary interventions to prevent them.

49.6 CASE 5. CASE OF ADMINISTRATION ERRORS

A man of 65 years of age arrived at the emergency department due to gastrointestinal bleeding caused by the consumption of a high dose of ibuprofen.

Medication safety name
Administration errors

Medication safety issue analysis
The dispensing of ibuprofen was intended for an older patient suffering from back pain; however, the patient mistakenly took ibuprofen 600 mg three times per day instead of ibuprofen 400 mg when necessary.

Recommendations
Healthcare professionals, including pharmacists, bear a responsibility for ensuring patient safety by safeguarding prescribed and dispensed medications. Communication between healthcare professionals during the management cycle is critical to achieve the desired treatment outcomes. Effective patient education and counseling are essential to achieving the desired clinical, economic, and humanistic outcomes when treating patients with anemia. Educating patients about adverse drug reactions (ADRs) and providing guidance on how to minimize or prevent them can prevent or minimize their occurrence during medication dispensing. However, if ADRs occur for any reason, identifying their potential causes is essential to managing them.

49.7 CONCLUSION

This chapter has discussed the real cases of patient care errors and problems. Patient safety case studies are an essential tool for improving healthcare quality and safety. They provide a detailed analysis of a specific patient safety incident or event, which can help identify the root causes, contributing factors, and possible solutions to prevent similar incidents from occurring in the future.

REFERENCES
Al-Worafi, Y.M. (Ed.). (2020a). Drug Safety in Developing Countries: Achievements and Challenges.

Al-Worafi, Y.M. (2020b). Evidence-based medications safety practice. In *Drug Safety in Developing Countries* (pp. 197–201). Academic Press.

Al-Worafi, Y.M. (2020c). Quality indicators for medications safety. In *Drug safety in Developing Countries* (pp. 229–242). Academic Press.

Al-Worafi, Y.M. (2020d). Drug safety: comparison between developing countries. In *Drug Safety in Developing Countries* (pp. 603–611). Academic Press.

Al-Worafi, Y.M. (2020e). Drug safety in developing versus developed countries. In *Drug Safety in Developing Countries* (pp. 613–615). Academic Press.

Al-Worafi, Y. (2022a). *A Guide to Online Pharmacy Education: Teaching Strategies and Assessment Methods*. CRC Press.

Al-Worafi, Y.M. (2022b). Patient care errors and related problems (part I): development and validation of the model. https://orcid.org/0000-0002-5752-2913

Al-Worafi, Y.M. (Ed.). (2023). *Clinical Case Studies on medication Safety*. Academic Press.

Vincent, C. (2011). *Patient safety*. John Wiley & Sons.

50 Patient Safety Case Studies

Nosocomial Infections Cases

50.1 IMPORTANCE OF PATIENT SAFETY & PATIENT CARE PLAN ERRORS AND RELATED PROBLEMS CASE STUDIES

Patient safety case studies are an essential tool for improving healthcare quality and safety. Prepare the future healthcare professionals with the necessary competencies related to the patient safety-related issues are the key to success in medication safety practice in the future, however, improving the current healthcare professionals' medication safety competencies is very important in order to improve the patients' treating outcomes in terms of efficacy and safety. They provide a detailed analysis of a specific patient safety incident or event, which can help identify the root causes, contributing factors, and possible solutions to prevent similar incidents from occurring in the future. Here are some of the key reasons why patient safety case studies are important:

1. Learning from mistakes: Patient safety case studies highlight the mistakes that were made in a specific incident, providing an opportunity for healthcare providers to learn from those mistakes and prevent them from happening again in the future.

2. Improving safety culture: By sharing patient safety case studies across healthcare organizations, staff can become more aware of the importance of safety culture, and how their actions and decisions can impact patient safety.

3. Identifying systemic issues: Patient safety case studies can reveal patterns or trends in safety incidents, which can help identify systemic issues that need to be addressed to improve patient safety.

4. Developing best practices: By analyzing patient safety case studies, healthcare providers can develop best practices for preventing similar incidents from occurring in the future. This can include changes to policies, procedures, or training programs.

5. Enhancing communication: Patient safety case studies can be used as a tool to enhance communication between healthcare providers, patients, and their families. Sharing these stories can help to build trust, foster transparency, and encourage open communication.

Overall, patient safety case studies are a critical component of any patient safety program. By examining specific incidents in detail, healthcare providers can learn from mistakes, improve safety culture, and ultimately improve patient outcomes (Al-Worafi et al., 2020a-e; Al-Worafi, 2022a,b; Al-Worafi, 2023; Vincent, 2011).

50.2 CASE 1. CASE OF HOSPITAL-ACQUIRED PNEUMONIA

A 71-year-old female who has been admitted to the hospital for an surgery. She had a history of hypertension and diabetes, for which he was taking medications. Following the surgery, she developed a fever, chills, and cough with sputum production. She also complained of shortness of breath and chest pain. Her vital signs were significant for fever, high blood pressure, pulse rate 105 beats per minute, respiratory rate 23 breaths per minute and oxygen saturation was 90% on room air.

Based on the patient's clinical presentation and risk factors, the diagnosis of hospital-acquired pneumonia (HAP) was suspected. A chest X-ray showed infiltrates in the right middle lobe of the lung. Sputum culture was obtained, and the patient was started on empiric antibiotic therapy with intravenous ceftriaxone and azithromycin. Oxygen therapy was initiated to maintain the oxygen saturation above 90%.

Over the next 24 hours, the patient's fever and respiratory symptoms improved. However, his oxygen saturation remained low, and he required supplemental oxygen therapy. Repeat chest X-ray showed persistent infiltrates in the right middle lobe. The sputum culture grew Klebsiella pneumoniae, which was sensitive to ceftriaxone and azithromycin.

The patient was continued on intravenous antibiotics, and his oxygen therapy was adjusted to maintain his oxygen saturation above 94%. She remained in the hospital for an additional 5 days, during which time he showed steady improvement. She was eventually discharged home with a course of oral antibiotics and was advised to follow up with his primary care physician.

DOI: 10.1201/9781003230465-54

Discussion:

HAP is a serious infection that can develop in patients who are hospitalized for an extended period, especially those who have undergone surgery or have a compromised immune system. Risk factors for HAP include age, comorbidities, prolonged hospitalization, mechanical ventilation, and the use of broad-spectrum antibiotics.

The diagnosis of HAP is based on the patient's clinical presentation, radiological findings, and microbiological cultures. Treatment involves the use of empiric antibiotics, which are selected based on the patient's risk factors and the suspected causative organism. Once the microbiological culture results are available, the antibiotic regimen can be adjusted accordingly.

The management of HAP also involves supportive care, such as oxygen therapy and airway clearance techniques, to maintain the patient's respiratory function. Close monitoring is required to assess the patient's response to treatment and to detect any complications that may arise.

In the case of this patient, the diagnosis of HAP was suspected based on his clinical presentation and risk factors. The initial empiric antibiotic therapy was effective in controlling his fever and respiratory symptoms, but his oxygen saturation remained low. Repeat chest X-ray and sputum culture confirmed the diagnosis of HAP and guided the choice of antibiotics. With appropriate antibiotic therapy and supportive care, the patient showed steady improvement and was eventually discharged home.

50.3 CASE 2. CASE OF HOSPITAL-ACQUIRED PNEUMONIA

- Age: 65 years

- Gender: Female

- Medical history: Type 2 Diabetes Mellitus, Hypertension, Chronic Obstructive Pulmonary Disease (COPD)

- Admitted to hospital for: Elective surgery for a hip replacement

- Length of stay in hospital before onset of symptoms: 5 days

Clinical Presentation: The patient presents with a fever, cough, shortness of breath, and increased sputum production. He also complains of chest pain when taking deep breaths.

Diagnostic Tests:

- Chest X-ray: Shows consolidation in the left lower lobe of the lung

- Sputum culture: Positive for Pseudomonas aeruginosa

Diagnosis: Hospital Acquired Pneumonia (HAP) caused by Pseudomonas aeruginosa

Treatment:

- Empirical antibiotic therapy started with intravenous ceftriaxone and levofloxacin.

- Once the sputum culture results were available, the antibiotic therapy was adjusted to target Pseudomonas aeruginosa with intravenous piperacillin-tazobactam.

- Inhaled bronchodilators and corticosteroids were also administered to improve breathing.

- Oxygen therapy was given to maintain oxygen saturation above 92%.

Outcome: The patient's symptoms improved gradually over the next few days. Repeat chest X-ray showed resolution of the consolidation in the left lower lobe. The patient was discharged after completing a 14-day course of antibiotics and follow-up appointments were scheduled to monitor her condition.

50.4 CASE 3. CASE OF HOSPITAL-ACQUIRED URINARY TRACT INFECTIONS

Patient Profile:

- Age: 68 years

- Gender: Female

- Medical history: Hypertension, Type 2 Diabetes Mellitus, Chronic Kidney Disease (CKD)

- Admitted to hospital for: Treatment of a fractured hip

- Length of stay in hospital before onset of symptoms: 7 days

Clinical Presentation: The patient presents with complaints of burning sensation during urination, increased frequency of urination, and lower abdominal pain. She also reports cloudy urine with a strong odor.

Diagnostic Tests:

- Urine culture: Positive for Escherichia coli (E.coli)

- Blood tests: Elevated white blood cell count and C-reactive protein levels

Diagnosis: Hospital Acquired Urinary Tract Infection caused by Escherichia coli (E.coli)

Treatment:

- Empirical antibiotic therapy started with oral trimethoprim-sulfamethoxazole

- Once the urine culture results were available, the antibiotic therapy was adjusted to target E.coli with intravenous ceftriaxone

- Intravenous fluids were administered to maintain hydration and to promote urine flow

- Bladder catheterization was done to drain the urine and to relieve any obstruction

- Regular monitoring of urine output, vital signs, and response to treatment

Outcome: The patient's symptoms improved gradually over the next few days. Repeat urine culture showed no growth of bacteria. The bladder catheter was removed after 72 hours of use. The patient was discharged after completing a 10-day course of antibiotics and follow-up appointments were scheduled to monitor her condition.

50.5 CASE 4. CASE OF HOSPITAL-ACQUIRED URINARY TRACT INFECTIONS

A 77-year-old female who was admitted to the hospital with a hip fracture following a fall at home. She had a history of hypertension and urinary incontinence, for which she was using pads. A urinary catheter was inserted on admission to the hospital to monitor her urine output and prevent urinary retention. On the third day of hospitalization, she developed a fever, abdominal discomfort, and cloudy urine output.

Based on the patient's clinical presentation and risk factors, the diagnosis of hospital-acquired urinary tract infection was suspected. A urine culture was obtained, which showed significant growth of Escherichia coli, a common causative organism of UTIs. The patient was started on empiric antibiotic therapy with intravenous ceftriaxone, pending the culture and sensitivity results.

Over the next 24 hours, the patient's fever and abdominal discomfort improved, and her urine output became clear. The urine culture confirmed the growth of E. coli, which was sensitive to ceftriaxone. The patient was continued on antibiotic therapy for a total of 7 days, and her urinary catheter was removed on the fourth day of treatment.

Discussion:

Hospital-acquired urinary tract infection is a common complication in hospitalized patients, especially those with indwelling urinary catheters. Risk factors for hospital-acquired urinary tract infection include older age, female gender, diabetes, and the duration of catheterization. The diagnosis of hospital-acquired urinary tract infection is based on the patient's clinical presentation, including fever, abdominal discomfort, and cloudy urine output, and the results of urine culture and sensitivity testing.

Treatment of hospital-acquired urinary tract infection involves the use of empiric antibiotics, pending the results of urine culture and sensitivity testing. Once the culture results are available, the antibiotic regimen can be adjusted accordingly. The duration of antibiotic therapy is generally 7–14 days, depending on the severity of the infection and the patient's response to treatment. Removal of the urinary catheter is recommended as soon as possible to reduce the risk of infection.

Prevention of hospital-acquired urinary tract infection involves a number of strategies, including the use of sterile techniques during catheter insertion, the use of catheters only when necessary, and the removal of catheters as soon as possible. Regular catheter care and maintenance are also important to reduce the risk of infection.

In the case of this patient, the diagnosis of hospital-acquired urinary tract infection was suspected based on her clinical presentation and risk factors, and confirmed by urine culture and sensitivity testing. Empiric antibiotic therapy was effective in controlling her fever and urinary symptoms, and the urinary catheter was removed as soon as possible. With appropriate antibiotic therapy and catheter care, the patient showed steady improvement and was eventually discharged home.

50.6 CASE 5. CASE OF HOSPITAL-ACQUIRED INFECTION AT THE SURGICAL SITE

- Age: 61 years
- Gender: Male
- Medical history: None
- Admitted to hospital for: surgery for a hernia repair
- Length of stay in hospital before onset of symptoms: 3 days

Clinical Presentation: The patient develops a fever, redness, swelling, and tenderness at the surgical site, and increased drainage from the wound.

Diagnostic Tests:

- Blood culture: Positive for Methicillin-resistant Staphylococcus aureus (MRSA)
- Wound culture: Positive for MRSA

Diagnosis: Hospital-Acquired Infection at the surgical site caused by Methicillin-resistant Staphylococcus aureus (MRSA)

Treatment:

- Empirical antibiotic therapy started with intravenous vancomycin and clindamycin
- The wound was opened, drained, and cleaned to remove infected tissues
- Negative pressure wound therapy was initiated to promote healing and reduce bacterial load
- Regular monitoring of wound status, vital signs, and response to treatment

Outcome: The patient's symptoms improved gradually over the next few days. Repeat wound culture showed no growth of bacteria. The patient was discharged after completing a 14-day course of antibiotics and follow-up appointments were scheduled to monitor his condition. He was advised to take precautions to prevent the spread of MRSA to others.

50.7 CONCLUSION

This chapter has discussed the real cases of hospital acquired infections. Patient safety case studies are an essential tool for improving healthcare quality and safety. They provide a detailed analysis of a specific patient safety incident or event, which can help identify the root causes, contributing factors, and possible solutions to prevent similar incidents from occurring in the future. The case studies provided above illustrate some of the common types of Hospital-Acquired Infections (HAIs) that patients can acquire during their hospital stay. Hospital-Acquired Pneumonia (HAP), Hospital-Acquired Urinary Tract Infections, and Hospital-Acquired Infections at surgical sites are some of the most frequent types of HAIs that can cause significant morbidity and mortality. These infections can occur due to a combination of factors, including weakened immune systems of patients, exposure to pathogens in the hospital environment, invasive procedures, and inappropriate use of antibiotics. It is essential to follow proper infection control practices, such as hand hygiene, proper use of personal protective equipment, and disinfection of hospital surfaces, to prevent HAIs. Early diagnosis, prompt and appropriate treatment, and proper infection control measures are critical to prevent the spread of HAIs and improve patient outcomes. It is also essential to monitor patients' response to treatment and perform regular follow-up to ensure complete recovery and prevent the recurrence of the infection.

REFERENCES

Al-Worafi, Y.M. (Ed.). (2020a). Drug Safety in Developing Countries: Achievements and Challenges.

Al-Worafi, Y.M. (2020b). Evidence-based medications safety practice. In *Drug Safety in Developing Countries* (pp. 197–201). Academic Press.

Al-Worafi, Y.M. (2020c). Quality indicators for medications safety. In *Drug safety in Developing Countries* (pp. 229–242). Academic Press.

Al-Worafi, Y.M. (2020d). Drug safety: comparison between developing countries. In *Drug Safety in Developing Countries* (pp. 603–611). Academic Press.

Al-Worafi, Y.M. (2020e). Drug safety in developing versus developed countries. In *Drug Safety in Developing Countries* (pp. 613–615). Academic Press.

Al-Worafi, Y. (2022a). *A Guide to Online Pharmacy Education: Teaching Strategies and Assessment Methods*. CRC Press.

Al-Worafi, Y.M. (2022b). Patient care errors and related problems (part I): development and validation of the model. https://orcid.org/0000–0002-5752-2913

Al-Worafi, Y.M. (Ed.). (2023). *Clinical Case Studies on medication Safety*. Academic Press.

Vincent, C. (2011). *Patient safety*. John Wiley & Sons.

51 Patient Safety Case Studies

Laboratory Medicine and Radiology

51.1 IMPORTANCE OF PATIENT SAFETY & PATIENT CARE PLAN ERRORS AND RELATED PROBLEMS CASE STUDIES

Patient safety case studies are an essential tool for improving healthcare quality and safety. Prepare the future healthcare professionals with the necessary competencies related to the patient safety-related issues are the key to success in medication safety practice in the future, however, improving the current healthcare professionals' medication safety competencies is very important in order to improve the patients' treating outcomes in terms of efficacy and safety. They provide a detailed analysis of a specific patient safety incident or event, which can help identify the root causes, contributing factors, and possible solutions to prevent similar incidents from occurring in the future. Here are some of the key reasons why patient safety case studies are important:

1. Learning from mistakes: Patient safety case studies highlight the mistakes that were made in a specific incident, providing an opportunity for healthcare providers to learn from those mistakes and prevent them from happening again in the future.

2. Improving safety culture: By sharing patient safety case studies across healthcare organizations, staff can become more aware of the importance of safety culture, and how their actions and decisions can impact patient safety.

3. Identifying systemic issues: Patient safety case studies can reveal patterns or trends in safety incidents, which can help identify systemic issues that need to be addressed to improve patient safety.

4. Developing best practices: By analyzing patient safety case studies, healthcare providers can develop best practices for preventing similar incidents from occurring in the future. This can include changes to policies, procedures, or training programs.

5. Enhancing communication: Patient safety case studies can be used as a tool to enhance communication between healthcare providers, patients, and their families. Sharing these stories can help to build trust, foster transparency, and encourage open communication.

Overall, patient safety case studies are a critical component of any patient safety program. By examining specific incidents in detail, healthcare providers can learn from mistakes, improve safety culture, and ultimately improve patient outcomes (Al-Worafi et al., 2020a–e; Al-Worafi, 2022a,b; Al-Worafi, 2023; Vincent, 2011).

51.2 CASE 1. CASE OF LABORATORY ERROR

- Age: 65 years
- Gender: Male
- Medical history: Hypertension, Diabetes Mellitus
- Complaint: Routine annual check-up

Clinical Presentation: The patient comes in for a routine annual check-up. His blood sample is collected for laboratory testing, which includes a Complete Blood Count (CBC), lipid profile, and HbA1c levels.

Diagnostic Tests:

- CBC results: Hemoglobin level of 8.0 g/dL (normal range: 13.5–17.5 g/dL), Red blood cell count of 3.5 million/μL (normal range: 4.5–5.5 million/μL)
- Lipid profile: Normal
- HbA1c levels: 6.2% (normal range: 4–5.6%)

Diagnosis: The laboratory report suggests that the patient has Anemia with normal Lipid profile and HbA1c levels.

Treatment: The laboratory report is reviewed by the healthcare provider, who orders additional diagnostic tests to determine the cause of the patient's anemia. The patient is referred to a hematologist for further evaluation.

However, upon further investigation, it is discovered that the laboratory had made an error in the CBC report, and the hemoglobin level was actually 12.0 g/dL, not 8.0 g/dL. The laboratory had accidentally transposed the patient's results with another patient's results.

Outcome: The healthcare provider immediately contacts the patient and informs him of the laboratory error. The patient is advised that he does not have anemia and that his hemoglobin levels are normal. The patient is reassured and advised to continue with his routine care. The laboratory error is reported and investigated to identify the cause and to implement measures to prevent such errors in the future. The patient is informed of the findings and provided with feedback about the laboratory's response to the error. The patient expresses satisfaction with the resolution of the issue and appreciation for the healthcare provider's prompt and transparent communication.

51.3 CASE 2. CASE OF LABORATORY ERROR

A 61-year-old male who underwent a routine physical exam that included a fasting lipid panel. The results of the lipid panel showed a total cholesterol level of 280 mg/dL, which was higher than the reference range of 125–200 mg/dL.

Based on the elevated cholesterol level, the patient was started on a low-fat diet and referred to a lipid specialist for further evaluation. The lipid specialist ordered a repeat lipid panel, which showed a total cholesterol level of 155 mg/dL, within the reference range.

Further investigation revealed that the first lipid panel was performed on a non-fasting blood sample, whereas the second lipid panel was performed on a fasting blood sample, which is required for accurate lipid measurements.

Discussion:
Laboratory errors can occur in any phase of the testing process, including pre-analytic, analytic, and post-analytic phases. Pre-analytic errors can include patient identification errors, specimen collection errors, and specimen transport errors. Analytic errors can include instrument malfunctions, calibration errors, and reagent errors. Post-analytic errors can include reporting errors, interpretation errors, and transcription errors.

In the case of this patient, the laboratory error was a pre-analytic error, specifically a specimen collection error. The first lipid panel was performed on a non-fasting blood sample, which resulted in an elevated cholesterol level. The second lipid panel, which was performed on a fasting blood sample, showed a normal cholesterol level.

To prevent laboratory errors, it is important to follow established protocols for specimen collection, handling, and transport. Patient identification should be verified at each step of the testing process, and samples should be collected and handled in a manner that minimizes the risk of contamination or degradation. In addition, it is important to perform quality control checks and to have established procedures for handling and reporting abnormal test results.

In this case, the laboratory error was identified and corrected, and the patient was able to receive appropriate treatment based on accurate test results.

51.4 CASE 3. CASE OF LABORATORY ERROR

A 30-year-old female presented to her primary care physician with symptoms of a urinary tract infection (UTI). The patient reported experiencing painful urination and frequent urination.

The patient's urine was collected for routine laboratory testing, including a urinalysis to evaluate for signs of infection. The laboratory reported that the patient's urine was negative for signs of infection.

Laboratory Error: Several days later, the laboratory reported that there had been a mix-up with the patient's sample and that the results had been reported in error. A repeat urinalysis showed that the patient did indeed have a UTI.

Clinical Outcome: The patient was notified of the laboratory error and was prescribed antibiotics to treat her UTI. She was advised to monitor her symptoms and to return to the clinic if her condition did not improve.

Lessons Learned: This case highlights the importance of accurate laboratory testing and reporting, as well as the need for proper quality control measures to prevent mix-ups and errors. The laboratory error delayed the patient's diagnosis and treatment, potentially prolonging her symptoms and increasing the risk of complications from the UTI.

51.5 CASE 4. CASE OF RADIOLOGY ERROR

A 42-year-old female presented to the emergency department with severe abdominal pain and vomiting. She reported having a history of endometriosis and had undergone a laparoscopic surgery a few years ago to remove endometrial tissue from her ovaries. The patient was also taking hormonal therapy for her condition.

Clinical Presentation: The patient's physical examination revealed tenderness in the lower abdomen and signs of bowel obstruction. Blood tests showed a high white blood cell count and elevated levels of inflammatory markers. The treating physician suspected that the patient had a bowel perforation and ordered a CT scan of the abdomen and pelvis to confirm the diagnosis.

Radiology Error: The radiologist who reviewed the CT scan reported that there was no evidence of bowel perforation, but did note the presence of a small mass in the patient's right ovary. Based on this finding, the radiologist recommended that the patient undergo a follow-up pelvic ultrasound to further evaluate the ovarian mass.

Clinical Outcome: The patient was discharged from the emergency department with a diagnosis of acute gastroenteritis and was advised to follow up with her gynecologist for the ovarian mass. She was given antibiotics for her symptoms and was told to return to the hospital if her condition worsened.

Several days later, the patient returned to the hospital with worsening abdominal pain and a high fever. A repeat CT scan showed that the patient did indeed have a bowel perforation, which had been missed on the initial scan. The patient underwent emergency surgery to repair the perforation and was found to have a large abscess in the pelvis, which was drained.

After the surgery, the patient's condition improved and she was eventually discharged from the hospital. However, she required additional medical treatment and had an extended recovery period due to the delayed diagnosis and treatment of her condition.

Lessons Learned: This case highlights the importance of thorough and accurate radiology interpretation, as well as the need for clear communication between radiologists and treating physicians. Had the radiologist correctly identified the bowel perforation on the initial CT scan, the patient could have received earlier treatment and potentially avoided the need for surgery and extended hospitalization. It also highlights the importance of considering the patient's full medical history and current clinical presentation when interpreting imaging studies, as the presence of a known condition like endometriosis could have influenced the interpretation of the ovarian mass.

51.6 CASE 5. CASE OF RADIOLOGY ERROR

A 63-year-old male with a history of chronic obstructive pulmonary disease (COPD) presented to the emergency department with shortness of breath and chest pain. The patient had recently undergone chemotherapy for lung cancer.

The treating physician suspected that the patient had a pulmonary embolism and ordered a computerized tomography (CT) angiogram of the chest to confirm the diagnosis. The radiologist who reviewed the scan reported that there was no evidence of a pulmonary embolism but did note the presence of a new mass in the patient's right lung.

Radiology Error: The radiologist recommended that the patient undergo a follow-up A positron emission tomography (PET) scan to further evaluate the lung mass. However, the radiologist failed to note that the CT scan also showed evidence of a small pulmonary embolism in the patient's left lung.

Clinical Outcome: The patient was discharged from the hospital with a diagnosis of COPD exacerbation and was advised to follow up with his oncologist for the lung mass. Several weeks later, the patient returned to the hospital with worsening shortness of breath and chest pain. A repeat CT scan showed that the patient did indeed have a pulmonary embolism, which had been missed on the initial scan. The patient was treated with anticoagulation therapy and was eventually discharged from the hospital.

Lessons Learned: This case highlights the importance of careful and thorough radiology interpretation, as well as the need to consider the full clinical picture when interpreting imaging studies. The radiologist's failure to note the presence of a pulmonary embolism on the initial CT scan delayed the patient's treatment and potentially contributed to his worsening condition.

51.7 CASE 6. CASE OF RADIOLOGY ERROR

A 49-year-old female presented to the emergency department with severe headache and confusion. The patient had a history of hypertension and had been taking antihypertensive medication for several years.

The treating physician suspected that the patient had suffered a stroke and ordered a CT scan of the head to confirm the diagnosis. The radiologist who reviewed the scan reported that there was no evidence of a stroke but did note the presence of a small brain tumor.

Radiology Error: The radiologist recommended that the patient undergo a follow-up MRI to further evaluate the brain tumor. However, the radiologist failed to note that the CT scan also showed evidence of a small subarachnoid hemorrhage.

Clinical Outcome: The patient was discharged from the hospital with a diagnosis of a brain tumor and was advised to follow up with a neurologist for further evaluation. Several weeks later, the patient returned to the hospital with worsening headache and confusion. A repeat CT scan showed that the patient did indeed have a subarachnoid hemorrhage, which had been missed on the initial scan. The patient underwent emergency treatment for the hemorrhage and was eventually discharged from the hospital.

Lessons Learned: This case highlights the importance of careful and thorough radiology interpretation, as well as the need to consider the full clinical picture when interpreting imaging studies. The radiologist's failure to note the presence of a subarachnoid hemorrhage on the initial CT scan delayed the patient's treatment and potentially contributed to her worsening condition.

51.8 CONCLUSION

This chapter has discussed the cases of laboratory and radiology errors. Laboratory medicine errors can occur at various stages, including specimen collection, testing, and reporting of results. The most common types of errors include misidentification of specimens, errors in labeling or processing specimens, transcription errors, and instrument or software malfunctions. Radiology errors can also occur at various stages, including image acquisition, interpretation, and reporting. The most common types of errors include misinterpretation of images, failure to detect abnormalities, and errors in communication of results. Both laboratory medicine errors and radiology errors can have serious consequences for patient safety, including delayed or incorrect diagnosis, unnecessary procedures or treatments, and even death. To reduce the risk of errors, healthcare providers must follow established protocols and procedures, use proper identification techniques, employ double-check systems, and report errors when they occur. Proper training and ongoing education can also help to prevent errors. Technology can also play a role in reducing errors, such as the use of electronic health records, barcoding, and other automated systems. In conclusion, preventing laboratory medicine errors and radiology errors is essential for ensuring patient safety and improving the quality of care. A combination of established protocols, proper identification techniques, double-check systems, education and training, and the use of technology can help reduce the risk of errors and improve patient outcomes.

REFERENCES

Al-Worafi, Y. M. (Ed.). (2020a). Drug Safety in Developing Countries: Achievements and Challenges.

Al-Worafi, Y.M. (2020b). Evidence-based medications safety practice. In *Drug Safety in Developing Countries* (pp. 197–201). Academic Press.

Al-Worafi, Y.M. (2020c). Quality indicators for medications safety. In *Drug safety in developing countries* (pp. 229–242). Academic Press.

Al-Worafi, Y.M. (2020d). Drug safety: comparison between developing countries. In *Drug Safety in Developing Countries* (pp. 603–611). Academic Press.

Al-Worafi, Y.M. (2020e). Drug safety in developing versus developed countries. In *Drug Safety in Developing Countries* (pp. 613–615). Academic Press.

Al-Worafi, Y. (2022a). *A Guide to Online Pharmacy Education: Teaching Strategies and Assessment Methods*. CRC Press.

Al-Worafi, Y.M. (2022b). Patient care errors and related problems (part I): development and validation of the model. https://orcid.org/0000–0002-5752-2913

Al-Worafi, Y.M. (Ed.). (2023). *Clinical Case Studies on medication Safety*. Academic Press.

Vincent, C. (2011). *Patient safety* . John Wiley & Sons.

52 Patient Safety Case Studies

Emergency Department

52.1 IMPORTANCE OF PATIENT SAFETY & PATIENT CARE PLAN ERRORS AND RELATED PROBLEMS CASE STUDIES

Patient safety case studies are an essential tool for improving healthcare quality and safety. Prepare the future healthcare professionals with the necessary competencies related to the patient safety-related issues are the key to success in medication safety practice in the future, however, improving the current healthcare professionals' medication safety competencies is very important in order to improve the patients' treating outcomes in terms of efficacy and safety. They provide a detailed analysis of a specific patient safety incident or event, which can help identify the root causes, contributing factors, and possible solutions to prevent similar incidents from occurring in the future. Here are some of the key reasons why patient safety case studies are important:

1. Learning from mistakes: Patient safety case studies highlight the mistakes that were made in a specific incident, providing an opportunity for healthcare providers to learn from those mistakes and prevent them from happening again in the future.

2. Improving safety culture: By sharing patient safety case studies across healthcare organizations, staff can become more aware of the importance of safety culture, and how their actions and decisions can impact patient safety.

3. Identifying systemic issues: Patient safety case studies can reveal patterns or trends in safety incidents, which can help identify systemic issues that need to be addressed to improve patient safety.

4. Developing best practices: By analyzing patient safety case studies, healthcare providers can develop best practices for preventing similar incidents from occurring in the future. This can include changes to policies, procedures, or training programs.

5. Enhancing communication: Patient safety case studies can be used as a tool to enhance communication between healthcare providers, patients, and their families. Sharing these stories can help to build trust, foster transparency, and encourage open communication.

Overall, patient safety case studies are a critical component of any patient safety program. By examining specific incidents in detail, healthcare providers can learn from mistakes, improve safety culture, and ultimately improve patient outcomes (Al-Worafi et al., 2020a–e; Al-Worafi, 2022a,b; Al-Worafi, 2023; Vincent, 2011).

52.2 CASE 1. CASE OF AN EMERGENCY DEPARTMENT ERROR

A 58-year-old male presented to the emergency department with severe chest pain and shortness of breath. The patient had a history of heart disease and had undergone a coronary artery bypass grafting (CABG) procedure several years prior.

The treating physician suspected that the patient was experiencing a heart attack and ordered an electrocardiogram (ECG) and a series of cardiac enzyme tests to confirm the diagnosis. The ECG showed evidence of ST-segment elevation, which is a sign of a heart attack.

Emergency Department Error: The physician who reviewed the ECG failed to recognize the significance of the ST-segment elevation and did not order urgent cardiac catheterization for the patient.

Clinical Outcome: The patient was admitted to the hospital and treated for a heart attack, but the delay in treatment potentially contributed to further damage to his heart muscle. The patient required a longer hospital stay and more intensive treatment due to the delayed diagnosis.

Lessons Learned: This case highlights the importance of prompt and accurate diagnosis in the emergency department, as well as the need for careful and thorough review of diagnostic tests. The physician's failure to recognize the significance of the ST-segment elevation delayed the patient's treatment and potentially contributed to worse outcomes.

DOI: 10.1201/9781003230465-56

52.3 CASE 2. CASE OF AN EMERGENCY DEPARTMENT ERROR

A 26-year-old female presented to the emergency department with severe abdominal pain and vomiting. The patient reported a history of irregular menstrual cycles and had previously been diagnosed with polycystic ovary syndrome (PCOS).

The treating physician suspected that the patient was experiencing an ovarian cyst rupture and ordered a pelvic ultrasound to confirm the diagnosis. The ultrasound showed evidence of a large ovarian cyst but did not show any signs of rupture.

Emergency Department Error: The physician who reviewed the ultrasound failed to recognize the significance of the size of the ovarian cyst and did not consider the possibility of torsion, which is a twisting of the ovary that can occur with large cysts.

Clinical Outcome: The patient was discharged from the emergency department with a diagnosis of an ovarian cyst and was advised to follow up with her gynecologist. Several hours later, the patient returned to the emergency department with worsening abdominal pain and was diagnosed with ovarian torsion. She underwent emergency surgery to remove the twisted ovary.

Lessons Learned: This case highlights the importance of considering the full clinical picture and potential complications when diagnosing patients in the emergency department. The physician's failure to consider the possibility of ovarian torsion delayed the patient's treatment and potentially contributed to worse outcomes.

52.4 CASE 3. CASE OF AN EMERGENCY DEPARTMENT ERROR

A 67-year-old male presented to the emergency department with complaints of chest pain and shortness of breath. The patient had a history of hypertension and hyperlipidemia.

Clinical Presentation: The treating physician suspected that the patient was experiencing a heart attack and ordered an electrocardiogram (ECG) and a series of cardiac enzyme tests to confirm the diagnosis. The ECG showed no evidence of acute ischemia.

Emergency Department Error: The physician who reviewed the ECG failed to recognize that the patient had a left bundle branch block, which can make it difficult to accurately diagnose acute myocardial infarction.

Clinical Outcome: The patient was discharged from the emergency department with a diagnosis of chest pain of unknown origin and was advised to follow up with his primary care physician. A few days later, the patient had a massive heart attack and died.

Lessons Learned: This case highlights the importance of recognizing the limitations of diagnostic tests and the need for careful interpretation of ECG results. The physician's failure to recognize the significance of the left bundle branch block potentially delayed the patient's diagnosis and contributed to worse outcomes.

52.5 CASE 4. CASE OF AN EMERGENCY DEPARTMENT ERROR

A 49-year-old female presented to the emergency department with complaints of severe abdominal pain and vomiting. The patient had a history of irritable bowel syndrome (IBS).

The treating physician suspected that the patient was experiencing an IBS flare-up and ordered a series of laboratory tests to rule out other potential causes of the symptoms. The laboratory tests showed no abnormalities.

Emergency Department Error: The physician failed to consider the possibility of ovarian torsion, which can present with symptoms similar to those of an IBS flare-up.

Clinical Outcome: The patient was discharged from the emergency department with a diagnosis of an IBS flare-up and was advised to follow up with her primary care physician. Several hours later, the patient returned to the emergency department with worsening abdominal pain and was diagnosed with ovarian torsion. She underwent emergency surgery to remove the twisted ovary.

Lessons Learned: This case highlights the importance of considering all potential diagnoses when evaluating patients in the emergency department, especially when the clinical picture does not fit with a typical presentation of a certain condition. The physician's failure to consider the possibility of ovarian torsion delayed the patient's treatment and potentially contributed to worse outcomes.

52.6 CASE 5. CASE OF AN EMERGENCY DEPARTMENT ERROR

A 57-year-old male with a history of hypertension and high cholesterol presented to the emergency department with severe chest pain and shortness of breath.

History: The patient had experienced chest pain for several hours before coming to the emergency department. He also reported feeling dizzy and nauseous. The patient had a history of heart disease in his family and was currently taking medication for his hypertension and high cholesterol.

Clinical Assessment: Upon arrival at the emergency department, the patient's vital signs were unstable, with a blood pressure of 160/100 mmHg, heart rate of 120 bpm, and oxygen saturation of 90% on room air. The physician on duty suspected a heart attack and ordered an electrocardiogram (ECG) and blood tests to confirm the diagnosis.

Diagnosis and Treatment: The ECG showed signs of myocardial infarction, and the blood tests showed elevated levels of cardiac enzymes. However, due to a communication error between the emergency department staff, there was a delay in interpreting the test results, and the patient was not given the appropriate treatment promptly.

Several hours later, the patient's condition worsened, and he developed cardiogenic shock. The physician then ordered an urgent cardiac catheterization, which revealed a complete blockage in one of the coronary arteries. The patient underwent emergency angioplasty and stent placement to open the blocked artery.

Outcome: The patient's condition stabilized after the angioplasty, but he suffered permanent damage to his heart muscle due to the delay in treatment. The hospital admitted the error and provided free medical treatment to the patient. The hospital also implemented measures to ensure that all test results were interpreted promptly and that patients received appropriate treatment in a timely manner.

Conclusion: Delayed diagnosis and treatment in the emergency department can lead to serious harm to patients, and communication errors can contribute to such delays. It is crucial for emergency department staff to have clear communication protocols and to prioritize prompt and accurate interpretation of test results to ensure that patients receive appropriate treatment in a timely manner.

52.7 CONCLUSION

This chapter has discussed the real cases of emergency department errors. Errors in emergency department care can have serious consequences for patient safety. Case studies has highlighted the various causes of errors, including communication breakdowns, system issues, and individual factors. However, strategies to prevent errors, such as improving communication, implementing protocols and guidelines, and enhancing teamwork and training, can significantly improve patient outcomes. It is also essential to create a culture of safety that promotes open communication, transparency, and continuous quality improvement. Involving patients and their families in the care process can also enhance patient safety by increasing their engagement and participation in decision-making. Overall, continued efforts to improve patient safety in emergency departments are necessary to ensure that patients receive the best possible care and minimize the risk of harm.

REFERENCES

Al-Worafi, Y.M. (Ed.). (2020a). Drug Safety in Developing Countries: Achievements and Challenges.

Al-Worafi, Y.M. (2020b). Evidence-based medications safety practice. In *Drug Safety in Developing Countries* (pp. 197–201). Academic Press.

Al-Worafi, Y.M. (2020c). Quality indicators for medications safety. In *Drug safety in developing countries* (pp. 229–242). Academic Press.

Al-Worafi, Y.M. (2020d). Drug safety: comparison between developing countries. In *Drug Safety in Developing Countries* (pp. 603–611). Academic Press.

Al-Worafi, Y.M. (2020e). Drug safety in developing versus developed countries. In *Drug Safety in Developing Countries* (pp. 613–615). Academic Press.

Al-Worafi, Y. (2022a). *A Guide to Online Pharmacy Education: Teaching Strategies and Assessment Methods*. CRC Press.

Al-Worafi, Y.M. (2022b). Patient care errors and related problems (part I): development and validation of the model. https://orcid.org/0000–0002-5752-2913

Al-Worafi, Y.M. (Ed.). (2023). *Clinical Case Studies on medication Safety*. Academic Press.

Vincent, C. (2011). *Patient safety*. John Wiley & Sons.

53 Patient Safety Case Studies

Intensive Care Unit

53.1 IMPORTANCE OF PATIENT SAFETY & PATIENT CARE PLAN ERRORS AND RELATED PROBLEMS CASE STUDIES

Patient safety case studies are an essential tool for improving healthcare quality and safety. Prepare the future healthcare professionals with the necessary competencies related to the patient safety-related issues are the key to success in medication safety practice in the future, however, improving the current healthcare professionals' medication safety competencies is very important in order to improve the patients' treating outcomes in terms of efficacy and safety. They provide a detailed analysis of a specific patient safety incident or event, which can help identify the root causes, contributing factors, and possible solutions to prevent similar incidents from occurring in the future. Here are some of the key reasons why patient safety case studies are important:

1. Learning from mistakes: Patient safety case studies highlight the mistakes that were made in a specific incident, providing an opportunity for healthcare providers to learn from those mistakes and prevent them from happening again in the future.

2. Improving safety culture: By sharing patient safety case studies across healthcare organizations, staff can become more aware of the importance of safety culture, and how their actions and decisions can impact patient safety.

3. Identifying systemic issues: Patient safety case studies can reveal patterns or trends in safety incidents, which can help identify systemic issues that need to be addressed to improve patient safety.

4. Developing best practices: By analyzing patient safety case studies, healthcare providers can develop best practices for preventing similar incidents from occurring in the future. This can include changes to policies, procedures, or training programs.

5. Enhancing communication: Patient safety case studies can be used as a tool to enhance communication between healthcare providers, patients, and their families. Sharing these stories can help to build trust, foster transparency, and encourage open communication.

Overall, patient safety case studies are a critical component of any patient safety program. By examining specific incidents in detail, healthcare providers can learn from mistakes, improve safety culture, and ultimately improve patient outcomes (Al-Worafi et al., 2020a–e; Al-Worafi, 2022a,b; Al-Worafi, 2023; Vincent, 2011).

53.2 CASE 1. INTENSIVE CARE UNIT (ICU) ERROR

A 65-year-old man who was admitted to the ICU with septic shock due to a urinary tract infection. He has a history of hypertension, diabetes, and heart disease. He is intubated and on a ventilator.

Case Overview: Despite receiving appropriate treatment for his condition, he experiences several errors in his care during his stay in the ICU.

Error 1: Medication Error On the first day of his admission, he is prescribed an antibiotic for his infection. However, the pharmacist dispenses the wrong medication, and he receives a medication that he is allergic to. He experiences an allergic reaction, which leads to a severe drop in his blood pressure, requiring additional medication and support.

Error 2: Delayed Diagnosis Despite receiving treatment for his septic shock, His condition does not improve as expected. It takes several days for the healthcare team to realize that he has developed a secondary infection in his lungs, which requires a different course of treatment. The delay in diagnosis leads to a delay in appropriate treatment, which prolongs Mr. Smith's stay in the ICU and increases his risk of complications.

Error 3: Communication Error On the third day of his admission, His ventilator tube becomes dislodged, and he experiences a period of inadequate oxygenation. However, the nursing staff does not immediately notice the problem, and He is not given prompt assistance. The delay in

DOI: 10.1201/9781003230465-57

recognizing and addressing the issue leads to a period of hypoxia, which can cause damage to his organs and increase his risk of mortality.

Error 4: Equipment Failure On the fifth day of his admission, his IV pump malfunctions, causing an overdose of medication. He experiences a seizure, which requires emergency intervention. The equipment failure leads to a dangerous situation for the patient, and highlights the importance of regular maintenance and monitoring of medical equipment in the ICU.

Outcome: Despite experiencing several errors in his care during his stay in the ICU, He is ultimately recovers and is discharged from the hospital. However, the errors in his care could have led to serious complications or even death, highlighting the importance of patient safety and quality improvement efforts in the ICU.

53.3 CASE 2. INTENSIVE CARE UNIT (ICU) ERROR

- Age: 42 years old
- Gender: Female
- Medical history: Type 1 Diabetes Mellitus, Hypertension, and Chronic Kidney Disease
- Reason for admission: Diabetic ketoacidosis

The patient was admitted to the ICU with complaints of increased thirst, frequent urination, and generalized weakness for the past 2 days. On examination, the patient was found to have tachycardia (heart rate of 110 beats/minute), hypotension (blood pressure of 80/50 mmHg), and ketotic breath odor. The patient was diagnosed with diabetic ketoacidosis and was started on intravenous insulin infusion and fluid resuscitation.

Error: On the second day of admission, the patient's insulin infusion was accidentally disconnected for 2 hours due to a nursing error. The error was not identified until the next nursing shift, resulting in a prolonged period of hyperglycemia and ketoacidosis. The patient's blood glucose level increased to 500 mg/dL, and the patient developed severe acidosis, requiring intubation and mechanical ventilation.

Diagnostic Workup: The following diagnostic tests were ordered:

- Arterial blood gas analysis: showed severe metabolic acidosis with a pH of 7.0 and a bicarbonate level of 5 mEq/L.
- Complete blood count: showed leukocytosis with a white blood cell count of 20,000 cells/mm3.
- Serum electrolytes: showed severe hyperkalemia with a potassium level of 7.0 mEq/L.
- Urinalysis: showed high ketone levels and glucose in the urine.

Treatment: The patient was started on intravenous bicarbonate and insulin infusion for the treatment of severe metabolic acidosis and hyperglycemia. The patient also received intravenous calcium gluconate for the treatment of hyperkalemia. The patient was intubated and mechanically ventilated due to the severity of acidosis and respiratory failure.

Outcome: The patient's metabolic parameters gradually improved over the next few days, and the patient was extubated after 3 days of mechanical ventilation. The patient's insulin infusion was restarted, and her blood glucose level was gradually brought under control. The patient was discharged from the ICU after 10 days of hospitalization with instructions for diabetes management and regular follow-up with an endocrinologist.

53.4 CASE 3. INTENSIVE CARE UNIT (ICU) ERROR

A 65-year-old woman who was admitted to the ICU after undergoing a cardiac surgery. She has a history of hypertension and hyperlipidemia. She is intubated and on a ventilator.

Case Overview: Despite receiving appropriate treatment for her condition, She experiences several errors in her care during her stay in the ICU.

Error 1: Delayed Diagnosis her condition does not improve as expected after her surgery. It takes several days for the healthcare team to realize that she has developed a postoperative infection, which requires a different course of treatment. The delay in diagnosis leads to a delay in appropriate treatment, which prolongs her stay in the ICU and increases her risk of complications.

Error 2: Communication Error On the fourth day of her admission, her family reports that she appears agitated and uncomfortable. However, the nursing staff does not immediately respond to their concerns, and she does not receive adequate pain management. The delay in recognizing and addressing the issue leads to unnecessary suffering for the patient and highlights the importance of effective communication and patient-centered care in the ICU.

Error 3: Medication Error She is prescribed a pain medication that is contraindicated with her medical history. The medication is administered, and she experiences an adverse reaction, which leads to respiratory distress and requires emergency intervention. The medication error highlights the importance of careful medication management and patient monitoring in the ICU.

Error 4: Staffing Shortage On the seventh day of her admission, her ventilator tube becomes dislodged, and she experiences a period of inadequate oxygenation. However, due to a staffing shortage, there are not enough healthcare professionals available to respond to the issue promptly. The delay in recognizing and addressing the problem leads to a period of hypoxia, which can cause damage to her organs and increase her risk of mortality.

Outcome: Despite experiencing several errors in her care during her stay in the ICU, she was ultimately recovers and is discharged from the hospital. However, the errors in her care could have led to serious complications or even death, highlighting the importance of patient safety and quality improvement efforts in the ICU.

53.5 CASE 4. INTENSIVE CARE UNIT (ICU) ERROR

- Age: 50 years old
- Gender: Male
- Medical history: Chronic obstructive pulmonary disease (COPD), Hypertension, and Obesity
- Reason for admission: Acute exacerbation of COPD

The patient was admitted to the ICU with complaints of increased shortness of breath, cough, and wheezing for the past 2 days. The patient had a history of COPD and was on home oxygen therapy. On examination, the patient was found to have tachypnea (respiratory rate of 35 breaths/minute), tachycardia (heart rate of 120 beats/minute), and hypoxemia (oxygen saturation of 88% on 4 L of supplemental oxygen). Chest X-ray revealed hyperinflation and bilateral infiltrates consistent with acute exacerbation of COPD.

Error: The patient was started on intravenous antibiotics, nebulized bronchodilators, and systemic corticosteroids for the treatment of acute exacerbation of COPD. However, due to a medication error, the patient was given a double dose of intravenous methylprednisolone (Solu-Medrol) instead of the prescribed dose. The error was not identified until several hours later, resulting in excessive corticosteroid exposure.

Diagnostic Workup: The following diagnostic tests were ordered:

- Arterial blood gas analysis: showed severe hypoxemia with a PaO2 of 55 mmHg on 4 L of supplemental oxygen.
- Complete blood count: showed leukocytosis with a white blood cell count of 18,000 cells/mm3.
- Chest X-ray: revealed hyperinflation and bilateral infiltrates consistent with acute exacerbation of COPD.
- Electrocardiogram (ECG): showed sinus tachycardia without any significant ST-T wave changes.

Treatment: The patient was initially started on nebulized bronchodilators, intravenous antibiotics, and systemic corticosteroids for the treatment of acute exacerbation of COPD. However, due to the medication error, the patient received a double dose of intravenous methylprednisolone, which resulted in excessive corticosteroid exposure. The patient was monitored closely for the development of steroid-induced adverse effects, such as hyperglycemia, hypertension, and electrolyte imbalances.

Outcome: The patient's respiratory distress improved over the next few days, and the patient was gradually weaned off supplemental oxygen. However, the patient developed steroid-induced hyperglycemia, which required insulin therapy to control. The patient's blood pressure also remained elevated, requiring the addition of antihypertensive medications. The patient was discharged from the ICU after 7 days of hospitalization and advised to continue with home oxygen therapy, nebulized bronchodilators, and oral corticosteroids for his COPD. The medication error was reported and investigated by the hospital's medication safety team to prevent similar incidents in the future.

53.6 CASE 5. INTENSIVE CARE UNIT (ICU) ERROR

A51-year-old man who was admitted to the ICU after a car accident that resulted in multiple injuries, including a traumatic brain injury. He has a history of hypertension and obesity. He is intubated and on a ventilator.

Case Overview: Despite receiving appropriate treatment for his condition, the patient experiences several errors in his care during his stay in the ICU.

Error 1: Equipment Failure On the second day of his admission, his ventilator malfunctions, causing a period of inadequate oxygenation. The nursing staff does not immediately notice the problem, and he does not receive prompt assistance. The delay in recognizing and addressing the issue leads to a period of hypoxia, which can cause damage to his organs and increase his risk of mortality. The equipment failure highlights the importance of regular maintenance and monitoring of medical equipment in the ICU.

Error 2: Communication Error On the fifth day of his admission, his family reports that he is experiencing severe pain. However, the nursing staff does not immediately respond to their concerns, and he does not receive adequate pain management. The delay in recognizing and addressing the issue leads to unnecessary suffering for the patient and highlights the importance of effective communication and patient-centered care in the ICU.

Error 3: Medication Error: he is prescribed a sedative medication to manage his pain. However, due to a miscommunication between the healthcare team, he receives an overdose of the medication, which leads to respiratory distress and requires emergency intervention. The medication error highlights the importance of careful medication management and patient monitoring in the ICU.

Error 4: Delayed Diagnosis: Despite receiving appropriate treatment for his injuries, his condition does not improve as expected. It takes several days for the healthcare team to realize that he has developed a secondary infection in his bloodstream, which requires a different course of treatment. The delay in diagnosis leads to a delay in appropriate treatment, which prolongs patient's stay in the ICU and increases his risk of complications.

Outcome: Despite experiencing several errors in his care during his stay in the ICU, the patient ultimately recovers and is discharged from the hospital. However, the errors in his care could have led to serious complications or even death, highlighting the importance of patient safety and quality improvement efforts in the ICU.

53.7 CONCLUSION

This chapter has discussed the real cases related to the intensive care unit errors. After analyzing multiple ICU error case studies, it is clear that medical errors can have devastating consequences for patients and their families. It is crucial for healthcare providers to prioritize patient safety and take steps to prevent errors from occurring. Some common factors that contribute to ICU errors include communication breakdowns between healthcare providers, inadequate staffing, lack of training and experience, and system failures. It is essential to address these issues and implement measures such as regular training and education, standardized protocols, and effective communication strategies to reduce the likelihood of errors. In addition, healthcare providers must be transparent and accountable when errors occur. This includes disclosing the error to the patient or their family, apologizing, and taking steps to prevent similar errors from happening in the future. Learning from mistakes and implementing changes to improve patient safety is essential to providing high-quality healthcare. Ultimately, preventing ICU errors requires a comprehensive approach that involves all members of the healthcare team, including physicians, nurses, pharmacists, and support staff.

By prioritizing patient safety and implementing effective strategies to prevent errors, healthcare providers can improve outcomes for critically ill patients and ensure that they receive the best possible care.

REFERENCES

Al-Worafi, Y.M. (Ed.). (2020a). *Drug Safety in Developing Countries: Achievements and Challenges.* Academic Press.

Al-Worafi, Y.M. (2020b). Evidence-based medications safety practice. In *Drug Safety in Developing Countries* (pp. 197–201). Academic Press.

Al-Worafi, Y.M. (2020c). Quality indicators for medications safety. In *Drug Safety in Developing Countries* (pp. 229–242). Academic Press.

Al-Worafi, Y.M. (2020d). Drug safety: Comparison between developing countries. In *Drug Safety in Developing Countries* (pp. 603–611). Academic Press.

Al-Worafi, Y.M. (2020e). Drug safety in developing versus developed countries. In *Drug Safety in Developing Countries* (pp. 613–615). Academic Press.

Al-Worafi, Y. (2022a). *A Guide to Online Pharmacy Education: Teaching Strategies and Assessment Methods.* CRC Press.

Al-Worafi, Y.M. (2022b). Patient care errors and related problems (part I): Development and validation of the model. https://orcid.org/0000-0002-5752-2913

Al-Worafi, Y.M. (Ed.). (2023). *Clinical Case Studies on Medication Safety.* Academic Press.

Vincent, C. (2011). *Patient Safety.* John Wiley & Sons.

54 Patient Safety Case Studies

Internal Medicine

54.1 IMPORTANCE OF PATIENT SAFETY & PATIENT CARE PLAN ERRORS AND RELATED PROBLEMS CASE STUDIES

Patient safety case studies are an essential tool for improving healthcare quality and safety. Prepare the future healthcare professionals with the necessary competencies related to the patient safety-related issues are the key to success in medication safety practice in the future, however, improving the current healthcare professionals' medication safety competencies is very important in order to improve the patients' treating outcomes in terms of efficacy and safety. They provide a detailed analysis of a specific patient safety incident or event, which can help identify the root causes, contributing factors, and possible solutions to prevent similar incidents from occurring in the future. Here are some of the key reasons why patient safety case studies are important:

1. Learning from mistakes: Patient safety case studies highlight the mistakes that were made in a specific incident, providing an opportunity for healthcare providers to learn from those mistakes and prevent them from happening again in the future.

2. Improving safety culture: By sharing patient safety case studies across healthcare organizations, staff can become more aware of the importance of safety culture, and how their actions and decisions can impact patient safety.

3. Identifying systemic issues: Patient safety case studies can reveal patterns or trends in safety incidents, which can help identify systemic issues that need to be addressed to improve patient safety.

4. Developing best practices: By analyzing patient safety case studies, healthcare providers can develop best practices for preventing similar incidents from occurring in the future. This can include changes to policies, procedures, or training programs.

5. Enhancing communication: Patient safety case studies can be used as a tool to enhance communication between healthcare providers, patients, and their families. Sharing these stories can help to build trust, foster transparency, and encourage open communication.

Overall, patient safety case studies are a critical component of any patient safety program. By examining specific incidents in detail, healthcare providers can learn from mistakes, improve safety culture, and ultimately improve patient outcomes (Al-Worafi et al., 2020a–e; Al-Worafi, 2022a,b; Al-Worafi, 2023; Vincent, 2011).

54.2 CASE 1. INTERNAL MEDICINE ERROR

A 65-year-old male with a history of hypertension, hyperlipidemia, and atrial fibrillation presented to the emergency department with complaints of chest pain and shortness of breath. He was admitted to the internal medicine service and started on heparin and nitroglycerin drip for suspected acute coronary syndrome.

On the second day of admission, the patient developed worsening shortness of breath and hypoxia. The resident on the team ordered a chest x-ray and started the patient on supplemental oxygen. The chest x-ray showed new bilateral infiltrates consistent with acute respiratory distress syndrome (ARDS).

The patient was transferred to the ICU and started on mechanical ventilation. However, the respiratory therapist noticed that the oxygen saturation levels were not improving despite increasing the oxygen delivery. Upon further investigation, it was discovered that the resident had ordered the oxygen at a flow rate of 1 L/min instead of the required 10 L/min. The patient's oxygen flow rate was increased to the appropriate level, and his oxygen saturation levels improved.

Diagnosis and Management:
The patient was diagnosed with acute respiratory distress syndrome (ARDS) likely secondary to pneumonia. He was started on broad-spectrum antibiotics and received supportive care in the ICU, including mechanical ventilation and fluid management. The resident's error in ordering the incorrect oxygen flow rate was addressed, and the patient's oxygen saturation levels were monitored closely.

Outcome:
Despite the initial error, the patient's condition gradually improved, and he was eventually weaned off mechanical ventilation and transferred to the medical-surgical floor. He continued to receive antibiotic therapy and close monitoring of his respiratory status. He was ultimately discharged home in stable condition with a follow-up appointment with his primary care physician.

Lessons Learned:
This case highlights the importance of careful attention to detail and communication between healthcare providers in the management of critically ill patients. The error in ordering the incorrect oxygen flow rate could have had serious consequences if not caught in a timely manner. It is essential for healthcare providers to double-check medication and treatment orders, especially when managing complex and acutely ill patients.

In addition, this case underscores the importance of early recognition and management of ARDS in patients with respiratory distress. Prompt initiation of appropriate treatment, such as antibiotics and mechanical ventilation, can improve outcomes in patients with ARDS.

Overall, this case underscores the need for healthcare providers to prioritize patient safety and quality of care. By learning from errors and implementing measures to prevent them from happening in the future, healthcare providers can improve outcomes and ensure that patients receive the best possible care.

54.3 CASE 2. INTERNAL MEDICINE ERROR

A 58-year-old female with a history of type 2 diabetes and hypertension was admitted to the internal medicine service for uncontrolled diabetes. Her blood glucose levels were consistently above 300 mg/dL despite increasing doses of insulin.

The resident on the team decided to switch the patient to an insulin infusion to achieve better glycemic control. However, the resident mistakenly ordered the insulin infusion at a rate of 100 units per hour instead of the intended rate of 10 units per hour. The error was not caught until several hours later when the patient's blood glucose levels dropped precipitously.

The patient was immediately started on a dextrose infusion to correct the hypoglycemia and closely monitored for signs of neuroglycopenia. Fortunately, the patient did not experience any adverse effects from the hypoglycemia.

Diagnosis and Management:
The patient was diagnosed with iatrogenic hypoglycemia due to an insulin infusion error. The insulin infusion was stopped, and the patient was started on a dextrose infusion to correct the hypoglycemia. The resident's error was addressed, and the patient's blood glucose levels were closely monitored to prevent further hypoglycemic episodes.

Outcome:
Despite the error, the patient's hypoglycemia was promptly identified and corrected, and she did not experience any adverse effects. The patient's insulin therapy was adjusted, and her blood glucose levels were brought under control. She was ultimately discharged home in stable condition with a follow-up appointment with her primary care physician.

Lessons Learned:
This case highlights the importance of medication safety and error prevention in the management of diabetes. Insulin therapy is a high-risk medication that requires careful dosing and monitoring to prevent adverse effects such as hypoglycemia. Healthcare providers must double-check medication orders and ensure that the correct dose and rate of administration are prescribed.

In addition, this case emphasizes the importance of prompt recognition and management of hypoglycemia in hospitalized patients. Hypoglycemia can have serious consequences, including neuroglycopenia, seizures, and even death. Healthcare providers must be vigilant in monitoring blood glucose levels and responding promptly to episodes of hypoglycemia.

Overall, this case underscores the need for healthcare providers to prioritize patient safety and quality of care. By learning from errors and implementing measures to prevent them from happening in the future, healthcare providers can improve outcomes and ensure that patients receive the best possible care.

54.4 CASE 3. INTERNAL MEDICINE ERROR

A 67-year-old male with a history of hypertension and diabetes presents to the emergency department with a three-day history of severe abdominal pain, nausea, vomiting, and diarrhea. He is admitted to the hospital with a working diagnosis of acute pancreatitis.

Medical Error: During his hospitalization, the patient's blood glucose levels were not properly managed, and he experienced multiple episodes of hypoglycemia. The medical team failed to adjust his insulin regimen properly, leading to a significant drop in his blood glucose levels.

Outcome: As a result of the medical error, the patient's condition deteriorated rapidly. He developed seizures, lost consciousness, and required intubation and mechanical ventilation. The patient was ultimately diagnosed with severe hypoglycemic encephalopathy, which resulted in permanent brain damage.

Root Cause Analysis: The medical error was due to a breakdown in communication between the healthcare team, inadequate monitoring of the patient's blood glucose levels, and a lack of adherence to established treatment guidelines for diabetes management.

Lessons Learned: To prevent similar errors in the future, it is essential to ensure effective communication and teamwork among healthcare providers, monitor patients' glucose levels closely, and follow established guidelines for diabetes management. Additional education and training may be necessary to improve clinicians' understanding of best practices for managing diabetes in hospitalized patients. Regular audits and reviews of treatment protocols and clinical outcomes may also help to identify areas for improvement and prevent future errors.

54.5 CASE 4. INTERNAL MEDICINE ERROR

A 73-year-old male with a history of chronic obstructive pulmonary disease (COPD) was admitted to the internal medicine service for worsening dyspnea and cough. The resident on the team started the patient on nebulized albuterol and ipratropium for symptomatic relief.

On the second day of admission, the patient's respiratory status worsened, and he was started on high-flow oxygen therapy. The resident ordered the oxygen at a flow rate of 15 L/min but failed to adjust the oxygen delivery device from a low-flow nasal cannula to a high-flow nasal cannula. As a result, the patient was receiving a fraction of the intended oxygen delivery, and his oxygen saturation levels remained low despite increasing the flow rate.

The error was caught by the nurse during routine rounds, and the oxygen delivery device was adjusted to a high-flow nasal cannula. The patient's oxygen saturation levels improved, and his respiratory status stabilized.

Diagnosis and Management:
The patient was diagnosed with acute exacerbation of COPD and started on nebulized broncho-dilators and high-flow oxygen therapy. The resident's error in ordering the incorrect oxygen delivery device was addressed, and the patient's oxygen saturation levels were closely monitored.

Outcome:
Despite the error, the patient's oxygen saturation levels were promptly corrected, and his respiratory status stabilized. He was continued on nebulized bronchodilators and high-flow oxygen therapy and received additional supportive care for his COPD exacerbation. He was ultimately discharged home in stable condition with a follow-up appointment with his primary care physician.

Lessons Learned:
This case highlights the importance of accurate and precise medication and treatment orders in the management of acutely ill patients. The error in ordering the incorrect oxygen delivery device could have had serious consequences if not caught in a timely manner. It is essential for healthcare providers to double-check medication and treatment orders, especially when managing complex and acutely ill patients.

In addition, this case emphasizes the importance of close monitoring of patients receiving high-flow oxygen therapy. High-flow oxygen therapy is a powerful tool for managing respiratory distress, but it must be used correctly to avoid adverse effects such as oxygen toxicity or carbon dioxide retention.

Overall, this case underscores the need for healthcare providers to prioritize patient safety and quality of care. By learning from errors and implementing measures to prevent them from happening in the future, healthcare providers can improve outcomes and ensure that patients receive the best possible care.

54.6 CASE 5. INTERNAL MEDICINE ERROR

A 63-year-old female with a history of congestive heart failure (CHF) and chronic kidney disease (CKD) was admitted to the internal medicine service for worsening edema and shortness of breath. The resident on the team started the patient on intravenous furosemide for diuresis and fluid management.

However, the resident mistakenly ordered the furosemide at a dose of 40 mg every 4 hours instead of the intended dose of 20 mg every 4 hours. The error was not caught until several doses had been administered, and the patient's renal function began to deteriorate.

The patient's serum creatinine levels increased from 1.5 mg/dL on admission to 2.5 mg/dL within 24 hours of starting the high-dose furosemide. The resident was alerted to the error by the nurse, and the furosemide dose was promptly reduced to the correct dose.

Diagnosis and Management:
The patient was diagnosed with iatrogenic acute kidney injury due to a medication error in the dosing of intravenous furosemide. The error in dosing was addressed, and the patient's renal function was closely monitored. The patient received additional supportive care for her CHF and CKD.

Outcome:
Despite the error, the patient's renal function improved with appropriate management, and she did not require dialysis. She was continued on a lower dose of furosemide and received additional diuretic and fluid management for her CHF and CKD. She was ultimately discharged home in stable condition with a follow-up appointment with her primary care physician.

Lessons Learned:
This case highlights the importance of medication safety and error prevention in the management of complex patients with multiple comorbidities. Furosemide is a high-risk medication that requires careful dosing and monitoring to prevent adverse effects such as acute kidney injury. Healthcare providers must double-check medication orders and ensure that the correct dose and frequency of administration are prescribed.

In addition, this case emphasizes the importance of prompt recognition and management of medication errors that can result in adverse patient outcomes. Healthcare providers must be vigilant in monitoring for adverse effects of medications and respond promptly to address any errors or complications.

Overall, this case underscores the need for healthcare providers to prioritize patient safety and quality of care. By learning from errors and implementing measures to prevent them from happening in the future, healthcare providers can improve outcomes and ensure that patients receive the best possible care.

54.7 CONCLUSION

This chapter has discussed the real cases of internal medicine errors and problems. Patient safety case studies are an essential tool for improving healthcare quality and safety. They provide a detailed analysis of a specific patient safety incident or event, which can help identify the root causes, contributing factors, and possible solutions to prevent similar incidents from occurring in the future. Case studies illustrate the potential impact of internal medicine errors on patient outcomes. In both cases, the medical errors were due to breakdowns in communication and inadequate monitoring of the patients' conditions. These errors led to serious complications, including permanent brain damage and patient death. To prevent similar errors in the future, it is important to prioritize effective communication and teamwork among healthcare providers, monitor patients' conditions closely, and follow established treatment guidelines. Additional education and training may be necessary to improve clinicians' understanding of best practices for managing complex medical conditions. Regular audits and reviews of treatment protocols and clinical outcomes can help identify areas for improvement and prevent future errors. Ultimately, preventing internal medicine errors requires a multifaceted approach that prioritizes patient safety, communication, and collaboration among healthcare providers. Healthcare organizations must invest in resources to ensure that clinicians have the knowledge, tools, and support they need to provide high-quality, safe patient care.

REFERENCES

Al-Worafi, Y.M. (Ed.). (2020a). *Drug Safety in Developing Countries: Achievements and Challenges.* Academic Press.

Al-Worafi, Y.M. (2020b). Evidence-based medications safety practice. In *Drug Safety in Developing Countries* (pp. 197–201). Academic Press.

Al-Worafi, Y.M. (2020c). Quality indicators for medications safety. In *Drug Safety in Developing Countries* (pp. 229–242). Academic Press.

Al-Worafi, Y.M. (2020d). Drug safety: Comparison between developing countries. In *Drug Safety in Developing Countries* (pp. 603–611). Academic Press.

Al-Worafi, Y.M. (2020e). Drug safety in developing versus developed countries. In *Drug Safety in Developing Countries* (pp. 613–615). Academic Press.

Al-Worafi, Y. (2022a). *A Guide to Online Pharmacy Education: Teaching Strategies and Assessment Methods.* CRC Press.

Al-Worafi, Y.M. (2022b). Patient care errors and related problems (part I): Development and validation of the model. https://orcid.org/0000-0002-5752-2913

Al-Worafi, Y.M. (Ed.). (2023). *Clinical Case Studies on Medication Safety.* Academic Press.

Vincent, C. (2011). *Patient Safety.* John Wiley & Sons.

55 Patient Safety Case Studies

Oncology

55.1 IMPORTANCE OF PATIENT SAFETY & PATIENT CARE PLAN ERRORS AND RELATED PROBLEMS CASE STUDIES

Patient safety case studies are an essential tool for improving healthcare quality and safety. Prepare the future healthcare professionals with the necessary competencies related to the patient safety-related issues are the key to success in medication safety practice in the future, however, improving the current healthcare professionals' medication safety competencies is very important in order to improve the patients' treating outcomes in terms of efficacy and safety. They provide a detailed analysis of a specific patient safety incident or event, which can help identify the root causes, contributing factors, and possible solutions to prevent similar incidents from occurring in the future. Here are some of the key reasons why patient safety case studies are important:

1. Learning from mistakes: Patient safety case studies highlight the mistakes that were made in a specific incident, providing an opportunity for healthcare providers to learn from those mistakes and prevent them from happening again in the future.

2. Improving safety culture: By sharing patient safety case studies across healthcare organizations, staff can become more aware of the importance of safety culture, and how their actions and decisions can impact patient safety.

3. Identifying systemic issues: Patient safety case studies can reveal patterns or trends in safety incidents, which can help identify systemic issues that need to be addressed to improve patient safety.

4. Developing best practices: By analyzing patient safety case studies, healthcare providers can develop best practices for preventing similar incidents from occurring in the future. This can include changes to policies, procedures, or training programs.

5. Enhancing communication: Patient safety case studies can be used as a tool to enhance communication between healthcare providers, patients, and their families. Sharing these stories can help to build trust, foster transparency, and encourage open communication.

Overall, patient safety case studies are a critical component of any patient safety program. By examining specific incidents in detail, healthcare providers can learn from mistakes, improve safety culture, and ultimately improve patient outcomes (Al-Worafi et al., 2020a–e; Al-Worafi, 2022a,b; Al-Worafi, 2023; Vincent, 2011).

55.2 CASE 1. ONCOLOGY ERROR

A 57-year-old female was diagnosed with breast cancer and was referred to a medical oncologist for further treatment. The oncologist reviewed the patient's medical records and prescribed a chemotherapy regimen that included doxorubicin and cyclophosphamide. The patient received six cycles of chemotherapy, and after completing the treatment, she underwent a A positron emission tomography (PET) scan which showed no evidence of disease.

However, six months later, the patient returned to the oncologist with complaints of fatigue and shortness of breath. The oncologist ordered a CT scan, which revealed a mass in the patient's lung. The patient underwent a biopsy, which confirmed the presence of lung cancer.

Upon further investigation, it was discovered that the oncologist had mistakenly prescribed the wrong dose of doxorubicin to the patient. The correct dose was 60 mg/m2, but the oncologist had prescribed 600 mg/m2, ten times the intended dose. This error had gone unnoticed by the nurse who administered the chemotherapy and the pharmacy that dispensed it.

The patient's lung cancer was result of the high dose of doxorubicin she received during her breast cancer treatment. She underwent treatment for the lung cancer, but her prognosis was poor due to the late detection of the cancer.

Lessons Learned:
This case highlights the importance of accurate dosing in oncology treatment. Errors in dosing can lead to serious consequences, including the development of secondary cancers. To prevent errors in

DOI: 10.1201/9781003230465-59

dosing, healthcare professionals must use accurate calculations and double-check their work. Additionally, systems should be in place to detect and prevent errors, such as independent double checks of medication orders and protocols for verifying medication dosages.

Finally, open communication between healthcare providers and patients is essential. Patients should be informed about their treatment plan, including the risks and benefits, and should be encouraged to ask questions and speak up if they have concerns about their treatment.

55.3 CASE 2. ONCOLOGY ERROR

Case Study:

A 48-year-old man with a history of colon cancer presented to his oncologist for follow-up care. The patient had undergone surgery to remove a tumor from his colon, followed by a course of chemotherapy with oxaliplatin and 5-fluorouracil (5-FU). He was now in remission and had been scheduled for routine surveillance scans.

The patient underwent a CT scan, which showed an enlarged lymph node in his abdomen. His oncologist ordered a biopsy, which confirmed the presence of cancer cells. The oncologist then prescribed a second-line chemotherapy regimen, which included irinotecan and cetuximab.

The patient received four cycles of chemotherapy but experienced significant side effects, including severe diarrhea, fatigue, and weight loss. He expressed his concerns to his oncologist, who reassured him that the side effects were expected and would improve over time.

However, the patient's condition continued to deteriorate, and he was eventually admitted to the hospital with dehydration and malnutrition. Further investigation revealed that the patient had received an incorrect dose of irinotecan. Instead of receiving 180 mg/m2, the patient had been given 280 mg/m2, which was a dose intended for patients with higher body weight.

The error had occurred due to a miscommunication between the oncologist and the pharmacist. The pharmacist had misinterpreted the patient's weight, and the error was not caught by the nurse who administered the chemotherapy.

The patient's condition stabilized after he received supportive care in the hospital, but he was left with permanent gastrointestinal damage due to the high dose of irinotecan.

Lessons Learned:

This case highlights the importance of accurate communication between healthcare providers and the need for independent double checks of medication orders. In addition, healthcare providers must be vigilant in monitoring their patients for adverse effects and responding promptly to any concerns raised by the patient.

Furthermore, healthcare providers should prioritize patient-centered care and be open to discussing the risks and benefits of treatment with their patients. Patients should also be encouraged to take an active role in their care, ask questions, and report any side effects or concerns to their healthcare providers.

55.4 CASE 3. ONCOLOGY ERROR

A 49-year-old woman with a history of breast cancer was referred to an oncologist for further treatment after undergoing a lumpectomy. The oncologist recommended radiation therapy and chemotherapy to ensure complete removal of the tumor. However, due to a miscommunication between the oncologist and the radiation therapist, the patient received a higher dose of radiation than what was prescribed, resulting in radiation toxicity.

Furthermore, during the chemotherapy administration, the oncologist failed to notice that the patient had developed neutropenia (a condition characterized by a low level of white blood cells), which is a common side effect of chemotherapy. As a result, the patient developed an infection and was admitted to the hospital. She eventually recovered from the infection, but her recovery was prolonged due to the delay in diagnosis and treatment.

After a thorough investigation, it was found that the oncologist had failed to document the patient's neutrophil count during chemotherapy administration, which could have prevented the infection. Moreover, the communication breakdown between the oncologist and radiation therapist had led to the administration of an incorrect dose of radiation.

This case highlights the importance of effective communication between healthcare providers and the need for rigorous documentation during treatment administration. Oncology errors can have severe consequences, and it is essential to follow proper protocols and guidelines to ensure patient safety.

55.5 CASE 4. ONCOLOGY ERROR

A 35-year-old woman was diagnosed with stage II breast cancer and underwent a mastectomy. Following the surgery, the oncologist recommended adjuvant chemotherapy to prevent the cancer from recurring. The patient received six cycles of chemotherapy, and during the last cycle, she developed severe neuropathy (nerve damage), which persisted even after the completion of chemotherapy.

After further investigation, it was found that the patient had received a higher dose of chemotherapy than what was recommended due to a calculation error. The patient's weight had been recorded incorrectly, leading to an incorrect dose calculation. The patient's medical records had also not been reviewed carefully, and there was no documentation of her history of neuropathy, which put her at higher risk for developing this complication.

This case highlights the importance of accurate dosing calculations and thorough documentation of medical history to prevent adverse events from chemotherapy. Oncology errors can have severe consequences, and it is ensuring accurate weight measurement and proper review of medical history.

55.6 CASE 5. ONCOLOGY ERROR

A 65-year-old man was diagnosed with stage III lung cancer and was referred to an oncologist for further management. The oncologist recommended chemotherapy and radiation therapy, followed by surgery to remove the tumor. The patient underwent six cycles of chemotherapy and radiation therapy and then underwent surgery.

During the post-operative period, the patient developed a wound infection, and a biopsy of the wound revealed that the cancer had spread to the surgical site. The patient underwent further treatment with radiation therapy and chemotherapy, but unfortunately, the cancer continued to progress, and the patient eventually succumbed to the disease.

After an investigation, it was found that the patient had received a lower dose of chemotherapy than what was prescribed due to an error in the calculation of the patient's weight. Moreover, the radiation therapy was not delivered to the targeted site due to a misalignment of the radiation beam.

This case highlights the importance of accurate dosing calculations and the need for precise delivery of radiation therapy. Oncology errors can have severe consequences, and it is essential to follow proper protocols and guidelines to ensure patient safety.

55.7 CONCLUSION

This chapter has discussed the real cases of oncology errors. Patient safety case studies are an essential tool for improving healthcare quality and safety. They provide a detailed analysis of a specific patient safety incident or event, which can help identify the root causes, contributing factors, and possible solutions to prevent similar incidents from occurring in the future. Errors in oncology care can have serious consequences for patients, including delayed diagnosis, ineffective treatments, and decreased quality of life. Oncology errors can occur at any stage of care, including diagnosis, treatment planning, and medication administration. Some common contributing factors to oncology errors include communication breakdowns, inadequate training, and system-level issues such as understaffing or inadequate resources.To mitigate the risk of oncology errors, healthcare providers should prioritize communication and collaboration among care teams, regularly review and update their knowledge and skills, and use technology and other tools to support safe and effective care. Additionally, patients and their families can play an important role in reducing the risk of errors by advocating for themselves and ensuring that they understand their diagnosis, treatment options, and medication regimen. By working together and taking proactive steps to address potential sources of error, healthcare providers and patients can improve the safety and quality of oncology care.

REFERENCES

Al-Worafi, Y.M. (Ed.). (2020a). Drug Safety in Developing Countries: Achievements and Challenges.

Al-Worafi, Y.M. (2020b). Evidence-based medications safety practice. In *Drug Safety in Developing Countries* (pp. 197–201). Academic Press.

Al-Worafi, Y.M. (2020c). Quality indicators for medications safety. In *Drug safety in developing countries* (pp. 229–242). Academic Press.

Al-Worafi, Y.M. (2020d). Drug safety: comparison between developing countries. In *Drug Safety in Developing Countries* (pp. 603–611). Academic Press.

Al-Worafi, Y.M. (2020e). Drug safety in developing versus developed countries. In *Drug Safety in Developing Countries* (pp. 613–615). Academic Press.

Al-Worafi, Y. (2022a). *A Guide to Online Pharmacy Education: Teaching Strategies and Assessment Methods*. CRC Press.

Al-Worafi, Y.M. (2022b). Patient care errors and related problems (part I): development and validation of the model. https://orcid.org/0000–0002-5752-2913

Al-Worafi, Y.M. (Ed.). (2023). *Clinical Case Studies on medication Safety*. Academic Press.

Vincent, C. (2011). *Patient safety*. John Wiley & Sons.

56 Patient Safety Case Studies

Antimicrobials

56.1 IMPORTANCE OF PATIENT SAFETY & PATIENT CARE PLAN ERRORS AND RELATED PROBLEMS CASE STUDIES

Patient safety case studies are an essential tool for improving healthcare quality and safety. Prepare the future healthcare professionals with the necessary competencies related to the patient safety-related issues are the key to success in medication safety practice in the future, however, improving the current healthcare professionals' medication safety competencies is very important in order to improve the patients' treating outcomes in terms of efficacy and safety. They provide a detailed analysis of a specific patient safety incident or event, which can help identify the root causes, contributing factors, and possible solutions to prevent similar incidents from occurring in the future. Here are some of the key reasons why patient safety case studies are important:

1. Learning from mistakes: Patient safety case studies highlight the mistakes that were made in a specific incident, providing an opportunity for healthcare providers to learn from those mistakes and prevent them from happening again in the future.

2. Improving safety culture: By sharing patient safety case studies across healthcare organizations, staff can become more aware of the importance of safety culture, and how their actions and decisions can impact patient safety.

3. Identifying systemic issues: Patient safety case studies can reveal patterns or trends in safety incidents, which can help identify systemic issues that need to be addressed to improve patient safety.

4. Developing best practices: By analyzing patient safety case studies, healthcare providers can develop best practices for preventing similar incidents from occurring in the future. This can include changes to policies, procedures, or training programs.

5. Enhancing communication: Patient safety case studies can be used as a tool to enhance communication between healthcare providers, patients, and their families. Sharing these stories can help to build trust, foster transparency, and encourage open communication.

Overall, patient safety case studies are a critical component of any patient safety program. By examining specific incidents in detail, healthcare providers can learn from mistakes, improve safety culture, and ultimately improve patient outcomes (Al-Worafi et al., 2020a–e; Al-Worafi, 2022a,b; Al-Worafi, 2023; Vincent, 2011).

56.2 CASE 1

A 62-year-old male patient was admitted to the hospital with a fever and severe abdominal pain. The patient was diagnosed with diverticulitis and prescribed antibiotics, including metronidazole and ciprofloxacin, for a 10-day course.

After four days of treatment, the patient developed a rash and reported feeling nauseous. The physician suspected a drug reaction and ordered a switch to clindamycin and doxycycline. The patient completed the 10-day course but continued to have abdominal pain and fever. A CT scan revealed a perforation in the colon and an abscess.

Further investigation revealed that the patient had a history of a severe allergy to ciprofloxacin, which was not documented in the medical record. The initial antibiotics prescribed caused an allergic reaction and worsened the patient's condition. The switch to clindamycin and doxycycline was appropriate, but the duration of the treatment was inadequate, resulting in a persistent infection.

This case study highlights the importance of obtaining a detailed patient history, including any drug allergies or adverse reactions. It also emphasizes the need for appropriate prescribing practices and vigilance in monitoring the patient's response to treatment. In this case, an antimicrobial error occurred due to incomplete documentation of the patient's medical history, resulting in an adverse reaction and inadequate treatment.

DOI: 10.1201/9781003230465-60

56.3 CASE 2

A 30-year-old female patient presented to her primary care physician with symptoms of a urinary tract infection (UTI), including dysuria and frequency. The physician prescribed a 3-day course of trimethoprim/sulfamethoxazole (TMP/SMX).

On the second day of treatment, the patient called the clinic and reported that she had developed a rash. The physician discontinued the TMP/SMX and prescribed ciprofloxacin for the remaining duration of the treatment.

The patient completed the 3-day course of ciprofloxacin but continued to have symptoms of a UTI. The physician prescribed another 3-day course of TMP/SMX.

On the second day of the second course of TMP/SMX, the patient developed severe abdominal pain and diarrhea. She was hospitalized and diagnosed with Clostridioides difficile (C. difficile) infection.

Further investigation revealed that the patient had a documented allergy to TMP/SMX, which was not noted in her medical record. The initial prescription of TMP/SMX caused an allergic reaction, and the subsequent prescription of ciprofloxacin was inappropriate for the treatment of a UTI. The second course of TMP/SMX further exacerbated the patient's condition by causing C. difficile infection.

This case study highlights the importance of obtaining a detailed patient history, including any drug allergies or adverse reactions, and verifying the patient's medication history before prescribing antibiotics. It also emphasizes the need for appropriate prescribing practices and vigilant monitoring of the patient's response to treatment. In this case, antimicrobial prescribing errors occurred due to incomplete documentation of the patient's medical history, resulting in adverse reactions and inadequate treatment.

56.4 CASE 3

A 62-year-old patient with a history of chronic obstructive pulmonary disease (COPD) presents to a pharmacy with a prescription for azithromycin, a commonly prescribed antibiotic. The pharmacy technician who receives the prescription is new and has not received sufficient training on dispensing medications, especially antibiotics.

The technician fills the prescription and gives it to the patient, who takes the medication as directed for the next five days. However, on the sixth day, the patient's symptoms worsen, and he develops a fever and shortness of breath. He goes to the emergency department, where he is diagnosed with pneumonia.

It is later discovered that the technician dispensed the wrong dosage of azithromycin to the patient. Instead of the prescribed dose of 500 mg once daily for three days, the patient was given 500 mg twice daily for five days.

This dispensing error led to the patient developing pneumonia and requiring hospitalization. The error was traced back to the technician's inadequate training, which resulted in a failure to double-check the prescription for accuracy and verify the dosage with the prescribing doctor.

This case study highlights the importance of proper training and diligence when dispensing antimicrobial medications. Antimicrobial stewardship programs and proper training for healthcare professionals can help prevent medication errors and ensure appropriate use of antibiotics to prevent the development of antibiotic-resistant bacteria.

56.5 CASE 4

A 45-year-old male patient with a history of diabetes presents to the emergency department with fever, chills, and a painful, swollen foot. The attending physician diagnoses the patient with a suspected foot infection and orders a blood test and an X-ray.

The blood test reveals an elevated white blood cell count, indicating an infection, and the X-ray shows evidence of osteomyelitis, a bone infection. The physician prescribes the patient with intravenous (IV) vancomycin and ciprofloxacin to treat the infection.

However, the physician does not adjust the dosage of the medications for the patient's impaired kidney function, as the patient's kidney function tests were not available at the time. The patient receives the prescribed antibiotics for five days, during which time his kidney function deteriorates, and he develops severe acute kidney injury.

The prescribing error is discovered, and the patient is immediately taken off the antibiotics and started on appropriate therapy for his kidney injury. The patient requires hospitalization for several weeks to recover from the acute kidney injury.

This case study highlights the importance of appropriate prescribing of antimicrobial medications, including adjusting dosages for patients with impaired kidney function. It also emphasizes the need for healthcare professionals to have access to patient information and test results to make informed decisions about prescribing medications. Antimicrobial stewardship programs and education for healthcare professionals can help prevent antimicrobial prescribing errors and reduce the risk of adverse events for patients.

56.6 CASE 5

A 73-year-old female patient with a history of recurrent urinary tract infections (UTIs) presents to the primary care physician with symptoms of a UTI. The physician prescribes the patient with ciprofloxacin for five days.

The patient takes the medication as prescribed but continues to experience symptoms after finishing the course of antibiotics. She returns to the physician, who prescribes another round of ciprofloxacin for another five days.

The patient completes the second course of antibiotics, but her symptoms persist. She returns to the physician again, who orders a urine culture and sensitivity test. The results show that the bacteria causing the infection are resistant to ciprofloxacin.

The physician then prescribes the patient with a different antibiotic, nitrofurantoin, but does not adjust the dosage for the patient's age and kidney function. The patient experiences adverse effects from the nitrofurantoin, including nausea and vomiting.

Upon review of the patient's medical history, it is discovered that the patient has been on multiple courses of antibiotics for recurrent UTIs, of antibiotic-resistant bacteria in her urinary tract.

This case study highlights the consequences of antimicrobial use errors, including the development of antibiotic resistance and adverse effects from inappropriate dosages. It emphasizes the importance of appropriate diagnosis and treatment of infections and the need to consider the patient's medical history, age, and kidney function when prescribing antibiotics.

Antimicrobial stewardship programs and education for healthcare professionals and patients can help prevent antimicrobial use errors and reduce the development of antibiotic resistance. Additionally, non-antibiotic strategies, such as probiotics and hygiene measures, may also be considered for preventing and managing recurrent UTIs.

56.7 CONCLUSION

This chapter has discussed the real cases of antimicrobials use errors and problems. Patient safety case studies are an essential tool for improving healthcare quality and safety. They provide a detailed analysis of a specific patient safety incident or event, which can help identify the root causes, contributing factors, and possible solutions to prevent similar incidents from occurring in the future. Promoting antimicrobial safety and reducing errors requires a comprehensive approach that involves various stakeholders, including healthcare providers, patients, and healthcare systems. This approach should focus on improving medication safety and reducing errors throughout the medication use process, from prescribing to monitoring, and should prioritize the appropriate use of antimicrobials to preserve their effectiveness and combat antibiotic resistance.

REFERENCES

Al-Worafi, Y.M. (Ed.). (2020a). Drug Safety in Developing Countries: Achievements and Challenges.

Al-Worafi, Y.M. (2020b). Evidence-based medications safety practice. In *Drug Safety in Developing Countries* (pp. 197–201). Academic Press.

Al-Worafi, Y.M. (2020c). Quality indicators for medications safety. In *Drug safety in developing countries* (pp. 229–242). Academic Press.

Al-Worafi, Y.M. (2020d). Drug safety: comparison between developing countries. In *Drug Safety in Developing Countries* (pp. 603–611). Academic Press.

Al-Worafi, Y.M. (2020e). Drug safety in developing versus developed countries. In *Drug Safety in Developing Countries* (pp. 613–615). Academic Press.

Al-Worafi, Y. (2022a). *A Guide to Online Pharmacy Education: Teaching Strategies and Assessment Methods*. CRC Press.

Al-Worafi, Y.M. (2022b). Patient care errors and related problems (part I): development and validation of the model. https://orcid.org/0000–0002-5752-2913

Al-Worafi, Y.M. (Ed.). (2023). *Clinical Case Studies on medication Safety*. Academic Press.

Vincent, C. (2011). *Patient safety*. John Wiley & Sons.

57 Patient Safety Case Studies

Special Population

57.1 IMPORTANCE OF PATIENT SAFETY & PATIENT CARE PLAN ERRORS AND RELATED PROBLEMS CASE STUDIES

Patient safety case studies are an essential tool for improving healthcare quality and safety. Prepare the future healthcare professionals with the necessary competencies related to the patient safety-related issues are the key to success in medication safety practice in the future, however, improving the current healthcare professionals' medication safety competencies is very important in order to improve the patients' treating outcomes in terms of efficacy and safety. They provide a detailed analysis of a specific patient safety incident or event, which can help identify the root causes, contributing factors, and possible solutions to prevent similar incidents from occurring in the future. Here are some of the key reasons why patient safety case studies are important:

1. Learning from mistakes: Patient safety case studies highlight the mistakes that were made in a specific incident, providing an opportunity for healthcare providers to learn from those mistakes and prevent them from happening again in the future.

2. Improving safety culture: By sharing patient safety case studies across healthcare organizations, staff can become more aware of the importance of safety culture, and how their actions and decisions can impact patient safety.

3. Identifying systemic issues: Patient safety case studies can reveal patterns or trends in safety incidents, which can help identify systemic issues that need to be addressed to improve patient safety.

4. Developing best practices: By analyzing patient safety case studies, healthcare providers can develop best practices for preventing similar incidents from occurring in the future. This can include changes to policies, procedures, or training programs.

5. Enhancing communication: Patient safety case studies can be used as a tool to enhance communication between healthcare providers, patients, and their families. Sharing these stories can help to build trust, foster transparency, and encourage open communication.

Overall, patient safety case studies are a critical component of any patient safety program. By examining specific incidents in detail, healthcare providers can learn from mistakes, improve safety culture, and ultimately improve patient outcomes (Al-Worafi et al., 2020a–e; Al-Worafi, 2022a,b; Al-Worafi, 2023; Vincent, 2011).

57.2 CASE 1. MEDICATION ERROR DURING PREGNANCY CASE STUDY

A 29-year-old pregnant woman, in her third trimester, was prescribed a medication to treat her hypertension by her obstetrician. The medication prescribed was Methyldopa, 500 mg twice daily. The woman had been on Methyldopa for the past 6 weeks without any side effects.

However, during a routine prenatal visit, the nurse mistakenly gave her Methotrexate, 10 mg orally, instead of Methyldopa. The nurse realized her error immediately after administering the medication and alerted the obstetrician.

The patient was immediately transferred to the hospital for monitoring and management. The patient was counseled on the potential effects of Methotrexate on the developing fetus and advised to consider termination of the pregnancy. The patient declined termination and opted for close monitoring.

The patient was started on folic acid supplementation and given intravenous fluids to help flush the medication out of her system. The patient was also closely monitored for any signs of toxicity, including gastrointestinal symptoms, liver and kidney dysfunction, and hematologic abnormalities. Regular fetal monitoring was also performed to ensure the well-being of the fetus.

The patient did not develop any signs of toxicity, and the fetus remained stable throughout the monitoring period. The patient continued on Methyldopa for the remainder of her pregnancy without any further incidents.

Discussion:
Medication errors are a significant problem in healthcare and can have serious consequences, especially during pregnancy. Medication errors during pregnancy can result in fetal malformations, growth restriction, miscarriage, stillbirth, and neonatal death.

DOI: 10.1201/9781003230465-61

Methotrexate is a known teratogen and can cause fetal malformations and miscarriage. Methotrexate inhibits DNA synthesis and cell division, leading to adverse effects on rapidly dividing cells, including fetal cells.

In this case study, the patient was fortunate not to experience any adverse effects from the medication error. The prompt identification of the error and immediate management likely contributed to the positive outcome. Folic acid supplementation and intravenous fluids were used to minimize the potential toxicity of Methotrexate.

It is important to establish a medication error reporting system to prevent future incidents and to improve patient safety. Healthcare professionals should also receive adequate training on medication administration and should double-check medications before administering them to patients.

Conclusion:
Medication errors during pregnancy can have serious consequences for both the mother and the fetus. Prompt identification and management of medication errors are critical to minimize the potential harm. The use of a medication error reporting system and adequate training of healthcare professionals can prevent future incidents and improve patient safety

57.3 CASE 2. MEDICATION ERROR DURING LACTATION CASE STUDY

A 28-year-old woman who recently gave birth was prescribed Metoclopramide to increase her milk production. The woman was instructed to take 10 mg orally three times daily.

However, the woman mistakenly took 10 mg of Metoprolol instead of Metoclopramide. The mistake was not immediately recognized, and the woman continued to take Metoprolol for the next two days.

The woman began to experience symptoms of dizziness, fatigue, and difficulty breathing. She went to the hospital, where it was discovered that she was taking Metoprolol instead of Metoclopramide.

The woman was advised to stop taking Metoprolol immediately and was given supportive treatment for her symptoms. The woman was also advised to pump and discard her breast milk for the next 24 hours.

The infant was monitored for any adverse effects. The infant did not show any signs of toxicity, and breastfeeding was resumed after 24 hours.

Discussion:
Medication errors during lactation can have serious consequences for both the mother and the infant. Medications can pass into breast milk and may cause harm to the infant. In this case, Metoprolol, a beta-blocker, was taken instead of Metoclopramide, a medication used to increase milk production.

Metoprolol can cause adverse effects in infants, including bradycardia, hypoglycemia, and respiratory depression. It is important to note that not all medications are safe to use during lactation. Healthcare professionals should consider the potential risks and benefits of medications before prescribing them to breastfeeding mothers.

In this case study, the prompt identification of the medication error and the cessation of Metoprolol prevented further harm to the infant. The woman was advised to pump and discard her breast milk for 24 hours to minimize the exposure of the infant to the medication.

Conclusion:
Medication errors during lactation can have serious consequences for both the mother and the infant. Healthcare professionals should consider the potential risks and benefits of medications before prescribing them to breastfeeding mothers. It is also essential to establish a medication error reporting system to prevent future incidents and improve patient safety. Prompt identification and management of medication errors are critical to minimizing the potential harm to both the mother and the infant.

57.4 CASE 3. MEDICATION ERROR GERIATRIC CASE STUDY

An 84-year-old male patient was admitted to the hospital with symptoms of pneumonia. The patient had a history of hypertension and was taking Lisinopril, 10 mg daily.

The patient's physician ordered Azithromycin, 500 mg orally, once daily, for the treatment of pneumonia. However, the nurse administering the medication accidentally gave the patient 500 mg of Levofloxacin instead of Azithromycin.

The error was not immediately recognized, and the patient began to experience symptoms of nausea, vomiting, and confusion. The physician was alerted, and the patient was immediately transferred to the intensive care unit for monitoring and management.

The patient was diagnosed with Levofloxacin toxicity and was given supportive treatment, including intravenous fluids and antiemetics. The patient's mental status gradually improved over the next few days, and the patient was discharged from the hospital after a week of monitoring.

Discussion:
Medication errors are common among older adults and can have serious consequences. Older adults are at an increased risk of medication errors due to polypharmacy, age-related changes in pharmacokinetics and pharmacodynamics, and comorbidities.

Levofloxacin is a broad-spectrum antibiotic that can cause adverse effects, including gastro-intestinal symptoms, central nervous system toxicity, and QT interval prolongation. Levofloxacin should be used with caution in older adults due to the risk of QT interval prolongation, which can lead to arrhythmias.

In this case study, the patient experienced Levofloxacin toxicity due to the medication error. The prompt identification of the error and the transfer to the intensive care unit likely contributed to the positive outcome. Supportive treatment, including intravenous fluids and antiemetics, was used to minimize the potential toxicity of Levofloxacin.

Conclusion:
Medication errors are common among older adults and can have serious consequences. Healthcare professionals should be aware of the potential risks and benefits of medications and should consider the age-related changes in pharmacokinetics and pharmacodynamics. It is important to establish a medication error reporting system to prevent future incidents and to improve patient safety. Prompt identification and management of medication errors are critical to minimizing the potential harm to older adults.

57.5 CASE 4. PAEDIATRIC CASE STUDY

A 3-year-old male child was brought to the emergency department with symptoms of fever and cough. The child was diagnosed with pneumonia and was prescribed Amoxicillin, 250 mg orally, three times daily.

The child's mother filled the prescription at the pharmacy and was instructed to give the child 5 ml of the medication three times daily. However, the mother mistakenly gave the child 5 ml of Azithromycin instead of Amoxicillin.

The error was not immediately recognized, and the child continued to take Azithromycin for the next two days. The child began to experience symptoms of diarrhea and vomiting, and the mother brought the child back to the hospital.

The medication error was identified, and the child was immediately given supportive treatment for the adverse effects of Azithromycin. The child's condition improved over the next few days, and the child was discharged from the hospital.

Discussion:
Medication errors in pediatric patients are common and can have serious consequences. Children are at an increased risk of medication errors due to their small size, weight, and immature organ systems. Medication errors in children can lead to adverse effects, including toxicity and death.

In this case study, the child was given Azithromycin instead of Amoxicillin, leading to adverse effects, including diarrhea and vomiting. Azithromycin is a broad-spectrum antibiotic that can cause gastrointestinal symptoms, including diarrhea, nausea, and vomiting.

The prompt identification of the medication error and the administration of supportive treatment were critical in minimizing the potential harm to the child. The child's mother was also advised on the importance of medication administration and the need to read and understand medication labels.

Conclusion:
Medication errors in pediatric patients can have serious consequences. Healthcare professionals should be aware of the potential risks and benefits of medications and should consider the age-related differences in pharmacokinetics and pharmacodynamics. It is essential to establish a medication error reporting system to prevent future incidents and to improve patient safety.

Parents and caregivers should also be educated on the importance of medication administration and the need to read and understand medication labels. Prompt identification and management of medication errors are critical to minimizing the potential harm to children.

57.6 CASE 5. ADOLESCENTS ERROR CASE STUDY

A 15-year-old girl who has been struggling with low mood and anxiety for several months. She is a high achiever in school and has always been very responsible and conscientious. However, lately, she has been making more mistakes than usual, and her grades have started to slip. Her parents have noticed that she has been more irritable and argumentative than usual and that she has been spending more time alone in her room.

Clinical Analysis:

This case presents several factors that suggest a potential mental health concern. Her change in mood and behavior may indicate depression or anxiety. Her academic performance decline suggests she might be experiencing difficulty concentrating or experiencing memory lapses. The increased irritability and arguments might indicate mood swings.

One possible explanation for these changes could be that she is experiencing significant stress or pressure in her life, which is impacting her emotional well-being and cognitive functioning. It is not uncommon for adolescents to struggle with academic or social pressure, which can lead to depressive symptoms or anxiety.

Another possibility is that she is experiencing a cognitive developmental shift. Adolescents typically experience a shift in cognitive abilities as they transition from concrete operational thinking to more abstract thinking. This can be accompanied by some confusion and difficulty applying new skills, which can result in mistakes and poorer academic performance.

It is also possible that Jenny is experiencing a combination of factors that are contributing to her changes. Given the complexity of her presentation, a comprehensive assessment by a qualified mental health professional would be necessary to determine the best course of treatment.

57.7 CONCLUSION

This chapter has discussed the real cases of special population care errors and problems, which could help medical and health students, identify the root causes, contributing factors, and possible solutions to prevent similar incidents from occurring in the future. Special populations, such as elderly patients, pediatric patients, and patients with chronic conditions or disabilities, may be more vulnerable to errors and adverse events due to their unique needs and requirements. Case studies have highlighted the need for healthcare providers to pay close attention to patient safety in special populations. Patient safety in special populations is an important area of focus for healthcare providers. It is essential to identify and address the unique needs and requirements of these populations to prevent errors and adverse events. Healthcare providers must be aware of the potential risks and take steps to mitigate them, including implementing best practices, utilizing technology and decision support tools, and providing ongoing education and training for healthcare staff.

REFERENCES

Al-Worafi, Y.M. (Ed.). (2020a). Drug Safety in Developing Countries: Achievements and Challenges.

Al-Worafi, Y.M. (2020b). Evidence-based medications safety practice. In *Drug Safety in Developing Countries* (pp. 197–201). Academic Press.

Al-Worafi, Y.M. (2020c). Quality indicators for medications safety. In *Drug safety in developing countries* (pp. 229–242). Academic Press.

Al-Worafi, Y.M. (2020d). Drug safety: comparison between developing countries. In *Drug Safety in Developing Countries* (pp. 603–611). Academic Press.

Al-Worafi, Y.M. (2020e). Drug safety in developing versus developed countries. In *Drug Safety in Developing Countries* (pp. 613–615). Academic Press.

Al-Worafi, Y. (2022a). *A Guide to Online Pharmacy Education: Teaching Strategies and Assessment Methods*. CRC Press.

Al-Worafi, Y.M. (2022b). Patient care errors and related problems (part I): development and validation of the model. https://orcid.org/0000–0002-5752-2913

Al-Worafi, Y.M. (Ed.). (2023). *Clinical Case Studies on medication Safety*. Academic Press.

Vincent, C. (2011). *Patient safety*. John Wiley & Sons.

58 Patient Safety Resources and Tools

58.1 BACKGROUND

Patient safety resources and tools are essential for improving the quality of care provided to patients and reducing the risk of adverse events. They are used by healthcare professionals, educators, researchers, and policymakers to identify and address patient safety issues, develop and implement interventions to prevent harm, and measure the impact of these interventions. In recent years, there has been a growing focus on patient safety in healthcare, as healthcare organizations and policymakers recognize the need to improve the safety and quality of care provided to patients. This has led to the development of a wide range of patient safety resources and tools that are designed to support healthcare professionals and other stakeholders in improving patient safety. Patient safety resources for education include training programs, courses, and educational materials that are designed to educate healthcare professionals on patient safety principles and best practices. These resources aim to increase awareness of patient safety issues, improve knowledge and skills related to patient safety, and encourage a culture of safety in healthcare organizations. Patient safety resources for practice include tools and guidelines that are designed to support healthcare professionals in implementing patient safety practices in their clinical work. These resources aim to improve the safety of care provided to patients by promoting the use of evidence-based practices, reducing the risk of adverse events, and supporting communication and collaboration between healthcare providers. Patient safety resources for research include journals, databases, and other resources that provide information on patient safety research, methods, and best practices. These resources aim to support researchers in conducting high-quality patient safety research, identifying gaps in the existing literature, and developing and testing interventions to improve patient safety. Overall, patient safety resources and tools are critical for improving the safety and quality of care provided to patients. They play an important role in promoting a culture of safety in healthcare organizations, supporting the implementation of evidence-based practices, and improving patient outcomes (Al-Worafi et al., 2020a–e; Al-Worafi, 2022a,b; Al-Worafi, 2023; Vincent, 2011).

58.2 PATIENT SAFETY RESOURCES FOR EDUCATION

There are many resources available to educate healthcare providers and patients on patient safety. Here are some examples:

1. Agency for Healthcare Research and Quality (AHRQ) - AHRQ offers a wide range of patient safety resources, including toolkits, webinars, and guides on topics such as reducing falls, medication safety, and healthcare-associated infections.

2. Institute for Healthcare Improvement (IHI) - IHI offers a variety of resources on patient safety, including online courses, toolkits, and white papers. Their resources cover a wide range of topics, such as preventing adverse drug events and improving communication between patients and providers.

3. National Patient Safety Foundation (NPSF) - NPSF provides educational resources and tools to help healthcare providers and patients improve patient safety. They offer courses and webinars, as well as resources on topics such as communication, teamwork, and patient engagement.

4. Joint Commission - The Joint Commission provides resources on a variety of patient safety topics, including hand hygiene, medication safety, and preventing falls. They offer webinars, newsletters, and other educational resources for healthcare providers.

5. Centers for Disease Control and Prevention (CDC) - The CDC provides resources on patient safety, including guidelines for infection prevention and control, as well as educational resources for healthcare providers and patients.

6. World Health Organization (WHO) - The WHO provides resources on patient safety, including a patient safety curriculum for healthcare providers, as well as guidelines on topics such as hand hygiene and preventing healthcare-associated infections.

7. MedlinePlus - MedlinePlus provides patient education resources on a variety of health topics, including patient safety. They offer easy-to-understand information on topics such as preventing falls, medication safety, and avoiding medical errors.

8. National Institute for Occupational Safety and Health (NIOSH) - NIOSH provides resources on preventing workplace violence in healthcare settings, as well as other workplace safety topics.

9. Patient Safety Movement Foundation (PSMF) - PSMF is a non-profit organization that provides educational resources and tools to help healthcare providers and patients improve patient safety. They offer a variety of resources on topics such as reducing medical errors, preventing infections, and improving communication.

10. American Nurses Association (ANA) - The ANA provides resources on patient safety for nurses, including webinars, toolkits, and guidelines on topics such as preventing falls, medication safety, and infection prevention.

11. American Medical Association (AMA) - The AMA provides resources on patient safety for physicians, including toolkits, guidelines, and educational modules on topics such as medication safety, communication, and teamwork.

12. Patient Safety and Quality Healthcare (PSQH) - PSQH provides a variety of resources on patient safety, including articles, webinars, and podcasts. Their resources cover a wide range of topics, such as patient engagement, medication safety, and quality improvement.

13. Health Research and Educational Trust (HRET) - HRET provides resources on patient safety and quality improvement, including toolkits, webinars, and guides on topics such as reducing healthcare-associated infections and improving communication.

14. National Association of Healthcare Quality (NAHQ) - NAHQ provides resources on healthcare quality and patient safety, including webinars, toolkits, and certification programs for healthcare quality professionals.

15. ECRI Institute - ECRI provides resources on patient safety and quality improvement, including toolkits, guidelines, and educational resources on topics such as medication safety, infection prevention, and falls prevention.

58.3 PATIENT SAFETY RESOURCES FOR PRACTICE

Ensuring patient safety is crucial in healthcare practice. Here are some resources that can help healthcare professionals improve patient safety:

1. Agency for Healthcare Research and Quality (AHRQ) - This is a government organization that offers resources and tools to improve patient safety, such as the Hospital Survey on Patient Safety Culture and the Comprehensive Unit-based Safety Program (CUSP).

2. National Patient Safety Foundation (NPSF) - This is a non-profit organization dedicated to improving patient safety. They offer a variety of resources and tools, such as the Patient Safety Curriculum for Medical Schools and the RCA2: Improving Root Cause Analyses and Actions to Prevent Harm.

3. Institute for Healthcare Improvement (IHI) - This organization offers various resources and tools, such as the IHI Open School, which provides online courses on patient safety and quality improvement, and the IHI Global Trigger Tool, which is a method for identifying adverse events and measuring harm.

4. Joint Commission - This is an independent, non-profit organization that accredits healthcare organizations and offers various resources for improving patient safety, such as the Sentinel Event Alert, which provides guidance on preventing sentinel events, and the National Patient Safety Goals, which are standards for improving patient safety.

5. Centers for Disease Control and Prevention (CDC) - This government organization provides resources for preventing healthcare-associated infections and improving antibiotic use, such as the CDC's Core Elements of Hospital Antibiotic Stewardship Programs.

6. World Health Organization (WHO) - This international organization offers resources for improving patient safety, such as the WHO Surgical Safety Checklist and the WHO Global Patient Safety Challenge on Medication Safety.

7. National Quality Forum (NQF) - This organization provides a framework for measuring and reporting on healthcare quality and patient safety, as well as tools and resources for improving quality, such as the NQF Safe Practices for Better Healthcare.

8. American Nurses Association (ANA) - This professional organization for nurses offers resources for improving patient safety, such as the ANA's Nursing's Social Policy Statement and the ANA's Principles for Nursing Practice.

9. American Medical Association (AMA) - This professional organization for physicians offers resources for improving patient safety, such as the AMA's Principles of Medical Ethics and the AMA's Physician's Guide to Medical Liability.

10. Institute for Safe Medication Practices (ISMP) - This non-profit organization provides resources for preventing medication errors, such as the ISMP Medication Safety Alert! newsletter and the ISMP Medication Safety Self Assessment.

11. The Leapfrog Group - This organization is focused on improving healthcare safety and quality through transparency and accountability. They provide a variety of resources, such as the Leapfrog Hospital Safety Grade and the Leapfrog Hospital Survey.

12. American Society of Health-System Pharmacists (ASHP) - This professional organization for pharmacists offers resources for improving medication safety, such as the ASHP Guidelines on Preventing Medication Errors in Hospitals and the ASHP Medication Safety Resource Center.

13. National Institute for Occupational Safety and Health (NIOSH) - This organization provides resources for preventing workplace injuries and illnesses in healthcare, such as the NIOSH Healthcare Wide Hazards and Controls resource and the NIOSH Safe Patient Handling and Mobility resource.

14. Patient Safety and Quality Healthcare (PSQH) - This is a publication and online resource that provides articles, case studies, and other resources for improving patient safety and quality in healthcare.

15. The Patient Safety Movement Foundation - This non-profit organization is dedicated to eliminating preventable patient deaths by promoting patient safety and healthcare transparency. They offer resources and tools, such as the Actionable Patient Safety Solutions (APSS) and the Patient Safety Curriculum.

16. The Society for Simulation in Healthcare (SSH) - This organization promotes the use of simulation in healthcare education and training to improve patient safety. They offer resources, such as the SSH Simulation Operations Handbook and the SSH Accreditation Standards for Healthcare Simulation Programs.

17. The National Council of State Boards of Nursing (NCSBN) - This organization provides resources for nursing practice, such as the NCSBN Model Nursing Practice Act and the NCSBN Guidelines for Delegation.

18. The American Board of Medical Specialties (ABMS) - This organization is responsible for certifying medical specialists in the United States. They offer resources for improving patient safety and quality, such as the ABMS Continuing Certification Directory and the ABMS Vision for the Future of Continuing Certification.

19. Diseases guidelines.

These resources can be useful for healthcare professionals looking to improve patient safety in their practice.

58.4 PATIENT SAFETY RESOURCES FOR RESEARCH

1. PubMed - PubMed is a free database maintained by the National Library of Medicine that includes over 30 million citations for biomedical literature, including research on patient safety. It is a useful resource for finding peer-reviewed journal articles on a wide range of topics related to patient safety.

2. Cochrane Library - The Cochrane Library is a collection of evidence-based reviews and meta-analyses of healthcare interventions, including interventions related to patient safety. It is a useful resource for finding systematic reviews and meta-analyses on patient safety topics.

3. Agency for Healthcare Research and Quality (AHRQ) - AHRQ is a government agency that conducts research and develops tools and resources to improve the quality and safety of healthcare. Their website includes a wide range of resources on patient safety, including research studies, guidelines, and tools.

4. National Patient Safety Foundation (NPSF) - NPSF is a non-profit organization dedicated to improving patient safety. Their website includes a wide range of resources on patient safety, including research studies, guidelines, and tools.

5. Institute for Healthcare Improvement (IHI) - IHI is a non-profit organization that focuses on improving healthcare quality and safety. Their website includes a wide range of resources on patient safety, including research studies, guidelines, and tools.

6. The Joint Commission - The Joint Commission is a non-profit organization that accredits healthcare organizations and develops standards for quality and safety. Their website includes a wide range of resources on patient safety, including research studies, guidelines, and tools.

7. World Health Organization (WHO) - The WHO is a United Nations agency that is responsible for international public health. Their website includes a wide range of resources on patient safety, including research studies, guidelines, and tools.

8. Health Services Research (HSR) - HSR is a peer-reviewed journal that publishes research on healthcare delivery, organization, and financing. It includes research studies on patient safety and other topics related to healthcare quality and safety.

9. BMJ Quality & Safety - BMJ Quality & Safety is a peer-reviewed journal that focuses on research, reviews, and analysis of healthcare quality and safety. It includes articles on patient safety, quality improvement, and healthcare systems.

10. Journal of Patient Safety - Journal of Patient Safety is a peer-reviewed journal that focuses on research, reviews, and analysis of patient safety issues. It includes articles on adverse events, medication safety, and quality improvement.

11. American Journal of Medical Quality - American Journal of Medical Quality is a peer-reviewed journal that focuses on research, reviews, and analysis of healthcare quality and safety. It includes articles on patient safety, healthcare systems, and quality improvement.

12. The Lancet - The Lancet is a peer-reviewed medical journal that covers a wide range of medical topics, including patient safety. It includes articles on medication safety, quality improvement, and healthcare systems.

13. National Quality Forum (NQF) - NQF is a non-profit organization that develops and endorses standards for healthcare quality and safety. Their website includes resources on patient safety, quality improvement, and healthcare systems.

14. Institute of Medicine (IOM) - The IOM is an independent organization that provides research and advice on healthcare issues. Their website includes reports on patient safety, healthcare quality, and healthcare systems.

15. The Leapfrog Group - The Leapfrog Group is a non-profit organization that advocates for healthcare safety and quality. Their website includes research on patient safety, quality improvement, and healthcare systems.

16. Scopus - Scopus is a large abstract and citation database of peer-reviewed literature, including research on patient safety. It includes articles from over 22,000 journals, conference proceedings, and books in a wide range of subject areas.

17. ResearchGate - ResearchGate is a social networking site for researchers that includes a large database of research publications, including research on patient safety. It allows researchers to share their work, collaborate with other researchers, and connect with peers in their field.

18. Google Scholar - Google Scholar is a free search engine that allows users to search for scholarly literature, including research on patient safety. It includes articles from a wide range of sources, including peer-reviewed journals, conference proceedings, and theses.

19. Web of Science - Web of Science is a large abstract and citation database of scholarly literature, including research on patient safety. It includes articles from over 20,000 journals, conference proceedings, and books in a wide range of subject areas.

20. CINAHL - CINAHL is a database of nursing and allied health literature, including research on patient safety. It includes articles from over 5,000 journals, as well as books, dissertations, and conference proceedings.

21. Medline - Medline is a database of biomedical literature, including research on patient safety. It includes articles from over 5,600 journals, as well as books, dissertations, and conference proceedings.

22. Embase - Embase is a database of biomedical literature, including research on patient safety. It includes articles from over 8,500 journals, as well as conference proceedings, books, and drug information.

58.5 PATIENT SAFETY TOOLS

There are many tools available to help healthcare providers improve patient safety. Here are some examples:

1. Root Cause Analysis (RCA) - RCA is a process used to identify the underlying causes of adverse events or near-misses. This tool helps healthcare providers understand what went wrong and how to prevent similar events from happening in the future.

2. Failure Mode and Effects Analysis (FMEA) - FMEA is a proactive risk assessment tool that helps healthcare providers identify and prioritize potential failures in a process or system. This tool is often used to prevent errors before they occur.

3. Trigger Tools - Trigger tools are used to identify potential adverse events by reviewing medical records for specific criteria or "triggers". This tool helps healthcare providers identify areas for improvement and prevent future errors.

4. Computerized Provider Order Entry (CPOE) - CPOE is a computer-based system that allows healthcare providers to enter orders for medications, tests, and other treatments electronically. This tool helps reduce errors related to handwriting or miscommunication.

5. Bar Coding and Scanning - Bar coding and scanning systems are used to ensure that the right medication or treatment is given to the right patient at the right time. This tool helps reduce errors related to medication administration.

6. Checklists - Checklists are used to standardize processes and ensure that all necessary steps are completed. This tool is often used in high-risk situations, such as surgery, to prevent errors and improve patient safety.

7. Clinical Decision Support Systems (CDSS) - CDSS are computer-based systems that provide healthcare providers with evidence-based guidelines and recommendations to support clinical decision-making. This tool helps improve patient safety by ensuring that patients receive the most appropriate and effective care.

8. Patient Safety Culture Surveys - Surveys are used to assess the culture of safety within a healthcare organization. This tool helps identify areas for improvement and monitor progress over time.

9. Standardized Order Sets - Standardized order sets are pre-designed templates for common medical conditions, which help standardize care and reduce the risk of errors. This tool is particularly helpful in complex medical situations, such as critical care.

10. Incident Reporting Systems - Incident reporting systems allow healthcare providers to report adverse events or near-misses. This tool helps healthcare organizations track and analyze incidents, and develop strategies to prevent future errors.

11. High-Reliability Organizing (HRO) - HRO is a management approach that emphasizes the importance of reliability, safety, and risk reduction. This tool helps healthcare organizations adopt a culture of safety and improve patient outcomes.

12. Simulation Training - Simulation training uses realistic scenarios to help healthcare providers practice critical skills and procedures. This tool helps improve performance and reduce the risk of errors in real-world situations.

13. Medication Reconciliation - Medication reconciliation is a process that involves comparing a patient's current medication regimen to their previous regimen, and identifying any discrepancies. This tool helps reduce medication errors related to prescribing, dispensing, and administering medications.

14. Patient Education - Patient education involves providing patients with information about their health condition, treatment options, and risks and benefits. This tool helps improve patient safety by ensuring that patients are informed and engaged in their care.

15. Handoff Communication Tools - Handoff communication tools are used to standardize communication during patient handoffs, which can be a high-risk time for errors. This tool helps ensure that critical information is transferred accurately and efficiently between healthcare providers.

16. Adverse Event Reporting Systems (AERS) - AERS is a system developed by the FDA for reporting ADRs associated with drugs and biologic products. Healthcare providers can report adverse events directly to the FDA through this system.

17. MedWatch - MedWatch is a voluntary reporting program run by the FDA that allows healthcare providers and patients to report adverse events associated with drugs, medical devices, and other healthcare products.

18. Institute for Safe Medication Practices (ISMP) - ISMP provides a voluntary reporting program called the Medication Errors Reporting Program (MERP). Healthcare providers can report medication errors and ADRs to this program, which provides information and recommendations for preventing future errors.

19. National Coordinating Council for Medication Error Reporting and Prevention (NCC MERP) - NCC MERP is a coalition of organizations that work together to promote medication safety. They provide tools and resources for reporting medication errors and ADRs, as well as guidelines for preventing future errors.

20. Joint Commission - The Joint Commission requires healthcare organizations to have a process for reporting and analyzing adverse events, including medication errors and ADRs. They provide guidelines and resources to help healthcare organizations implement effective reporting systems.

21. Safety Reporting Portal - The Safety Reporting Portal is a system developed by the FDA for reporting safety concerns related to medical products. Healthcare providers and patients can report ADRs, medication errors, and other safety concerns through this system.

22. Vaccine Adverse Event Reporting System (VAERS) - VAERS is a system developed by the CDC and FDA for reporting adverse events associated with vaccines. Healthcare providers and patients can report vaccine-related adverse events through this system.

23. Yellow Card Scheme - The Yellow Card Scheme is a program run by the Medicines and Healthcare products Regulatory Agency (MHRA) in the UK for reporting ADRs associated with drugs and vaccines. Healthcare providers and patients can report adverse events through this program.

58.6 CONCLUSION

This chapter has discussed the patient safety resources and tools for education, practice and research. Patient safety is a critical issue that affects millions of patients worldwide every year. Patient safety resources and tools are essential for improving the safety and quality of care provided to patients and reducing the risk of adverse events. These resources and tools are designed to support healthcare professionals, educators, researchers, and policymakers in identifying and addressing patient safety issues, implementing evidence-based practices, and measuring the impact of interventions. Patient safety resources for education, practice, and research play a vital role in promoting a culture of safety in healthcare organizations and improving patient outcomes. By leveraging patient safety resources and tools, healthcare professionals and other stakeholders can work together to ensure that patients receive safe and high-quality care.

REFERENCES

Al-Worafi, Y.M. (Ed.). (2020a). Drug Safety in Developing Countries: Achievements and Challenges.

Al-Worafi, Y.M. (2020b). Evidence-based medications safety practice. In *Drug Safety in Developing Countries* (pp. 197–201). Academic Press.

Al-Worafi, Y.M. (2020c). Quality indicators for medications safety. In *Drug safety in developing countries* (pp. 229–242). Academic Press.

Al-Worafi, Y.M. (2020d). Drug safety: comparison between developing countries. In *Drug Safety in Developing Countries* (pp. 603–611). Academic Press.

Al-Worafi, Y.M. (2020e). Drug safety in developing versus developed countries. In *Drug Safety in Developing Countries* (pp. 613–615). Academic Press.

Al-Worafi, Y. (2022a). *A Guide to Online Pharmacy Education: Teaching Strategies and Assessment Methods.* CRC Press.

Al-Worafi, Y.M. (2022b). Patient care errors and related problems (part I): development and validation of the model. https://orcid.org/0000-0002-5752-2913

Al-Worafi, Y.M. (Ed.). (2023). *Clinical Case Studies on medication Safety.* Academic Press.

Vincent, C. (2011). *Patient safety.* John Wiley & Sons.

Index

3d printing, 319

Active lecture, 14
Acupuncture, 78
Acute respiratory distress syndrome (ARDS), 461
Adherence, 119
Administration errors, 27
Adolescents, 270–273
    causes of, 271
    challenges and recommendations, 272–273
    errors and related problems, 270–271
    prevention of, 271–272
Adverse Drug reactions (ADRs), 2, 3, 7, 12, 22, 24, 27,
    101, 104, 113, 123, 138, 140, 144, 183, 217,
    229, 235–237, 272, 273, 287, 288, 337, 344,
    407, 408, 436–438, 441
Adverse Event Reporting Systems (AERS), 484
Affordable Care Act, 4
AG assessment tool, 44–45
Agency for Healthcare Research and Quality (AHRQ),
    151, 479, 480, 482
Alcohol consumption, 52
Allergies, 44
The American Board of Medical Specialties
    (ABMS), 481
American College of Surgeons (ACS), 3
American Journal of Medical Quality, 482
American Medical Association (AMA), 345, 480,
    481
American Nurses Association (ANA), 480, 481
American Society of Health- System Pharmacists
    (ASHP), 7, 481
Antimicrobial resistance (AMR), 139, 298–299
    causes of, 299–300
    challenges and recommendations, 301–303
    in developing countries, 299
    interventions, 300–301
    prevention of, 300
Antimicrobial safety interventions, 300–301
Artificial intelligence (AI), 319, 322
Association of American Medical Colleges (AAMC), 4
Augmented Reality (AR) Technology, 321
Auscultation-act, 46
Automated alert systems, 320
Ayurveda, 78, 80–81

Bar coding and scanning, 483
Barcode Medication Administration (BCMA), 320
Beauty and cosmetic medicine, 309–310
Biofields. *See* Energy medicine
Biologically-based practices, 78, 82–83
Black Death, 278
Blended teaching strategy, 16
Bloodstream infections, 158
BMJ quality & safety, 482
Bogdanich, Walt, 3

Breast cancer, 216
Breastfeeding, 261–265

Caregivers, 270
Centers for Disease Control and Prevention (CDC),
    479, 480
Central Drugs Standard Control Organization
    (CDSCO), 138
Checklists, 483
Chief Complaint (CC), 43
Chiropractic, 78
Chronic Kidney Disease (CKD), 443, 464
Chronic Obstructive Pulmonary Disease (COPD), 443,
    449, 458, 463, 471
Chronic pain, 78
CINAHL, 483
Clinical Decision Support Systems (CDSS), 320, 483
Clinical pathology. *See* Laboratory medicine
Clinical trials
    advantages of, 397–398
    barriers of, 399–400
    in developing countries, 400–402
    disadvantages of, 398
    facilitators of, 399
    history of, 395–396
    importance of, 396–397
    phases of, 397
    quality of, 400
    rationality of, 396
Cochrane Library, 482
Cognitive Behavioral Therapy (CBT), 52
Cohen, Michael, 3
Colon cancer, 216
Communication, 42, 335
Community services-based learning, 16
Competencies and learning outcomes, 10
    cognitive, 10–11
    communication, education, and collaboration, 11
    ethical, legal, and professional responsibilities, 12
    health promotion and community services, 12
    knowledge, 10
    leadership and management, 11
    learning and personal/professional
        development, 11
    medication safety, 11–12
    patient care, 11
    patient safety, 12
    prescribing, 12
    research, 12
    technology, 12
Complementary and alternative medicines (CAM),
    24, 29
Complete Blood Count (CBC), 447
Comprehensive Unit-based Safety Program (CUSP), 480
Computerized Provider Order Entry (CPOE), 483
Computerized tomography (CT), 449

Congestive heart failure (CHF), 464
Consolidated Standards of Reporting Trials (CONSORT), 400
Continuous Professional Development (CPD), 8
Coronary artery bypass grafting (CABG), 452
Coronary artery disease, 78
COVID-19 pandemic, 278, 279
Cultural competence, 332
Cushing, Harvey, 3, 24

Davis, Neil, 3
Delphi method, 25
Dermatology, beauty and cosmetic medicine, 308–314
  causes of, 311
  in developing countries, 312–313
  errors and related problems, 310–311
  prevention of, 311–312
Diagnostic errors, 335
Diagnostic-Related Groups (DRGs), 3
Diet challenges, 55
Diethylstilbestrol (DES), 2
Direct assessment methods, 17
Discharge medication errors, 28
Dispensing and administration errors, 110–114
  causes and factors, 110–111
  challenges of, 112–114
  prevention of, 111–112
Dispensing errors, 27–28
Drug abuse and misuse, 138
Drug interactions, 28
Drug safety education, 2
Drug Use Evaluation (DUE), 111
Drug-Related Problems (DRPs), 7, 138

Educating healthcare professionals, 5
Education and counseling errors, 28
Efficacy of medications, 119
Electrocardiogram (ECG), 452–454, 458
Electronic health records (EHRs), 208, 210, 319, 320, 322
Electronic Medical Records (EMRs), 319
Electronic medication administration systems (eMARs), 322
Embase, 483
Emergency department (ED), 183–186
  causes of, 184
  challenges and recommendations, 186–187
  errors and related problems, 183–184
  prevention of, 184–185
Energy medicine, 79, 85–86
Energy therapies, 78
Enteral nutrition, 94–95
Epidemiology and pharmacoepidemiology research
  advantages of, 408–409
  barriers of, 410
  in developing countries, 411–412
  disadvantages of, 409
  facilitators of, 409–410
  importance of, 408

quality of, 410–411
rationality of, 407–408
Evidence-based medicine (EBM), 332
Evidence-based patient safety
  barriers for the, 335
  in developing countries, challenges and recommendations, 336–338
  errors and related problems, 335–336
  facilitators for the, 334–335
  importance of, 333–334
  rationality of, 332–333
Exercise challenges, 55

Failure Mode and Effects Analysis (FMEA), 483
Fall prevention systems, 319
Falls, 335
Family-centered care, 243
Fecal occult blood test (FOBT), 430
Flipped classroom, 15
Florence Nightingale, 3
Focused Assessment. See Rapid trauma assessment
Food and Drug Administration (FDA), 2, 3

Geriatrics, 235–238
  causes of, 236
  challenges and recommendations, 237–238
  errors and related problems, 235–236
  prevention of, 236–237
Global Patient Safety Action Plan, 4
Global Patient Safety Challenge, 4
Google Scholar, 483

Hand hygiene monitoring systems, 320
Handoff communication tools, 484
The Hawthorne Studies, 345
Headaches, 78
Health care, 2
Health education, 35
Health information technology (HIT), 332
Health pandemics, 278
Health Research and Educational Trust (HRET), 480
Health screening, 34–35
Health Services Research (HSR), 482
Healthcare outcomes, 5
Healthcare professionals, 5, 288
Healthcare systems, 46, 55
Healthcare-associated infections (HAIs), 335, 417
Healthy pregnancy, 252
Hephaestus, 3
Herbal medicines, 78, 142
Herd immunity, 34
High-Reliability Organizing (HRO), 484
History of Present Illness (HPI), 43
Homeopathy, 78, 81
Hooker, Worthington, 3, 18, 24
Hopkins, Johns, 4
Hormone oxytocin, 261
Hospital-acquired. See Nosocomial infections
Hospital Acquired Pneumonia (HAP), 442, 443

Hypertension, 443, 458

Imaging tests, 174
Immunization, 34, 37
Incident Reporting Systems, 483
Indirect assessment methods, 17–18
Insomnia, 78
Institute for Healthcare Improvement (IHI), 4, 479, 480, 482
Institute for Safe Medication Practices (ISMP), 481, 484
Institute of Medicine (IoM), 3, 345, 482
Institute of Safe Medicine Practices (ISMP), 110
Integrative medicine, 79
Intensive care unit (ICU), 192–195
    causes of, 192–193
    challenges and recommendations, 194
    errors and related problems, 192
    prevention of, 193
Interactive lecture-based teaching strategy, 15
Interactive vodcast, 14
Interactive web-based learning, 14
Interactive-spaced education, 14
Internal medicine (IM), 208–211
    causes of, 208–209
    challenges and recommendations, 211
    errors and related problems, 208
    prevention of, 209–210
Internists, 208
Irritable bowel syndrome (IBS), 453
Isolation and cohorting, 278

The Joint Commission, 479, 480, 482, 484
The Joint Commission on Accreditation of Healthcare Organizations (JCAHO), 345
Joint Commission for Accreditation of Hospitals (JCAH), 3
Journal of Patient Safety, 482

Kiani, Joe, 4

Laboratory medicine, 165–169
    causes of, 166
    challenges and recommendations, 168–169
    prevention of, 166–167
Lactation, 261–265
    causes of, 262
    challenges and recommendations, 263–265
    errors and related problems, 261–262
    prevention of, 262–263
The Lancet, 482
The Leapfrog Group, 481, 482
Literature review
    advantages of, 350–351
    barriers to, 352
    in developing countries, 353–354
    disadvantages of, 351
    facilitators of, 351–352
    importance of, 349–350
    quality of, 353
    rationality of, 349

Lung cancer, 216

Manipulative and body-based practices, 78–79, 83–85
Massage therapy, 78
Mastitis, 262
Maternal and infant mortality rates, 254–256
Medical education, 2
Medical errors, 5, 29
Medical errors prevention, 61–62
    challenges of, 62–64
    facilitators and barriers, 62
Medical imaging, 319
Medication abuse and misuse, 7, 28, 140
Medication error reporting program (MERP), 4, 484
Medication errors, 7, 138, 335
Medication management systems, 319
Medication reconciliation errors, 28, 484
Medication Safety Certificate, 7
Medication safety issues, 138–144
    adverse drug reactions (ADRs) and medication errors, 138–139
    challenges of, 143–144
    counterfeit and substandard medications, 140
    herbal medicines, 142
    medication abuse and misuse, 140
    nutraceuticals, 142–143
    pharmacovigilance, 138
    self-care and self-medications, 139
    self-medication with antimicrobials, 139
    storage and disposal of medicines, 141–142
    substance abuse, 140–141
Medication therapy management (MTM), 225
Medications safety, 2
Medicines and Healthcare products Regulatory Agency (MHRA), 484
Medicines Control Council (MCC), 138
Medline, 483
MedlinePlus, 479
MedWatch, 484
Menopausal, 78
Methicillin-resistant Staphylococcus aureus (MRSA), 445
Methotrexate, 475
Migration of healthcare professionals, 47, 57
Mind-body medicine, 78, 81–82
Mixed method research
    advantages of, 386
    barriers of, 387–388
    in developing countries, 389–390
    disadvantages of, 386
    facilitators of, 387
    importance of, 385–386
    online, 388–389
    quality of, 388
    rationality of, 384–385
Monitoring errors
    causes and factors, 120–121
    challenges of, 122–124
    prevention of, 121–122

treatment evaluation, 119

National Academy of Medicine (NAM), 3
National Association of Healthcare Quality
    (NAHQ), 480
National Coordinating Council for Medication Error
    Reporting and Prevention (NCC
    MERP), 484
The National Council of State Boards of Nursing
    (NCSBN), 481
National Institute for Occupational Safety and Health
    (NIOSH), 480, 481
National medication errors, 46
National Patient Safety Foundation (NPSF), 4, 479,
    480, 482
National Quality Forum (NQF), 481, 482
Naturopathy, 78, 81
Non-pharmacological errors, 27
Nosocomial infections, 158–160
Nutraceuticals, 142–143
Nutrition care plan, 93–94
Nutrition Care Process (NCP), 93
Nutrition routes, 92–93
Nutrition support, 92
Nutrition-related errors, 29

Obesity, 458
Objective structured clinical examination (OSCE), 18
Oncology, 216–220
    causes of, 217
    challenges and recommendations, 219–220
    errors and related problems, 216–217
    prevention of, 217–218
Online patient safety education, 7
Over-the-counter (OTC) medications, 139

Palpation assessment, 46
Pandemic, 278–282
    causes of, 279–280
    challenges and recommendations, 280–282
    errors and related problems, 279
    prevention of, 280
Parenteral nutrition, 95
Patient assessment and diagnosis errors, 27
Patient assessment errors, 44
Patient care errors and related problems, 24–29
    complementary and alternative medicine (CAM)
        errors, 78–88
    dispensing and administration errors, 110–114
    medical errors, 61–64
    monitoring errors, 119–124
    non-pharmacological errors, 52–57
    nutrition errors, 92–97
    patient assessment and diagnostic errors, 42–47
    patient education and counseling errors, 129–134
    pharmacological errors, 101–105
    preventive medicine errors, 34–37
    surgical errors, 69–73
Patient care plan errors and related problems (Part I)
    health education error, 429–430

health screening error, 430
patient education error, 430–431, 432–434
prescribing error, 431–432
preventive medicine errors, 428–429
Patient care plan errors and related problems (Part II))
    administration errors, 441
    dispensing error, 440–441
    mild adverse drug reaction, 436–437
    prescribing errors, 439–440
    therapeutic evaluation error, 437–439
Patient confidence, 5
Patient education, 484
Patient education and counseling errors, 129–134
    causes and factors, 130–131
    challenges of, 132–133
    prevention of, 131–132
Patient engagement tools, 321
Patient identification systems, 319
Patient monitoring systems, 319, 320
Patient portals, 320
Patient Safety and Quality Healthcare (PSQH),
    480, 481
Patient safety case studies
    antimicrobials, 470–472
    emergency department, 452–454
    intensive care unit, 456–450
    internal medicine, 461–464
    laboratory medicine and radiology, 447–450
    nosocomial infections cases, 442–445
    oncology, 466–468
    patient care plan errors and related problems (Part I),
        428–434
    patient care plan errors and related problems
        (Part II)), 435–441
    special population, 474–477
Patient safety culture, 149–153
    dimensions of, 150
    factors affecting, 152
    field of, 149
    importance of, 151
    measurement of, 151
    perceptions and attitudes of healthcare providers,
        152–153
    rationality of, 150
    recommendations for, 153
Patient safety culture surveys, 483
Patient safety curriculum guide, 4
Patient safety education
    assessment methods, 16–18
    history of, 2–4
    importance of, 4–5
    issues, 2
    teaching strategies, 14–16
Patient safety in developing countries
    challenges of, 8
    curriculum, 7
    degrees and programs, 7
    online education, 7
    quality and accreditation, 7–8
Patient Safety Movement Foundation (PSMF), 480, 481

Patient safety research
    clinical trials, 395–402
    in developing countries, 418–422
    epidemiology and pharmacoepidemiology,
        407–412
    history of, 344–345
    importance of, 345–347
    literature review, 349–354
    mixed methods, 384–390
    qualitative methods, 359–366
    quantitative methods, 371–379
Patient safety resources
    for education, 479–480
    for practice, 480–481
    for research, 481–483
Patient safety-related issues, 22
    culture, 149–153
    emergency department (ED), 183–186
    intensive care unit (ICU), 192–195
    internal medicine (IM), 208–211
    laboratory medicine, 165–169
    medication safety issues, 138–144
    oncology, 216–220
    pharmacies, 225–230
    radiology, 174–178
    surgery, 200–204
Patient safety tools, 483–484
Patient safety training, 287–293
    barriers for, 290
    challenges and recommendations, 291–293
    facilitators of, 289–290
    for healthcare professionals, 288
    importance of, 289
    for medical students, 287–288
    online, 290–291
    rational for, 288–289
Pediatrics, 243–247
    issues, causes of, 244
    in developing countries, 245–247
    errors and related problems, 243–244
    prevention of, 245
Percussion-act, 46
Personal protective equipment (PPE), 278, 279, 282
Pharmacies errors, 225–230
    causes of, 226–227
    challenges and recommendations, 228–230
    errors and related problems, 226
    prevention of, 227
    safety culture, 227–228
Pharmacological errors, 27, 101–105
    causes and factors, 101–102
    challenges of, 103–105
    prevention of, 102–103
Pharmacovigilance Program of India (PvPI), 138
Pharmacovigilance, 7
PICO framework (Patient, Intervention, Comparison,
    Outcome)333
Polycystic ovary syndrome (PCOS), 453
Positron emission tomography (PET), 466, 449
Pregnancy, 252–256

issues, causes of, 253
    challenges and recommendations, 254–256
    errors and problems related, 252–253
    prevention of, 253–254
Prescribing errors, 27
Prescription writing errors, 28
Pressure injuries, 335
Preventive medicine errors, 27, 36–37
Problem-Based Learning (PBL), 14, 15
Process-oriented guided inquiry learning (POGIL), 14
Project-based learning, 16
Pronovost, Peter, 4
Prostate cancer, 216
PubMed, 481

Qualitative research
    advantages of, 361–362
    barriers of, 363
    in developing countries, 364–366
    disadvantages of, 362
    facilitators of, 362
    importance of, 360–361
    online, 363–364
    quality of, 363
    rationality of, 359–360
Quantitative research
    advantages of, 373–374
    barriers of, 375
    in developing countries, 377–379
    disadvantages of, 374
    facilators of, 374–375
    importance of, 372–373
    online, 376–377
    quality of, 376
    rationality of, 371–372

Radiology, 174–178
    errors, causes of, 175–176
    challenges and recommendations, 177–178
    prevention of, 176
Randomized controlled trial (RCT), 395
Rapid medical assessment, 43
Rapid trauma assessment, 43
Registered dietitian nutritionists (RDNs), 93
Remote patient monitoring, 319, 320
ResearchGate, 482
Robotic surgery, 319
Root Cause Analysis (RCA), 483

Safety of medications, 119
Safety reporting portal, 484
Scopus, 482
Self-care related problems, 27
Self-directed learning, 16
Sepsis. *See* Bloodstream infections
Simulation Training, 484
Sleep hygiene, 52
Smoking cessation, 52, 55, 56
Social distancing, 278
The Society for Simulation in Healthcare (SSH), 481

Spanish flu, 278
Special Population
    adolescents error, 477
    medication error during lactation, 475
    medication error during pregnancy, 474–475
    medication error geriatric, 475–476
    paediatric, 476–477
Standard Operating Procedures (SOPs), 71
Standardized order sets, 483
Stress management, 52
Substance abuse, 140–141
Surgery
    errors, causes of, 201
    challenges and recommendations, 203
    errors and related problems, 201
    prevention of, 202
Surgical errors, 27
    causes and factors, 69–70
    challenges of, 72–73
    facilitators and barriers, 71
    prevention of, 70–71
Surgical navigation systems, 320
Surgical site infections (SSIs), 69, 158

Team-Based Learning (TBL), 14
Technology for patient safety
    advantages of, 322–323
    applications of, 320–322
    Artificial Intelligence (AI) in, 322
    barriers, 324

in developing countries, challenges and
        recommendations, 324–326
    disadvantages of, 323
    facilitators, 323–324
Technology-Enhanced Active Learning (TEAL), 15
Telehealth, 320
Telemedicine, 319, 320, 322
Traditional Chinese medicine, 78, 81
Transcribing and orders errors, 27
Treatment evaluation and monitoring errors, 28
Trigger tools, 483
Trimesters, 252
Type, 2 Diabetes Mellitus, 443

United States Pharmacopeia (USP), 3, 4, 110
Urinary tract infection (UTI), 448, 471, 472

Vaccination, 35, 246, 282. *See also* Immunization
Vaccine Adverse Event Reporting System
        (VAERS), 484
Video-based learning, 16
Virtual Reality (VR) Technology, 321

Wearable technology, 319
Web of Science, 483
Weight management, 55, 56
Workforce challenges, 47, 55–56
World Health Organization (WHO), 4, 22, 138, 158,
        344, 345, 479, 480, 482

Yellow Card Scheme, 484

For Product Safety Concerns and Information please contact our EU
representative GPSR@taylorandfrancis.com
Taylor & Francis Verlag GmbH, Kaufingerstraße 24, 80331 München, Germany